5
FIFTH EDITION

NETTER'S CLINICAL ANATOMY

JOHN T. HANSEN, PhD

Emeritus Professor of Neuroscience
and former Schmitt Chair of Neurobiology and Anatomy
and Associate Dean for Admissions
University of Rochester Medical Center
Rochester, New York

Illustrations by

FRANK H. NETTER, MD

Contributing Illustrators

CARLOS A.G. MACHADO, MD

JOHN A. CRAIG, MD

JAMES A. PERKINS, MS, MFA

KRISTEN WIENANDT MARZEJON, MS, MFA

TIFFANY S. DAVANZO, MA, CMI

ELSEVIER

Elsevier

1600 John F. Kennedy Blvd.
Ste. 1800
Philadelphia, PA 19103-2899

Previous editions copyrighted 2019, 2014, 2009, 2005.

Library of Congress Control Number: 2021948448

Executive Content Strategist: Elyse O'Grady
Senior Content Development Specialist: Marybeth Thiel
Publishing Services Manager: Deepthi Unni
Senior Project Manager: Beula Christopher
Design: Renee Duenow

Printed in India

9 8 7 6 5 4 3 2

I dedicate this book to my wife
Paula,

and to my children
Amy and Sean,

and to my grandchildren
Abigail, Benjamin, and Jonathan.

Without their unconditional love, presence, and encouragement,
little would have been accomplished either personally or professionally.
Because we've shared so much, this effort, like all the others,
was multiauthored.

About the Artists

Frank H. Netter, MD

Frank H. Netter was born in 1906, in New York City. He studied art at the Art Students' League and the National Academy of Design before entering medical school at New York University, where he received his medical degree in 1931. During his student years, Dr. Netter's notebook sketches attracted the attention of the medical faculty and other physicians, allowing him to augment his income by illustrating articles and textbooks. He continued illustrating as a sideline after establishing a surgical practice in 1933, but he ultimately opted to give up his practice in favor of a full-time commitment to art. After service in the United States Army during World War II, Dr. Netter began his long collaboration with the CIBA Pharmaceutical Company (now Novartis Pharmaceuticals). This 45-year partnership resulted in the production of the extraordinary collection of medical art so familiar to physicians and other medical professionals worldwide.

In 2005, Elsevier, Inc. purchased the Netter Collection and all publications from Icon Learning Systems. More than 50 publications featuring the art of Dr. Netter are available through Elsevier, Inc. (in the US: www.us.elsevierhealth.com/Netter and outside the US: www.elsevierhealth.com).

Dr. Netter's works are among the finest examples of the use of illustration in the teaching of medical concepts. The 14-book *Netter Collection of Medical Illustrations*, which includes the greater part of the more than 20,000 paintings created by Dr. Netter, became and remains one of the most famous medical works ever published. *The Netter Atlas of Human Anatomy*, first published in 1989, presents the anatomic paintings from the Netter Collection. Now translated into 16 languages, it is the anatomy atlas of choice among medical and health professions students the world over.

The Netter illustrations are appreciated not only for their aesthetic qualities but, more important, for their intellectual content. As Dr. Netter wrote in 1949, ". . . clarification of a subject is the aim and goal of illustration. No matter how beautifully painted, how delicately and subtly rendered a subject may be, it is of little value as a *medical illustration* if it does not serve to make clear some medical point." Dr. Netter's planning, conception, point of view, and approach are what inform his paintings and what make them so intellectually valuable.

Frank H. Netter, MD, physician and artist, died in 1991.

Learn more about the physician-artist whose work has inspired the Netter Reference collection: https://netterimages.com/artist-frank-h-netter.html.

Carlos A. G. Machado, MD

Carlos A. G. Machado was chosen by Novartis to be Dr. Netter's successor. He continues to be the main artist who contributes to the Netter collection of medical illustrations.

Self-taught in medical illustration, cardiologist Carlos Machado has contributed meticulous updates to some of Dr. Netter's original plates and has created many paintings of his own in the style of Netter as an extension of the Netter collection. Dr. Machado's photorealistic expertise and his keen insight into the physician/patient relationship inform his vivid and unforgettable visual style. His dedication to researching each topic and subject he paints places him among the premier medical illustrators at work today.

Learn more about his background and see more of his art at: https://netterimages.com/artist-carlos-a-g-machado.html.

About the Author

John T. Hansen, PhD, is Emeritus Professor of Neuroscience, the former Killian J. and Caroline F. Schmitt Professor and Chair of Neurobiology and Anatomy, and the Associate Dean for Admissions at the University of Rochester Medical Center, Rochester, New York.

Dr. Hansen is the recipient of numerous teaching awards from students at three different medical schools. From 1995–1998, he was Professor and a Robert Wood Johnson Dean's Senior Teaching Scholar. In 1999, he was the recipient of the *Alpha Omega Alpha* Robert J. Glaser Distinguished Teacher Award given annually by the Association of American Medical Colleges to nationally recognized medical educators. From 2004–2005, Dr. Hansen was Chair of the Northeast Group on Student Affairs for the Association of American Medical Colleges. He also was selected twice by Rochester's graduating medical school class to give their Faculty Commencement Address. In 2013, he was selected as an Honored Member of the American Association of Clinical Anatomists, that organization's highest recognition. In 2018, he was elected to membership in *Alpha Omega Alpha* by the Rochester Medical Class of 2018, and in 2020 was the recipient of the Alumni Service Award from the University of Rochester School of Medicine and Dentistry.

Dr. Hansen has served on the USMLE Step Anatomy Test Material Development Committee, and has given numerous Faculty Development Workshops on lecturing skills, exam writing, and basic science curriculum development at Rochester. He also has been invited to consult on basic science curricular development at a number of U.S. and foreign medical schools.

In 2010, Dr. Hansen was the first recipient of the *University of Rochester's Presidential Diversity Award* in recognition of his "advocacy, support, mentoring, planning, and leading the medical school's initiatives to increase the recruitment, retention, excellence, and graduation of students from diverse backgrounds."

Dr. Hansen's investigative research career encompassed the study of the peripheral and central nervous system's dopaminergic pathways, neural plasticity, and central nervous system inflammation. He is the recipient of a prestigious five-year National Institutes of Health Research Career Development Award, a number of foundation and NIH research grants, and has presented his research findings at major U.S. universities and national meetings, as well as at a number of international meetings. In addition to over 100 full-length research publications, he also is the co-author of the 2002 edition of the *Netter's Atlas of Human Physiology*, the lead consulting editor of the 3rd through the 7th editions of the *Netter's Atlas of Human Anatomy* (from 2003–2021), author of *Netter's Anatomy Flash Cards*, the *Essential Anatomy Dissector*, *Netter's Anatomy Coloring Book*, and is the co-author of the *TNM Staging Atlas with Oncoanatomy*, selected from 630 world wide entries as the Book of the Year in 2008 by the British Medical Association.

Acknowledgments

Compiling the illustrations, researching, and writing *Netter's Clinical Anatomy*, fifth edition, has been both enjoyable and educational, confirming again the importance of lifelong learning in the health professions.

Netter's Clinical Anatomy is for all my students, and I am indebted to all of them who, like many others, yearn for a better view to help them learn the relevant essential anatomy that informs the practice of medicine. Anatomy is a visual science, and Netter's illustrations are the gold standard of medical illustration.

Thanks and appreciation belong to my colleagues and reviewers who provided encouragement and constructive comments that clarified many aspects of the book. Especially, I wish to acknowledge David Lambert, MD, Senior Associate Dean for Undergraduate Medical Education at Rochester, who co-authored the first edition of this book with me and remains a treasured colleague and friend.

At Elsevier, it has been a distinct pleasure to work with dedicated, professional people who massaged, molded, and ultimately nourished the dream beyond even my wildest imagination. I owe much to the efforts of Marybeth Thiel, Senior Content Development Specialist, and Beula Christopher, Senior Project Manager, both of whom kept me organized, focused, and on time. Without them, little would have been accomplished. Thanks and appreciation also to Renee Duenow, Designer and Karen Giacomucci, Illustration Manager. A special thank you to Madelene Hyde, Publishing Director, and Elyse O'Grady, Executive Content Strategist, for believing in the idea and always supporting my efforts. This competent team defines the word "professionalism," and it has been an honor to work with all of them.

Special thanks to Carlos Machado, MD, for his beautiful artistic renderings that superbly complemented, updated, and extended the Netter anatomy collection. Also, I wish to express my thanks to my faculty colleagues at Rochester for their generous and constructive feedback.

Finally, I remain indebted to Frank H. Netter, MD, whose creative genius lives on in generations of biomedical professionals who have learned clinical anatomy from his rich collection of medical illustrations.

To all of these remarkable people, and others, "Thank you."

JOHN T. HANSEN, PHD

Preface

Human anatomy is the foundation upon which the education of our medical, dental, and allied health science students is built. However, today's biomedical science curriculum must cover an ever-increasing body of scientific knowledge, often in fewer hours, as competing disciplines and new technologies emerge. Many of these same technologies, especially those in the imaging science fields, have made understanding anatomy even more important and have moved our discipline firmly into the realm of clinical medicine. It is fair to say that competent clinicians and allied health professionals can no longer simply view their anatomical training in isolation from the clinical implications related to that anatomy.

In this context, I am proud to introduce the fifth edition of *Netter's Clinical Anatomy*. Generations of students have used Dr. Frank H. Netter's elegant anatomical illustrations to learn anatomy, and this book combines his beautiful anatomical and embryological renderings with numerous clinical illustrations to help students bridge the gap between normal anatomy and its clinical application across each region of the human body. Additional anatomical images are provided by Carlos Machado, MD. These newly created images by Dr. Machado are based on the latest clinical approaches and provide exquisite examples of the importance of clinical anatomy.

This fifth edition provides succinct text, key bulleted points, and ample summary tables, which offer students a concise textbook description of normal human anatomy, as well as a quick reference and review guide for clinical practitioners. Additionally, over 200 *Clinical Focus* boxes representing some of the more commonly encountered clinical conditions seen in medical practice are integrated with the normal anatomy throughout the textbook. These clinical correlations are drawn from a wide variety of medical fields including emergency medicine, radiology, orthopedics, and surgery, but also include relevant clinical anatomy related to the fields of cardiology, endocrinology, infectious diseases, neurology, oncology, reproductive biology, and urology. By design, the text and clinical correlations are not exhaustive, but are meant to help students focus on the essential elements of anatomy and begin to appreciate some of the clinical manifestations related to that anatomy. Other features of this edition include:

- An updated Introduction to the Human Body chapter designed to introduce students to anatomical terminology and orient them to the body's organ systems
- A set of end-of-chapter clinically oriented multiple choice review questions
- Basic embryology of each system that provides a contextual framework for human postnatal anatomy and several common congenital defects
- Online access with additional *Clinical Focus* boxes

My intent in writing this updated fifth edition of *Netter's Clinical Anatomy* is to provide a concise and focused introduction to clinical anatomy as a viable alternative to the more comprehensive anatomy textbooks, which few students read and/or often find too difficult to navigate when looking for the "essential" anatomical details. Moreover, this textbook serves as an excellent review text for students studying for their Step 1 USMLE examinations, or beginning their clinical clerkships and elective programs. It also serves as an excellent reference text that clinicians will find useful for their own review and for patient education.

The text is by no means comprehensive, but does provide the essential anatomy needed by the generalist physician-in-training that is commonly encountered in the first year of medical school. I have intentionally focused on the anatomy that a first-year student might be expected to grasp and carry forward into his or her clerkship training, especially in this day and age when anatomy courses are often streamlined and laboratory dissection exercises abbreviated. Those students, who by choice, choose to enter specialties where advanced anatomical training is required (e.g., surgical specialties, radiology, physical therapy, etc.) may encounter a need for additional anatomical expertise that will be provided by their graduate medical or allied health education. By meeting the needs of the beginning student and providing ample detail for subsequent review or handy reference, my hope is that *Netter's Clinical Anatomy* will be the anatomy textbook of choice that will actually be read and used by students throughout their undergraduate medical or allied health careers.

I hope that you, the health science student-in-training or the physician-in-practice, will find *Netter's Clinical Anatomy* the valuable link you've searched for to enhance your understanding of clinical anatomy as only Frank Netter can present it.

JOHN T. HANSEN, PhD

Contents

Clinical Focus Boxes

chapter 5

Pelvis and Perineum

chapter 6   # Lower Limb

chapter 8 · Head and Neck

Introduction to the Human Body

1. TERMINOLOGY

Anatomical Position

The study of anatomy requires a clinical vocabulary that defines position, movements, relationships, and planes of reference, as well as the systems of the human body. The study of anatomy can be by **body region** or by **body organ systems**. Generally, courses of anatomy in the United States approach anatomical study by regions, integrating all applicable body systems into the study of a particular region. This textbook therefore is arranged regionally, and for those studying anatomy for the first time, this initial chapter introduces you to the major body systems that you will encounter in your study of anatomy. You will find it extremely helpful to refer back to this introduction as you encounter various body systems in your study of regional anatomy.

By convention, anatomical descriptions of the human body are based on a person in the **anatomical position** (Fig. 1.1), as follows:
- Standing erect and facing forward
- Arms hanging at the sides with palms facing forward
- Legs placed together with feet facing forward

Terms of Relationship and Body Planes

Anatomical descriptions often are referenced to one or more of three distinct body planes (Fig. 1.2 and Table 1.1), as follows:
- **Sagittal plane:** a vertical plane that divides the body into equal right and left halves (median or midsagittal plane) or a plane parallel to the median sagittal plane (parasagittal) that divides the body into unequal right and left portions.
- **Frontal (coronal) plane:** a vertical plane that divides the body into anterior and posterior portions (equal or unequal); this plane is at right angles to the median sagittal plane.
- **Transverse (axial) plane:** a horizontal plane that divides the body into superior and inferior portions (equal or unequal) and is at right angles to both the median sagittal and the frontal planes (sometimes called *cross sections*).

Key terms of relationship used in anatomy and the clinic are summarized in Table 1.1. A structure or feature closer to the front of the body is considered *anterior* (ventral), and one closer to the back is termed *posterior* (dorsal). The terms *medial* and *lateral* are used to distinguish a structure or feature in relationship to the midline; the nose is medial to the ear, and in anatomical position, the nose also is anterior to the ear. Sometimes these terms of relationship are used in combination (e.g., *superomedial,* meaning closer to the head and nearer the median sagittal plane).

Movements

Body movements usually occur at the joints where two or more bones or cartilages articulate with one another. Muscles act on joints to accomplish these movements and may be described as follows: "The biceps muscle flexes the forearm at the elbow." Fig. 1.3 summarizes the terms of movement.

Anatomical Variability

The human body is remarkably complex and remarkably consistent anatomically, but normal variations do exist, often related to size, gender,

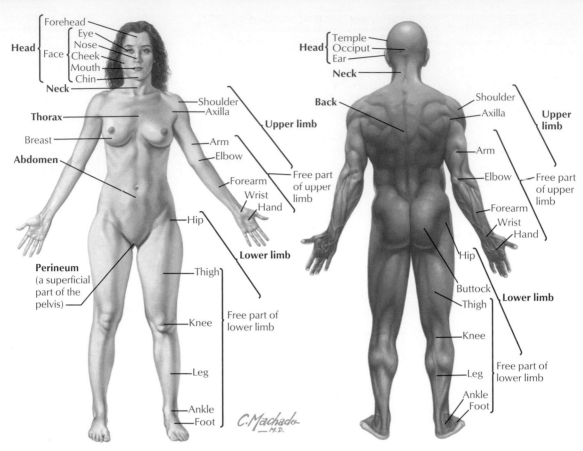

FIGURE 1.1 Surface Anatomy: Regions. (From *Netter's atlas of human anatomy*, ed 8, Plates 2 and 3; S-2 and S-3.)

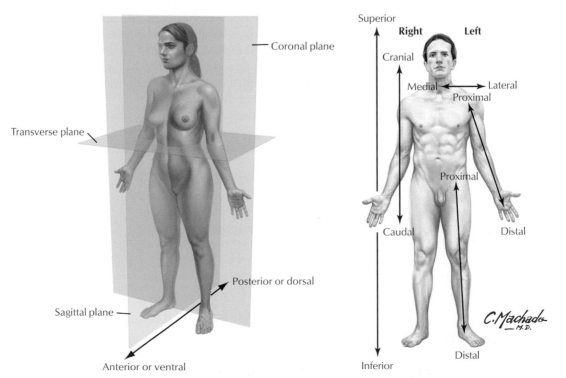

FIGURE 1.2 Body Planes and Terms of Anatomical Relationship. (From *Netter's atlas of human anatomy*, ed 8, Plate 1; S-1.)

TABLE 1.1 General Terms of Anatomical Relationship

TERM	DEFINITION	TERM	DEFINITION
Anterior (ventral)	Near the front	Median plane	Divides body into equal right and left parts
Posterior (dorsal)	Near the back		
Superior (cranial)	Upward, or near the head	Midsagittal plane	Median plane
Inferior (caudal)	Downward, or near the feet	Sagittal plane	Divides body into unequal right and left parts
Medial	Toward the midline or median plane		
Lateral	Farther from the midline or median plane	Frontal (coronal) plane	Divides body into equal or unequal anterior and posterior parts
Proximal	Near a reference point	Transverse plane	Divides body into equal or unequal superior and inferior parts (cross sections)
Distal	Away from a reference point		
Superficial	Closer to the surface		
Deep	Farther from the surface		

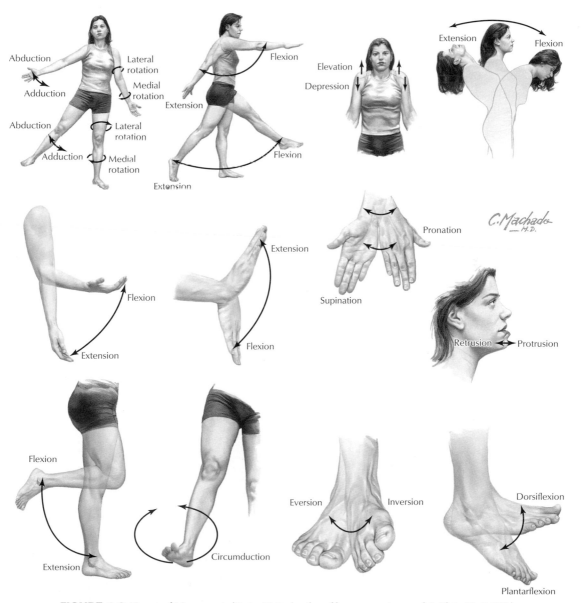

FIGURE 1.3 Terms of Movement. (From *Netter's atlas of human anatomy*, ed 8, Plate 11; S-265.)

age, number, shape, and attachment. Variations are particularly common in the following structures:

- **Bones:** the fine features of bones (processes, spines, articular surfaces) may be variable depending on the forces working on a bone.
- **Muscles:** they vary with size and fine details of their attachments (it is better to learn their actions and general attachments rather than focus on detailed exceptions).
- **Organs:** the size and shape of some organs will vary depending on their normal physiology or pathophysiologic changes that have occurred previously.
- **Arteries:** they are surprisingly consistent, although some variation is seen in the branching patterns, especially in the lower neck (subclavian branches) and in the pelvis (internal iliac branches).
- **Veins:** they are consistent, although variations, especially in size and number of veins, can occur and often can be traced to their complex embryologic development; veins generally are more numerous than arteries, larger, and more variable.

2. SKIN

The skin is the largest organ in the body, accounting for about 15% to 20% of the total body mass, and has the following functions:

- *Protection:* against mechanical abrasion and in immune responses, as well as prevention of dehydration.
- *Temperature regulation:* largely through vasodilation, vasoconstriction, fat storage, or activation of sweat glands.
- *Sensations:* to touch by specialized mechanoreceptors such as pacinian and Meissner's corpuscles; to pain by nociceptors; and to temperature by thermoreceptors.
- *Endocrine regulation:* by secretion of hormones, cytokines, and growth factors, and by synthesis and storage of vitamin D.
- *Exocrine secretions:* by secretion of sweat and oily sebum from sebaceous glands.

The skin consists of two layers (Fig. 1.4):

- **Epidermis:** is the outer protective layer consisting of a keratinized stratified squamous epithelium derived from the embryonic ectoderm.
- **Dermis:** is the dense connective tissue layer that gives skin most of its thickness and support, and is derived from the embryonic mesoderm.

Fascia is a connective tissue sheet that may contain variable amounts of fat. It can interconnect structures, provide a conduit for vessels and nerves (termed **neurovascular bundles**), and provide a sheath around structures (e.g., muscles) that permits them to slide over one another easily. **Superficial**

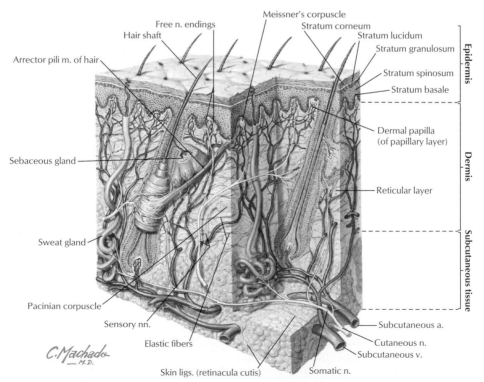

FIGURE 1.4 Layers of the Skin. (From *Netter's atlas of human anatomy*, ed 8, Plate 12; S-4.)

Clinical Focus 1.1

Psoriasis

Psoriasis is a chronic inflammatory skin disorder that affects approximately 1% to 3% of the population (women and men equally). It is characterized by defined red plaques capped with a surface scale of desquamated epidermis. Although the pathogenesis is unknown, psoriasis seems to involve a genetic predisposition.

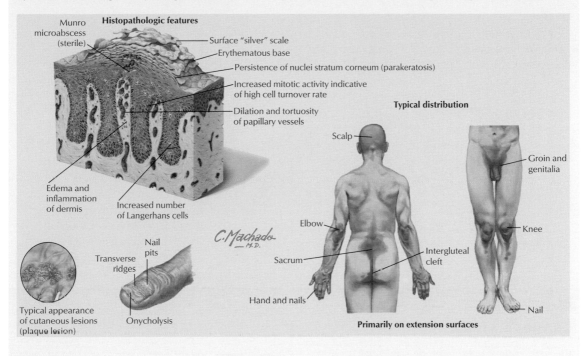

Histopathologic features

Munro microabscess (sterile)

Surface "silver" scale

Erythematous base

Persistence of nuclei stratum corneum (parakeratosis)

Increased mitotic activity indicative of high cell turnover rate

Dilation and tortuosity of papillary vessels

Edema and inflammation of dermis

Increased number of Langerhans cells

Typical appearance of cutaneous lesions (plaque lesion)

Onycholysis

Transverse ridges

Nail pits

C. Machado — M.D.

Typical distribution

Scalp

Groin and genitalia

Elbow

Knee

Sacrum

Intergluteal cleft

Hand and nails

Nail

Primarily on extension surfaces

fascia is attached to and lies just beneath the dermis of the skin and can vary in thickness and density; it acts as a cushion, contains variable amounts of fat, and allows the skin to glide over its surface. **Deep fascia** usually consists of a dense connective tissue, is attached to the deep surface of the superficial fascia, and often ensheathes muscles and divides them into functional groupings. Extensions of the deep fascia encasing muscles also may course inward and attach to the skeleton, dividing groups of muscles with **intermuscular septa.** Common injuries to the skin include abrasions, cuts (lacerations), and burns. Burns are classified as follows:

- **First-degree:** burn damage that is limited to the superficial layers of the epidermis; termed a *superficial* burn, clinically it causes erythema (redness of the skin).
- **Second-degree:** burn damage that includes all of the epidermis and extends into the superficial dermis; termed a *partial-thickness* burn, it causes blisters but spares the hair follicles and sweat glands.

- **Third-degree:** burn damage that includes all the epidermis and dermis and may even involve the subcutaneous tissue and underlying deep fascia and muscle; termed a *full-thickness* burn, it causes charring.

3. SKELETAL SYSTEM

Descriptive Regions

The human skeleton is divided into two descriptive regions (Fig. 1.5):

- **Axial skeleton:** includes the bones of the skull, vertebral column (spine), ribs, and sternum, which form the "axis" or central line of the body (80 bones).
- **Appendicular skeleton:** includes the bones of the limbs, including the pectoral and pelvic girdles, which attach the limbs to the body's axis (134 bones).

Shapes and Function of Bones

The skeleton is composed of a living, dynamic, rigid connective tissue that forms the bones and cartilages.

Clinical Focus 1.2

Burns

Burns to the skin are classified into three degrees of severity based on the depth of the burn:

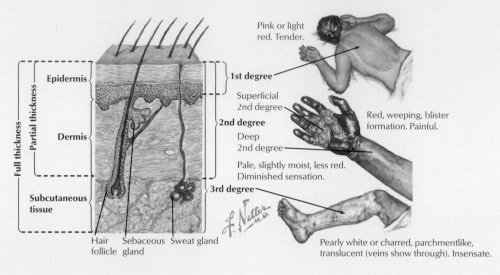

Epidermis
Partial thickness
Full thickness
Dermis
Subcutaneous tissue
Hair follicle
Sebaceous gland
Sweat gland

Pink or light red. Tender.
1st degree
Superficial 2nd degree
2nd degree
Red, weeping, blister formation. Painful.
Deep 2nd degree
Pale, slightly moist, less red. Diminished sensation.
3rd degree
Pearly white or charred, parchmentlike, translucent (veins show through). Insensate.

Clinical Focus 1.3

Langer's Lines

Collagen in the skin creates tension lines called *Langer's lines*. Surgeons sometimes use these lines to make skin incisions; other times, they may use the natural skin folds. The resulting incision wounds tend to gape less when the incision is parallel to Langer's lines, resulting in a smaller scar after healing. However, skin fold incisions also may conceal the scar following healing of the incision.

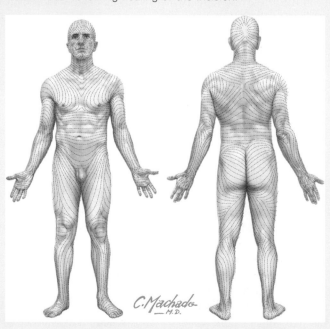

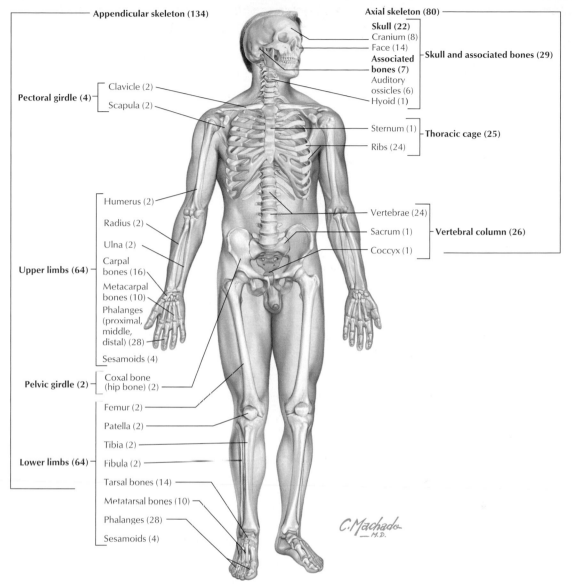

Appendicular skeleton (134)

Clavicle (2) — Pectoral girdle (4)
Scapula (2)

Humerus (2)
Radius (2)
Ulna (2)
Carpal bones (16)
Metacarpal bones (10)
Phalanges (proximal, middle, distal) (28)
Sesamoids (4)   Upper limbs (64)

Coxal bone (hip bone) (2) — Pelvic girdle (2)

Femur (2)
Patella (2)
Tibia (2)
Fibula (2)
Tarsal bones (14)
Metatarsal bones (10)
Phalanges (28)
Sesamoids (4)   Lower limbs (64)

Axial skeleton (80)

Skull (22)
Cranium (8)
Face (14)   Skull and associated bones (29)
Associated bones (7)
Auditory ossicles (6)
Hyoid (1)

Sternum (1) — Thoracic cage (25)
Ribs (24)

Vertebrae (24)
Sacrum (1)   Vertebral column (26)
Coccyx (1)

C. Machado M.D.

FIGURE 1.5 Axial and Appendicular Regions of Skeleton. (From *Netter's atlas of human anatomy*, ed 8, Plate 8; S-120.)

Generally, humans have about 214 bones, although this number varies, particularly in the number of small sesamoid bones that may be present. (Typically, we have 8 sesamoid bones of the hands and feet.) Cartilage is attached to some bones, especially where flexibility is important, or covers the surfaces of bones at points of articulation. About 99% of the body's calcium is stored in bone, and many bones possess a central cavity that contains bone marrow—a collection of hemopoietic (blood-forming) cells. Most of the bones can be classified into one of the following five shapes (Fig. 1.6):

- Long.
- Short.
- Flat.
- Irregular.
- Sesamoid.
  The functions of the skeletal system include:
- Support.
- Protection of vital organs.
- A mechanism, along with muscles, for movement.
- Storage of calcium and other salts, growth factors, and cytokines.
- A source of blood cells.

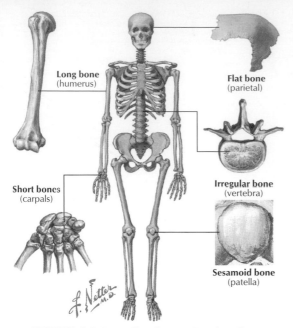

FIGURE 1.6 Bone Classification Based on Shape.

There are two types of bone:
- **Compact:** is a relatively solid mass of bone, commonly seen as a superficial layer of bone, that provides strength.
- **Spongy** (trabecular or cancellous): is a less dense trabeculated network of bone spicules making up the substance of most bones and surrounding an inner marrow cavity.

Long bones also are divided into the following descriptive regions (Fig. 1.7):
- **Epiphysis:** the ends of long bones, which develop from secondary ossification centers.
- **Epiphysial plate:** the site of growth in length; it contains cartilage in actively growing bones.
- **Metaphysis:** the site where the bone's shaft joins the epiphysis and epiphysial plate.
- **Diaphysis:** the shaft of a long bone, which represents the primary ossification center and the site where growth in width occurs.

As a living, dynamic tissue, bone receives a rich blood supply from:
- *Nutrient arteries:* usually one or several larger arteries that pass through the diaphysis and supply the compact and spongy bone, as well as the bone marrow.
- *Metaphysial and epiphysial arteries:* usually arise from articular branches supplying the joint.
- *Periosteal arteries:* numerous small arteries from adjacent vessels that supply the compact bone.

Markings on the Bones

Various surface features of bones (ridges, grooves, and bumps) result from the tension placed on them by the attachment of tendons, ligaments, and fascia, as well as by neurovascular bundles or other structures that pass along the bone. Descriptively, these features include the following:
- **Condyle:** a rounded articular surface covered with articular (hyaline) cartilage.
- **Crest:** a ridge (narrow or wide) of bone.
- **Epicondyle:** a prominent ridge or eminence superior to a condyle.
- **Facet:** a flat, smooth articular surface, usually covered with articular (hyaline) cartilage.
- **Fissure:** a very narrow "slitlike" opening in a bone.
- **Foramen:** a round or oval "hole" in the bone for passage of another structure (nerve or vessel).
- **Fossa:** a "cuplike" depression in the bone, usually for articulation with another bone.
- **Groove:** a furrow in the bone.
- **Line:** a fine linear ridge of bone, but less prominent than a crest.
- **Malleolus:** a rounded eminence.
- **Meatus:** a passageway or canal in a bone.
- **Notch:** an indentation along the edge of a bone.
- **Process:** a bony prominence that may be sharp or blunt.
- **Protuberance:** a protruding eminence on an otherwise smooth surface.
- **Ramus:** a thin part of a bone that joins a thicker process of the same bone.
- **Spine:** a sharp process projecting from a bone.
- **Trochanter:** large, blunt process for muscle tendon or ligament attachment.
- **Tubercle:** a small, elevated process.
- **Tuberosity:** a large, rounded eminence that may be coarse or rough.

Bone Development

Bones develop in one of the following two ways:
- **Intramembranous formation:** most flat bones develop in this way by direct calcium deposition into a mesenchymal (primitive mesoderm) precursor or model of the bone.
- **Endochondral formation:** most long and irregularly shaped bones develop by calcium deposition into a cartilaginous model of the bone that provides a scaffold for the future bone.

The following sequence of events defines endochondral bone formation (Fig. 1.7, *A-F*):
- Formation of a thin collar of bone around a hyaline cartilage model.

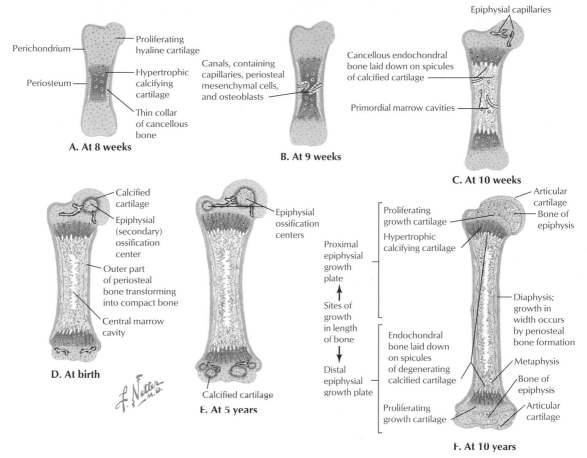

FIGURE 1.7 Growth and Ossification of Long Bones (Midfrontal Sections).

- Cavitation of the primary ossification center and invasion of vessels, nerves, lymphatics, red marrow elements, and osteoblasts.
- Formation of spongy (cancellous) endochondral bone on calcified spicules.
- Diaphysis elongation, formation of the central marrow cavity, and appearance of the secondary ossification centers in the epiphyses.
- Long bone growth during childhood.
- Epiphysial fusion occurring from puberty into maturity (early to mid-20s).

Types of Joints

Joints are the sites of union or articulation of two or more bones or cartilages, and are classified into one of the following three types (Fig. 1.8):

- **Fibrous** (synarthroses): bones joined by fibrous connective tissue.
- **Cartilaginous** (amphiarthroses): bones joined by cartilage, or by cartilage and fibrous tissue.
- **Synovial** (diarthroses): in this most common type of joint, the bones are joined by a joint cavity filled with a small amount of synovial fluid and surrounded by a capsule; the bony articular surfaces are covered with hyaline cartilage.

Fibrous joints include **sutures** (flat bones of the skull), **syndesmoses** (two bones connected by a fibrous membrane), and **gomphoses** (teeth fitting into fibrous tissue-lined sockets).

Cartilaginous joints include **primary** (synchondrosis) joints between surfaces lined by hyaline cartilage (epiphysial plate connecting the diaphysis with the epiphysis), and **secondary** (symphysis) joints between hyaline-lined articular surfaces and an intervening fibrocartilaginous disc. Primary joints allow for growth and some bending, whereas secondary joints allow for strength and some flexibility.

Synovial joints generally allow for considerable movement and are classified according to their shape and the type of movement that they permit (uniaxial, biaxial, or multiaxial movement) (Fig. 1.9), as follows:

- **Hinge** (ginglymus): are uniaxial joints for flexion and extension.
- **Pivot** (trochoid): are uniaxial joints for rotation.

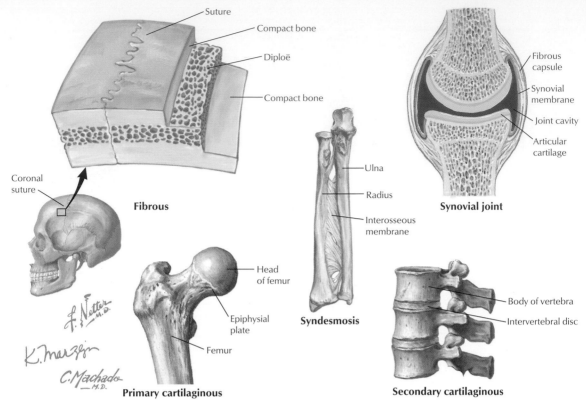

FIGURE 1.8 Types of Joints.

- **Saddle:** are biaxial joints for flexion, extension, abduction, adduction, and circumduction.
- **Condyloid** (ellipsoid; sometimes classified separately): are biaxial joints for flexion, extension, abduction, adduction, and circumduction.
- **Plane** (gliding): are joints that only allow simple gliding movements.
- **Ball-and-socket** (spheroid): are multiaxial joints for flexion, extension, abduction, adduction, mediolateral rotation, and circumduction.

4. MUSCULAR SYSTEM

Muscle cells (fibers) produce contractions (shortenings in length) that result in movement, maintenance of posture, changes in shape, or the propulsion of fluids through hollow tissues or organs. There are three different types of muscle:

- **Skeletal:** striated muscle fibers that are attached to bone and are responsible for movements of the skeleton (sometimes simplistically referred to as *voluntary muscle*).
- **Cardiac:** striated muscle fibers that make up the walls of the heart and proximal portions of the great veins where they enter the heart.

- **Smooth:** nonstriated muscle fibers that line various organ systems (gastrointestinal, urogenital, respiratory), attach to hair follicles, and line the walls of most blood vessels (sometimes simplistically referred to as *involuntary muscle*).

Skeletal muscle is divided into **fascicles** (bundles), which are composed of muscle fibers (muscle cells) (Fig. 1.10). The muscle fiber cells contain longitudinally oriented **myofibrils** that run the full length of the cell. Each myofibril is composed of many **myofilaments,** which are composed of individual **myosin** (thick filaments) and **actin** (thin filaments) that slide over one another during muscle contraction.

Skeletal muscle moves bones at their joints and possesses an **origin** (the muscle's fixed or proximal attachment) and an **insertion** (the muscle's movable or distal attachment). In a few instances, the muscle's origin moves more than its insertion. At the gross level, anatomists classify muscle on the basis of its shape:

- **Flat:** muscle that has parallel fibers, usually in a broad flat sheet with a broad tendon of attachment called an *aponeurosis.*
- **Quadrate:** muscle that has a four-sided appearance.

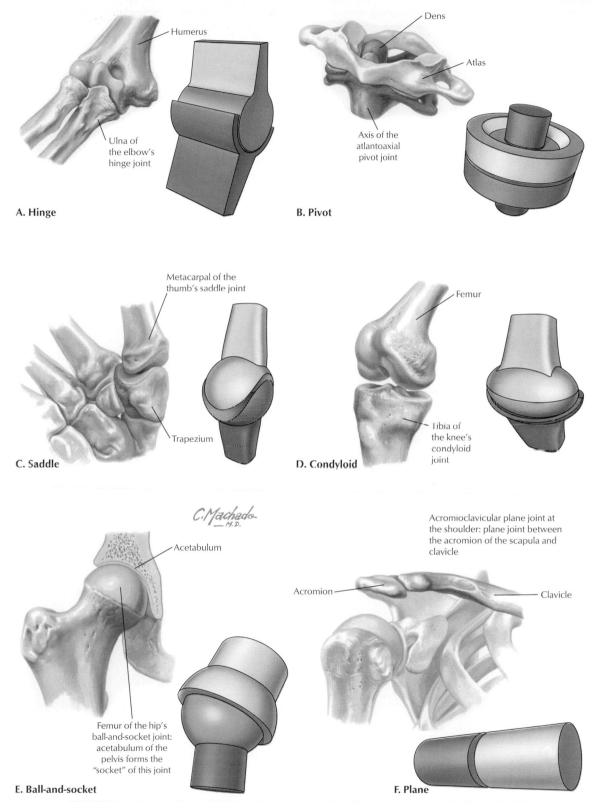

FIGURE 1.9 Types of Synovial Joints. (From *Netter's atlas of human anatomy*, ed 8, Plate 9; S-121.)

Clinical Focus 1.4

Fractures

Fractures are classified as either **closed** (the skin is intact) or **open** (the skin is perforated; often referred to as a *compound fracture*). Additionally, the fracture may be classified with respect to its anatomical appearance (e.g., transverse, spiral).

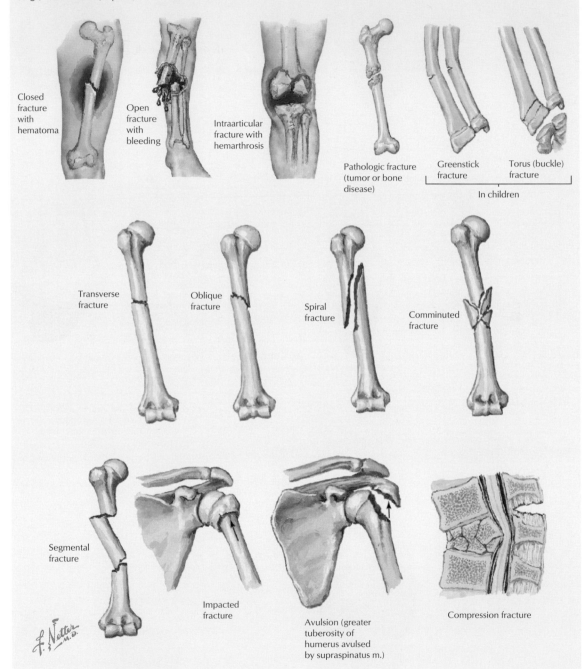

Closed fracture with hematoma

Open fracture with bleeding

Intraarticular fracture with hemarthrosis

Pathologic fracture (tumor or bone disease)

Greenstick fracture

Torus (buckle) fracture

In children

Transverse fracture

Oblique fracture

Spiral fracture

Comminuted fracture

Segmental fracture

Impacted fracture

Avulsion (greater tuberosity of humerus avulsed by supraspinatus m.)

Compression fracture

Clinical Focus 1.5

Degenerative Joint Disease

Degenerative joint disease is a catch-all term for osteoarthritis, degenerative arthritis, osteoarthrosis, or hypertrophic arthritis; it is characterized by progressive loss of articular cartilage and failure of repair. **Osteoarthritis** can affect any synovial joint but most often involves the foot, knee, hip, spine, and hand. As the articular cartilage is lost, the joint space (the space between the two articulating bones) becomes narrowed, and the exposed bony surfaces rub against each other, causing significant pain.

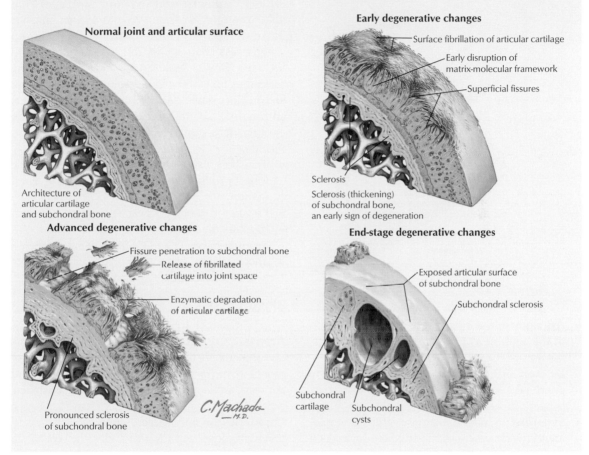

Normal joint and articular surface

Architecture of articular cartilage and subchondral bone

Early degenerative changes

Surface fibrillation of articular cartilage

Early disruption of matrix-molecular framework

Superficial fissures

Sclerosis

Sclerosis (thickening) of subchondral bone, an early sign of degeneration

Advanced degenerative changes

Fissure penetration to subchondral bone

Release of fibrillated cartilage into joint space

Enzymatic degradation of articular cartilage

Pronounced sclerosis of subchondral bone

End-stage degenerative changes

Exposed articular surface of subchondral bone

Subchondral sclerosis

Subchondral cartilage

Subchondral cysts

C. Machado —M.D.

- **Circular:** muscle that forms sphincters that close off tubes or openings.
- **Digastric:** two muscles in series and connected by a common tendon.
- **Fusiform:** muscle that has a wide center and tapered ends.
- **Pennate:** muscle that has a feathered appearance (unipennate, bipennate, or multipennate forms).

Muscle contraction shortens the muscle. Generally, skeletal muscle contracts in one of three ways:

- *Reflexive:* involuntary or through automatic contraction; seen in the diaphragm during respiration or in the reflex contraction elicited by tapping a muscle's tendon with a reflex hammer.
- *Tonic:* maintains "muscle tone," a slight contraction that may not cause movement but allows the muscle to maintain firmness necessary for stability of a joint and important in maintaining posture.
- *Phasic:* includes two types of contraction: **isometric contraction**, where no movement occurs but the muscle maintains tension to hold a position (stronger than tonic contraction); and **isotonic contraction**, where the muscle shortens to produce movement.

Muscle contraction that produces movements can act in several ways, depending on the conditions:

- **Agonist:** the main muscle responsible for a specific movement (the "prime mover").

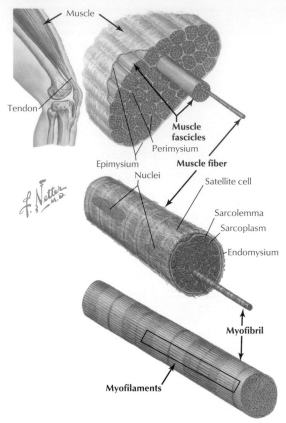

FIGURE 1.10 Structure of Skeletal Muscle.

- **Antagonist:** the muscle that opposes the action of the agonist; as an agonist muscle contracts, the antagonistic muscle relaxes.
- **Fixator:** one or more muscles that steady the proximal part of a limb when a more distal part is being moved.
- **Synergist:** a muscle, or muscles, that complements (works synergistically with) the contraction of the agonist, either by assisting with the movement generated by the agonist or by reducing unnecessary movements that would occur as the agonist contracts.

5. CARDIOVASCULAR SYSTEM

The cardiovascular system consists of (1) the **heart**, which pumps blood into the *pulmonary circulation* for gas exchange and into the *systemic circulation* to supply the body tissues; and (2) the **vessels** that carry the blood, including the arteries, arterioles, capillaries, venules, and veins. The blood passing through the cardiovascular system consists of the following formed elements (Fig. 1.11):

- Platelets.
- White blood cells (WBCs).
- Red blood cells (RBCs).
- Plasma.

Blood is a fluid connective tissue that circulates through the arteries to reach the body's tissues and then returns to the heart through the veins. When blood is "spun down" in a centrifuge tube, the RBCs precipitate to the bottom of the tube, where they account for about 45% of the blood volume. This is called the **hematocrit** and normally ranges from 40% to 50% in males and 35% to 45% in females. The next layer is a **"buffy coat,"** which makes up slightly less than 1% of the blood volume and includes WBCs (leukocytes) and platelets. The remaining 55% of the blood volume is the **plasma** and includes water, plasma proteins, clotting factors, and various solutes (**serum** is plasma with the clotting factors removed). The functions of blood include:

- Transport of dissolved gases, nutrients, metabolic waste products, and hormones to and from tissues.
- Prevention of fluid loss via clotting mechanisms.
- Immune defense.
- Regulation of pH and electrolyte balance.
- Thermoregulation through blood vessel constriction and dilation.

Blood Vessels

Blood circulates through the blood vessels (Fig. 1.12). **Arteries** carry blood away from the heart, and **veins** carry blood back to the heart. Arteries generally have more smooth muscle in their walls than veins and are responsible for most of the vascular resistance, especially the small muscular arteries and arterioles. **Capillaries** are simple microscopic tubes with very thin walls connecting arteries to veins; they constitute more that 90% of all the blood vessels in the human body. At any point in time, most of the blood resides in the veins (about 64%) and is returned to the right side of the heart; thus veins are the capacitance vessels, capable of holding most of the blood, and are far more variable and numerous than their corresponding arteries.

The major arteries are illustrated in Fig. 1.13. At certain points along the pathway of the systemic arterial circulation, large and medium-sized arteries lie near the body's surface and can be used to take a **pulse** by compressing the artery against a hard underlying structure (usually a bone). The most distal pulse from the heart is usually taken over the dorsalis pedis artery on the dorsum of the foot or by the posterior tibial artery pulse, at the medial aspect of the ankle.

FIGURE 1.11

Composition of Blood.

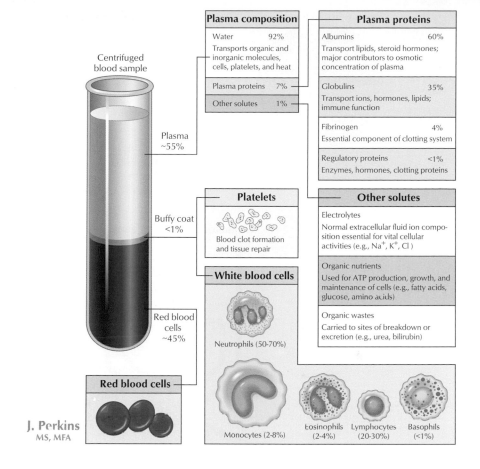

The following labels appear on the figure:

Centrifuged blood sample

Plasma ~55%

Buffy coat <1%

Red blood cells ~45%

Red blood cells

J. Perkins MS, MFA

Plasma composition

Water	92%
Transports organic and inorganic molecules, cells, platelets, and heat	
Plasma proteins	7%
Other solutes	1%

Plasma proteins

Albumins	60%
Transport lipids, steroid hormones; major contributors to osmotic concentration of plasma	
Globulins	35%
Transport ions, hormones, lipids; immune function	
Fibrinogen	4%
Essential component of clotting system	
Regulatory proteins	<1%
Enzymes, hormones, clotting proteins	

Platelets

Blood clot formation and tissue repair

Other solutes

Electrolytes
Normal extracellular fluid ion composition essential for vital cellular activities (e.g., Na^+, K^+, Cl^-)

Organic nutrients
Used for ATP production, growth, and maintenance of cells (e.g., fatty acids, glucose, amino acids)

Organic wastes
Carried to sites of breakdown or excretion (e.g., urea, bilirubin)

White blood cells

Neutrophils (50-70%)

Monocytes (2-8%) Eosinophils (2-4%) Lymphocytes (20-30%) Basophils (<1%)

The major veins are illustrated in Fig. 1.14. Veins are capacitance vessels because they are distensible and numerous and can serve as reservoirs for the blood. Because veins carry blood at low pressure and often against gravity, larger veins of the limbs and lower neck region have numerous valves that aid in venous return to the heart (several other veins throughout the body may also contain valves). Both the presence of valves and the contractions of adjacent skeletal muscles help to "pump" the venous blood against gravity and toward the heart. In most of the body, the veins occur as a superficial set of veins in the subcutaneous tissue that connects with a deeper set of veins that parallel the arteries. Types of veins include:

- *Venules:* these are very small veins that collect blood from the capillary beds.
- *Veins:* these are small, medium, and large veins that contain some smooth muscle in their walls, but not as much as their corresponding arteries.
- *Portal venous systems:* these are veins that transport blood between two capillary beds (e.g., the hepatic portal system draining the GI tract).

Heart

The heart is a hollow muscular (cardiac muscle) organ that is divided into four chambers (Figs. 1.12, 1.15):

- **Right atrium:** receives the blood from the systemic circulation via the superior and inferior venae cavae.
- **Right ventricle:** receives the blood from the right atrium and pumps it into the pulmonary circulation via the pulmonary trunk and pulmonary arteries.
- **Left atrium:** receives the blood from the lungs via pulmonary veins.
- **Left ventricle:** receives the blood from the left atrium and pumps it into the systemic circulation via the aorta.

The atria and ventricles are separated by atrioventricular valves (**tricuspid** on the right side and **mitral** on the left side) that prevent the blood from refluxing into the atria when the ventricles contract. Likewise, the two major outflow vessels, the pulmonary trunk from the right ventricle and the ascending aorta from the left ventricle, possess the

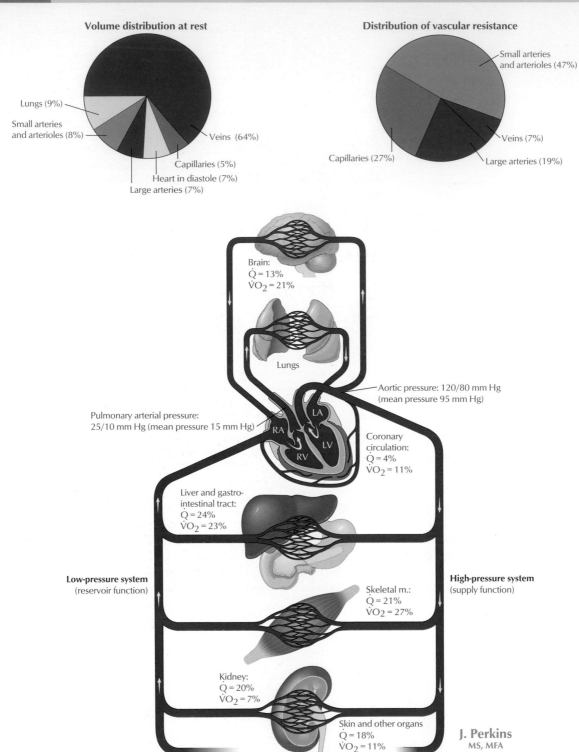

FIGURE 1.12 General Organization of Cardiovascular System. The amount of blood flow per minute ($\dot{Q}$), as a percentage of the cardiac output, and the relative percentage of oxygen used per minute ($\dot{V}O_2$) by the various organ systems are noted.

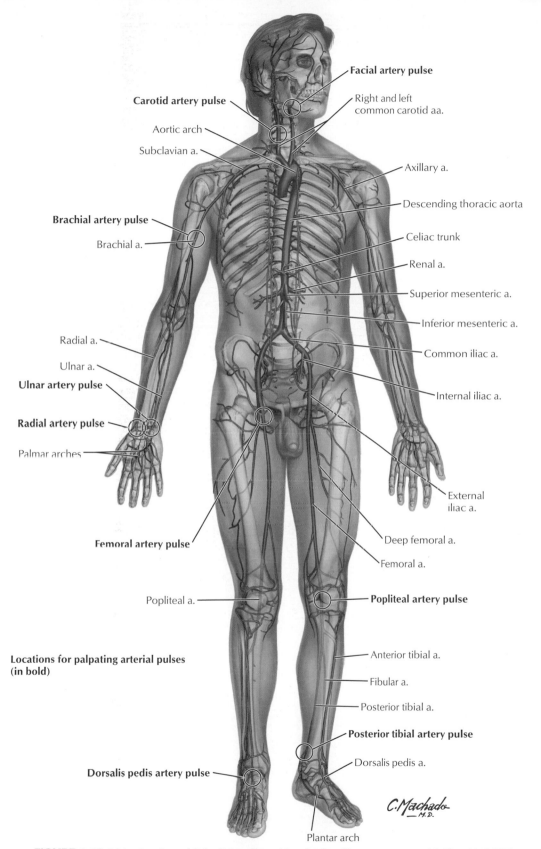

Facial artery pulse

Carotid artery pulse

Right and left
common carotid aa.

Aortic arch

Subclavian a.

Axillary a.

Descending thoracic aorta

Brachial artery pulse

Celiac trunk

Brachial a.

Renal a.

Superior mesenteric a.

Inferior mesenteric a.

Radial a.

Common iliac a.

Ulnar a.

Ulnar artery pulse

Internal iliac a.

Radial artery pulse

Palmar arches

External
iliac a.

Femoral artery pulse

Deep femoral a.

Femoral a.

Popliteal a.

Popliteal artery pulse

**Locations for palpating arterial pulses
(in bold)**

Anterior tibial a.

Fibular a.

Posterior tibial a.

Posterior tibial artery pulse

Dorsalis pedis a.

Dorsalis pedis artery pulse

Plantar arch

FIGURE 1.13 Major Arteries and Pulse Points. (From *Netter's atlas of human anatomy*, ed 8, Plate 14; S-303.)

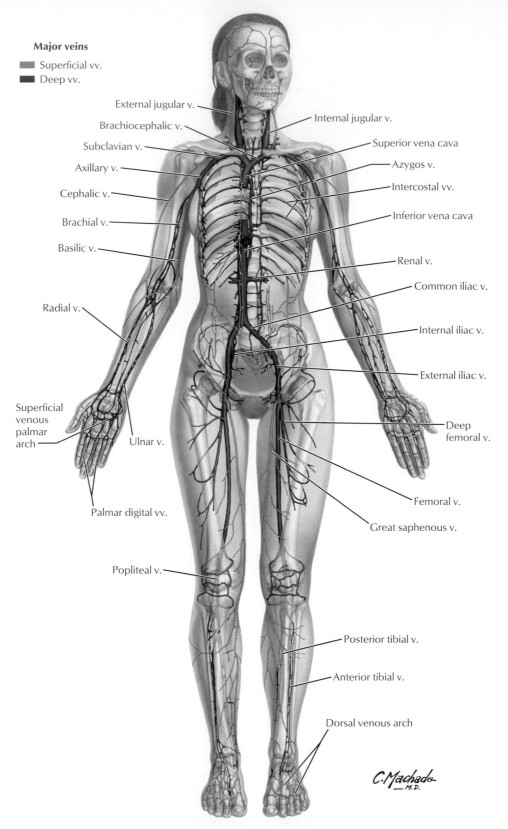

FIGURE 1.14 Major Veins. (From *Netter's atlas of human anatomy*, ed 8, Plate 15; S-304.)

Clinical Focus 1.6

Atherogenesis

Thickening and narrowing of the arterial wall and eventual deposition of lipid into the wall can lead to one form of **atherosclerosis.** The narrowed artery may not be able to meet the metabolic needs of the adjacent tissues, which may become ischemic. Multiple factors, including focal inflammation of the arterial wall, may result in this condition. When development of a plaque is such that it is likely to rupture and lead to thrombosis and arterial occlusion, the atherogenic process is termed **unstable plaque formation.**

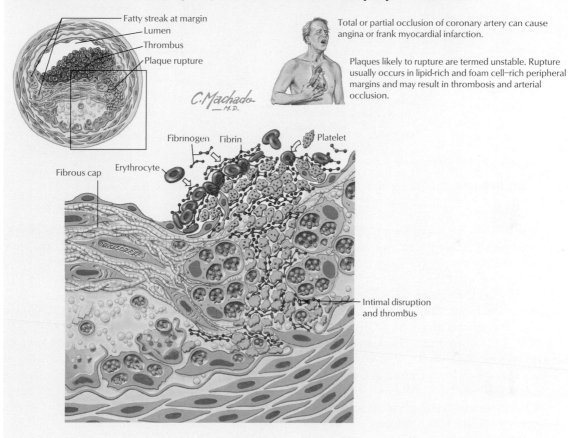

Fatty streak at margin
Lumen
Thrombus
Plaque rupture

Total or partial occlusion of coronary artery can cause angina or frank myocardial infarction.

Plaques likely to rupture are termed unstable. Rupture usually occurs in lipid-rich and foam cell–rich peripheral margins and may result in thrombosis and arterial occlusion.

C. Machado
_M.D._

Fibrinogen   Fibrin

Platelet

Fibrous cap   Erythrocyte

Intimal disruption and thrombus

pulmonary (**pulmonic**) valve and the **aortic** valve (both semilunar valves), respectively.

6. LYMPHATIC SYSTEM

General Organization

The lymphatic system is intimately associated with the cardiovascular system, both in the development of its lymphatic vessels and in its immune function. The lymphatic system functions to:

- Protect the body against infection by activating defense mechanisms of the immune system.
- Collect tissue fluids, solutes, hormones, and plasma proteins and return them to the circulatory system (bloodstream).
- Absorb fat (chylomicrons) from the small intestine.

Components of the lymphatic system include the following:

- **Lymph:** a watery fluid that resembles plasma but contains fewer proteins and may contain fat, together with cells (mainly lymphocytes and a few RBCs).
- **Lymphocytes:** the cellular components of lymph, including T cells, B cells, and NK cells ("natural killer" cells).
- **Lymph vessels:** an extensive network of vessels and capillaries in the peripheral tissues that transport lymph and lymphocytes.
- **Lymphoid organs:** these are collections of lymphoid tissue, including lymph nodes, aggregates

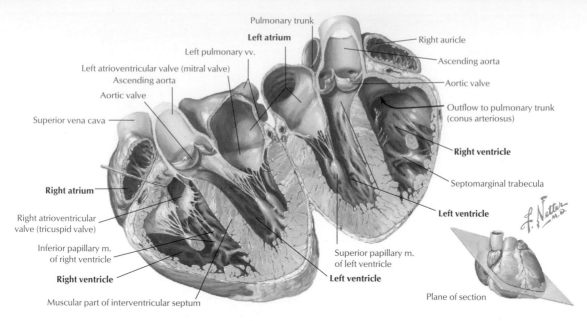

FIGURE 1.15 Chambers of the Heart. (From *Netter's atlas of human anatomy*, ed 8, Plate 245; S-316.)

of lymphoid tissue along the respiratory and gastrointestinal passageways, tonsils, thymus, spleen, and bone marrow.

Lymphatic Drainage

The body is about 60% fluid by weight, with 40% located in the intracellular fluid (ICF) compartment (inside the cells) and the remaining 20% in the extracellular fluid (ECF) compartment. The lymphatics are essential for returning ECF, solutes, and protein (lost via the capillaries into the ECF compartment) back to the bloodstream, thus helping to maintain a normal blood volume. On average, the lymphatics return about 3.5 to 4.0 liters of fluid per day back to the bloodstream. The lymphatics also distribute various hormones, nutrients (fats from the bowel and proteins from the interstitium), and waste products from the ECF to the bloodstream.

Lymphatic vessels transport lymph from everywhere in the body via major lymphatic channels. The majority of lymph (about 75-80%) ultimately collects in the **thoracic duct** for delivery back to the venous system (joins the veins at the union of the left internal jugular and left subclavian veins) (Fig. 1.16). A much smaller **right lymphatic duct** drains the right upper quadrant of the body lymphatics to a similar site on the right side. Along the route of these lymphatic vessels, encapsulated **lymph nodes** are strategically placed to "filter" the lymph as it moves toward the venous system. Lymph

nodes form a key site for phagocytosis of microorganisms and other particulate matter, and they can initiate the body's immune responses.

Immune Response

When a foreign microorganism, virus-infected cell, or cancer cell is detected within the body, the lymphatic system mounts what is called an *immune response.* The detected pathogens are distinguished from the body's own normal cells, and then a response is initiated to neutralize the pathogen. The human body has evolved three major responses to protect against foreign invaders:

- **Nonspecific barriers:** this first line of defense is composed of physical barriers to invasion. These include the skin and mucous membranes that line the body's exterior (skin) or its respiratory, gastrointestinal, urinary, and reproductive systems (mucosa and its secretions, which may include enzymes, acidic secretions, flushing mechanisms such as tear secretion or the voiding of urine, sticky mucus to sequester pathogens, and physical coughing and sneezing to remove pathogens and irritants).
- **Innate immunity:** this second line of defense (if the nonspecific barrier is breached) is composed of a variety of cells and antimicrobial secretions, and manifests itself by producing inflammation and fever.
- **Adaptive immunity:** this third line of defense is characterized by specific pathogen recognition,

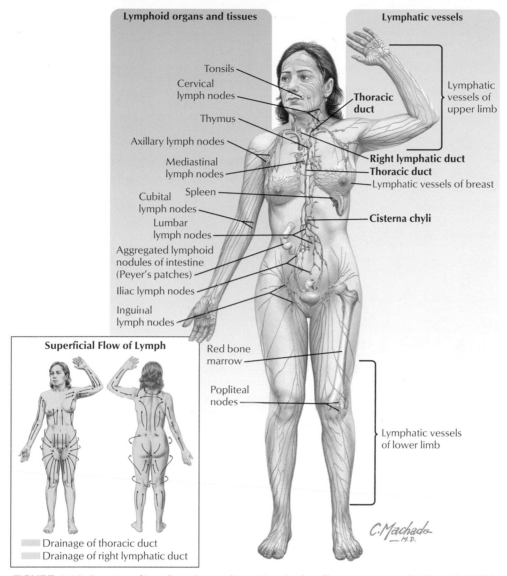

Lymphoid organs and tissues

- Tonsils
- Cervical lymph nodes
- Thymus
- Axillary lymph nodes
- Mediastinal lymph nodes
- Cubital lymph nodes
- Spleen
- Lumbar lymph nodes
- Aggregated lymphoid nodules of intestine (Peyer's patches)
- Iliac lymph nodes
- Inguinal lymph nodes

Lymphatic vessels

- Thoracic duct
- Lymphatic vessels of upper limb
- **Right lymphatic duct**
- **Thoracic duct**
- Lymphatic vessels of breast
- **Cisterna chyli**

Superficial Flow of Lymph

- Red bone marrow
- Popliteal nodes
- Lymphatic vessels of lower limb

Drainage of thoracic duct
Drainage of right lymphatic duct

C. Machado — M.D.

FIGURE 1.16 Overview of Lymphatic System. (From *Netter's atlas of human anatomy*, ed 8, Plate 16; S-343.)

immunologic memory, amplification of immune responses, and rapid response against pathogens that reinvade the body.

7. RESPIRATORY SYSTEM

The respiratory system provides oxygen to the body for its metabolic needs and eliminates carbon dioxide. Structurally, the respiratory system includes the following (Fig. 1.17):
- **Nose and paranasal sinuses.**
- **Pharynx** and its subdivisions (nasopharynx, oropharynx, and laryngopharynx).
- **Larynx**, continuous with the trachea inferiorly.

- **Trachea.**
- **Lungs** (a right lung and a left lung) and their bronchi, bronchioles, alveolar ducts/sacs, and alveoli.

Functionally, the respiratory system performs five basic functions:
- Filters and humidifies the air and moves it in and out of the lungs.
- Provides a large surface area for gas exchange with the blood.
- Helps to regulate the pH of body fluids.
- Participates in vocalization.
- Assists the olfactory system with the detection of smells.

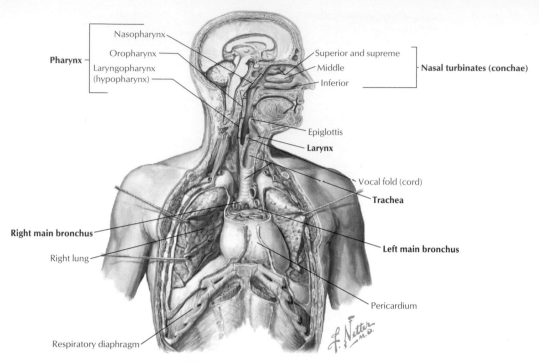

Pharynx — {
  Nasopharynx
  Oropharynx
  Laryngopharynx (hypopharynx)
}

Nasal turbinates (conchae) — {
  Superior and supreme
  Middle
  Inferior
}

Epiglottis
Larynx
Vocal fold (cord)
Trachea
Right main bronchus
Left main bronchus
Right lung
Pericardium
Respiratory diaphragm

FIGURE 1.17 Respiratory System.

8. NERVOUS SYSTEM

General Organization

The nervous system integrates and regulates many body activities, sometimes at discrete locations (specific targets) and sometimes more globally. The nervous system usually acts quite rapidly and can also modulate effects of the endocrine and immune systems. The nervous system is separated into two structural divisions (Fig. 1.18):

- **Central nervous system** (CNS): includes the brain and spinal cord.
- **Peripheral nervous system** (PNS): includes the somatic, autonomic, and enteric nerves outside the CNS.

Neurons

Nerve cells are called **neurons,** and their structure reflects the functional characteristics of an individual neuron (Fig. 1.19). Information comes to the neuron largely through treelike processes called **axons,** which terminate on the neuron at specialized junctions called **synapses.** Synapses can occur on neuronal processes called **dendrites** or on the neuronal cell body, called a **soma** or *perikaryon.*

Neurons convey efferent (motor or output) information via action potentials that course along a *single axon* arising from the soma that then

synapses on a selective target, usually another neuron or target cells, such as muscle cells. Common types of neurons include the following:

- *Unipolar* (often called *pseudounipolar*): a neuron with one axon that divides into two long processes (sensory neurons found in the spinal ganglia of a spinal nerve).
- *Bipolar:* a neuron that possesses one axon and one dendrite (rare but found in the retina and olfactory epithelium).
- *Multipolar:* a neuron that possesses one axon and two or more dendrites (the most common type).

Although the human nervous system contains billions of neurons, all neurons can be classified largely into one of three functional types:

- **Motor neurons:** they convey **efferent** impulses from the CNS or ganglia (collections of neurons outside the CNS) to target (effector) cells; *somatic* efferent axons target skeletal muscle, and *visceral* efferent axons target smooth muscle, cardiac muscle, and glands.
- **Sensory neurons:** they convey **afferent** impulses from peripheral receptors to the CNS; *somatic afferent axons* convey pain, temperature, touch, pressure, and proprioception (nonconscious) sensations; *visceral afferent axons* convey pain and other sensations (e.g., nausea) from organs, glands, and blood vessels to the CNS.

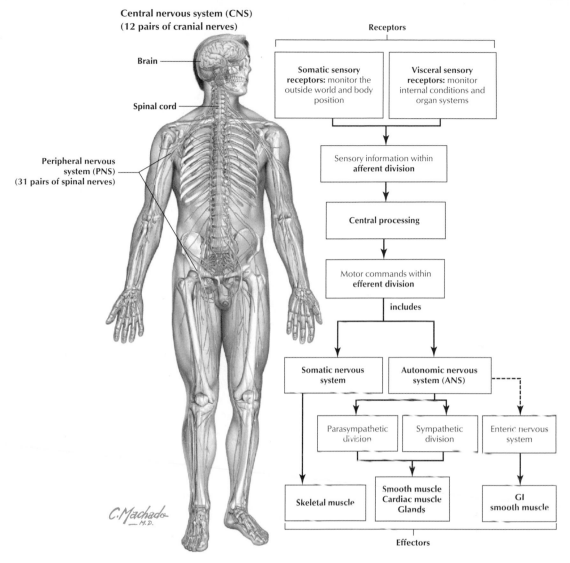

FIGURE 1.18 General Organization of Nervous System. (From *Netter's atlas of human anatomy*, ed 8, Plate 4; S-15.)

- **Interneurons:** they convey impulses between sensory and motor neurons in the CNS, thus forming integrated networks between cells; interneurons probably account for more than 99% of all neurons in the body.

Neurons can vary considerably in size, ranging from several micrometers to more than 100 μm in diameter. Neurons may possess numerous branching dendrites, studded with dendritic spines that increase the receptive area of the neuron many-fold. The neuron's axon may be quite short or over 1 meter long. The axonal diameter may vary. Axons that are larger than 1 to 2 μm in diameter are insulated by **myelin** sheaths. In the CNS, axons are myelinated by a special glial cell called an

oligodendrocyte, whereas in the PNS they are surrounded by a glial cell called a **Schwann cell**, which often also myelinates the PNS axons. Some Schwann cells do not produce myelin and simply invest a group of nerve fibers separately within their cytoplasm, e.g. most cutaneous (sensory) nerves to the skin.

Glia

Glia are the cells that support neurons, within both the CNS (neuroglia) and the PNS. Glial cells far outnumber the neurons in the nervous system and contribute to most of the postnatal growth, along with axonal myelination, seen in the CNS. Functionally, glia:

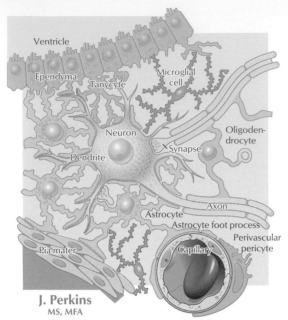

J. Perkins
MS, MFA

FIGURE 1.19 Cell Types Found in Central Nervous System.

- Provide structural isolation of neurons and their synapses.
- Sequester ions in the extracellular compartment.
- Provide trophic support to the neurons and their processes.
- Support growth and secrete growth factors.
- Support some of the signaling functions of neurons.
- Myelinate axons.
- Phagocytize debris and participate in inflammatory responses.
- Play a dynamic role in pruning or preserving neuronal connections.
- Rid the brain of metabolites and dump them into the CSF.
- Participate in the formation of the blood-brain barrier.

The different types of glial cells include the following (see Fig. 1.19):

- **Astrocytes:** these are the most numerous of the glial cells; provide physical and metabolic support for CNS neurons, can become reactive during CNS injury, release growth factors and other bioactive molecules, and contribute to the formation of the *blood-brain barrier*.
- **Oligodendrocytes:** these are smaller glial cells; responsible for the formation and maintenance of myelin in the CNS.
- **Microglia:** these are smallest and rarest of CNS glia, although more numerous than neurons in

CNS; these phagocytic cells participate in inflammatory reactions, remodel and remove synapses, and respond to injury.
- **Ependymal cells:** these cells line the ventricles of the brain and the central canal of the spinal cord, which contains **cerebrospinal fluid (CSF)**.
- **Schwann cells:** these are the glial cells of the PNS; surround all axons (myelinating many of them) and provide trophic support, facilitate regrowth of PNS axons, and clean away cellular debris (Fig. 1.20).

Peripheral Nerves

The peripheral nerves observed grossly in the human body are composed of bundles of thousands of nerve fibers enclosed within a connective tissue covering and supplied by small blood vessels. The nerve "fibers" consist of axons (efferent and afferent) individually separated from each other by the cytoplasmic processes of Schwann cells or myelinated by a multilayered wrapping of continuous Schwann cell membrane (the *myelin sheath*).

The peripheral nerve resembles an electrical cable of axons that is further supported by three connective tissue sleeves or coverings (Fig. 1.20):

- **Endoneurium:** a thin connective tissue sleeve that surrounds the axons and Schwann cells.
- **Perineurium:** a dense layer of connective tissue that encircles a bundle (fascicle) of nerve fibers.
- **Epineurium:** an outer thick connective tissue sheath that encircles bundles of fascicles; this is the "nerve" typically seen grossly coursing throughout the human body.

Peripheral nerves include the 12 pairs of **cranial nerves** arising from the brain or brainstem and the 31 pairs of **spinal nerves** arising from the spinal cord.

Meninges

The brain and spinal cord are surrounded by three membranous connective tissue layers called the *meninges*. These three layers include the following (Fig. 1.21):

- **Dura mater:** the thick, outermost meningeal layer, richly innervated by sensory nerve fibers.
- **Arachnoid mater**: the fine, weblike avascular membrane directly beneath the dural surface.
- **Pia mater:** the delicate membrane of connective tissue that intimately envelops the brain and spinal cord.

The space between the arachnoid and the underlying pia is called the **subarachnoid space** and contains **cerebrospinal fluid** (CSF), which bathes and protects the CNS.

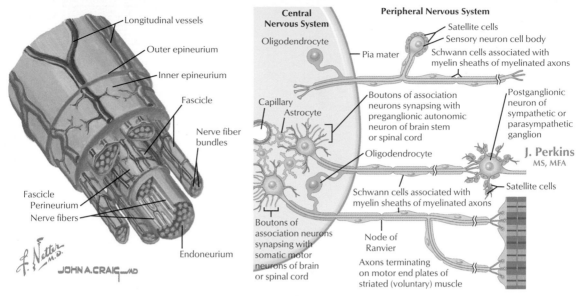

FIGURE 1.20 Features of Typical Peripheral Nerve.

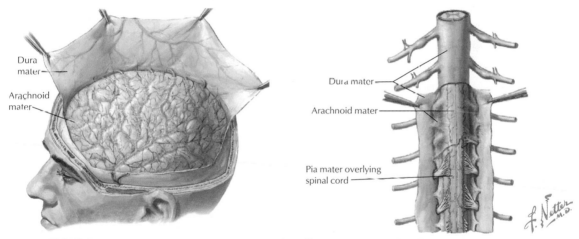

FIGURE 1.21 CNS Meninges. (From *Netter's atlas of human anatomy*, ed 8, Plates 129 and 189; S-28 and S-19.)

Cranial Nerves

Twelve pairs of cranial nerves arise from the brain, and they are identified both by their names and by Roman numerals I to XII (Fig. 1.22). The cranial nerves are somewhat unique and can contain multiple functional components:

- **General:** same general functions as spinal nerves.
- **Special:** functions found only in cranial nerves.
- **Afferent** and **efferent:** sensory and motor functions, respectively.
- **Somatic** and **visceral:** related to skin and skeletal muscle (somatic) or to smooth muscle, cardiac muscle, and glands (visceral).

Therefore, each cranial nerve (CN) may possess multiple functional components, such as the following:

- *General somatic afferents* (GSAs): they contain nerve fibers that are sensory from the skin, such as those of a spinal nerve.
- *General visceral efferents* (GVEs): they contain motor fibers to visceral structures (smooth muscle and/or glands), such as a parasympathetic fiber from the sacral spinal cord (spinal cord levels S2 to S4 give rise to parasympathetics).
- *Special somatic afferents* (SSAs): they contain special sensory fibers, such as those for vision and hearing.

In general, **CN I** and **CN II** arise from the forebrain and are really tracts of the brain for the special senses of smell and sight. The other cranial nerves arise from the brainstem. Cranial nerves **III**, **IV**, and **VI** move the extraocular skeletal muscles

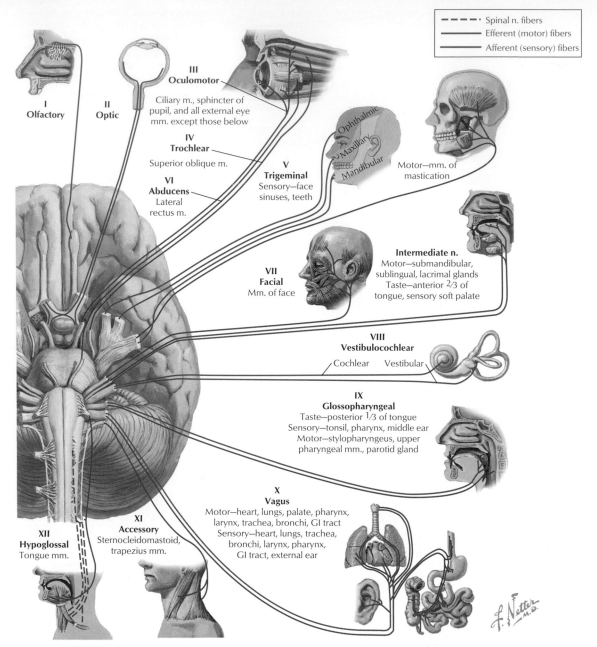

FIGURE 1.22 Overview of Cranial Nerves. (From *Netter's atlas of human anatomy*, ed 8, Plate 145; S-53.)

of the eyeball. **CN V** has three divisions: V_1 and V_2 are sensory, and V_3 is both motor to skeletal muscle and sensory. Cranial nerves **VII, IX,** and **X** are both motor and sensory. **CN VIII** is the special sense of hearing and balance. **CN XI** and **CN XII** are motor to skeletal muscle. Cranial nerves **III, VII, IX,** and **X** also contain parasympathetic fibers of origin (visceral), although many of the autonomic fibers will "jump" onto the branches of **CN V** to reach their targets. Table 1.2 summarizes the types of fibers in each cranial nerve.

Spinal Nerves

The spinal cord gives rise to 31 pairs of spinal nerves (Figs. 1.23, 1.24, 2.13, and Chapter 2 – Section 5. Spinal Cord), which then form two major branches (rami):

- **Posterior (dorsal) ramus:** a small ramus that courses dorsally to the back; it conveys motor and sensory information to and from the skin, intrinsic back skeletal muscles (erector spinae, transversospinales), and synovial joints of the vertebral column.
- **Anterior (ventral) ramus:** a much larger ramus that courses laterally and ventrally; it innervates

TABLE 1.2 Cranial Nerve Fibers

CRANIAL NERVE	FUNCTIONAL COMPONENT*
I Olfactory	SVA (Special sense of smell)
II Optic	SSA (Special sense of sight)
III Oculomotor	GSE (Motor to extraocular muscles)
	GVE (Parasympathetic to smooth muscle in eye)
IV Trochlear	GSE (Motor to one extraocular muscle)
V Trigeminal	GSA (Sensory to face, orbit, nose, anterior tongue)
	SVE (Motor to skeletal muscles)
VI Abducens	GSE (Motor to one extraocular muscle)
VII Facial	GSA (Sensory to skin of ear)
	SVA (Special sense of taste to anterior tongue)
	GVE (Motor to glands—salivary, nasal, lacrimal)
	SVE (Motor to facial muscles)
VIII Vestibulocochlear	SSA (Special sense of hearing and balance)
IX Glossopharyngeal	GSA (Sensory to posterior tongue)
	SVA (Special sense of taste—posterior tongue)
	GVA (Sensory from middle ear, pharynx, carotid body, sinus)
	GVE (Motor to parotid gland)
	SVE (Motor to one muscle of pharynx)
X Vagus	GSA (Sensory external ear)
	SVA (Special sense of taste—epiglottis)
	GVA (Sensory from pharynx, larynx, thoracoabdominal organs)
	GVE (Motor to thoracoabdominal organs)
	SVE (Motor to muscles of pharynx/larynx)
XI Accessory	GSE (Motor to two muscles)
XII Hypoglossal	GSE (Motor to tongue muscles)

*GSA, General somatic afferent; GSE, general somatic efferent; GVA, general visceral afferent; GVE, general visceral efferent; SSA, special somatic afferent; SVA, special visceral afferent; SVE, special visceral efferent.

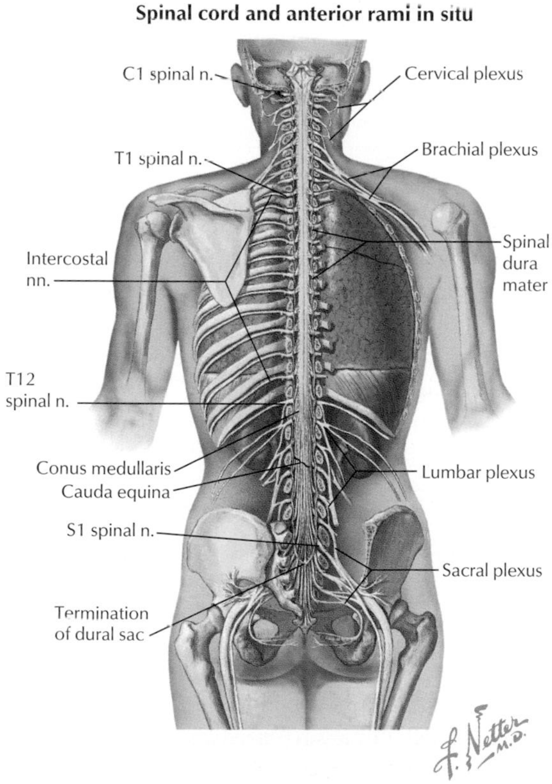

Spinal cord and anterior rami in situ

FIGURE 1.23 Overview of Spinal Cord and Spinal Nerves. (From *Netter's atlas of human anatomy*, ed 8, Plate 186; S-16.)

all the remaining skin and skeletal muscles of the neck, limbs, and trunk.

Once nerve fibers (sensory or motor) are beyond, or peripheral to, the spinal cord proper, the fibers (axons) then reside in nerves of the PNS. Components of the PNS include the following (Fig. 1.24):

- **Somatic nervous system:** sensory and motor fibers to skin, skeletal muscle, and joints (Fig. 1.24, left side).
- **Autonomic nervous system** (ANS): sensory and motor fibers to all smooth muscle (viscera, vasculature), cardiac muscle (heart), and glands (Fig. 1.24, right side).
- **Enteric nervous system:** plexuses and ganglia of the GI tract that regulate bowel secretion, absorption, and motility (originally considered part of ANS); they are linked to the ANS for optimal regulation.

Features of the *somatic nervous system* include the following:

- It is a one-neuron motor system.
- The motor (efferent) neuron is in the CNS, and an axon projects to a peripheral target (e.g., skeletal muscle).
- The sensory (afferent) neuron (pseudounipolar) resides in a peripheral ganglion called a *spinal ganglion* and conveys sensory information from

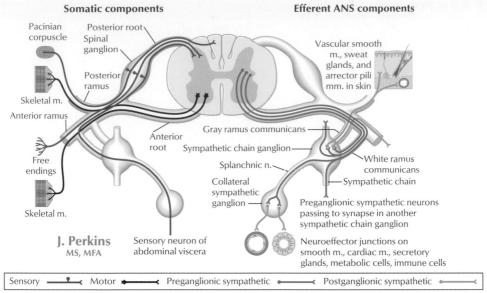

FIGURE 1.24 Elements of Peripheral Nervous System. For clarity, this schematic shows the arrangement of the efferent and afferent somatic nerve components of a typical spinal nerve on the left side and the efferent components of the ANS of a typical spinal nerve on the right side.

the skin, muscle, or joint to the CNS (in this case the spinal cord).

The unilateral area of skin innervated by the somatic sensory fibers from a single spinal nerve root is called a **dermatome**. The nerve roots to neighboring dermatomes overlap. Therefore, damage to a single dorsal root would produce *hypoesthesia* (diminished sensation), not anesthesia (complete loss of sensation), to the region supplied predominately by that dermatome level. Complete dermatomal anesthesia would result if three contiguous dorsal roots were damaged. Clinically, dermatome maps of the body can be helpful in localizing spinal cord or peripheral nerve lesions (see Chapter 2).

Features of the *ANS division of the PNS* include the following:

- It is a two-neuron motor system; the first neuron resides in the CNS and the second neuron in a peripheral autonomic ganglion.
- The axon of the first neuron is termed *preganglionic* and of the second neuron, *postganglionic*.
- The ANS has two divisions, sympathetic and parasympathetic.
- The *sensory neuron* (pseudounipolar) resides in a spinal ganglion (similar to the somatic system) and conveys sensory information from the viscera to the CNS (not shown in Fig. 1.24).

Autonomic Nervous System

The ANS is divided into sympathetic and parasympathetic divisions. In contrast to the somatic division of the PNS, the ANS is a *two-neuron system* with

a **preganglionic neuron** in the CNS that sends its axon into a peripheral nerve to synapse on a **postganglionic neuron** in a peripheral autonomic ganglion (Fig. 1.25). The postganglionic neuron then sends its axon to the target (*smooth muscle, cardiac muscle, and glands*). The ANS is a visceral system, since many of the body's organs are composed of smooth muscle walls or contain secretory glandular tissue.

Sympathetic Division

The **sympathetic division** of the ANS is also known as the *thoracolumbar division* because:

- Its preganglionic neurons are found only within the intermediolateral gray matter of the T1-L2 spinal cord levels.

Preganglionic axons exit the T1-L2 spinal cord in an anterior root, then enter a spinal nerve, and then via a white **ramus communicans** enter the **sympathetic chain.** The sympathetic chain is a bilateral chain of ganglia just lateral to the vertebral bodies that runs from the base of the skull to the coccyx. Once in the sympathetic chain, the preganglionic axon may take one of three synaptic routes (Fig. 1.25):

1. Synapse on a postganglionic sympathetic neuron at the T1-L2 level, or ascend or descend to synapse on a **sympathetic chain neuron** at any of the 31 spinal nerve levels.
2. Pass through the sympathetic chain, enter a **splanchnic (visceral) nerve,** and synapse in a **collateral (prevertebral) ganglion** in the abdominopelvic

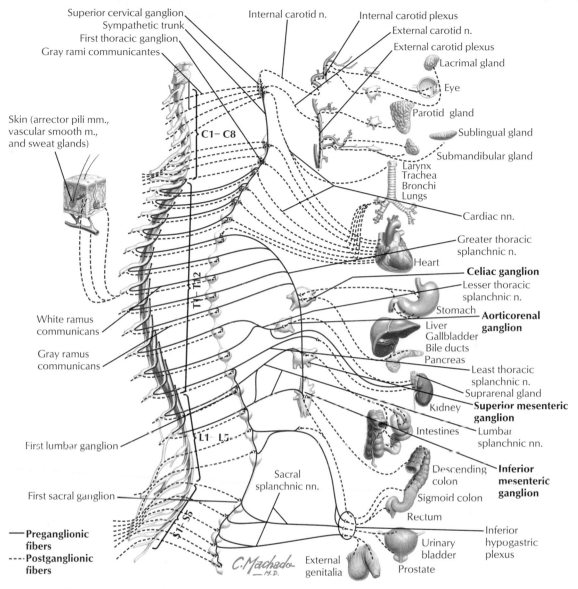

FIGURE 1.25 Sympathetic Division of Autonomic Nervous System. (From *Netter's atlas of human anatomy*, ed 8, Plate 6; S-21.)

cavity (celiac, aorticorenal, superior mesenteric or inferior mesenteric ganglia).

3. Pass through the sympathetic chain, enter a splanchnic nerve, pass through a collateral ganglion (aorticorenal), and synapse on the cells of the **adrenal medulla** (the central portion of the adrenal gland).

Axons of the postganglionic sympathetic neurons (which greatly outnumber preganglionic neurons) may act in one of four ways (Fig. 1.25):

1. Reenter the spinal nerve via a **gray ramus communicans** and join any one of the 31 spinal nerves (anterior and posterior rami) as they distribute widely throughout the body. These fibers innervate sweat glands (sudomotor), arrector pili muscles of hair (pilomotor resulting in "goose bumps"), and blood vessels (vasomotor).

2. Reenter the spinal nerve but course along blood vessels in the head, or join cardiopulmonary or hypogastric plexuses of nerves to distribute to the head, thorax, and pelvic viscera.

3. Arise from postganglionic neurons in abdominopelvic **collateral ganglia** and course with blood vessels to abdominopelvic viscera.

4. Cells of the **adrenal medulla** are differentiated neuroendocrine cells **(paraneurons)** that do not

TABLE 1.3 Effects of Sympathetic Stimulation on Various Structures

STRUCTURE	EFFECTS	STRUCTURE	EFFECTS
Eye	Dilates the pupil	Liver	Causes glycogen breakdown, glucose synthesis and release
Lacrimal glands	Reduces secretion slightly (vasoconstriction)	Salivary glands	Reduces and thickens secretion via vasoconstriction
Skin	Causes goose bumps (arrector pili muscle contraction)	Genital system	Causes ejaculation and orgasm, and remission of erection
Sweat glands	Increases secretion		Constricts male internal urethral sphincter muscle
Peripheral vessels	Causes vasoconstriction		
Heart	Increases heart rate and force of contraction	Urinary system	Decreases urine production via vasoconstriction
Coronary arteries	Vasoconstriction (metabolic vasodilation overrides this effect)		Constricts male internal urethral sphincter muscle
Lungs	Assists in bronchodilation and reduced secretion	Adrenal medulla	Increases secretion of epinephrine or norepinephrine
Digestive tract	Decreases peristalsis, contracts internal anal sphincter muscle, causes vasoconstriction to shunt blood elsewhere		

have axons but release hormones directly into the bloodstream. They are innervated directly by preganglionic sympathetic fibers.

Preganglionic axons release acetylcholine (ACh) at their synapses, and norepinephrine (NE) is the transmitter released by postganglionic axons (except ACh is released on *sweat glands*). The cells of the adrenal medulla (modified postganglionic sympathetic neurons) release epinephrine and some NE into the blood, not as neurotransmitters but as *hormones*. The sympathetic system acts globally throughout the body to mobilize it in "fright-flight-fight" situations (Table 1.3).

Parasympathetic Division

The parasympathetic division of the ANS also is a two-neuron system with its preganglionic neuron in the CNS and postganglionic neuron in a peripheral ganglion (Fig. 1.26). The **parasympathetic division** also is known as the *craniosacral division* because:

- Its preganglionic neurons are found in cranial nerves III, VII, IX, and X and in the sacral spinal cord at levels S2-S4.
- Its preganglionic neurons reside in the four cranial nuclei associated with the four cranial nerves listed earlier or in the lateral gray matter of the sacral spinal cord at levels S2-S4.

Preganglionic parasympathetic axons exit the CNS in one of three ways:

1. Exit the brainstem in the **cranial nerve** (except CN X) and pass to a **peripheral ganglion** in the head (ciliary, pterygopalatine, submandibular, or otic ganglia) to synapse on the parasympathetic postganglionic neurons residing in these ganglia.

2. *CN X preganglionic fibers* exit the brainstem and provide preganglionic parasympathetic fibers **to terminal ganglia** (microscopically small postganglionic neurons) in the neck, thorax, and proximal two-thirds of the abdominal viscera.

3. Exit the sacral spinal cord via an anterior root and then enter the **pelvic splanchnic nerves**, to synapse on postganglionic neurons in **terminal ganglia** located in or near the viscera to be innervated.

Axons of the postganglionic parasympathetic neurons take one of two courses:

1. Pass from the **parasympathetic ganglion in the head** (ciliary, pterygopalatine, otic, and submandibular) on existing nerves or blood vessels, to innervate smooth muscle and glands of the head.

2. Pass from terminal ganglia in or near the viscera innervated and then synapse on smooth muscle, cardiac muscle, or glands in the neck, thorax, and abdominopelvic cavity.

As noted above, the vagus nerve (CN X) is unique. Its preganglionic axons exit the brainstem and synapse on terminal ganglia in or near the targets in the neck, thorax (heart, lungs, glands, smooth muscle), and abdominal cavity (proximal two thirds of the GI tract and its accessory organs). Short axons of the terminal ganglia neurons then synapse on their targets.

Parasympathetic axons *do not pass* into the limbs as do sympathetic axons. Therefore, the vascular smooth muscle, arrector pili muscles of the skin (attached to hair follicles), and sweat glands are all innervated only by the sympathetic system. ACh is the *neurotransmitter* at all parasympathetic

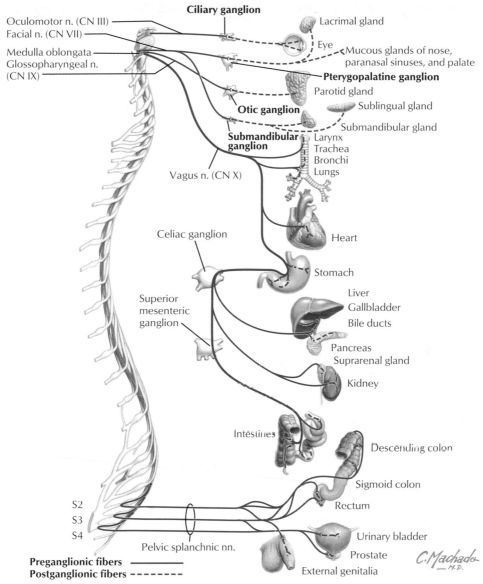

Ciliary ganglion
Oculomotor n. (CN III)
Facial n. (CN VII)
Lacrimal gland
Eye
Mucous glands of nose, paranasal sinuses, and palate
Medulla oblongata
Glossopharyngeal n. (CN IX)
Pterygopalatine ganglion
Parotid gland
Otic ganglion
Sublingual gland
Submandibular gland
Submandibular ganglion
Larynx
Trachea
Bronchi
Lungs
Vagus n. (CN X)
Celiac ganglion
Heart
Stomach
Liver
Gallbladder
Bile ducts
Superior mesenteric ganglion
Pancreas
Suprarenal gland
Kidney
Intestines
Descending colon
Sigmoid colon
S2
S3
S4
Rectum
Pelvic splanchnic nn.
Urinary bladder
Prostate
Preganglionic fibers ————
Postganglionic fibers --------
External genitalia
C. Machado —M.D.

FIGURE 1.26 Parasympathetic Division of Autonomic Nervous System. (From *Netter's atlas of human anatomy*, ed 8, Plate 7; S-22.)

synapses, both preganglionic and postganglionic synapses.

The parasympathetic system is involved in feeding and sexual arousal functions and acts more slowly and focally than the sympathetic system. For example, CN X can slow the heart rate without affecting input to the stomach. In general, the sympathetic and parasympathetic systems maintain homeostasis, although as a protective measure, the body maintains a low level of "sympathetic tone" and can activate this division on a moment's notice. ANS function is regulated ultimately by the hypothalamus. Most presynaptic parasympathetic axons are long, extending to their peripheral targets, while the postsynaptic

fibers are short because the parasympathetic ganglia often reside near or in the organs they innervate. Table 1.4 summarizes the specific functions of the parasympathetic division of the ANS.

Although the ANS uses classic neurotransmitters such as NE and ACh at its synapses, its neurons also co-release a wide variety of neuroactive peptides and other neuromodulators that "fine-tune" their functions at the level of their respective targets.

Enteric Nervous System

The enteric nervous system was formally considered the third division of the ANS. The word *enteric* refers to the bowel. This component of the PNS consists

TABLE 1.4 Effects of Parasympathetic Stimulation on Various Structures

STRUCTURE	EFFECTS	STRUCTURE	EFFECTS
Eye	Constricts pupil	Digestive tract	Increases peristalsis, increases secretion, inhibits internal anal sphincter for defecation
Ciliary body	Constricts muscle for accommodation (near vision)		
Lacrimal glands	Increase secretion	Liver	Aids glycogen synthesis and storage
Heart	Decreases heart rate and force of contraction	Salivary glands	Increase secretion
		Genital system	Promotes engorgement of erectile tissues
Coronary arteries	Vasodilation (of little importance)		
Lungs	Cause bronchoconstriction and increased secretion	Urinary system	Contracts bladder (detrusor muscle) for urination, inhibits contraction of male internal urethral sphincter, increases urine production

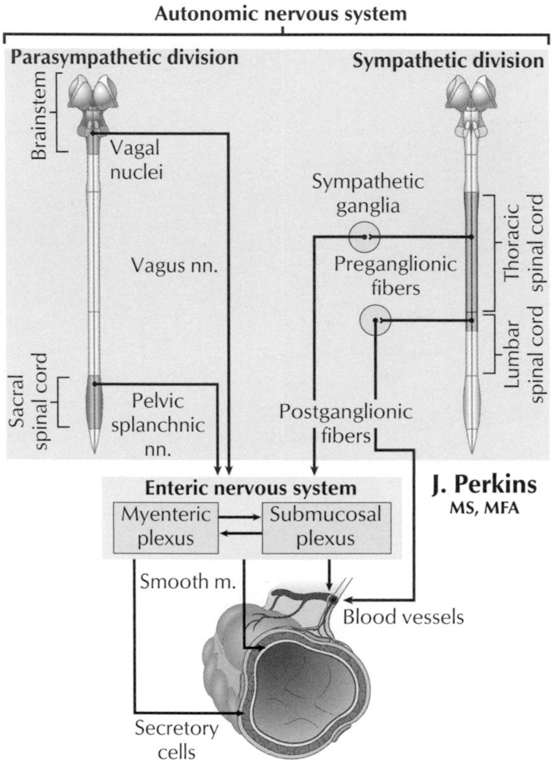

FIGURE 1.27 Relationship of Enteric Nervous System to Sympathetic and Parasympathetic ANS Divisions.

of ganglia and nerve plexuses in the walls and mesenteries of the GI tract. These ganglia and their neural networks include the following (Fig. 1.27):

- **Myenteric (Auerbach's) plexuses:** ganglia and nerves located between the circular and longitudinal smooth muscle layers of the muscularis externa of the bowel wall.
- **Submucosal (Meissner's) plexuses:** ganglia and nerves located in the submucosa of the bowel wall.

The enteric nervous system has important links to both divisions of the ANS, which are critical for optimal regulation of bowel secretion, absorption, and motility. More than 20 different transmitter substances have been identified in the intrinsic neurons of the enteric nervous system, pointing to the fine degree of regulation that occurs at the level of the bowel wall. Optimal GI functioning requires coordinated interactions of the ANS, the enteric nervous system, and the endocrine system.

9. ENDOCRINE SYSTEM

The endocrine system, along with the nervous and immune systems, facilitates communication, integration, and regulation of many of the body's functions (Fig. 1.28). Specifically, the endocrine system interacts with target sites (cells and tissues), some that are quite a distance from a gland, by releasing hormones into the bloodstream. Generally, endocrine glands and hormones also share the following features:

- Secretion is controlled by feedback mechanisms.
- Hormones bind target receptors on cell membranes or within the cells (cytoplasmic or nuclear).
- Hormone action may be slow to appear but may have long-lasting effects.
- Hormones are chemically diverse molecules (amines, peptides/proteins, steroids).

Hormones can communicate through a variety of cell-to-cell interactions, including:

- *Autocrine:* interacts on another cell as well as on itself.
- *Paracrine:* interacts directly on an adjacent or nearby cell.
- *Endocrine:* interacts at a great distance by traveling in the bloodstream.
- *Neurocrine:* interacts similar to a neurotransmitter, except released into the bloodstream.

Table 1.5 summarizes the major hormones and the tissues responsible for their release.

Additionally, other organs have paracrine or endocrine functions. For example, the **placenta** releases human chorionic gonadotropin (hCG), estrogens, progesterone, and human placental lactogen

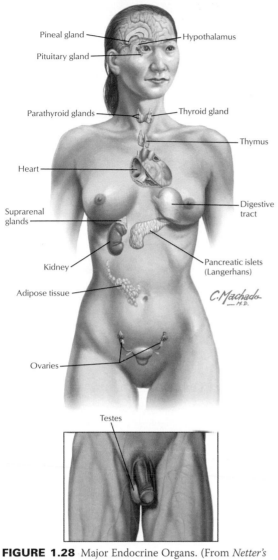

FIGURE 1.28 Major Endocrine Organs. (From *Netter's atlas of human anatomy*, ed 8, Plate 21; S-522.)

TABLE 1.5 Major Hormones*	
TISSUE/ ORGAN	**HORMONE**
Hypothalamus	Antidiuretic hormone (ADH), oxytocin, thyrotropin-releasing hormone (TRH), corticotropin-releasing hormone (CRH), growth hormone–releasing hormone (GHRH), gonadotropin-releasing hormone (GnRH), somatostatin (SS), dopamine (DA)
Pineal gland	Melatonin
Anterior pituitary gland	Adrenocorticotropic hormone (ACTH), thyroid-stimulating hormone (TSH), growth hormone (GH), prolactin, follicle-stimulating hormone (FSH), luteinizing hormone (LH), melanocyte-stimulating hormone (MSH)
Posterior pituitary gland	Oxytocin, vasopressin (ADH)
Thyroid gland	Thyroxine (T_4), triiodothyronine (T_3), calcitonin
Parathyroid glands	Parathyroid hormone (PTH, parathormone)
Thymus gland	Thymopoietin, thymulin, thymosin, thymic humoral factor, interleukins, interferons
Heart	Atrial natriuretic peptide (ANP)
Digestive tract	Gastrin, secretin, cholecystokinin (CCK), motilin, gastric inhibitory peptide (GIP), glucagon, SS, vasoactive intestinal peptide (VIP), ghrelin, leptin, and many more
Liver	Insulin-like growth factors (IGFs)
Suprarenal (adrenal) glands	Cortisol, aldosterone, androgens, epinephrine (E), norepinephrine (NE)
Pancreatic islets	Insulin, glucagon, SS, VIP, pancreatic polypeptide
Kidneys	Erythropoietin (EPO), calcitriol, renin, urodilatin
Fat	Leptin
Ovaries	Estrogens, progestins, inhibin, relaxin
Testes	Testosterone, inhibin
White blood cells and some connective tissue cells	Various cytokines; interleukins, colony-stimulating factors, interferons, tumor necrosis factor (TNF)

*This list is not comprehensive; only the more commonly found hormones are listed.

(hPL), whereas other cells release a variety of growth factors. The mesenteries of the GI tract also release various substances, and they contain a variable amount of fat, which itself releases the hormone leptin. Again, the endocrine system is widespread and critically important in regulating bodily functions. Each year, researchers find additional paracrine and endocrine substances, and many of their regulatory functions continue to be elucidated.

10. GASTROINTESTINAL SYSTEM

The GI system includes the epithelial-lined tube that begins with the oral cavity and extends to the anal canal, as well as GI-associated glands, including the following:

- **Salivary glands:** three major glands and hundreds of microscopic minor salivary glands scattered throughout the oral mucosa.
- **Liver:** the largest solid gland in the body
- **Gallbladder:** functions to store and concentrate bile needed for fat digestion.
- **Pancreas:** crucial exocrine (digestive enzymes) and endocrine organ.

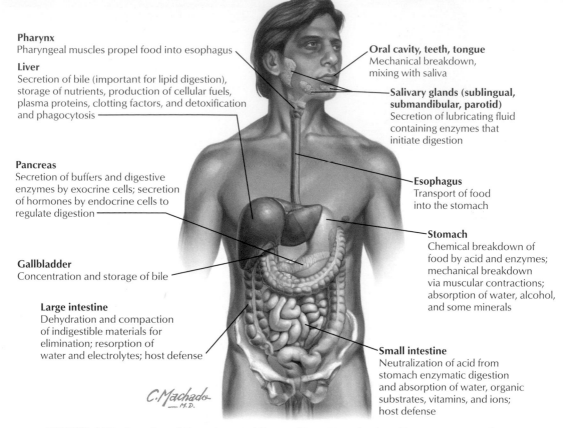

Pharynx
Pharyngeal muscles propel food into esophagus

Liver
Secretion of bile (important for lipid digestion), storage of nutrients, production of cellular fuels, plasma proteins, clotting factors, and detoxification and phagocytosis

Pancreas
Secretion of buffers and digestive enzymes by exocrine cells; secretion of hormones by endocrine cells to regulate digestion

Gallbladder
Concentration and storage of bile

Large intestine
Dehydration and compaction of indigestible materials for elimination; resorption of water and electrolytes; host defense

Oral cavity, teeth, tongue
Mechanical breakdown, mixing with saliva

Salivary glands (sublingual, submandibular, parotid)
Secretion of lubricating fluid containing enzymes that initiate digestion

Esophagus
Transport of food into the stomach

Stomach
Chemical breakdown of food by acid and enzymes; mechanical breakdown via muscular contractions; absorption of water, alcohol, and some minerals

Small intestine
Neutralization of acid from stomach enzymatic digestion and absorption of water, organic substrates, vitamins, and ions; host defense

C. Machado
_M.D.

FIGURE 1.29 Overview of Gastrointestinal System. (From *Netter's atlas of human anatomy*, ed 8, Plate 18; S-394.)

The epithelial-lined tube that is the GI tract measures about 28 feet (8 m) in length (from mouth to anal canal) and includes the following cavities and visceral structures (Fig. 1.29):

- **Oral cavity:** tongue, teeth, and salivary glands.
- **Pharynx:** throat, subdivided into the nasopharynx, oropharynx, and laryngopharynx.
- **Esophagus:** passing from the pharynx to the stomach.
- **Stomach:** the expandable saclike portion of the GI tract.
- **Small intestine:** subdivided into the duodenum, jejunum, and ileum.
- **Large intestine:** subdivided into the cecum, ascending colon, transverse colon, descending colon, sigmoid colon, rectum, and anal canal.

11. URINARY SYSTEM

The urinary system includes the following components (Fig. 1.30):

- **Kidneys:** paired retroperitoneal organs that filter the plasma and produce urine; located high in the posterior abdominal wall just anterior to the muscles of the posterior wall.
- **Ureters:** course retroperitoneally from the kidneys to the pelvis and convey urine from the kidneys to the urinary bladder.
- **Urinary bladder:** lies subperitoneally in the anterior pelvis, stores urine, and, when appropriate, discharges the urine through the urethra.
- **Urethra:** courses from the urinary bladder to the exterior.
  The **kidneys** function to:
- Filter the plasma and begin the process of urine formation.
- Reabsorb important electrolytes, organic molecules, vitamins, and water from the filtrate.
- Excrete metabolic wastes, metabolites, and foreign chemicals (e.g., drugs).
- Regulate fluid volume, composition, and pH.
- Secrete hormones that regulate blood pressure, erythropoiesis, and calcium metabolism.
- Convey urine to the ureters, which then pass the urine to the bladder.

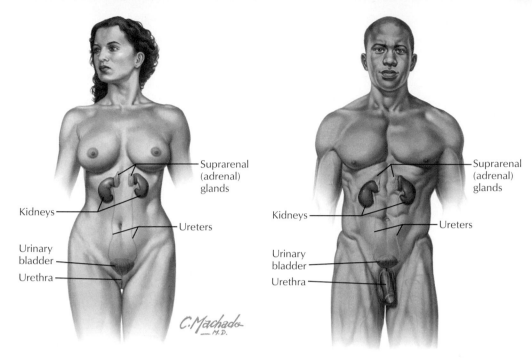

FIGURE 1.30 Urinary System. (From *Netter's atlas of human anatomy*, ed 8, Plate 19; S-458.)

The *kidneys* filter about 180 liters of fluid each day. Grossly, each kidney measures about 12 cm long × 6 cm wide × 3 cm thick and weighs about 150 grams, although variability is common. Approximately 20% of the blood pumped by the heart passes to the kidney each minute for plasma filtration, although most of the fluid and important plasma constituents are returned to the blood as the filtrate courses down the tubules of the *kidney's nephrons* (the nephrons are the kidney's filtration units; they are microscopically small and number about 1 million in each kidney).

Each ureter is about 24 to 34 cm long, lies in a retroperitoneal position, and contains a thick smooth muscle wall. The *urinary bladder* serves as a reservoir for the urine and is a smooth muscle "bag" that expels the urine when appropriate. The *female urethra* is short (3-4 cm), whereas the *male urethra* is long (~20 cm), coursing through the prostate gland, external urethral sphincter, and corpus spongiosum of the penis.

12. REPRODUCTIVE SYSTEM

Female Reproductive System

The female reproductive system is composed of the following structures (Fig. 1.31):

- **Ovaries:** the paired gonads of the female reproductive system; produce the female germ cells called *ova* (oocytes, eggs) and secrete the hormones estrogen and progesterone.
- **Uterine tubes** (fallopian tubes): paired tubes that extend from the superolateral walls of the uterus and open as fimbriated funnels into the pelvic cavity adjacent to the ovary, to "capture" the oocyte as it is ovulated.
- **Uterus:** hollow, pear-shaped muscular (smooth muscle) organ that protects and nourishes a developing fetus.
- **Vagina:** distensible fibromuscular tube (also called *birth canal*) approximately 8 to 9 cm long that extends from the uterine cervix (neck) to the vestibule.

Male Reproductive System

The male reproductive system is composed of the following structures (see Fig. 1.31):

- **Testes:** the paired gonads of the male reproductive system, egg shaped and about the size of a chestnut; produce the male germ cells, *spermatozoa,* and reside in the scrotum (externalized from the abdominopelvic cavity).
- **Epididymis:** a convoluted tubule that receives the spermatozoa and stores them as they mature.
- **Ductus (vas) deferens:** a muscular (smooth muscle) tube about 40 to 45 cm long that conveys sperm from the epididymis to the ejaculatory duct (seminal vesicle).

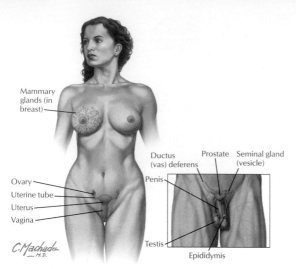

FIGURE 1.31 Reproductive System. (From *Netter's atlas of human anatomy*, ed 8, Plate 20; S-472.)

- **Seminal vesicles:** paired tubular glands that lie posterior to the prostate gland, about 15 cm long; produce seminal fluid and join the ductus deferens at the ejaculatory duct.
- **Prostate gland:** a walnut-sized gland that surrounds the urethra as it leaves the urinary bladder; produces prostatic fluid, which is added to semen (sperm are suspended in glandular secretions).
- **Urethra:** a canal that passes through the prostate gland, enters the penis, and conveys the semen for expulsion from the body during ejaculation.

13. BODY CAVITIES

Organ systems and other visceral structures are often segregated into body cavities. These cavities can protect the viscera and also may allow for some expansion and contraction in size. Two major collections of body cavities are recognized (Fig. 1.32):

- **Posterior cavities:** include the brain, surrounded by the meninges and bony cranium, and the spinal cord, surrounded by the same meninges as the brain and the bony vertebral column.
- **Anterior cavities:** include the thoracic and abdominopelvic cavities, separated by the respiratory diaphragm (a skeletal muscle important in respiration).

The CNS (brain and spinal cord) is surrounded by three membranes (see Fig. 1.21):
- Pia mater.
- Arachnoid mater.
- Dura mater.

The thoracic cavity contains two **pleural cavities** (right and left) and a single midline space called the **mediastinum** (middle space) that contains the heart and structures lying posterior to it, including the thoracic descending aorta and esophagus. The heart itself resides in the **pericardial sac,** which has a parietal and a visceral layer.

The abdominopelvic cavity also is lined by a serous membrane, the **peritoneum,** which has a parietal layer (which lines the interior abdominopelvic walls) and a visceral layer (which envelopes the viscera).

14. OVERVIEW OF EARLY DEVELOPMENT

Week 1: Fertilization and Implantation

Fertilization occurs in the ampulla of the uterine tube (fallopian tube) usually within 24 hours after ovulation (Fig. 1.33). The fertilized ovum (the union of sperm and egg nuclei, with a diploid number of chromosomes) is termed a **zygote.** Subsequent cell division (cleavage) occurs at the two-, four-, eight-, and 16-cell stages and results in formation of a ball of cells that travels down the uterine tube toward the uterine cavity. When the cell mass reaches days 3 to 4 of development, it resembles a mulberry and is called a **morula** (16-cell stage). As the growing morula enters the uterine cavity at about day 5, it contains hundreds of cells and it develops a fluid-filled cyst in its interior; it is now known as a **blastocyst**. At about days 5 to 6, implantation occurs as the blastocyst literally erodes or burrows its way into the uterine wall (endometrium) (see Fig. 1.33).

Week 2: Formation of the Bilaminar Embryonic Disc

As the blastocyst implants, it forms an inner cell mass (future embryo, **embryoblast**) and a larger fluid-filled cavity surrounded by an outer cell layer called the **trophoblast** (Figs. 1.33 and 1.34). The trophoblast undergoes differentiation and complex cellular interactions with maternal tissues to initiate formation of the primitive

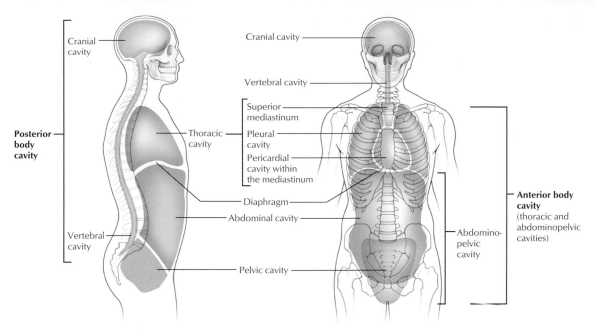

FIGURE 1.32 Major Body Cavities. (From *Netter's atlas of human anatomy*, ed 8, Plate BP 2; S-BP 2.)

uteroplacental circulation. Simultaneously, the inner cell mass develops into the following two cell types (bilaminar disc formation):

- **Epiblast:** formation of a sheet of columnar cells on the dorsal surface of the embryoblast.
- **Hypoblast:** a sheet of cuboidal cells on the ventral surface of the embryoblast.

The epiblast forms a cavity on the dorsal side that gives rise to the *amniotic cavity*. The blastocyst cavity on the ventral side becomes the *primitive yolk sac*, which is lined by simple squamous epithelium derived from the hypoblast. About day 12,

further hypoblast cell migration forms the true yolk sac, and the old blastocyst cavity becomes coated with extraembryonic mesoderm.

Week 3: Gastrulation

Gastrulation (development of a trilaminar embryonic disc) begins with the appearance of the **primitive streak** on the dorsal surface of the epiblast (Fig. 1.35). This streak forms a groove demarcated at its cephalic end (head) by the **primitive node**. The node forms a midline cord of mesoderm that becomes the **notochord**. Migrating epiblast cells

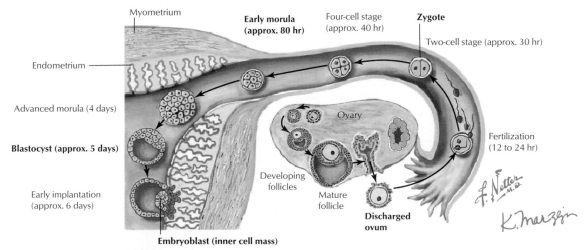

FIGURE 1.33 Schematic of Key Events: Week 1 of Human Development.

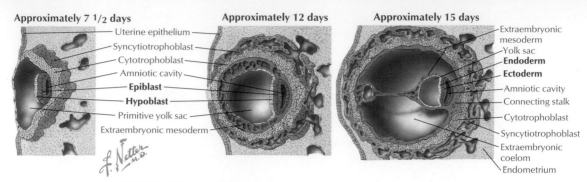

FIGURE 1.34 Bilaminar Disc Formation: Week 2 of Human Development.

Clinical Focus 1.7

Potential Spaces

Each of these spaces—pleural, pericardial, and peritoneal—is considered a "potential" space, because between the parietal and visceral layers, there is usually only a small amount of serous lubricating fluid, to keep organ surfaces moist and slick and thus reduce friction from movements such as respiration, heartbeats, and peristalsis. However, during inflammation or trauma (when pus or blood can accumulate), fluids can collect in these spaces and restrict movement of the viscera. In such situations, these "potential" spaces become real spaces, and the offending fluids may have to be removed so they do not compromise organ function or exacerbate an ongoing infection.

move toward the primitive streak, invaginate, and replace the underlying hypoblast cells to become the **endoderm** germ layer. Other invaginating epiblast cells develop between the endoderm and overlying epiblast and become the **mesoderm.** Finally, the surface epiblast cells form the **ectoderm**, the third germ layer. All body tissues are derived from one of these three embryonic germ layers.

Embryonic Germ Layer Derivatives

Figs. 1.36 to 1.38 and the accompanying tables provide a general overview of the adult derivatives of the *three embryonic germ layers* that are formed during gastrulation. As you study each region of the body, refer to these summary pages to review the embryonic origins of the various tissues. Many clinical problems arise during the development *in utero* of these germ layer derivatives.

In general, **ectodermal** derivatives include the following (Fig. 1.36):

- Epidermis and various appendages associated with the skin (hair, nails, glands).

- Components of the central and peripheral nervous systems.
- Some bones, muscles, and connective tissues of the head and neck (neural crest).

In general, **mesodermal** derivatives include the following (Fig. 1.37):

- Notochord.
- Skeletal, smooth, and cardiac muscle.
- Parenchyma or reticular structures and connective tissues of many organ systems.
- Reproductive and urinary systems.
- Most skeletal structures.
- Dermis of the skin.

In general, **endodermal** derivatives include the following (Fig. 1.38):

- Lining of GI tract and accessory GI organs.
- Lining of the airway.
- Various structures derived from the pharyngeal pouches.
- Embryonic blood cells.
- Derivatives associated with the development of the cloaca.

15. IMAGING THE INTERNAL ANATOMY

General Introduction

In 1895, Wilhelm Roentgen (Würzburg, Germany) used x-rays generated from a cathode ray tube to make the first radiographic image, for which he ultimately was awarded the first Nobel Prize in Physics in 1901. As the x-rays (a form of electromagnetic radiation) pass through the body, they lose energy to the tissues, and only the photons with sufficient energy to penetrate the tissues then expose a sheet of photographic film. Radiographic images are now largely collected as digital information (Table 1.6).

Plain (Conventional) Radiographs

A plain radiograph, also known as a conventional or plain film radiograph, provides an image in which the

Formation of intraembryonic mesoderm from the primitive streak and node (knot)

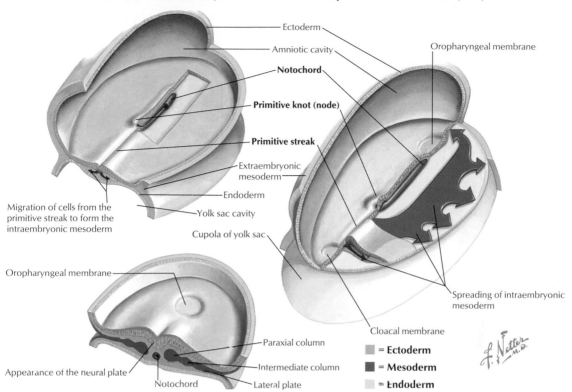

FIGURE 1.35 Gastrulation Formation: Week 3 of Human Development.

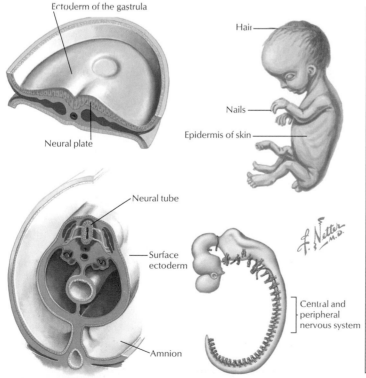

Primordia	Derivatives or fate
Surface ectoderm	Epidermis of the skin Sweat, sebaceous, and mammary glands Nails and hair Tooth enamel Lacrimal glands Conjunctiva External auditory meatus
(Stomodeum and nasal placodes) (Otic placodes) (Lens placodes)	Oral and nasal epithelium Anterior pituitary gland Inner ear Lens of eye
Neural tube	Central nervous system Somatomotor neurons Branchiomotor neurons Presynaptic autonomic neurons Retina/optic nerves Posterior pituitary gland

Neural crest	Peripheral sensory neurons
	Postsynaptic autonomic
	  neurons
	All ganglia
	Adrenal medulla cells
	Melanocytes
	Bone, muscle,
	  and connective tissue
	  in the head and neck

Amnion	Protective bag (with chorion) around fetus

FIGURE 1.36 Ectodermal Derivatives.

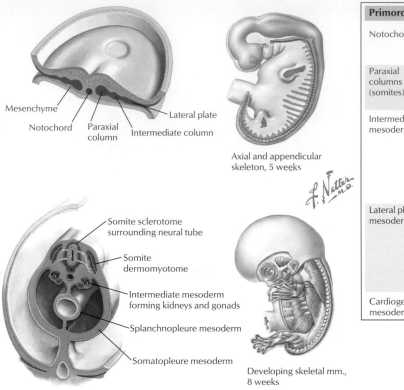

Primordia	Derivatives or fate
Notochord	Nucleus pulposus of an intervertebral disc Induces neurulation
Paraxial columns (somites)	Skeletal muscle Bone Connective tissue (e.g., dorsal dermis, meninges)
Intermediate mesoderm	Gonads Kidneys and ureters Uterus and uterine tubes Upper vagina Ductus deferens, epididymis, and related tubules Seminal vesicles and ejaculatory ducts
Lateral plate mesoderm	Dermis (ventral) Superficial fascia and related tissues (ventral) Bones and connective tissues of limbs Pleura and peritoneum GI tract connective tissue stroma
Cardiogenic mesoderm	Heart Pericardium

Mesenchyme

Notochord

Paraxial column

Intermediate column

Lateral plate

Axial and appendicular skeleton, 5 weeks

Somite sclerotome surrounding neural tube

Somite dermomyotome

Intermediate mesoderm forming kidneys and gonads

Splanchnopleure mesoderm

Somatopleure mesoderm

Developing skeletal mm., 8 weeks

FIGURE 1.37 Mesodermal Derivatives.

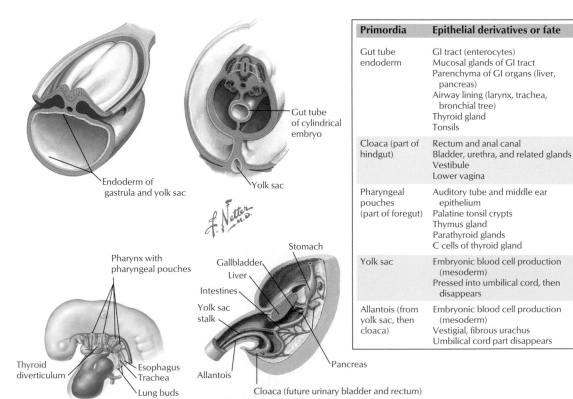

Primordia	Epithelial derivatives or fate
Gut tube endoderm	GI tract (enterocytes) Mucosal glands of GI tract Parenchyma of GI organs (liver, pancreas) Airway lining (larynx, trachea, bronchial tree) Thyroid gland Tonsils
Cloaca (part of hindgut)	Rectum and anal canal Bladder, urethra, and related glands Vestibule Lower vagina
Pharyngeal pouches (part of foregut)	Auditory tube and middle ear epithelium Palatine tonsil crypts Thymus gland Parathyroid glands C cells of thyroid gland
Yolk sac	Embryonic blood cell production (mesoderm) Pressed into umbilical cord, then disappears
Allantois (from yolk sac, then cloaca)	Embryonic blood cell production (mesoderm) Vestigial, fibrous urachus Umbilical cord part disappears

Endoderm of gastrula and yolk sac

Gut tube of cylindrical embryo

Yolk sac

Pharynx with pharyngeal pouches

Gallbladder

Liver

Intestines

Yolk sac stalk

Stomach

Thyroid diverticulum

Esophagus

Trachea

Lung buds

Allantois

Pancreas

Cloaca (future urinary bladder and rectum)

FIGURE 1.38 Endodermal Derivatives.

TABLE 1.6 Attenuation of X-rays Passing Through the Body*

MEDIUM	GRAY SCALE
Bone	White
Soft tissue	Light gray
Water (reference)	Gray
Fat	Dark gray
Lung	Very dark gray
Air	Black

*Greatest to least attenuation.

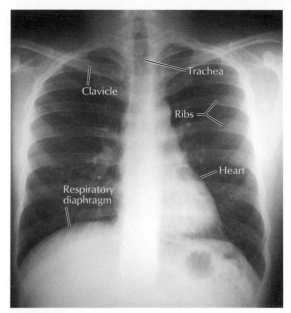

A. PA projection of chest.

patient is positioned either anterior (anteroposterior, AP) to or posterior (posteroanterior, PA) to the x-ray source (Fig. 1.39, *A*). The x-ray tube also may be placed in a lateral or oblique position in reference to the patient. Contrast media (radiopaque fluids such as barium sulfate or iodine compounds) can be administered to study tubular structures such as the bowel or vessels. A *double contrast* study uses barium and air to image the lumen of structures such as the distal colon (Fig. 1.39, *B*). X-rays now are collected digitally in real time by producing a stream of x-rays. Techniques are now available that can even image moving structures in the body using angiography (contrast medium in the heart and larger vessels) and fluoroscopy.

Computed Tomography

Computed tomography (CT) was invented in 1972 by Sir Godfrey Hounsfield (at EMI Labs, Hayes, England), who received the Nobel Prize in Medicine or Physiology in 1979 (shared with Allen McLeod Cormack of Tufts University, Medford, Massachusetts). A CT scanner uses x-rays generated by a tube that passes around the body and collects a series of images in the axial (transverse slices) plane. A sophisticated computer program then transforms the multiple images into a single slice (Fig. 1.40, *A*).

In the 1980s, multislice (multidetector) CT scanners were developed that capture many slices as the tube rotates in a helical pattern around the patient, who is moving through the scanner on a table. Three-dimensional (3-D) images can be recreated by the computer from these slices. Bone is well imaged by CT, and contrast media may be employed to enhance the imaging of hollow viscera (e.g., GI tract). Additionally, CT angiography (CTA) can image larger blood vessels in 2-D and 3-D after intravascular administration of contrast material (Fig. 1.40, *B*).

Advantages of CT include lower costs than magnetic resonance imaging (MRI), greater availability, 3-D capabilities, ability to image bony

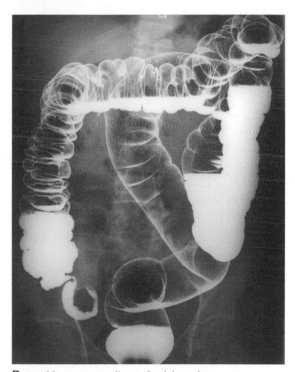

B. Double contrast radiograph of the colon.

FIGURE 1.39 Plain (Conventional) Radiographs. *PA,* Posteroanterior. (From Major NM: *A practical approach to radiology,* Philadelphia, 2006, Saunders.)

features, and faster speed than MRI. Disadvantages of CT include the high dose of x-rays compared with plain films, artifacts (motion, scattering), and relatively poor tissue definition compared with MRI.

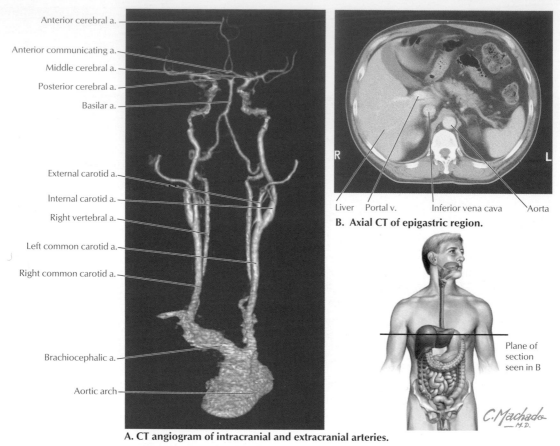

Anterior cerebral a.
Anterior communicating a.
Middle cerebral a.
Posterior cerebral a.
Basilar a.
External carotid a.
Internal carotid a.
Right vertebral a.
Left common carotid a.
Right common carotid a.
Brachiocephalic a.
Aortic arch

A. CT angiogram of intracranial and extracranial arteries.

Liver   Portal v.   Inferior vena cava   Aorta

B. Axial CT of epigastric region.

Plane of section seen in B

FIGURE 1.40 Computed Tomography (CT). (From Kelley LL, Petersen C: *Sectional anatomy for imaging professionals,* St Louis, 2007, Mosby.)

Positron Emission Tomography/ Computed Tomography

Glucose uptake in tissues (following 18-fluorodeoxy-D-glucose administration) can be imaged by positron emission tomography (PET/CT), an especially useful technique for detecting tissues or structures with a higher metabolic rate, such as malignant tumors and inflammatory lesions.

Magnetic Resonance Imaging

Paul Lauterbur (Illinois) and Sir Peter Mansfield (Nottingham, England) were awarded the Nobel Prize in Medicine or Physiology in 2003 for their contributions to the development of MRI. Since the first MR image of a human subject was produced in 1977, this process has become a versatile and safe diagnostic tool. Strong magnets align hydrogen's free protons (the hydrogen in molecules of water present in almost all biologic tissues). Then a radio wave pulse passes through the patient and deflects the protons, which return to their aligned state but emit small radio pulses whose strength, frequency, and time produce distinct signals. Computers then analyze these signals and create axial, coronal, and sagittal images (Fig. 1.41).

Advantages of MRI include the lack of ionizing radiation, the ability to image all planes, and the capability to image soft tissues at very high resolution compared with CT. Disadvantages include high cost, inability to image patients with metallic implants or foreign bodies, inability to image bone well, longer procedure time than CT, potential for patients to become claustrophobic in the scanner, and the tendency for artifacts (movement).

Ultrasound

Ultrasound uses very-high-frequency longitudinal sound waves that are generated by a transducer. The waves produced by the transducer are reflected or refracted as they collide with the soft tissue interfaces. The proportion of sound reflected is measured as acoustic impedance and represents different densities of soft tissue. A computer then interprets these signals and produces a real-time image (Fig. 1.42).

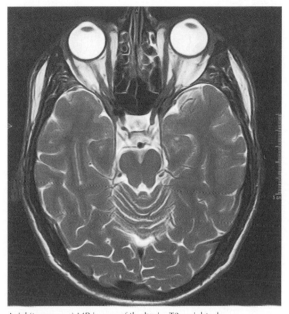

Axial (transverse) MR image of the brain, T2-weighted

FIGURE 1.41 Magnetic Resonance Imaging (MRI). (From Wicke L: *Atlas of radiologic anatomy,* ed 7, Philadelphia, 2004, Saunders.)

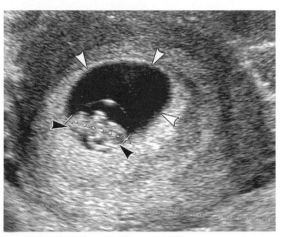

A viable 9-week-old fetus (*black arrowheads*) is seen, surrounded by the gestational sac (*white arrowheads*)

FIGURE 1.42 Ultrasound. (Reprinted with permission from Jackson S, Thomas R: *Cross-sectional imaging made easy,* Philadelphia, 2004, Churchill Livingstone.)

Clinical Focus

Available Online

1.8 Myasthenia Gravis

 Additional figures available online (see inside front cover for details).

Challenge Yourself Questions

1. A radiologist is examining a computer-generated series of MR scans in the frontal plane. Which of the following terms is synonymous with the frontal plane?
   - **A.** Axial
   - **B.** Coronal
   - **C.** Cross section
   - **D.** Sagittal
   - **E.** Transverse

2. Clinically, the bones can be classified by their shape. Which of the following shapes is used to define the patella (kneecap)?
   - **A.** Flat
   - **B.** Irregular
   - **C.** Long
   - **D.** Sesamoid
   - **E.** Short

3. Long bones are responsible for most of our height. Which of the following portions of the long bone is most important in lengthening the bone?
   - **A.** Diaphysis
   - **B.** Epiphysis
   - **C.** Epiphysial plate
   - **D.** Metaphysis
   - **E.** Shaft

4. An elderly woman falls and fractures her femoral neck ("breaks her hip"). Which of the following type of synovial joints was involved in the fracture?
   - **A.** Ball-and-socket (spheroid)
   - **B.** Condyloid (ellipsoid)
   - **C.** Hinge (ginglymus)
   - **D.** Plane (gliding)
   - **E.** Saddle (biaxial)

5. When examining your musculoskeletal system, the orthopedist may check the strength of a contracting muscle at a joint. As this is done, another muscle relaxes and would be designated by which of the following terms?
   - **A.** Agonist
   - **B.** Antagonist
   - **C.** Extensor
   - **D.** Fixator
   - **E.** Synergist

6. During cardiac catheterization, the physician watches the blood flow from the right ventricle into which of the following vessels?
   - **A.** Aorta
   - **B.** Coronary arteries
   - **C.** Inferior vena cava
   - **D.** Pulmonary trunk
   - **E.** Superior vena cava

7. The lymphatic and immune systems are vitally important in defense of the body. Most of the lymph ultimately drains back into the venous system by which of the following structures?
   - **A.** Arachnoid granulations
   - **B.** Choroid plexus
   - **C.** Cisterna chyli
   - **D.** Right lymphatic duct
   - **E.** Thoracic duct

8. A patient experiencing a central nervous system (CNS) inflammatory process will be activating which of the following phagocytic glial cells?
   - **A.** Astrocytes
   - **B.** Ependymal cells
   - **C.** Microglia
   - **D.** Oligodendrocytes
   - **E.** Schwann cells

Multiple-choice and short-answer review questions available online; see inside front cover for details.

44

9. The brain and spinal cord are surrounded by membranous connective tissue layers. The pain associated with most CNS inflammatory processes is mediated by sensory nerves in which of these tissue layers?

   A. Arachnoid mater
   B. Dura mater
   C. Endoneurium
   D. Ependyma
   E. Pia mater

10. A neurologist is concerned about a patient's inability to walk without a distinct limp (movement disorder). Which of the following portions of the peripheral nervous system (PNS) will the neurologist examine first?

   A. Autonomic
   B. Enteric
   C. Myenteric
   D. Somatic
   E. Submucosal

11. In response to a perceived threat of danger, which of the following PNS components will be globally activated?

   A. Enteric
   B. Parasympathetic
   C. Postganglionic
   D. Preganglionic
   E. Sympathetic

12. In designing a novel pharmaceutical agonist for use in controlling blood pressure, the scientists must be cognizant of which of the following distinguishing features of the autonomic nervous system?

   A. It is a one-neuron efferent system.
   B. It is a two-neuron efferent system.
   C. It is associated with 10 cranial nerves.
   D. It releases only neuropeptides as transmitters.
   E. It releases only norepinephrine as a transmitter.

13. A kidney stone becomes lodged in the portion of the urinary system between the kidney and bladder. In which of the following structures will the stone be found?

   A. Bile duct
   B. Oviduct
   C. Thoracic duct
   D. Ureter
   E. Urethra

14. A patient has difficulty digesting fats (e.g., french fries) and experiences pain after a heavy meal, which then subsides. Of the following organs of the gastrointestinal tract, which would most likely be the culprit?

   A. Colon
   B. Gallbladder
   C. Pancreas
   D. Salivary glands
   E. Stomach

15. A patient who presents with an autoimmune disease characterized by loss of weight, rapid pulse, sweating, shortness of breath, bulging eyes (exophthalmos), and muscle wasting likely has oversecretion of a hormone produced and stored by which endocrine organ?

   A. Ovary
   B. Pancreas
   C. Pineal gland
   D. Posterior pituitary gland
   E. Thyroid gland

16. Bleeding into the pericardial sac would also suggest that blood would be present in which of the following cavities?

   A. Abdominal
   B. Left pleural
   C. Mediastinum
   D. Right pleural
   E. Vertebral

17. A congenital defect of the spinal cord occurs during the third week of embryonic development. Which of the following events characterizes this critical period of embryonic development?

   A. Blastocyst formation
   B. Embryoblast formation
   C. Gastrulation
   D. Morula formation
   E. Zygote formation

18. Malformation of the primitive heart would most likely point to a problem with the development of which embryonic tissue?

   A. Amnion
   B. Chorion
   C. Ectoderm
   D. Endoderm
   E. Mesoderm

19. Of the following types of medical imaging approaches, which is the least invasive and least expensive?

   A. Computed tomography
   B. Magnetic resonance imaging
   C. Plain radiograph
   D. Positron emission tomography
   E. Ultrasound

20. As an x-ray beam passes through the human body, which of the following is the correct order of attenuation of the photons, from greatest to least attenuation?

   A. Bone-fat-lung–soft tissue–water-air
   B. Bone-fat–soft tissue–lung-water-air
   C. Bone-lung–soft tissue–fat-water-air
   D. Bone–soft tissue–lung-fat-water-air
   E. Bone–soft tissue–water-fat-lung-air

21. A physician will know what the term *dorsiflexion of the foot* means, but a patient being tested may not be familiar with the term. Therefore, the physician might instruct a patient to do what when she wants the patient to dorsiflex the foot?

   A. Point your foot downward
   B. Point your foot upward
   C. Stand on your toes
   D. Turn your foot to the inside
   E. Turn your foot to the outside

22. Burns are typically classified according to how deep into the tissue the burn injury extends. When a burn has been classified as a second-degree burn, how deep has the burn penetrated the tissue?

   A. Through the epidermis and dermis of the skin
   B. Through the epidermal level only
   C. Through to the level of the investing fascia
   D. Through to the level of the subcutaneous tissue
   E. Through the skin to the underlying muscle

23. Notes on a patient's chart indicate that the patient has had multiple fractures of the axial skeleton. Which of the following bones is part of the axial skeleton?

   A. Clavicle
   B. Fibula
   C. Humerus
   D. Scapula
   E. Sternum

24. When a nurse takes a patient's pulse during a routine examination, the nurse will typically feel the pulse in which of the following arteries?

   A. Brachial artery
   B. Carotid artery
   C. Dorsalis pedis artery
   D. Femoral artery
   E. Radial artery

25. When fluids are lost to the extracellular space, which of the following systems or organs is critical in returning the fluids to the vascular system?

   A. Arachnoid granulations
   B. Gallbladder
   C. Lymphatic system
   D. Respiratory system
   E. Thyroid gland

26. In a patient with a resorption problem, the physician diagnoses the problem as being associated with the large intestine. Which of the following portions of the GI system can be excluded from further examination of the patient?

   A. Ascending colon
   B. Cecum
   C. Ileum
   D. Rectum
   E. Sigmoid colon

27. A patient is having difficulty becoming pregnant. Her physician suspects a problem associated with the portion of her reproductive system that receives the ovulated oocyte. Which of the following structures is the focus of the physician's concern?

   A. Ductus deferens
   B. Urethra
   C. Uterine tube
   D. Uterus
   E. Vagina

28. Following fertilization, how long docs it usually take for the blastocyst to become implanted in the uterine wall?

   A. Twenty-four hours
   B. Forty-eight hours
   C. Three days
   D. Six days
   E. Nine days

29. A physician diagnoses a congenital malformation in a tissue that is a derivative of the embryonic endoderm. Which of the following tissues or structures is most likely the malformed one?

    A. Biceps muscle
    B. Dermis of the hand
    C. Epidermis of the arm
    D. Epithelium of the trachea
    E. Femur

30. Which of the following approaches is the best one for imaging bony structures because it subjects the patient to the lowest dosage of x-rays but is still highly accurate?

    A. Computed tomography (CT)
    B. Magnetic resonance imaging (MRI)
    C. Plain radiography
    D. Positron emission tomography (PET)
    E. Ultrasound

Answers to Challenge Yourself Questions

1. **B.** The coronal plane is named for the coronal suture on the skull and is a plane that is parallel to that suture and synonymous with frontal plane. Axial, transverse, and cross section also are synonymous terms and divide the body into superior and inferior portions.

2. **D.** The patella is a round bone and the largest of the sesamoid bones. Two sesamoid bones also usually exist at the base of each thumb and base of each large toe.

3. **C.** Bone growth in length occurs at the epiphysial plate, where hyaline cartilage undergoes proliferation and ossification. Growth in width occurs at the diaphysis.

4. **A.** The hip is a perfect example of a ball-and-socket joint and is one of the more stable synovial joints in the body. The shoulder joint also is a ball-and-socket joint but is more mobile and less stable than the hip joint.

5. **B.** The antagonist is the muscle that opposes the action of the agonist, the muscle that is contracting and in this case the muscle being tested by the orthopedist.

6. **D.** Venous blood from the body passes through the right side of the heart (right atrium and ventricle) and then passes into the pulmonary trunk, which divides into a right pulmonary artery and a left pulmonary artery carrying blood away from the heart and to the lungs for gas exchange.

7. **E.** The thoracic duct drains lymph from about three-quarters of the body and returns it to the venous system at the junction of the left internal jugular and left subclavian veins. The cisterna chyli is the beginning of the thoracic duct in the upper abdomen.

8. **C.** Microglia are the endogenous glial cells in the CNS that are phagocytic and respond to any breach in the blood-brain barrier or to infection.

9. **B.** The dura mater is heavily innervated by sensory nerve fibers, whereas the arachnoid and pia mater are not innervated.

10. **D.** The neurologist will examine the somatic division of the PNS first to determine if the problem is associated with a peripheral nerve and/or skeletal muscle. Skeletal muscle is innervated by the somatic nervous system.

11. **E.** The sympathetic division of the ANS is functionally the "fight or flight" responder to any threat, perceived or real, and mobilizes the body globally.

12. **B.** This is the only answer that accurately reflects the ANS. It is a two-neuron efferent system, and different transmitters are co-localized and released. Because of this, ACh, NE, and neuropeptides can be targeted at different synaptic sites pharmacologically to alter the response of the system. The only exception is the neuroendocrine cells of the adrenal medulla, which are modified postganglionic sympathetic neurons innervated by preganglionic sympathetic fibers.

13. **D.** The ureter is the duct connecting the kidney (renal pelvis) to the urinary bladder.

14. **B.** The gallbladder stores and concentrates bile, which is necessary for the emulsification of fats in our diet. When fats enter the GI tract, the gallbladder is stimulated, contracts, and releases concentrated bile into the second portion of the duodenum.

15. **E.** These signs and symptoms are characteristic of Graves' disease (hyperthyroidism), an excess synthesis and release of thyroid hormone, which upregulates metabolism.

16. **C.** The pericardium and the heart reside in the mediastinum (middle space), the region between the two pleural cavities, all of which are in the thoracic cavity.

17. **C.** Gastrulation is the defining event of the third week of embryonic development. This is when the trilaminar disc (ectoderm, mesoderm, endoderm) develops and when the ectoderm begins to migrate medially and fold along the midline axis to form the future neural tube and spinal cord.

18. **E.** The heart (cardiac muscle) is a derivative largely of the mesoderm. Later in its development, the neural crest (neural folds of ectoderm) also plays an important role.

19. **E.** Ultrasound uses very-high-frequency longitudinal sound waves, is relatively safe, and is cost effective compared with the other imaging modalities. Unfortunately, it is not suitable for all imaging; its resolution is limited and it cannot penetrate bone.

20. **E.** The densest structure in the body is bone, with the greatest attenuation of photons, followed by soft tissues, water (the reference medium), fat, lung (mostly air), and then air itself. On a plain radiograph, a very dense tissue like bone appears white, while air appears black.

21. **B.** Dorsiflexion of the foot at the ankle occurs when one points the foot upward. This movement is the same as extension and is the opposite of flexion (plantarflexion). Most patients will not be familiar with the term *dorsiflexion* (or *extension*), so the physician must phrase the instruction in words that are easily understood.

22. **A.** A second-degree burn penetrates both the epidermis and the dermis, but does not go further. A third-degree burn includes the subcutaneous tissue below the dermis.

23. **E.** The sternum is part of the central axis of the body and the axial skeleton. All the other bones listed are part of the appendicular skeleton (bones associated with the limbs).

24. **E.** Typically, the radial artery pulse is taken at the wrist and is easily felt. The dorsalis pedis pulse is also important because it is the pulse farthest from the heart; it is detected on the dorsal surface of the foot.

25. **C.** A considerable amount of fluid is lost to the extracellular compartment at the level of the capillaries. The fluid can be recaptured by the lymphatic vessels and returned to the venous system. Important proteins not easily reabsorbed by the venous system also can be captured by the lymphatic system. The arachnoid granulations allow cerebrospinal fluid in the nervous system to return to the venous system.

26. **C.** The ileum is part of the small intestine, and therefore it can be excluded by the physician. All of the other listed options arc part of the large intestine and must be considered in his examination.

27. **C.** The ovulated oocyte is usually captured and passes into the uterine (fallopian) tube, where fertilization could normally occur if sperm were present. The resulting zygote would undergo cell divisions and travel into the uterine cavity, where it would normally become implanted.

28. **D.** Implantation of the blastocyst usually occurs around the fifth to sixth day after fertilization in the uterine tube.

29. **D.** The only tissue listed that is derived from the embryonic endoderm is the epithelial lining of the trachea. The epidermis is derived from the ectoderm, and all the other options are derived from the mesoderm.

30. **C.** Plain radiography uses the lowest dosage of x-rays. CT is often a good way to image bony structures but uses a higher dosage of x-rays. None of the other imaging modalities use x-rays. and none are as accurate as CT or plain radiography at delineating the fine features of bony structures.

Back

1. INTRODUCTION

The back forms the axis (central line) of the human body and consists of the vertebral column, spinal cord, supporting muscles, and associated tissues (skin, connective tissues, vasculature, and nerves). A hallmark of human anatomy is the concept of "segmentation," and the back is a prime example. **Segmentation** and **bilateral symmetry** of the back will become obvious as you study the vertebral column, the distribution of the spinal nerves, the muscles of the back, and its vascular supply. Functionally, the back is involved in three primary tasks, as follows:

- *Support.* The vertebral column forms the axis of the body and is critical for upright posture (standing or sitting), as a support for the head, as an attachment point and brace for movements of the upper limbs, and as a support for transferring the weight of the trunk to the lower limbs.
- *Protection.* The vertebral column protects the spinal cord and proximal portions of the spinal nerves before they distribute throughout the body.
- *Movements.* Muscles of the back function in movements of the head and upper limbs and in support and movements of the vertebral column.

2. SURFACE ANATOMY

Fig. 2.1 shows key surface landmarks of the back, including the following bony landmarks:

- **Vertebrae prominens:** the spinous process of the C7 vertebra, usually the most prominent process in the midline at the posterior base of the neck.
- **Scapula:** a part of the pectoral girdle that supports the upper limb; note its spine, inferior angle, and medial border.
- **Iliac crests:** felt best when you place your hands "on your hips." An imaginary horizontal line connecting the iliac crests passes through the spinous process of vertebra L4 and the intervertebral disc of L4-L5, providing a useful landmark for a lumbar puncture or an epidural block (see Clinical Focus 2.11).
- **Posterior superior iliac spines:** an imaginary horizontal line connecting these two points passes through the spinous process of S2 (second sacral segment).

3. VERTEBRAL COLUMN

The vertebral column (spine) forms the central axis of the human body, highlighting the segmental nature of all vertebrates, and usually is composed of 33 vertebrae distributed as follows (Fig. 2.2):

- **Cervical:** seven vertebrae; the first two called the atlas (C1) and axis (C2).
- **Thoracic:** 12 vertebrae; each articulates with a pair of ribs.
- **Lumbar:** five vertebrae; large vertebrae for support of the body's weight.
- **Sacral:** five fused vertebrae for stability in the transfer of weight from the trunk to the lower limbs.
- **Coccyx:** four vertebrae, but variable; Co1 often is not fused, but Co2-Co4 are fused (a remnant of the embryonic tail).

The actual number of vertebrae can vary, especially the number of coccygeal vertebrae.

Viewed from the lateral aspect (Fig. 2.2), one can identify the following:

- **Cervical curvature** (cervical lordosis): a secondary curvature acquired when the infant can support the weight of the head.
- **Thoracic curvature** (thoracic kyphosis): a primary curvature present in the fetus (imagine the spine in the "fetal position").
- **Lumbar curvature** (lumbar lordosis): a secondary curvature acquired when the infant assumes an upright posture and supports its own weight.

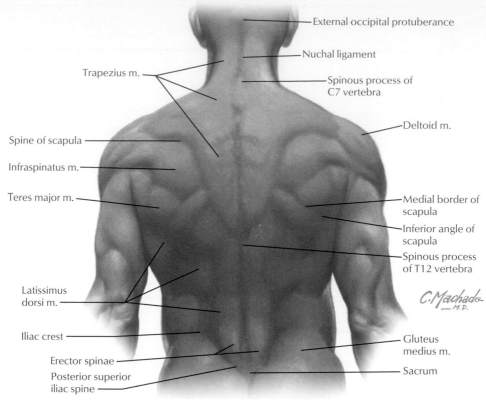

FIGURE 2.1 Key Bony and Muscular Landmarks of the Back. (From *Netter's atlas of human anatomy*, ed 8, Plate 178; S-6.)

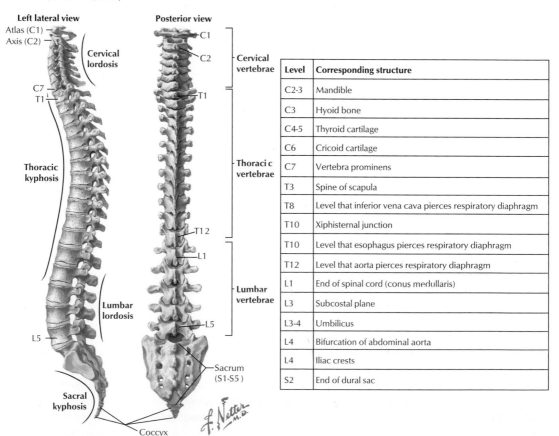

Level	Corresponding structure
C2-3	Mandible
C3	Hyoid bone
C4-5	Thyroid cartilage
C6	Cricoid cartilage
C7	Vertebra prominens
T3	Spine of scapula
T8	Level that inferior vena cava pierces respiratory diaphragm
T10	Xiphisternal junction
T10	Level that esophagus pierces respiratory diaphragm
T12	Level that aorta pierces respiratory diaphragm
L1	End of spinal cord (conus medullaris)
L3	Subcostal plane
L3-4	Umbilicus
L4	Bifurcation of abdominal aorta
L4	Iliac crests
S2	End of dural sac

FIGURE 2.2 Vertebral Column. (From *Netter's atlas of human anatomy*, ed 8, Plate 179; S-137.)

Clinical Focus 2.1

Scoliosis

Scoliosis is an abnormal lateral curvature of the spine, which also includes an abnormal rotation of one vertebra upon another. In addition to scoliosis, accentuated curvatures of the spine include **kyphosis** (hunchback) and **lordosis** (swayback).

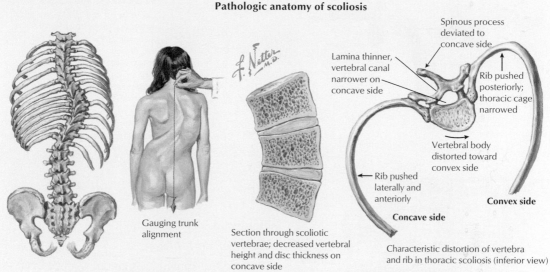

Pathologic anatomy of scoliosis

Gauging trunk alignment

Section through scoliotic vertebrae; decreased vertebral height and disc thickness on concave side

Lamina thinner, vertebral canal narrower on concave side

Spinous process deviated to concave side

Rib pushed posteriorly; thoracic cage narrowed

Vertebral body distorted toward convex side

Rib pushed laterally and anteriorly

Concave side

Convex side

Characteristic distortion of vertebra and rib in thoracic scoliosis (inferior view)

Several Common Abnormal Curvatures of the Spine		
Disorder	**Definition**	**Etiology**
Scoliosis (illustrated)	Accentuated lateral and rotational curve of thoracic or lumbar spine	Genetic, trauma, idiopathic; occurs in adolescent girls more than boys
Kyphosis	Hunchback, accentuated flexion of thoracic spine	Poor posture, osteoporosis
Lordosis	Swayback, accentuated extension of lumbar spine	Weakened trunk muscles, late pregnancy, obesity

- **Sacral curvature**: (sacral kyphosis) a primary curvature present in the fetus.

Typical Vertebra

A "typical" vertebra has the following features (Fig. 2.3):
- **Arch:** a projection formed by paired pedicles and laminae and the spinous processes; the arch serves as the site for articulation with adjacent vertebrae and also as the attachment point for ligaments and muscles.
- **Articular processes** (facets): two superior and two inferior facets for articulation with adjacent vertebrae.
- **Body:** the weight-bearing portion of a vertebra that tends to increase in size as one descends the spine.
- **Intervertebral foramen** (foramina): the opening formed by the vertebral notches that is traversed by spinal nerve roots and associated vessels.
- **Lamina** (laminae): paired portions of the vertebral arch that connect the transverse processes to the spinous process.
- **Pedicle:** paired portions of the vertebral arch that attach the transverse processes to the body.
- **Transverse foramina:** apertures that exist in transverse processes of cervical vertebrae only and transmit the vertebral vessels; C7 transmits only the vertebral vein and is usually smaller.
- **Transverse processes:** the lateral extensions from the union of the pedicle and lamina.
- **Spinous process:** a projection that extends posteriorly from the union of two laminae.

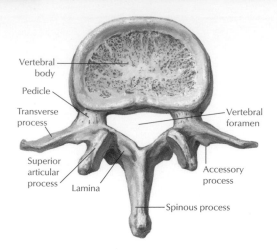

Vertebral body
Pedicle
Transverse process
Vertebral foramen
Superior articular process
Lamina
Accessory process
Spinous process

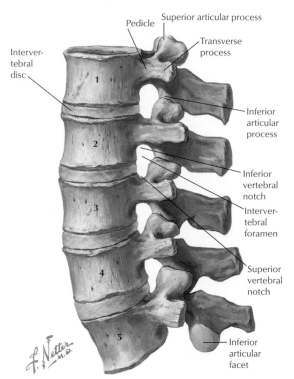

Intervertebral disc
Pedicle
Superior articular process
Transverse process
Inferior articular process
Inferior vertebral notch
Intervertebral foramen
Superior vertebral notch
Inferior articular facet

FIGURE 2.3 Features of Typical Vertebra, as Represented by L2 Vertebra (superior view) and Articulated Lumbar Vertebrae (L1-L5). (From *Netter's atlas of human anatomy*, ed 8, Plate 181; S-145.

TABLE 2.1 Key Features of the Cervical Vertebrae (C1-C7)	
VERTEBRAE	**DISTINGUISHING CHARACTERISTICS**
Atlas (C1)	Ringlike bone; superior facet articulates with occipital bone. Two lateral masses with facets No body or spinous process C1 rotates on articular facets of C2. Vertebral artery runs in groove on posterior arch.
Axis (C2)	Dens projects superiorly. Strongest cervical vertebra
C3 to C7	Large, triangular vertebral foramen Transverse foramen through which vertebral artery passes (except C7) Narrow intervertebral foramina Nerve roots at risk of compression
C3 to C5	Short, bifid spinous process
C6 to C7	Long spinous process
C7	Vertebra prominens; nonbifid

Regional Vertebrae

Cervical Vertebrae

The cervical spine is composed of seven cervical vertebrae. The first two cervical vertebrae are unique and called the atlas and axis (Fig. 2.4). The **atlas** (C1) holds the head on the neck (the titan Atlas of Greek mythology held the heavens on his shoulders as punishment by Zeus). The **axis** (C2) is the point of articulation where the head turns on the neck, providing an "axis of rotation."

Table 2.1 summarizes key features of the cervical vertebrae. The cervical region is a fairly mobile portion of the spine, allowing for flexion and extension as well as rotation and lateral bending.

Thoracic and Lumbar Vertebrae

The thoracic spine is composed of 12 thoracic vertebrae (Fig. 2.5 and Table 2.2). The 12 pairs of ribs articulate with the thoracic vertebrae. This region of the spine is more rigid and inflexible than the cervical region.

The lumbar spine is composed of five lumbar vertebrae (see Figs. 2.3 and 2.5 and Table 2.2). The lumbar vertebrae are comparatively large for bearing the weight of the trunk and are fairly mobile, but not nearly as mobile as the cervical vertebrae.

Sacrum and Coccyx

The sacrum is composed of five fused vertebrae that form a single, wedge-shaped bone (Fig. 2.5 and Table 2.2). The sacrum provides support for the pelvis. The coccyx is a remnant of the embryonic

- **Vertebral foramen** (canal): a triangular foramen formed from the vertebral arch and body that contains the spinal cord and its meningeal coverings.
- **Vertebral notches:** superior and inferior semicircular features that in articulated vertebrae form an intervertebral foramen (two semicircular notches form a circle).

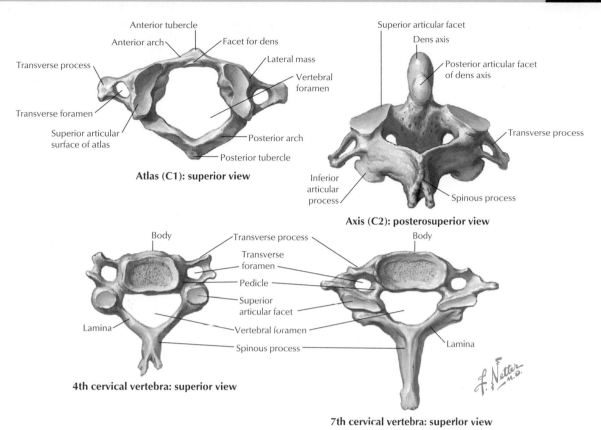

Anterior tubercle

Anterior arch — Facet for dens

Transverse process

Lateral mass

Vertebral foramen

Transverse foramen

Superior articular surface of atlas

Posterior arch

Posterior tubercle

Atlas (C1): superior view

Superior articular facet

Dens axis

Posterior articular facet of dens axis

Transverse process

Inferior articular process

Spinous process

Axis (C2): posterosuperior view

Body

Transverse process

Transverse foramen

Pedicle

Superior articular facet

Lamina

Vertebral foramen

Spinous process

4th cervical vertebra: superior view

Body

Lamina

7th cervical vertebra: superior view

FIGURE 2.4 Representative Cervical Vertebrae. (From *Netter's atlas of human anatomy*, ed 8, Plate 43; S-140.)

Clinical Focus 2.2

Cervical Fractures

Fractures of the axis (C2) often involve the dens and are classified as types I, II, and III. Type I fractures are usually stable, type II fractures are unstable, and type III fractures, which extend into the body, usually reunite well when immobilized. The **hangman fracture,** a pedicle fracture of the axis, can be stabilized, if survived, with or without spinal cord damage. A **Jefferson fracture** is a burst fracture of the atlas (C1), often caused by a blow to the top of the head.

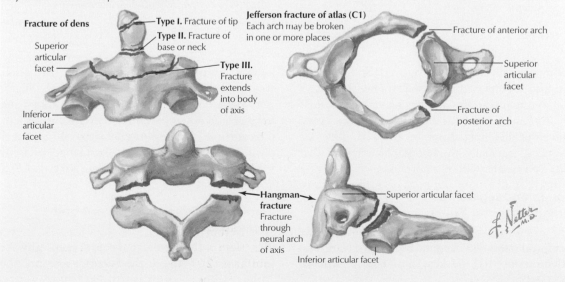

Fracture of dens

Superior articular facet

Inferior articular facet

Type I. Fracture of tip

Type II. Fracture of base or neck

Type III. Fracture extends into body of axis

Jefferson fracture of atlas (C1)
Each arch may be broken in one or more places

Fracture of anterior arch

Superior articular facet

Fracture of posterior arch

Hangman fracture
Fracture through neural arch of axis

Superior articular facet

Inferior articular facet

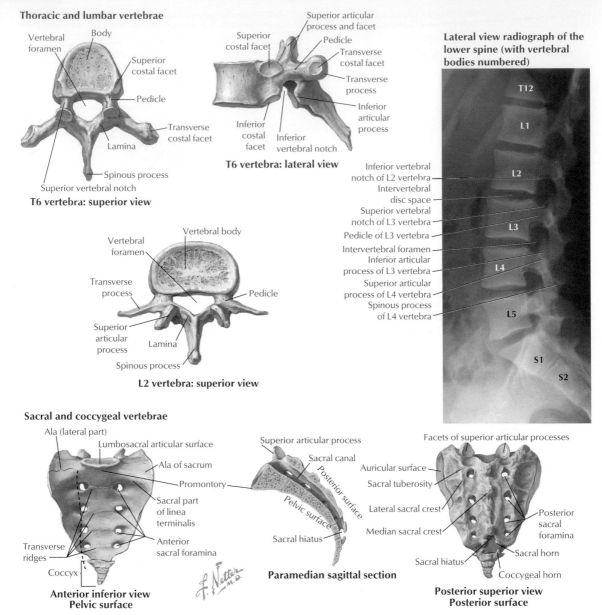

Thoracic and lumbar vertebrae

T6 vertebra: superior view labels: Vertebral foramen, Body, Superior costal facet, Pedicle, Transverse costal facet, Lamina, Spinous process, Superior vertebral notch

T6 vertebra: superior view

T6 vertebra lateral view labels: Superior costal facet, Superior articular process and facet, Pedicle, Transverse costal facet, Transverse process, Inferior articular process, Inferior costal facet, Inferior vertebral notch

T6 vertebra: lateral view

L2 vertebra superior view labels: Vertebral foramen, Vertebral body, Transverse process, Pedicle, Superior articular process, Lamina, Spinous process

L2 vertebra: superior view

Lateral view radiograph of the lower spine (with vertebral bodies numbered)

Radiograph labels: T12, L1, L2, L3, L4, L5, S1, S2, Inferior vertebral notch of L2 vertebra, Intervertebral disc space, Superior vertebral notch of L3 vertebra, Pedicle of L3 vertebra, Intervertebral foramen, Inferior articular process of L3 vertebra, Superior articular process of L4 vertebra, Spinous process of L4 vertebra

Sacral and coccygeal vertebrae

Anterior inferior view labels: Ala (lateral part), Lumbosacral articular surface, Ala of sacrum, Promontory, Sacral part of linea terminalis, Anterior sacral foramina, Transverse ridges, Coccyx

Anterior inferior view Pelvic surface

Paramedian sagittal section labels: Superior articular process, Sacral canal, Posterior surface, Pelvic surface, Sacral hiatus

Paramedian sagittal section

Posterior superior view labels: Facets of superior articular processes, Auricular surface, Sacral tuberosity, Lateral sacral crest, Median sacral crest, Posterior sacral foramina, Sacral horn, Coccygeal horn, Sacral hiatus

Posterior superior view Posterior surface

FIGURE 2.5 Representative Vertebrae. (From *Netter's atlas of human anatomy*, ed 8, Plates 180 and 183; S-144 and S-146.

tail and usually consists of four vertebrae, with the last three often fused into a single bone. The coccyx lacks vertebral arches and has no vertebral canal.

The features and number of vertebrae can vary, and clinicians must always be aware of subtle differences, especially on radiographic imaging, that may be variants within a normal range.

Joints and Ligaments of Craniovertebral Spine

The craniovertebral joints include the **atlanto-occipital** (atlas and occipital bone of the skull) and **atlantoaxial** (atlas and axis) joints. Both are synovial

joints that provide a relatively wide range of motion compared with other joints of the vertebral column. The atlantooccipital joint permits one to nod the head up and down (flexion and extension), as if to indicate "yes," whereas the atlantoaxial joint is a pivot joint that permits one to rotate the head from side to side, as if to indicate "no" (Fig. 2.6 and Table 2.3).

Joints and Ligaments of Vertebral Arches and Bodies

The joints of the vertebral arches (**zygapophysial joints**) occur between the superior and inferior

TABLE 2.2 Key Features of Thoracic, Lumbar, Sacral, and Coccygeal Vertebrae

VERTEBRAE	DISTINGUISHING CHARACTERISTICS	VERTEBRAE	DISTINGUISHING CHARACTERISTICS
Thoracic (T1-T12)	Heart-shaped body, with facets for rib articulation Small circular vertebral foramen Long transverse processes, with facets for rib articulation in T1-T10 Long spinous processes, which slope posteriorly and overlap next vertebra	Sacrum (S1-S5)	Large, wedge-shaped bone that transmits body weight to pelvis Five fused vertebrae, with fusion complete by puberty Four pairs of sacral foramina on dorsal and ventral (pelvic) side Sacral hiatus, the opening of sacral vertebral foramen
Lumbar (L1-L5)	Kidney-shaped body, massive for support Midsized triangular vertebral foramen Facets face medial or lateral direction, which permits good flexion and extension Spinous process is short and strong. L5: largest vertebra with massive transverse processes	Coccyx (Co1-Co4)	Co1 often is not fused. Co2 to Co4 are fused. No pedicles, laminae, or spines Remnant of our embryonic tail

Clinical Focus 2.3

Osteoarthritis

Osteoarthritis is the most common form of arthritis and often involves erosion of the articular cartilage of weight-bearing joints, such as those of the vertebral column.

Cervical spine involvement

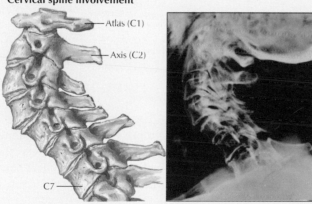

Atlas (C1)

Axis (C2)

C7

Extensive thinning of cervical discs and hyperextension deformity. Narrowing of intervertebral foramina. Lateral radiograph reveals similar changes.

Lumbar spine involvement

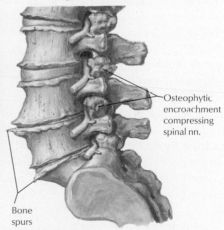

Osteophytic encroachment compressing spinal nn.

Bone spurs

Degeneration of lumbar intervertebral discs and hypertrophic changes at vertebral margins with spur formation. Osteophytic encroachment on intervertebral foramina compresses spinal nerves.

Characteristics of Osteoarthritis	
Characteristic	**Description**
Etiology	Progressive erosion of cartilage in joints of spine, fingers, knee, and hip most commonly
Prevalence	Significant after age 65 years
Risk factors	Age, female sex, joint trauma, repetitive stress, obesity, genetic, race, previous inflammatory joint disease
Complications	In spine, involves intervertebral disc and facet joints, leading to hyperextension deformity and spinal nerve impingement

TABLE 2.3 Key Features of Atlantooccipital and Atlantoaxial Joints

LIGAMENT	ATTACHMENT	COMMENT
Atlantooccipital (Biaxial Condyloid Synovial) Joint		
Articular capsule	Surrounds facets and occipital condyles	Allows flexion and extension
Anterior and posterior membranes	Anterior and posterior arches of C1 to foramen magnum	Limit movement of joint
Atlantoaxial (Uniaxial Synovial) Joint		
Tectorial membrane	Axis body to margin of foramen magnum	Is continuation of posterior longitudinal ligament
Apical	Dens to occipital bone	Is very small
Alar	Dens to occipital condyles	Limits rotation
Cruciate	Dens to lateral masses	Resembles a cross; allows rotation

TABLE 2.4 Features of the Zygapophysial and Intervertebral Joints

LIGAMENT	ATTACHMENT	COMMENT
Zygapophysial (Plane Synovial) Joints		
Articular capsule	Surrounds facets	Allows gliding motion C5-C6 is most mobile. L4-L5 permits most flexion.
Intervertebral (Secondary Cartilaginous [Symphyses]) Joints		
Anterior longitudinal (AL)	Anterior bodies and intervertebral discs	Is strong and prevents hyperextension
Posterior longitudinal (PL)	Posterior bodies and intervertebral discs	Is weaker than AL and prevents hyperflexion
Ligamenta flava	Connect adjacent laminae of vertebrae	Limit flexion and are more elastic
Interspinous	Connect spines	Are weak
Supraspinous	Connect spinous tips	Are stronger and limit flexion
Ligamentum nuchae	C7 to occipital bone	Is cervical extension of supraspinous ligament and is strong
Intertransverse	Connect transverse processes	Are weak ligaments
Intervertebral discs	Between adjacent bodies	Are secured by AL and PL ligaments

articular processes (facets) of adjacent vertebrae and allow for some gliding or sliding movement (Fig. 2.7 and Table 2.4). These joints slope inferiorly in the cervical spine (facilitate flexion and extension), are more vertically oriented in the thoracic region (limit flexion and extension but allow for rotation), and are interlocking in the lumbar spine (they do allow flexion and extension, but not to the degree present in the cervical spine). Corresponding ligaments connect the spinous processes, laminae, and bodies of adjacent vertebrae (see Tables 2.3 and 2.4). Strong **anterior** and **posterior longitudinal ligaments** run along most of the length of the vertebral column. Of these two ligaments, the anterior longitudinal ligament is stronger and prevents hyperextension (see Figs. 2.6 and 2.7 and Table 2.4).

The joints of the vertebral bodies (intervertebral joints) occur between the adjacent vertebral bodies (see Fig. 2.7 and Table 2.4). The intervertebral joints are lined by a thin layer of hyaline cartilage with an intervening **intervertebral disc** (except between the first two cervical vertebrae). These stable, weight-bearing joints also absorb pressure because the intervertebral disc is between the bodies. Intervertebral discs are composed of a central nuclear zone of collagen and hydrated proteoglycans

called the **nucleus pulposus,** which is surrounded by concentric lamellae of collagen fibers that compose the **anulus fibrosus** (see Clinical Focus 2.6). The inner gelatinous nucleus pulposus (remnant of the embryonic notochord) is hydrated and acts as a "shock absorber," compressing when load bearing and relaxing when the load is removed. The outer fibrocartilaginous anulus fibrosus, arranged in concentric lamellae, is encircled by a thin ring of collagen and resists compression and shearing forces.

The lumbar intervertebral discs are the thickest and the upper thoracic ones are the thinnest intervertebral discs. The anterior and posterior longitudinal ligaments help to stabilize these joints (see Table 2.4).

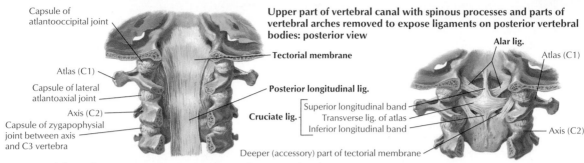

Capsule of atlantooccipital joint

Atlas (C1)

Capsule of lateral atlantoaxial joint

Axis (C2)

Capsule of zygapophysial joint between axis and C3 vertebra

Upper part of vertebral canal with spinous processes and parts of vertebral arches removed to expose ligaments on posterior vertebral bodies: posterior view

Tectorial membrane

Posterior longitudinal lig.

Cruciate lig.
- Superior longitudinal band
- Transverse lig. of atlas
- Inferior longitudinal band

Deeper (accessory) part of tectorial membrane

Alar lig.

Atlas (C1)

Axis (C2)

Tectorial membrane removed to expose deeper ligs.: posterior view

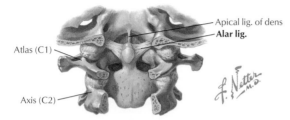

Apical lig. of dens
Alar lig.

Atlas (C1)

Axis (C2)

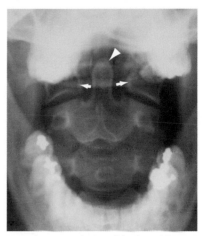

Normal open-mouth view of the dens of C2 (*arrowhead*) and the lateral masses of C1 (*arrows*).

Cruciate lig. removed to show deepest ligs.: posterior view

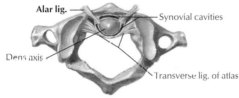

Alar lig.

Synovial cavities

Dens axis

Transverse lig. of atlas

Median atlantoaxial joint: superior view

FIGURE 2.6 Craniovertebral Joints and Ligaments. (From *Netter's atlas of human anatomy*, ed 8, Plate 47; S-142; radiograph from Major N: *A practical approach to radiology*, Philadelphia, Saunders-Elsevier, 2006.)

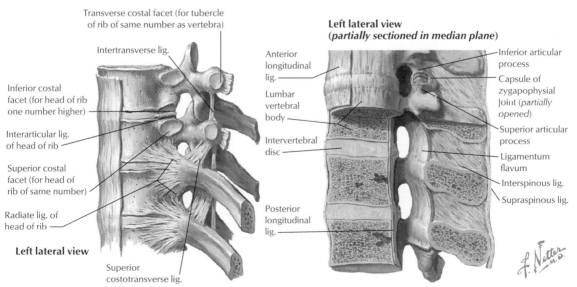

Transverse costal facet (for tubercle of rib of same number as vertebra)

Intertransverse lig.

Inferior costal facet (for head of rib one number higher)

Interarticular lig. of head of rib

Superior costal facet (for head of rib of same number)

Radiate lig. of head of rib

Left lateral view

Superior costotransverse lig.

Left lateral view (*partially sectioned in median plane*)

Anterior longitudinal lig.

Lumbar vertebral body

Intervertebral disc

Posterior longitudinal lig.

Inferior articular process

Capsule of zygapophysial joint (*partially opened*)

Superior articular process

Ligamentum flavum

Interspinous lig.

Supraspinous lig.

FIGURE 2.7 Joints of Vertebral Arches and Bodies. (From *Netter's atlas of human anatomy*, ed 8, Plate 185; S-148.)

Clinical Focus 2.4

Osteoporosis

Osteoporosis (porous bone) is the most common bone disease and results from an imbalance in bone resorption and formation, which places bones at a great risk for fracture.

Axial

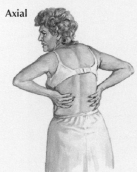

Vertebral compression fractures cause continuous (acute) or intermittent (chronic) back pain from midthoracic to midlumbar region, occasionally to lower lumbar region.

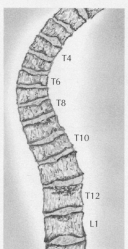

Multiple compression fractures of lower thoracic and upper lumbar vertebrae in patient with severe osteoporosis

Characteristics of Osteoporosis	
Characteristic	Description
Etiology	Postmenopausal women, genetics, vitamin D synthesis deficiency, idiopathic
Risk factors	Family history, white female, increasing age, estrogen deficiency, vitamin D deficiency, low calcium intake, smoking, excessive alcohol use, inactive lifestyle
Complications	Vertebral compression fractures, fracture of proximal femur or humerus, ribs, and distal radius (Colles' fracture)

A change in backbone strength over time

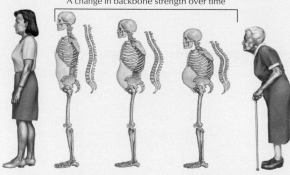

Osteoporosis is the thinning of the bones. Bones become fragile, and loss of height is common as the back bones begin to collapse.

Appendicular fractures caused by minimal trauma

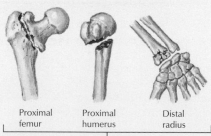

Proximal femur   Proximal humerus   Distal radius

Most common types

Clinical Focus 2.5

Spondylolysis and Spondylolisthesis

Spondylolysis is a congenital defect or an acquired stress fracture of the lamina that presents with no slippage of adjacent articulating vertebrae (most common at L5-S1). Its radiographic appearance suggests a "Scottie dog" (terrier) with a collar (fracture site shown as red collar).

Spondylolisthesis is a bilateral defect (complete dislocation, or luxation) resulting in an anterior displacement of the L5 body and transverse process. The posterior fragment (vertebral laminae and spinous process of L5) remains in proper alignment over the sacrum (S1). This defect has the radiographic appearance of a dog with a broken neck (highlighted in yellow, with the fracture in red). Pressure on spinal nerves often leads to low back and lower limb pain.

Posterior oblique views: Scottie dog profile in yellow and fracture site in red

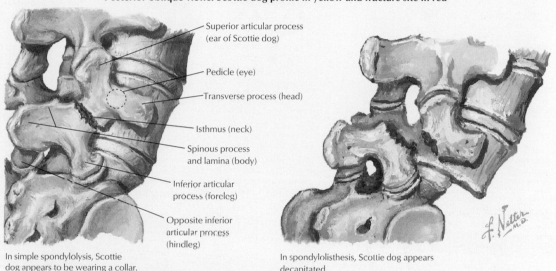

Superior articular process (ear of Scottie dog)

Pedicle (eye)

Transverse process (head)

Isthmus (neck)

Spinous process and lamina (body)

Inferior articular process (foreleg)

Opposite inferior articular process (hindleg)

In simple spondylolysis, Scottie dog appears to be wearing a collar.

In spondylolisthesis, Scottie dog appears decapitated.

Clinical Focus 2.6

Intervertebral Disc Herniation

The intervertebral discs are composed of a central nuclear zone of collagen and hydrated proteoglycans called the **nucleus pulposus**, which is surrounded by concentric lamellae of collagen fibers that compose the **anulus fibrosus**. The nucleus pulposus is hydrated and acts as a "shock absorber," compressing when load bearing and relaxing when the load is removed. Over time, the repeated compression-relaxation cycle of the intervertebral discs can lead to peripheral tears of the anulus fibrosus that allow for the extrusion and herniation of the more gelatinous nucleus pulposus. This often occurs with age, and the nucleus pulposus becomes more dehydrated, thus transferring more of the compression forces to the anulus fibrosus. This added stress may cause thickening of the anulus and tears. Most disc herniations occur in a posterolateral direction because the anulus fibrosus tears often occur at the posterolateral margins of the disc (rim lesions). Moreover, the posterior longitudinal ligament reinforces the anulus such that posterior herniations are much less common; otherwise, the disc would herniate into the vertebral canal and compress the spinal cord or its nerve roots.

Continued

Clinical Focus 2.6

Intervertebral Disc Herniation—cont'd

The most common sites for disc herniation in the cervical region are the **C5-C6 and C6-C7 levels,** resulting in shoulder and upper limb pain. In the lumbar region the primary sites are the **L4-L5 and L5-S1 levels**. Lumbar disc herniation is much more common than cervical herniation and results in pain over the sacroiliac joint, hip, posterior thigh, and leg.

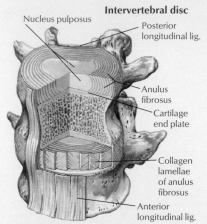

Intervertebral disc

Nucleus pulposus
Posterior longitudinal lig.
Anulus fibrosus
Cartilage end plate
Collagen lamellae of anulus fibrosus
Anterior longitudinal lig.

Intervertebral disc composed of central nuclear zone of collagen and hydrated proteoglycans surrounded by concentric lamellae of collagen fibers

Disc rupture and nuclear herniation

Nucleus pulposus
Rim lesion
Tears in internal anular lamellae
Shortened disc space
Herniated nucleus pulposus

Peripheral tear of anulus fibrosus and cartilage end plate (rim lesion) initiates sequence of events that weaken and tear internal anular lamellae, allowing extrusion and herniation of nucleus pulposus.

Clinical features of herniated lumbar disc					
Level of herniation	Pain	Numbness	Weakness	Atrophy	Reflexes
L4-L5 disc; 5th lumbar n. root	Over sacro-iliac joint, hip, lateral thigh, and leg	Lateral leg, first 3 toes	Dorsiflexion of great toe and foot; difficulty walking on heels; foot-drop may occur	Minor	Changes uncommon in knee and ankle jerks, but internal hamstring reflex diminished or absent
L5-S1 disc; 1st sacral n. root	Over sacro-iliac joint, hip, postero-lateral thigh, and leg to heel	Back of calf, lateral heel, foot to toe	Plantar-flexion of foot and great toe may be affected; difficulty walking on toes	Gastrocnemi-us and soleus	Ankle jerk diminished or absent

Sagittal MRI of an intervertebral disc herniation

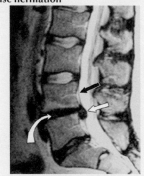

Herniation of L4–L5 intervertebral disc (*white arrows*) with some displacement of the posterior longitudinal ligament (*black arrow*). The two discs above this site show the normal hydrated appearance of the nucleus pulposus.
Reprinted with permission from Jackson S, Thomas R: Cross-Sectional Imaging Made Easy. Philadelphia, Churchill Livingstone, 2004.

Herniation of a lumbar disc

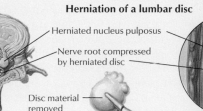

Herniated nucleus pulposus
Nerve root compressed by herniated disc
Portion of lamina and facet removed
Disc material removed

Disc material removed to decompress nerve root

Clinical Focus 2.7

Back Pain Associated With the Zygapophysial (Facet) Joints

Although changes in the vertebral facet joints are not the most common cause of back pain (~15%), such alterations can lead to chronic pain. Although the articular surfaces of the synovial facet joints are not directly innervated, sensory nerve fibers derived from the posterior rami of spinal nerves do supply the synovial linings of the capsules surrounding the joints. Two examples of painful conditions associated with facet joints are degeneration of the articular cartilage and osteophyte overgrowth of the articular processes.

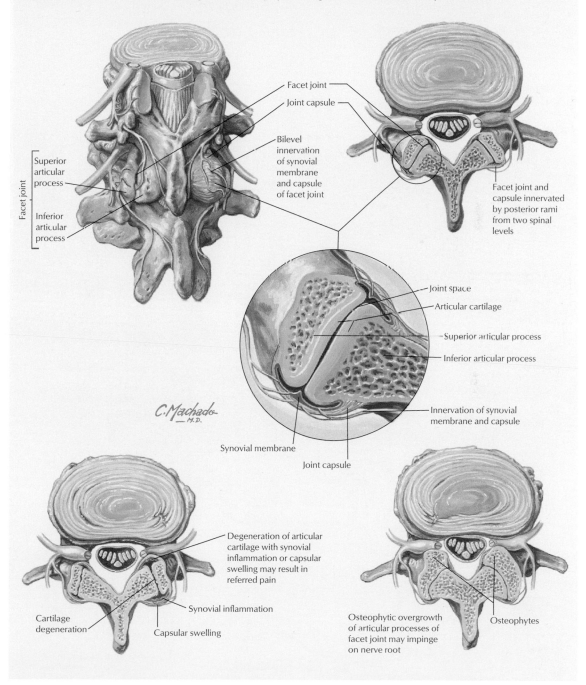

Facet joint

Joint capsule

Bilevel innervation of synovial membrane and capsule of facet joint

Superior articular process

Facet joint

Inferior articular process

Facet joint and capsule innervated by posterior rami from two spinal levels

Joint space

Articular cartilage

Superior articular process

Inferior articular process

Innervation of synovial membrane and capsule

Synovial membrane

Joint capsule

Degeneration of articular cartilage with synovial inflammation or capsular swelling may result in referred pain

Synovial inflammation

Cartilage degeneration

Capsular swelling

Osteophytic overgrowth of articular processes of facet joint may impinge on nerve root

Osteophytes

Clinical Focus 2.8

Low Back Pain

Low back pain, the **most common musculoskeletal disorder**, can have various causes. Physical examination, although not always revealing a definite cause, may provide clues to the level of spinal nerve involvement and relative sensitivity to pain. The following causes are identified most often:

- Intervertebral disc rupture and herniation
- Nerve inflammation or compression
- Degenerative changes in vertebral facet joints
- Sacroiliac joint and ligament involvement
- Metabolic bone disease
- Psychosocial factors
- Abdominal aneurysm
- Metastatic cancer
- Myofascial disorders

A. Standing

Body build
Posture
Deformities
Pelvic obliquity
Spine alignment
Palpate for:
   muscle spasm
   trigger zones
   myofascial nodes
   sciatic nerve tenderness
Compress iliac crests
for sacroiliac tenderness

Walking on heels (tests foot
and great toe dorsiflexion)

Walking on toes
(tests calf muscles)

Spinal column
movements:
   flexion
   extension
   side bending
   rotation

B. Kneeling on chair

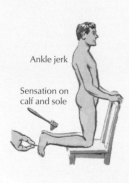

Ankle jerk

Sensation on
calf and sole

C. Seated on table

Straight leg raising

Knee jerk

Measure calf circumference

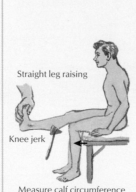

D. Supine

Straight leg raising: flex
thigh on pelvis and then
extend knee with foot
dorsiflexed (sciatic
nerve stretch)

Palpate for
peripheral
pulses and skin
temperature

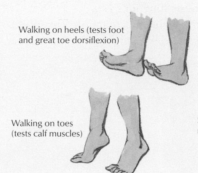

Palpate abdomen; listen for
bruit (abdominal and inguinal)

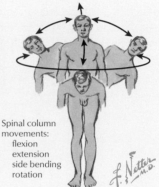

Palpate for flattening
of lumbar lordosis
during leg raising

Measure leg lengths (anterior superior
iliac spine to medial malleolus) and thigh
circumferences

Test sensation and motor power

E. Prone

Test for renal tenderness

Spine
extension

Palpate for local
tenderness or spasm

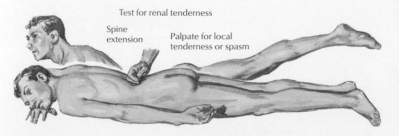

F. Rectal and/or pelvic examination

G. MRI and/or CT and/or myelogram of
1. lumbosacral spine
2. abdomen/pelvis

H. Laboratory studies
Serum Ca^{2+} and PO_4^{-}, alkaline
phosphatase, prostate-specific
antigen (males over 40), CBC,
ESR, and urinalysis

Movements of the Spine

The essential movements of the spine are flexion, extension, lateral flexion (lateral bending), and rotation (Fig. 2.8). The greatest freedom of movement occurs in the cervical and lumbar spine, with the neck having the greatest range of motion. Flexion is greatest in the cervical region, and extension is greatest in the lumbar region. The thoracic region is relatively stable, as is the sacrum.

Again, the atlantooccipital joint permits flexion and extension (e.g., nodding in acknowledgment), and the atlantoaxial joint allows side-to-side movements (rotation; e.g., indicating "no"). This is accomplished by a uniaxial synovial joint between the dens of the axis and its articulation with the anterior arch of the atlas. The **dens** functions as a pivot that permits the atlas and attached occipital bone of the skull to rotate on the axis. **Alar ligaments** limit this side-to-side movement so that rotation of the atlantoaxial joint occurs with the skull and atlas rotating as a single unit on the axis (see Fig. 2.6).

Movements of the spine are a function of the following features:

- Size and compressibility of the intervertebral discs.
- Tightness of the joint capsules.
- Orientation of the articular facets (zygapophysial joints).
- Muscle and ligament function.
- Articulations with the thoracic cage.
- Limitations imposed by the adjacent tissues and increasing age.

Blood Supply to the Spine

The spine receives blood from spinal arteries derived from branches of larger arteries that serve each

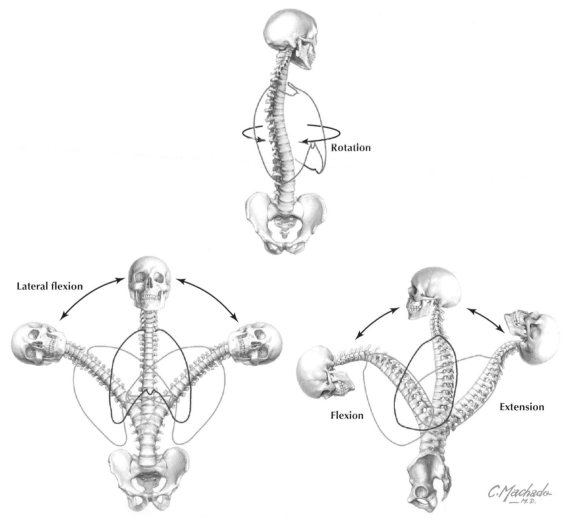

FIGURE 2.8 Movements of the Spine.

Clinical Focus 2.9

Whiplash Injury

"Whiplash" is a nonmedical term for a **cervical hyperextension** injury, which is usually associated with a rear-end vehicular crash. The relaxed neck is thrown backward, or hyperextended, as the vehicle accelerates rapidly forward. Rapid recoil of the neck into extreme flexion occurs next. Properly adjusted headrests can greatly reduce the occurrence of this hyperextension injury, which often results in stretched or torn cervical muscles and, in severe cases, ligament, bone, and nerve damage.

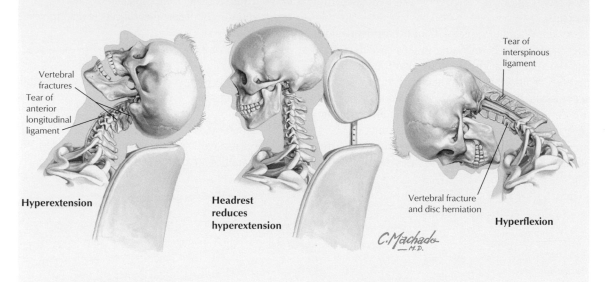

midline region of the body (Fig. 2.9). These major arteries include the following:

- **Vertebral arteries:** arising from the subclavian arteries in the neck.
- **Ascending cervical arteries:** arising from a branch of the subclavian arteries.
- **Posterior intercostal arteries:** arising from the thoracic aorta.
- **Lumbar arteries:** arising from the abdominal aorta.
- **Lateral sacral arteries:** arising from pelvic internal iliac arteries.

Spinal arteries arise from these branches and divide into small *posterior branches* that supply the vertebral arch and small *anterior branches* that supply the vertebral body (see Fig. 2.9). Also, longitudinal branches of **radicular arteries,** which arise from these spinal arteries, course along the inside aspect of the vertebral canal and supply the vertebral column. (Do not confuse these arteries with those that supply the spinal cord, discussed later. In some cases, arteries that do supply the spinal cord also contribute branches that supply the vertebrae.)

Radicular veins receive tributaries from the spinal cord and the internal vertebral veins that course within the vertebral canal; this **internal**

venous plexus also anastomoses with a network of **external vertebral veins** (see Fig. 2.9). The internal vertebral venous plexus lacks valves, whereas the external vertebral venous plexus has recently been shown to possess some valves, directing blood flow toward the internal venous plexus. The radicular veins then drain blood from the vertebral venous plexus to *segmental* and *intervertebral veins,* with the blood ultimately collecting in the segmental branches of the following major venous channels:

- **Superior vena cava:** drains cervical vertebral region.
- **Azygos venous system:** drains thoracic region.
- **Inferior vena cava:** this large vein drains lumbosacral regions of the spine.

Innervation of the Spine

The spine is innervated by meningeal branches of the spinal nerves. The zygapophysial (facet) joints are innervated by medial branches of the posterior rami (see Clinical Focus 2.7).

4. MUSCLES OF THE BACK

Although the spine is the axis of the human body and courses down the body's midline, dividing it

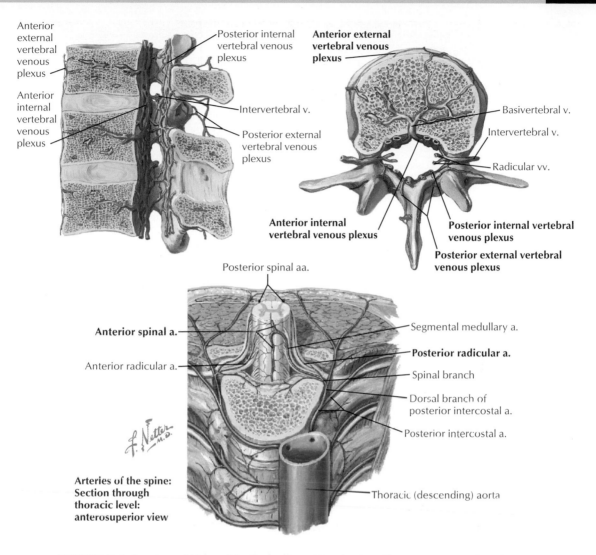

FIGURE 2.9 Arteries and Veins of the Spine. (From *Netter's atlas of human anatomy*, ed 8, Plates 192 and 193; S-24 and S-25.)

into approximately equal right and left halves, it is not midway between the anterior and posterior halves of the body. In fact, most of the body's weight lies anterior to the more posteriorly aligned vertebral column. Consequently, to support the body and spine, most of the muscles associated with the spine attach to its lateral and posterior processes, assisting the spine in maintaining an upright posture that offsets the uneven weight distribution.

The muscles of the back are divided into two major groups, as follows:

Extrinsic back muscles: involved in movements of the upper limb and with respiration.

Intrinsic back muscles: involved in movements of the spine and maintenance of posture.

Extrinsic Back Muscles

The extrinsic muscles of the back are considered "extrinsic" because embryologically they arise from *hypaxial myotomes* (see Fig. 2.22). The extrinsic back muscles are divided into the following two functional groups (Fig. 2.10 and Table 2.5):

- **Superficial muscles:** involved in movements of the upper limb (trapezius, latissimus dorsi, levator scapulae, two rhomboids), and attach the pectoral girdle (clavicle, scapula, humerus) to the axial skeleton (skull, ribs, spine).
- **Intermediate muscles:** thin accessory muscles of respiration (serratus posterior superior and inferior) that assist with movements of the rib cage lie deep to the superficial muscles and extend from the spine to the ribs.

TABLE 2.5 Muscles of the Back

MUSCLE	SUPERIOR ATTACHMENT	INFERIOR ATTACHMENT	INNERVATION	MAIN ACTIONS
Extrinsic Back Muscles				
Trapezius	Superior nuchal line, external occipital protuberance, nuchal ligament, and spinous processes of C7-T12	Lateral third of clavicle, acromion, and spine of scapula	Accessory nerve (cranial nerve XI)	Elevates, retracts, and rotates scapula; lower fibers depress scapula
Latissimus dorsi	Spinous processes of T7-L5, sacrum, thoracolumbar fascia, iliac crest, and last three ribs	Humerus (intertubercular sulcus)	Thoracodorsal nerve (C6-C8)	Extends, adducts, and medially rotates humerus
Levator scapulae	Posterior tubercles of transverse processes of C1-C4	Medial border of scapula from superior angle to spine	C3-C4 and dorsal scapular (C5) nerve	Elevates scapula medially and tilts glenoid cavity inferiorly
Rhomboid minor and major	*Minor:* nuchal ligament and spinous processes of C7-T1 *Major:* spinous processes of T2-T5	Medial border of scapula at spine Medial border of scapula below base of spine	Dorsal scapular nerve (C4-C5)	Retract scapula, rotate it to depress glenoid cavity, and fix scapula to thoracic wall
Serratus posterior superior	Ligamentum nuchae and spinous processes of C7-T3	Superior aspect of ribs 2-5	T1-T4 anterior rami	Elevates ribs
Serratus posterior inferior	Spinous processes of T11-L3	Inferior border of ribs 9-12	T9-T12 anterior rami	Depresses ribs
Intrinsic Back Muscles				
Splenius capitis	Nuchal ligament, spinous processes of C7-T4	Mastoid process of temporal bone and lateral third of superior nuchal line	Middle cervical nerves*	Bilaterally: extends head Unilaterally: laterally bends (flexes) and rotates face to same side
Splenius colli	Spinous processes of T3-T6	Transverse processes of C1-C3	Lower cervical nerves*	Bilaterally: extends neck Unilaterally: laterally bends (flexes) and rotates neck toward same side
Erector spinae	Posterior sacrum, iliac crest, sacrospinous ligament, supraspinous ligament, and spinous processes of lower lumbar and sacral vertebrae	*Iliocostalis:* angles of lower ribs and cervical transverse processes *Longissimus:* between tubercles and angles of ribs, transverse processes of thoracic and cervical vertebrae, mastoid process *Spinalis:* spinous processes of upper thoracic and midcervical vertebrae	Respective spinal nerves of each region*	Extends and laterally bends vertebral column and head
Semispinalis	Transverse processes of C4-T12	Spinous processes of cervical and thoracic regions	Respective spinal nerves of each region*	Extends head, neck, and thorax and rotates them to opposite side
Multifidi	Sacrum, ilium, and transverse processes of T1-T12 and articular processes of C4-C7	Spinous processes of vertebrae above, spanning two to four segments	Respective spinal nerves of each region*	Stabilizes spine during local movements
Rotatores	Transverse processes of cervical, thoracic, and lumbar regions	Lamina and transverse process of spine above, spanning one or two segments	Respective spinal nerves of each region*	Stabilize, extend, and rotate spine

*Posterior rami of spinal nerves.
Variations in spinal nerve contributions to the innervation of muscles, their attachments, and their actions are common in human anatomy. Therefore, expect differences between texts and realize that anatomical variation is normal.

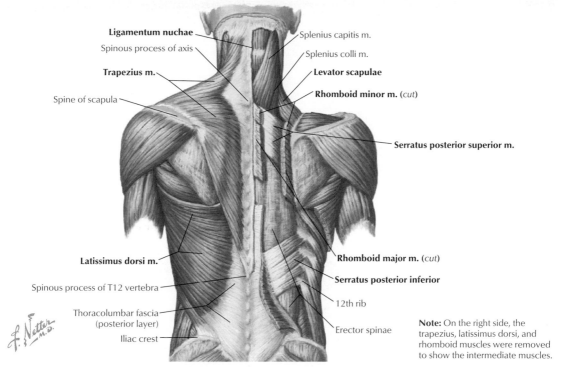

Ligamentum nuchae
Spinous process of axis
Trapezius m.
Spine of scapula
Splenius capitis m.
Splenius colli m.
Levator scapulae
Rhomboid minor m. (*cut*)
Serratus posterior superior m.
Latissimus dorsi m.
Spinous process of T12 vertebra
Thoracolumbar fascia (posterior layer)
Iliac crest
Rhomboid major m. (*cut*)
Serratus posterior inferior
12th rib
Erector spinae

Note: On the right side, the trapezius, latissimus dorsi, and rhomboid muscles were removed to show the intermediate muscles.

FIGURE 2.10 Extrinsic Muscles of the Back. (From *Netter's atlas of human anatomy*, ed 8, Plate 195; S-199.)

Intrinsic Back Muscles

The intrinsic back muscles are the "true" muscles of the back because they develop from *epaxial myotomes* (see Fig. 2.22), function in movements of the spine, and help maintain posture. The intrinsic muscles are enclosed within a deep fascial layer that extends in the midline from the medial crest of the sacrum to the **ligamentum nuchae** (a broad extension of the supraspinous ligament that extends from the spinous process of the C7 vertebra to the external occipital protuberance of the skull) (Fig. 2.10) and skull, and that spreads laterally to the transverse processes and angles of the ribs. In the thoracic and lumbar regions, the deep fascia makes up a distinct sheath known as the **thoracolumbar fascia** (Figs. 2.10 and 2.11; see also Fig 4.31).

In the lumbar region, this fascial sheath has the following three layers (see also Fig. 4.31):

- **Posterior layer:** extending from the lumbar and sacral spinous processes laterally over the surface of the erector spinae muscles.
- **Middle layer:** extending from the lumbar transverse processes to the iliac crest inferiorly and to the 12th rib superiorly.
- **Anterior layer:** covering the quadratus lumborum muscle of the posterior abdominal wall and extending to the lumbar transverse processes,

and iliac crest, and superiorly, forming the lateral arcuate ligament for attachment of the respiratory diaphragm.

The intrinsic back muscles also are among the few muscles of the body that are innervated by posterior rami of a spinal nerve. From superficial to deep, the intrinsic muscles include the following three layers (Fig. 2.11 and Table 2.5):

- **Superficial layer:** including the splenius muscles that occupy the lateral and posterior neck (*spinotransversales muscles*).
- **Intermediate layer:** including the erector spinae muscles that mainly extend and laterally bend the spine.
- **Deep layer:** including the transversospinales muscles that fill the spaces between the transverse processes and spinous processes.

The intermediate, or **erector spinae,** layer of muscles is the largest group of the intrinsic back muscles and is important for maintaining posture, extending the spine, and laterally bending the spine. These muscles are divided into three major groups, as follows (Fig. 2.11 and Table 2.5):

- **Iliocostalis:** most laterally located and associated with attachments to the ribs and cervical transverse processes.

The superficial and intermediate (erector spinae) layers of the intrinsic back muscles

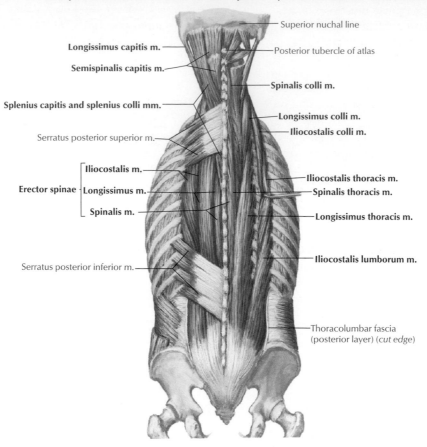

Superior nuchal line

Longissimus capitis m.

Semispinalis capitis m.

Posterior tubercle of atlas

Spinalis colli m.

Splenius capitis and splenius colli mm.

Longissimus colli m.

Iliocostalis colli m.

Serratus posterior superior m.

Iliocostalis thoracis m.

Erector spinae — **Iliocostalis m.**

Longissimus m.

Spinalis m.

Spinalis thoracis m.

Longissimus thoracis m.

Iliocostalis lumborum m.

Serratus posterior inferior m.

Thoracolumbar fascia
(posterior layer) (*cut edge*)

The deep (transversospinal) layer of the intrinsic back muscles

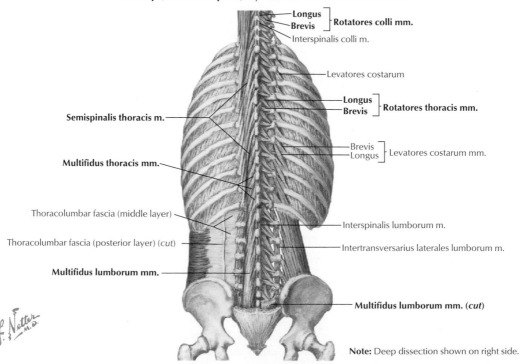

Longus
Brevis } **Rotatores colli mm.**

Interspinalis colli m.

Levatores costarum

Longus
Brevis } **Rotatores thoracis mm.**

Semispinalis thoracis m.

Brevis
Longus } Levatores costarum mm.

Multifidus thoracis mm.

Thoracolumbar fascia (middle layer)

Interspinalis lumborum m.

Thoracolumbar fascia (posterior layer) (*cut*)

Intertransversarius laterales lumborum m.

Multifidus lumborum mm.

Multifidus lumborum mm. (*cut*)

Note: Deep dissection shown on right side.

FIGURE 2.11 Intrinsic Muscles of the Back. (From *Netter's atlas of human anatomy*, ed 8, Plate 196 and 197; S-200 and S-201.)

- **Longissimus:** intermediate and largest column of the erector spinae muscles.
- **Spinalis:** most medially located and smallest of the erector spinae group, with attachments to the vertebral spinous processes.

These three groups are further subdivided into regional divisions—lumborum, thoracis, colli, and capitis—based on their attachments as one proceeds superiorly (Fig. 2.11).

The transversospinales (transversospinal) muscles (deep layer) are often simply called the "paravertebral" muscles because they form a solid mass of muscle tissue interposed and running obliquely between the transverse and spinous processes (Fig. 2.11). The transversospinal muscles comprise the following three groups:

- **Semispinalis group:** thoracis, colli, and capitis muscles; the most superficial transversospinal muscles, found in the thoracic and cervical regions superior to the occipital bone.
- **Multifidus group:** the muscles found deep to the semispinalis group and in all spinal regions, but most prominently in the lumbar region.
- **Rotatores group:** deepest transversospinal muscles; present in all spinal regions, but most prominently in the thoracic region.

Deep to the transversospinal muscles lies a relatively small set of segmental muscles that assist in elevating the ribs (*levatores costarum*) and stabilizing adjacent vertebrae while larger muscle groups act on the spine (*interspinales, intertransversarii*) (Fig. 2.11).

Suboccipital Muscles

In the back of the neck, deep to the trapezius, splenius, and semispinalis muscles, lie several small muscles that move the head; they are attached to the skull, the atlas, and the axis (Fig. 2.12 and Table 2.6). These muscles are the **suboccipital muscles**, innervated by the suboccipital nerve (posterior ramus of C1) and forming a *suboccipital* triangle with the following muscle boundaries:

- **Rectus posterior major capitis.**
- **Obliquus superior capitis** (superior oblique muscle of head).
- **Obliquus inferior capitis** (inferior oblique muscle of head).

Deep within the suboccipital triangle, the **vertebral artery**, a branch of the subclavian artery in the lower anterior neck, passes through the transverse foramen of the atlas and loops medially to enter the foramen magnum of the skull to supply

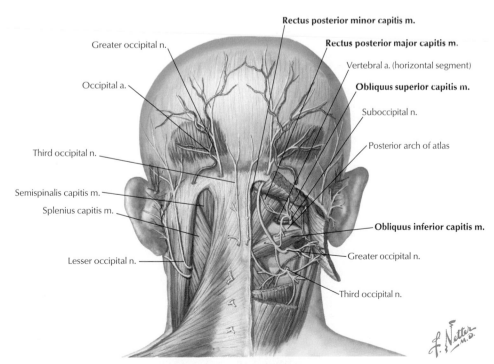

FIGURE 2.12 Suboccipital Triangle and Associated Musculature. (From *Netter's atlas of human anatomy*, ed 8, Plate 199; S-202.)

TABLE 2.6 Suboccipital Muscles

MUSCLE	SUPERIOR ATTACHMENT	INFERIOR ATTACHMENT	INNERVATION	MAIN ACTIONS
Rectus posterior major capitis	Spine of axis	Lateral inferior nuchal line	Suboccipital nerve (C1)	Extends head and rotates to same side
Rectus posterior minor capitis	Tubercle of posterior arch of atlas	Median inferior nuchal line	Suboccipital nerve (C1)	Extends head
Obliquus superior capitis	Atlas transverse process	Occipital bone	Suboccipital nerve (C1)	Extends head and bends it laterally
Obliquus inferior capitis	Spine of axis	Atlas transverse process	Suboccipital nerve (C1)	Rotates head to same side

Variations in spinal nerve contributions to the innervation of muscles, their attachments, and their actions are common in human anatomy. Therefore, expect differences between texts and realize that anatomical variation is normal.

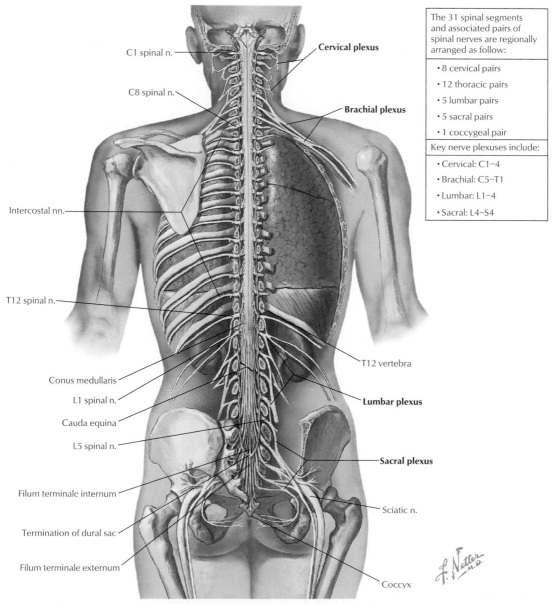

The 31 spinal segments and associated pairs of spinal nerves are regionally arranged as follow:

- 8 cervical pairs
- 12 thoracic pairs
- 5 lumbar pairs
- 5 sacral pairs
- 1 coccygeal pair

Key nerve plexuses include:

- Cervical: C1–4
- Brachial: C5–T1
- Lumbar: L1–4
- Sacral: L4–S4

FIGURE 2.13 Spinal Cord and Nerves In Situ. (From *Netter's atlas of human anatomy*, ed 8, Plate 186; S-16.)

the brainstem. The first three pairs of spinal nerves are also found in this region (Fig. 2.12).

5. SPINAL CORD

The spinal cord is a direct continuation of the medulla oblongata, extending below the foramen magnum at the base of the skull and passing through the vertebral (spinal) canal formed by the articulated vertebrae (Fig. 2.13).

The spinal cord has a slightly larger diameter in the cervical and lumbar regions, primarily because of increased numbers of neurons and axons in these regions for innervation of the muscles in the upper and lower limbs. The spinal cord ends as a tapered region called the **conus medullaris,** which is situated at about the L1-L2 vertebral level (or L3 in neonates). From this point inferiorly, the nerve rootlets course to their respective levels and form a bundle called the **cauda equina** ("horse's tail"). The spinal cord is anchored inferiorly by the **terminal filum,** which is attached to the coccyx. The terminal filum is a pial extension that picks up a layer of arachnoid and dura mater after passing through the dural sac (at the L2 vertebral level) and before attaching to the coccyx (see Spinal Meninges). Features of the spinal cord include the following:

- The 31 pairs of spinal nerves (8 cervical, 12 thoracic, 5 lumbar, and 5 sacral pairs and 1 coccygeal pair).
- Each spinal nerve is formed by a posterior (dorsal) and anterior (ventral) root. (C1 lacks a posterior root in about 50% of people)
- Motor neurons reside in the spinal cord gray matter (anterior horn).
- Sensory neurons reside in the spinal ganglia.
- Anterior rami of spinal nerves often converge to form **plexuses** (mixed networks of nerve axons organized into a **cervical, brachial, lumbar, or sacral plexus)** or segmental thoracic nerves **(intercostal nerves and the subcostal nerve [T12])**.
- Posterior rami of spinal nerves are small and only innervate the zygapophysial (facet) joints, the deep intrinsic back muscles, the muscles of the suboccipital region (epaxial muscles of embryo); and a narrow strip of skin above the intrinsic muscles that extends down the back about 3 to 4 cm lateral to the midline.

Typical Spinal Nerve

The typical scheme for a **somatic** (innervates skin and skeletal muscle) peripheral nerve shows a motor neuron in the spinal cord anterior horn (gray matter) sending a myelinated axon through an anterior (ventral) **root** and a **spinal nerve,** and then into posterior and anterior rami of a peripheral nerve, which ends at a neuromuscular junction on a skeletal muscle (Figs. 2.14 and 2.15). Likewise, a nerve ending in the skin sends a sensory axon toward the spinal cord in a peripheral nerve. (Sensory axons also arise from the muscle spindles and joints and are similarly conveyed back to the spinal cord.) Thus, each peripheral nerve contains hundreds or thousands of motor and sensory axons. The sensory neuron is a pseudounipolar neuron with its cell body in a **spinal ganglion** (a ganglion in the periphery is a collection of neuronal cell bodies, just as a "nucleus" is in the brain) and sends its central axon into the posterior horn (gray matter) of the spinal cord. At each level of the spinal cord, the gray matter is visible as a butterfly-shaped central collection of neurons that possesses a posterior and an anterior horn (Fig. 2.14).

The spinal cord gives rise to 31 pairs of spinal nerves, which then form two major branches (rami), as follows:

- **Posterior ramus:** a small ramus (branch) that courses dorsally to the back and conveys motor and sensory information to and from the skin and the intrinsic back muscles and suboccipital skeletal muscles.
- **Anterior ramus:** a much larger ramus (branch) that courses laterally and ventrally and innervates all the remaining skin and skeletal muscles of the neck, limbs, and trunk.

Once nerve fibers (sensory or motor) are beyond, or peripheral to, the spinal cord proper, the fibers then reside in nerves of the peripheral nervous system (PNS). Components of the PNS include the following (see Nervous System, Chapter 1):

- **Somatic nervous system:** sensory and motor fibers to skin, skeletal muscle, and joints (Fig. 2.15, left side).
- **Autonomic nervous system** (ANS): sensory and motor fibers to all smooth muscle (including viscera and vasculature), cardiac muscle (heart), and glands (Fig. 2.15, right side).
- **Enteric nervous system:** intrinsic plexuses and ganglia of the gastrointestinal tract that regulate bowel secretion, absorption, and motility (originally, considered part of the ANS); linked to the ANS for optimal regulation (see Fig. 1.27).

Thus, most peripheral nerves arising from the spinal cord contains hundreds or thousands of three types of axons (Fig. 2.15, left and right sides):

Segment of the spinal cord showing the dorsal and ventral roots, membranes removed: anterior view (*greatly magnified*)

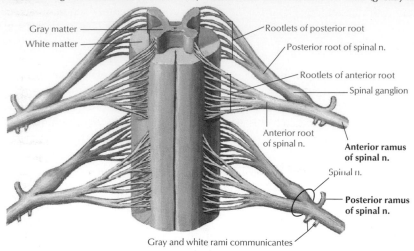

Schematic of a typical peripheral nerve showing the somatic axons (autonomic axons not shown)

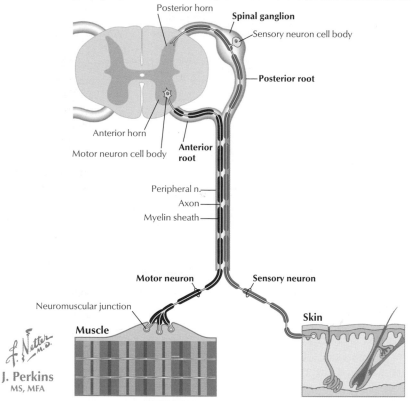

J. Perkins
MS, MFA

FIGURE 2.14 Typical Spinal Nerve.

- **Somatic efferent** (motor) axons to skeletal muscle.
- **Afferent** (sensory) axons from the skin, skeletal muscle, and joints or viscera.
- **Autonomic** axons to smooth muscle (vascular smooth muscle and arrector pili muscles in the skin), cardiac muscle, and glands.

Each of the 31 pairs of spinal nerves exits the spinal cord and passes through an opening in the vertebral column (intervertebral foramen) to gain access to the periphery. The C1 nerve pair passes between the skull and the atlas, with subsequent cervical nerve pairs exiting the intervertebral foramen above the vertebra of the same number;

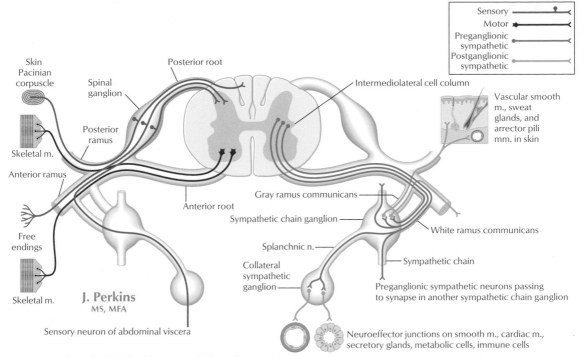

Note: For simplicity, the left side of the figure only shows the somatic components while the right side only shows the sympathetic efferent components.

FIGURE 2.15 Structural Anatomy of a Thoracic Spinal Nerve.

the C2 nerve exits via the intervertebral foramen superior to the C2 vertebra, and so on, until one reaches the C8 nerve, which then exits the intervertebral foramen above the T1 vertebra. All the remaining thoracic, lumbar, and sacral nerves exit via the intervertebral foramen below the vertebra of the same number (Fig. 2.16).

As it divides into its smaller **posterior ramus** and larger **anterior ramus**, the spinal nerve's smaller posterior ramus also gives off several small *recurrent meningeal branches* that reenter the intervertebral foramen and innervate the dura mater, intervertebral discs, ligaments, and blood vessels associated with the spinal cord and vertebral column (see Fig. 2.18).

Dermatomes

The region of skin innervated by the somatic sensory nerve axons associated with a single spinal ganglion at a single spinal cord level is called a **dermatome.** (Likewise, over the anterolateral head, the skin is innervated by one of the three divisions of the trigeminal cranial nerve, as discussed later.) The neurons that give rise to these sensory fibers are pseudounipolar neurons that reside in the single spinal ganglion associated with the specific spinal cord level (Figs. 2.14 and 2.15). (Note that for each level, we are speaking of a pair of nerves, roots,

and ganglia, with 31 pairs of spinal nerves, one pair for each spinal cord level.) The first cervical spinal cord level, C1, does possess sensory fibers, but these provide minimal if any contribution to the skin, so at the top of the head the dermatome pattern begins with the C2 dermatome (Fig. 2.17 and Table 2.7).

The dermatomes encircle the body in segmental fashion, corresponding to the spinal cord level that receives sensory input from that segment of skin (touch, pain, temperature, and position). The sensation conveyed by touching the skin is largely that of pressure and pain. Knowledge of the dermatome pattern is useful in localizing specific spinal cord segments and in assessing the integrity of the spinal cord at that level (intact or "lesioned").

The sensory nerve fibers that innervate a segment of skin and constitute the "dermatome" exhibit some overlap of nerve fibers. Consequently, a segment of skin is innervated primarily by fibers from a single spinal cord level, but there will be some overlap with sensory fibers from the level above and below the primary cord level. For example, dermatome T5 will have some overlap with sensory fibers associated with the T4 and T6 spinal levels. Thus, dermatomes provide a good approximation of spinal cord levels, but variation is common and overlap exists (Table 2.7).

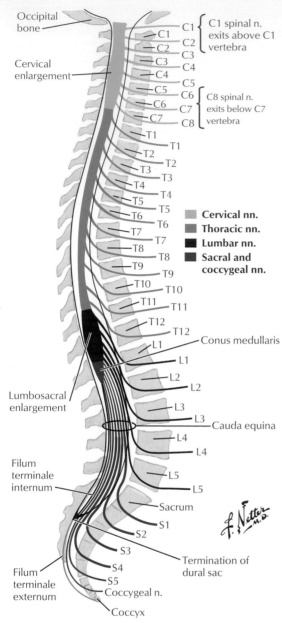

FIGURE 2.16 Relationship of Spinal Nerves to Vertebrae. (From *Netter's atlas of human anatomy*, ed 8, Plate 187; S-18.)

Labels in Figure 2.16:
- Occipital bone
- Cervical enlargement
- C1 spinal n. exits above C1 vertebra
- C8 spinal n. exits below C7 vertebra
- Cervical nn.
- Thoracic nn.
- Lumbar nn.
- Sacral and coccygeal nn.
- Conus medullaris
- Lumbosacral enlargement
- Cauda equina
- Filum terminale internum
- Sacrum
- Termination of dural sac
- Filum terminale externum
- Coccygeal n.
- Coccyx

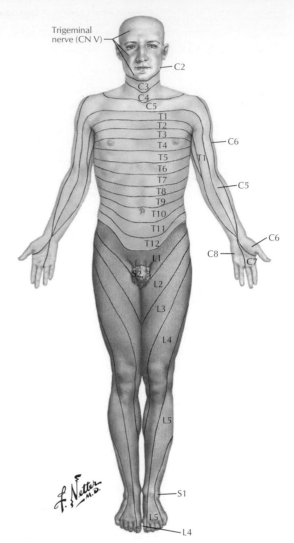

FIGURE 2.17 Distribution of Dermatomes.

Spinal Meninges

The brain and spinal cord are covered by three membranes called the **meninges** and are bathed in **cerebrospinal fluid** (CSF) (Fig. 2.18). The three meningeal layers are the dura, arachnoid, and pia mater.

Dura Mater

The dura mater ("tough mother") is a thick outer covering that is richly innervated by sensory nerve

TABLE 2.7 Key Dermatomes as Related to Body Surface	
VERTEBRA(E)	**BODY SURFACE**
C5	Clavicles
C5-C7	Lateral upper limb
C6	Thumb
C7	Middle finger
C8	Little finger
C8-T2	Medial upper limb
T4	Nipple
T10	Umbilicus (navel)
T12-L1	Inguinal/groin region
L1-L4	Anterior and inner surfaces of lower limbs
L4	Knee; medial side of big toe
L5	2nd to 4th toes
L4-S1	Foot
S1-S2	Posterior lower limb
S2-S4	Perineum

Clinical Focus 2.10

Herpes Zoster

Herpes zoster, or *shingles,* is the most common infection of the peripheral nervous system. It is an acute neuralgia confined to the dermatome distribution of a specific spinal or cranial sensory nerve root.

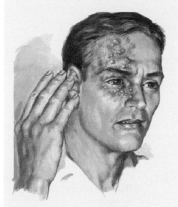

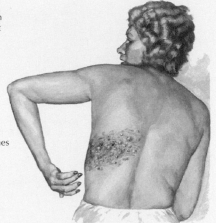

Painful erythematous vesicular eruption in distribution of ophthalmic division of right trigeminal (V) n.

Herpes zoster following course of 6th and 7th left thoracic dermatomes

Features of Shingles	
Characteristic	**Description**
Etiology	Reactivation of previous infection of dorsal root or sensory ganglion by varicella-zoster virus (which causes chickenpox)
Presentation	Vesicular rash confined to a radicular or cranial nerve sensory distribution; initial intense, burning, localized pain; vesicles appear 72-96 hours later
Sites affected	Usually one or several contiguous unilateral dermatomes (T5-L2), CN V (semilunar ganglion), or CN VII (geniculate ganglion)

endings and that extends around the spinal cord down to the level of the S2 vertebra, where the dural sac ends. The **epidural (extradural) space** lies between the vertebral canal walls and the spinal dural sac and contains fat, small nerves, and blood vessels (Fig. 2.18).

Arachnoid Mater

The fine, weblike arachnoid membrane is avascular and lies directly beneath, but is not attached to, the dura mater. The arachnoid mater also ends at the level of the S2 vertebra. Wispy threads of connective tissue extend from this layer to the underlying pia mater and span the **subarachnoid space,** which is filled with cerebrospinal fluid (CSF). The subarachnoid space ends at the S2 vertebral level.

Pia Mater

The pia mater is a delicate, transparent inner layer that intimately covers the spinal cord. At the cervical and thoracic levels, extensions of pia form approximately 21 pairs of triangular **denticulate** ("having small teeth") **ligaments** that extend laterally and help to anchor the spinal cord by inserting into the dura mater. At the conus medullaris, the pia mater forms the **terminal filum,** a single cord of thickened pia mater that pierces the dural sac at the S2 vertebral level, acquires an arachnoid and dural covering, and then passes through the sacral hiatus to attach to the tip of the coccyx, thus anchoring the spinal cord inferiorly.

Subarachnoid Space and Choroid Plexus

Cerebrospinal fluid fills the **subarachnoid space,** which lies between the arachnoid and pia meningeal layers (Figs. 2.18 and 2.19). Thus, CSF circulates through the brain ventricles and then gains access to the subarachnoid space through the lateral and median apertures, where it flows around and over the brain and inferiorly along the spinal cord to

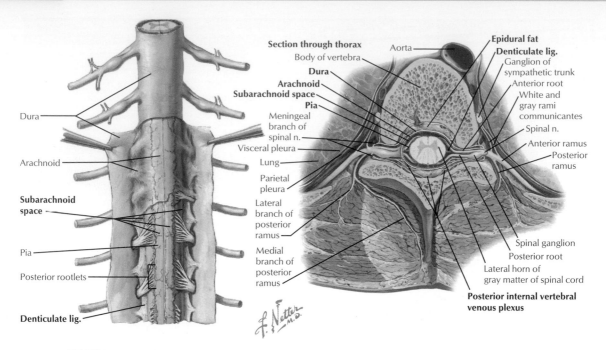

FIGURE 2.18 Spinal Meninges and Relationship to Spine. (From *Netter's atlas of human anatomy*, ed 8, Plates 189 and 190; S-17 and S-22.)

the most caudal extent of the dural sac, which ends at about the S2 vertebral level.

Cerebrospinal fluid is secreted by the **choroid plexus,** and most CSF is absorbed primarily by the **arachnoid granulations** (associated with the superior sagittal dural venous sinus) (Figs. 2.19 and 8.8), and secondarily by small veins that also contain microscopic arachnoid granulations on the surface of the pia mater throughout the central nervous system (CNS) (Fig. 2.19). With about 500-700 mL produced daily, CSF supports and cushions the spinal cord and brain, fulfills some of the functions normally provided by the lymphatic system, and fills the 150 mL volume of the brain's ventricular system and the subarachnoid space.

It should be noted that recent microscopic evidence provides support for the claim that some CNS regions do possess lymphatics. Future studies may elucidate a larger role for lymphatic drainage in some regions of the CNS.

Blood Supply to Spinal Cord

The spinal cord receives blood from spinal arteries derived from branches of larger arteries that serve each midline region of the body (Fig. 2.20). These major arteries include the following:

- **Vertebral arteries:** arising from the subclavian arteries in the neck.
- **Ascending cervical arteries:** arising from a branch of the subclavian arteries.
- **Posterior intercostal arteries:** arising from the thoracic aorta.
- **Lumbar arteries:** arising from the abdominal aorta.
- **Lateral sacral arteries:** arising from pelvic internal iliac arteries.

A single **anterior spinal artery** and two **posterior spinal arteries,** originating intracranially from the vertebral arteries, run longitudinally along the length of the cord and are joined segmentally in each region by segmental arteries (Fig. 2.20). The largest of these segmental branches is the **major anterior segmental medullary artery** (of Adamkiewicz), found in the lower thoracic or upper lumbar region; it is the major blood supply for the lower two thirds of the spinal cord. The posterior and anterior roots are supplied by segmental **radicular** (medullary) **arteries.**

Multiple **anterior** and **posterior spinal veins** run the length of the cord and drain into segmental (medullary) radicular veins (see Fig. 2.9). **Radicular veins** receive tributaries from the internal vertebral plexus veins that course within the vertebral canal in the epidural space. This plexus of veins drains superiorly through the foramen magnum and then into the dural venous sinuses. This plexus also drains into an external venous plexus that ultimately drains into the following veins:

- Superior vena cava.
- Azygos venous system of the thorax.
- Inferior vena cava.

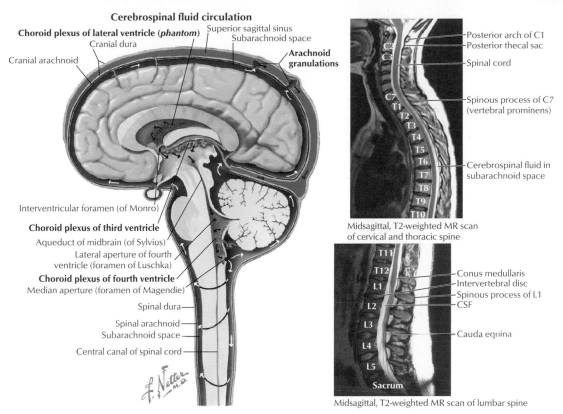

Cerebrospinal fluid circulation

Choroid plexus of lateral ventricle (*phantom*)
Cranial dura
Cranial arachnoid
Superior sagittal sinus
Subarachnoid space
Arachnoid granulations

Interventricular foramen (of Monro)
Choroid plexus of third ventricle
Aqueduct of midbrain (of Sylvius)
Lateral aperture of fourth ventricle (foramen of Luschka)
Choroid plexus of fourth ventricle
Median aperture (foramen of Magendie)
Spinal dura
Spinal arachnoid
Subarachnoid space
Central canal of spinal cord

Posterior arch of C1
Posterior thecal sac
Spinal cord
Spinous process of C7 (vertebral prominens)
Cerebrospinal fluid in subarachnoid space

Midsagittal, T2-weighted MR scan of cervical and thoracic spine

Conus medullaris
Intervertebral disc
Spinous process of L1
CSF
Cauda equina

Midsagittal, T2-weighted MR scan of lumbar spine

FIGURE 2.19 Cerebrospinal Fluid Circulation. (From *Netter's atlas of human anatomy,* ed 8, Plate 136; S-35; MR images from Kelley LL, Petersen C: *Sectional anatomy for imaging professionals,* St Louis, 2007, Mosby-Elsevier.)

Clinical Focus 2.11

Lumbar Puncture and Epidural Anesthesia

Cerebrospinal fluid may be sampled and examined clinically by performing a lumbar puncture (spinal tap). A spinal needle is inserted into the subarachnoid space of the lumbar cistern, in the midline between the L3 and L4 or the L4 and L5 vertebral spinal processes. Because the spinal cord ends at approximately the L1 or L2 vertebral level, the needle will not pierce and damage the cord. Anesthetic agents may be directly delivered into the epidural space (above the dura mater) to anesthetize the nerve fibers of the cauda equina; this common form of anesthesia is used during childbirth in most Western countries. The epidural anesthetic infiltrates the dural sac to reach the nerve roots and is usually administered at the same levels as the lumbar puncture.

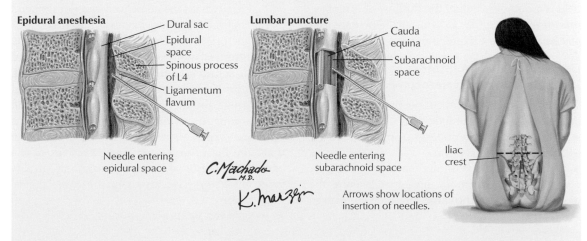

Epidural anesthesia
Dural sac
Epidural space
Spinous process of L4
Ligamentum flavum
Needle entering epidural space

Lumbar puncture
Cauda equina
Subarachnoid space
Needle entering subarachnoid space

Iliac crest

Arrows show locations of insertion of needles.

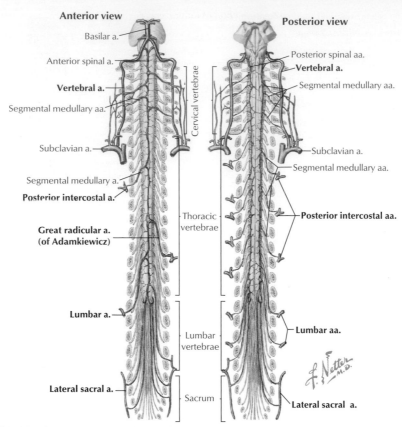

FIGURE 2.20 Blood Supply to Spinal Cord. (From *Netter's atlas of human anatomy*, ed 8, Plate 191; S-23.)

6. EMBRYOLOGY

Most of the bones inferior to the skull form by **endochondral** bone formation, that is, from a cartilaginous precursor that becomes ossified. The embryonic development of the musculoskeletal components of the back represents a classic example of segmentation, with each segment corresponding to the distribution of peripheral nerves. This process begins around the end of the third week of embryonic development (day 19), during the period called gastrulation (see Chapter 1).

Development of Myotomes, Dermatomes, and Sclerotomes

The bones, muscles, and connective tissues of the embryo arise from the following sources:
- Primitive streak mesoderm (somites).
- Lateral plate mesoderm.
- Diffuse collections of mesenchyme.

As the neural groove invaginates along the posterior midline of the embryonic disc, it is flanked on either side by masses of mesoderm called **somites.** About 42 to 44 pairs of somites develop along this central axis and subsequently develop into the following (Fig. 2.21):
- **Dermomyotomes:** divide further to form **dermatomes,** which become the dermis of the skin, and **myotomes,** which differentiate into segmental masses of skeletal muscle.
- **Sclerotomes:** the medial part of each somite that, along with the notochord, migrates around the neural tube and forms the cartilaginous precursors of the axial skeleton.

Myotomes have a segmental distribution, just like the somites from which they are derived. Each segment is innervated by a pair of nerves originating from the spinal cord segment. A small dorsal portion of the myotome becomes an **epimere** (epaxial) mass of skeletal muscle that will form the true intrinsic muscles of the back (e.g., erector spinae muscles) and are innervated by a posterior ramus of the spinal nerve (Fig. 2.22).

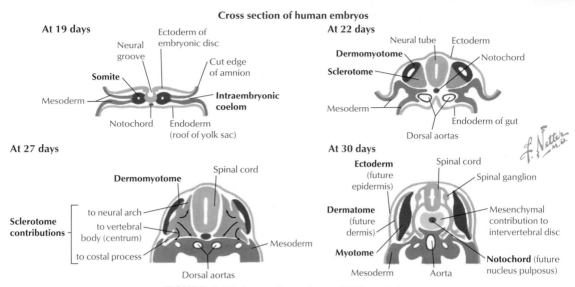

FIGURE 2.21 Somite Formation and Differentiation.

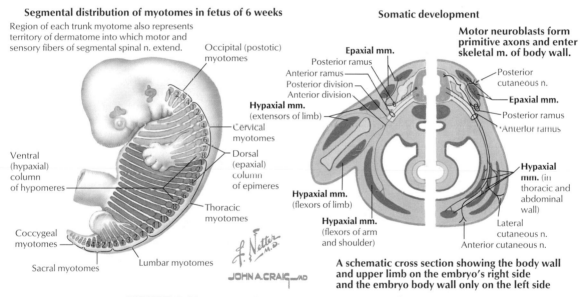

FIGURE 2.22 Myotome Segmentation into Epimeres and Hypomeres.

A much larger anterior segment becomes the **hypomere** (hypaxial) mass of skeletal muscle, which will form the muscles of the trunk wall and limb muscles, all innervated by an anterior ramus of the spinal nerve. Adjacent myotome segments often merge so that an individual skeletal muscle derived from those myotomes is innervated by more than one spinal cord segment. For example, the latissimus dorsi muscle is innervated by the thoracodorsal nerve, which is composed of nerves

from the anterior rami of spinal cord segments C6-C8.

Vertebral Column Development

Each vertebra first appears as a hyaline cartilage model that then ossifies, beginning in a **primary ossification center** (Fig. 2.23). Ossification centers include the following:

- **Body:** forms the vertebral body; important for support of body weight.

Fate of body, costal process, and neural arch components of vertebral column, with sites and time of appearance of ossification centers

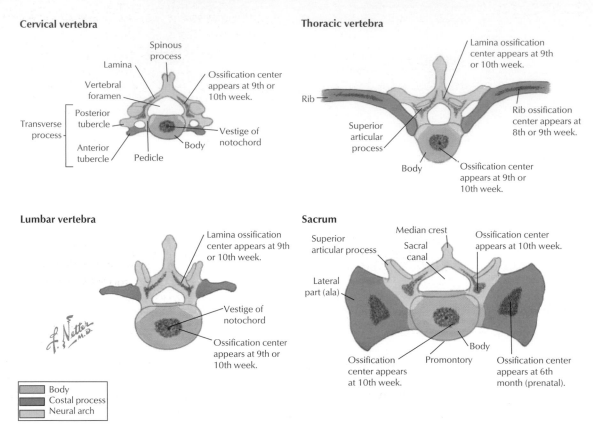

FIGURE 2.23 Ossification of Vertebral Column.

- **Costal process:** forms the ribs, or in vertebrae without rib articulation, part of the transverse process; important for movement and muscle attachment.
- **Neural arch:** includes the pedicle and lamina, for protection of the spinal cord, and the spinous process, for muscle attachment.

The body of the vertebra does not develop from a single sclerotome but rather from the fusion of two adjacent sclerotomes (i.e., fusion of caudal half of sclerotome above with cranial half of sclerotome below). The intervertebral foramen thus lies over this fusion and provides the opening for the spinal roots that will form the spinal nerve that will innervate the myotome at that particular segment.

The **notochord** initially is in the central portion of each vertebral body but disappears. The notochord persists only as the central portion (**nucleus pulposus**) of each intervertebral disc, surrounded by concentric lamellae of fibrocartilage.

Neurulation and Development of the Spinal Cord

Neurulation (neural tube formation) begins concurrently with **gastrulation** (formation of the trilaminar embryonic disc during the third week of development). As the primitive streak recedes caudally, the midline surface ectoderm thickens to form the **neural plate,** which then invaginates to form the **neural groove** (Fig. 2.24, *A*). The **neural crest** forms at the dorsal aspect of the neural groove (Fig. 2.24, *B*) and fuses in the midline as the groove sinks below the surface and pinches off to form the **neural tube** (Fig. 2.24, *C*). The neural tube forms the following:

- Neurons of central nervous system (CNS: brain, spinal cord).
- Supporting cells of CNS.
- Somatomotor neurons (innervate skeletal muscle) of PNS.

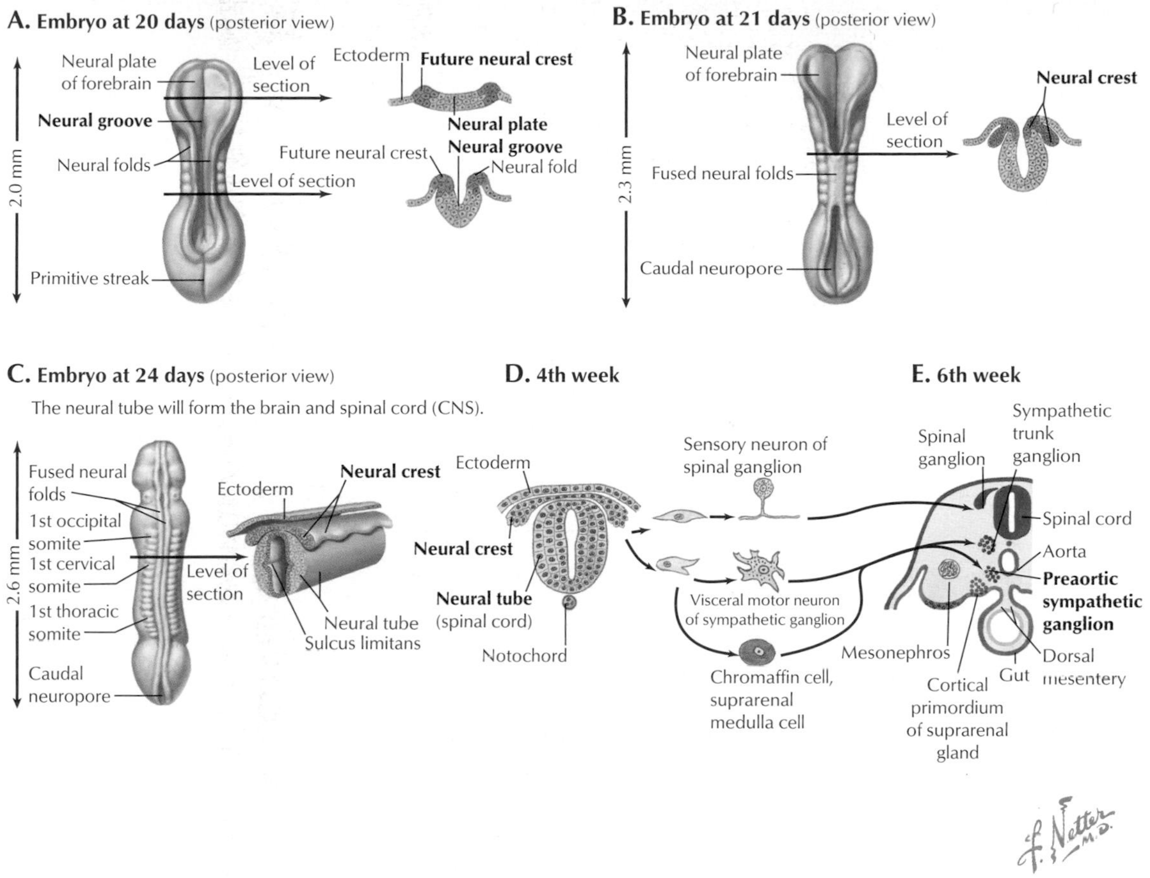

A. Embryo at 20 days (posterior view)

Neural plate of forebrain

Level of section

Ectoderm **Future neural crest**

Neural groove

Neural plate

Neural folds

Future neural crest

Neural groove

Neural fold

Level of section

2.0 mm

Primitive streak

B. Embryo at 21 days (posterior view)

Neural plate of forebrain

Neural crest

Level of section

Fused neural folds

2.3 mm

Caudal neuropore

C. Embryo at 24 days (posterior view)

The neural tube will form the brain and spinal cord (CNS).

Fused neural folds

Ectoderm

Neural crest

Ectoderm

1st occipital somite

1st cervical somite

Level of section

Neural crest

1st thoracic somite

Neural tube

Sulcus limitans

Neural tube (spinal cord)

2.6 mm

Caudal neuropore

Notochord

D. 4th week

Sensory neuron of spinal ganglion

Visceral motor neuron of sympathetic ganglion

Chromaffin cell, suprarenal medulla cell

E. 6th week

Spinal ganglion

Sympathetic trunk ganglion

Spinal cord

Aorta

Preaortic sympathetic ganglion

Mesonephros

Cortical primordium of suprarenal gland

Gut

Dorsal mesentery

FIGURE 2.24 Neurulation.

- Presynaptic autonomic neurons of PNS.
  The **neural crest** gives rise to the following (Fig. 2.24, D and E):
- Sensory neurons of PNS found in dorsal root ganglia.
- Unipolar sensory neurons of cranial nerves V, VII, IX, and X
- Bipolar cells of ganglia of CN VIII
- Postsynaptic autonomic neurons (sympathetic and parasympathetic systems)
- Pia and arachnoid mater cells
- Microglial cells
- Cells of the enteric (gut) nervous system
- Various paraganglion chromaffin cells associated with the central and peripheral nervous system (carotid body chemoreceptors, small intensely fluorescent [SIF] cells of ganglia, etc.)
- Schwann cells of PNS.
- Adrenal medullary chromaffin cells, in each adrenal gland.
- Head mesenchyme and portions of heart.
- Melanocytes in skin.

- Arachnoid mater and pia mater meninges (dura mater is formed from mesenchyme).
  The cells in the walls of the neural tube compose the **neuroepithelium,** which develops into three zones, as follows:
- **Ependymal zone:** inner layer lining central canal of spinal cord (also lines ventricles of brain).
- **Mantle:** intermediate zone that develops into gray matter of spinal cord.
- **Marginal zone:** outer layer that becomes white matter of spinal cord.
  Glial cells are found primarily in the mantle and marginal zone. The neural tube is distinguished by a longitudinal groove on each side that forms the **sulcus limitans** and divides the tube into a dorsal **alar plate** and a ventral **basal plate** (Fig. 2.25). The dorsal alar plate forms the sensory derivatives of the spinal cord, and the ventral basal plate gives rise to the somatic and autonomic motor neurons, whose axons will leave the spinal cord and pass into the peripheral tissues. The sensory neurons of the spinal ganglia are formed from neural crest cells.

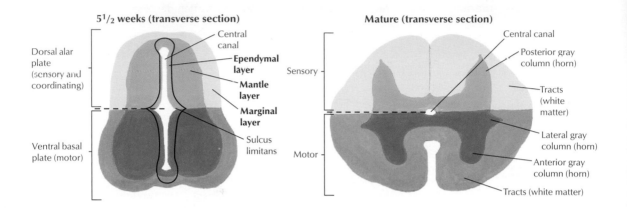

5¹/₂ weeks (transverse section)

Dorsal alar plate (sensory and coordinating)

Ventral basal plate (motor)

Central canal

Ependymal layer

Mantle layer

Marginal layer

Sulcus limitans

Mature (transverse section)

Sensory

Motor

Central canal

Posterior gray column (horn)

Tracts (white matter)

Lateral gray column (horn)

Anterior gray column (horn)

Tracts (white matter)

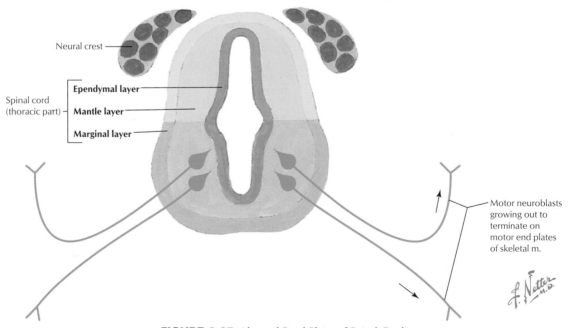

Differentiation and growth of neurons at 26 days

Neural crest

Spinal cord (thoracic part)

Ependymal layer

Mantle layer

Marginal layer

Motor neuroblasts growing out to terminate on motor end plates of skeletal m.

FIGURE 2.25 Alar and Basal Plates of Spinal Cord.

Clinical Focus 2.12

Spina Bifida

Spina bifida, one of several neural tube defects, is linked to low folic acid ingestion during the first trimester of pregnancy. Spina bifida is a congenital defect in which the neural tube remains too close to the surface such that the sclerotome cells do not migrate over the tube and form the neural arch of the vertebra **(spina bifida occulta).** This defect occurs most often at the L5 or S1 vertebral level and may present with neurologic findings. If the meninges and CSF protrude as a cyst **(meningocele)** or if the meninges and the cord itself reside in the cyst **(meningomyelocele),** significant neurologic problems often develop.

Spina bifida occulta

Types of spina bifida cystica with protrusion of spinal contents

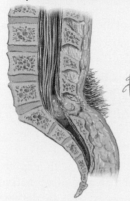
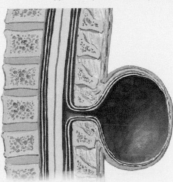
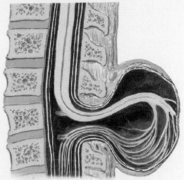
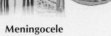

Meningocele

Meningomyelocele

Clinical Focus

Available Online

2.13 Myofascial Pain

2.14 Acute Spinal Syndromes

Additional figures available online (see inside front cover for details).

Challenge Yourself Questions

1. Besides his apparent mental deficits, the "hunchback of Notre Dame" also suffered from which of the following conditions?

   A. Halitosis
   B. Kyphosis
   C. Lordosis
   D. Osmosis
   E. Scoliosis

2. You are asked to assist a resident with a lumbar puncture procedure to withdraw a cerebrospinal fluid sample for analysis. Which of the following surface landmarks will help you determine where along the midline of the spine you will insert the spinal needle?

   A. An imaginary line crossing the two iliac crests
   B. An imaginary line crossing the two posterior superior iliac spines
   C. At the level of the 5th lumbar spinous process
   D. At the level of the umbilicus
   E. At the level of the vertebra prominens

3. A 56-year-old man presents with a history of pain for the last 18 months over the right buttock and radiating down the posterior aspect of the thigh and leg. A radiographic examination reveals a herniated disc between the L5 and the S1 vertebral levels. Which of the following nerves is most likely affected by this herniated disc?

   A. L3
   B. L4
   C. L5
   D. S1
   E. S2

4. A 19-year-old man sustained an apparent cervical spine hyperextension ("whiplash") injury after a rear-end roller-coaster crash at a local amusement park. Radiographic examination reveals several cervical vertebral body fractures and the rupture of an adjacent vertebral ligament. Which of the following vertebral ligaments was most likely ruptured during this hyperextension injury?

   A. Anterior longitudinal ligament
   B. Cruciate ligament
   C. Interspinous ligament
   D. Ligamentum flavum
   E. Nuchal ligament

5. A 34-year-old woman presents with a spider bite and a circumscribed area of inflammation on the back of her neck over the C4 dermatome region. Which of the following types of nerve fibers mediate this sensation?

   A. Somatic afferents in C4 anterior root
   B. Somatic afferents in C4 posterior root
   C. Somatic afferents in C4 anterior ramus
   D. Somatic efferents in C4 anterior root
   E. Somatic efferents in C4 posterior root
   F. Somatic efferents in C4 anterior ramus

6. A newborn female presents with a congenital neural tube defect likely caused by a folic acid deficiency and characterized by the failure of the sclerotome to form the neural arch. Which of the following conditions is consistent with this congenital defect?

   A. Osteophyte overgrowth
   B. Osteoporosis
   C. Scoliosis
   D. Spina bifida
   E. Spondylolysis

Multiple-choice and short-answer review questions available online; see inside front cover for details.

84

7. After an automobile crash, a 39-year-old man presents with a headache and midback pain. A radiographic examination reveals trauma to the thoracic spine and bleeding from the anterior and posterior internal vertebral venous plexus. In which of the following regions is the blood most likely accumulating?

   A. Central spinal canal
   B. Epidural space
   C. Lumbar triangle
   D. Subarachnoid space
   E. Subdural space

8. A high school football player receives a helmet-to-helmet blow to his head and neck and is brought into the emergency department. A radiographic examination reveals a mild dislocation of the atlantoaxial joint. When you examine his neck, you notice his range of motion is decreased. Which of the following movements of the head would most likely be affected?

   A. Abduction
   B. Adduction
   C. Extension
   D. Flexion
   E. Rotation

9. A patient is admitted to the emergency department with a sharp penetrating wound in the upper back region just lateral to the thoracic spine. Based on a quick examination, the physician concludes that several of the spinal ganglia are clearly damaged. Which of the following neural elements are most likely compromised by this injury?

   A. Postganglionic efferents
   B. Somatic afferents only
   C. Somatic afferents and efferents
   D. Somatic and visceral afferents
   E. Somatic efferents only

10. A congenital defect that involves the neural crest cells would potentially involve the normal development of which of the following structures?

   A. Anterior spinal artery
   B. Choroid plexus
   C. Dura mater
   D. Intrinsic back muscles
   E. Schwann cells

For each of the following conditions (11-20), select the muscle (A-K) most likely responsible.

A. Erector spinae
B. Latissimus dorsi
C. Levator scapulae
D. Obliquus inferior capitis
E. Rectus posterior major capitis
F. Rhomboid major
G. Rotatores
H. Semispinalis
I. Serratus posterior superior
J. Splenius capitis
K. Trapezius

____ 11. A work-related injury results in a weakness against resistance in elevation of the scapula and atrophy of one of the lateral neck muscles. The physician suspects damage to a cranial nerve.

____ 12. An injury results in significant weakness in extension and lateral rotation along the entire length of the spine.

____ 13. After an automobile crash, a patient presents with radiating pain around the shoulder blades and weakness in elevating the ribs on deep breathing.

____ 14. An injury to the back results in a weakened ability to extend and medially rotate the upper limb.

____ 15. Sharp trauma to the back of the neck damages the suboccipital nerve, resulting in a weakened ability to extend and rotate the head to the same side against resistance.

____ 16. Malformation of the craniocervical portion of the embryonic epaxial (epimere) muscle group that attaches to the ligamentum nuchae results in a weakened ability to extend the neck bilaterally.

____ 17. Trauma to the lateral neck results in a lesion to the dorsal scapular nerve and a weakened ability to shrug the shoulders.

____ 18. The loss of innervation to this pair of hypaxial (hypomere) muscles results in a bilateral weakened ability to retract the scapulae but does not affect the ability to elevate the scapulae.

_____ 19. During spinal surgery, these small intrinsic back muscles must be retracted from the lamina and transverse processes of one or two vertebral segments.

_____ 20. During surgery in the neck, the vertebral artery is observed passing just deep to this muscle prior to the artery entering the foramen magnum.

21. A woman presents with a painful neck. Imaging reveals spinal stenosis (narrowing of the vertebral foramen). Hypertrophy of which of the following ligaments would most likely result in this syndrome?
    A. Anterior longitudinal ligament
    B. Interspinous ligament
    C. Ligamentum flavum
    D. Nuchal ligament
    E. Supraspinous ligament

22. A 51-year-old man is admitted to the emergency department following a bicycle accident. His physical examination reveals weakened medial rotation, extension, and adduction of an upper limb. Which of the following nerves is most likely injured?
    A. Accessory nerve (CN XI)
    B. Axillary nerve
    C. Dorsal scapular nerve
    D. Radial nerve
    E. Thoracodorsal nerve

23. A 54-year-old woman presents with a case of shingles (herpes zoster infection) that affects the sensory spinal nerve roots innervating the skin on her back overlying the inferior angle of her scapula. Which of the following dermatomes is most likely involved?
    A. C5-C6
    B. T1-T2
    C. T6-T7
    D. T10-T11
    E. L1-L2

24. During a routine lumbar puncture to sample the CSF, which of the following ligaments normally would be penetrated by the spinal needle?
    A. Anterior longitudinal ligament
    B. Denticulate ligament
    C. Nuchal ligament
    D. Posterior longitudinal ligament
    E. Supraspinous ligament

25. A 26-year-old woman involved in an automobile crash presents with a headache and back pain. Imaging reveals a hematoma from rupture of her internal vertebral venous plexus. The blood is most likely present in which of the following areas or spaces?
    A. Central canal
    B. Epidural space
    C. 4th ventricle
    D. Subarachnoid space
    E. Subdural space

26. The erector spinae muscles are derived from which of the following embryonic tissues?
    A. Ectoderm
    B. Endoderm
    C. Epimeres
    D. Hypomeres
    E. Neural crest

27. During surgery involving the posterior abdominal wall, it is important to not damage the primary blood supply to the lower two-thirds of the spinal cord, which usually is supplied by which of the following arteries?
    A. Lateral sacral arteries
    B. Lumbar arteries
    C. Major anterior segmental medullary artery
    D. Posterior intercostal arteries
    E. Vertebral arteries

28. Extreme exercise and/or physical trauma may easily damage the spinal cord. However, it is tethered laterally by several important structures that prevent side-to-side excursions of the cord. Which of the following structures is responsible for this stabilization of the cord?
    A. Denticulate ligaments
    B. Interspinous ligament
    C. Ligamentum flavum
    D. Supraspinous ligament
    E. Terminal filum

29. Trauma involving the intervertebral foramen between the C3 and C4 vertebrae results in damage to the anterior root of a spinal nerve. Which of the following nerve fibers are damaged?

    A. Motor fibers of the C3 spinal cord level
    B. Motor fibers of the C4 spinal cord level
    C. Sensory fibers of the C3 spinal cord level
    D. Sensory fibers of the C4 spinal cord level
    E. Motor and sensory fibers of the C3 spinal cord level
    F. Motor and sensory fibers of the C4 spinal cord level

For questions 30 to 35, refer to the midsagittal MRI of the lumbar spine and provide the letter that correctly answers the question or identifies the structure described.

30. Which letter points to the cauda equina?

31. Where is the nucleus pulposus?

32. Where is the CSF located?

33. Where is the spinous process of the L3 vertebra located?

34. Identify the supraspinous ligament.

35. Identify the ligamentum flavum.

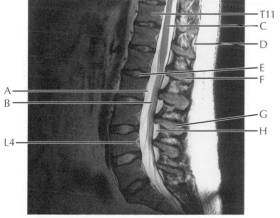

From Kelley LL, Petersen C: *Sectional anatomy for imaging professionals*, ed 3, St Louis, 2012, Elsevier.

Answers to Challenge Yourself Questions

1. **B.** Kyphosis, or "humpback (hunchback)," is one of several accentuated spinal curvatures. It is commonly observed in the thoracic spine. Halitosis refers to bad breath, and lordosis to the lumbar curvature, either the normal curvature or an accentuated lordosis similar to that observed in women during the third trimester of pregnancy. Osmosis is the passage of a solvent through a semipermeable membrane based on solute concentration, and scoliosis is an abnormal lateral curvature of the spine.

2. **A.** An imaginary line connecting the two iliac crests demarcates the space between the L3 and L4 spinous processes with patients on their side and the spine flexed. Lumbar punctures are usually performed between the L3-L4 or L4-L5 levels to avoid injury to the spinal cord proper, which usually ends as the conus medullaris at the L1-L2 vertebral levels. Below the L2 vertebral level, the nerve roots comprise the cauda equina, and are suspended in the CSF-filled subarachnoid space.

3. **D.** The nucleus pulposus of the intervertebral discs usually herniates in a posterolateral direction, where it can impinge on the nerve roots passing through the intervertebral foramen. A disc herniating at the L4-L5 level usually impinges on the L5 roots, and herniation at the L5-S1 level usually involves the S1 roots.

4. **A.** Hyperextension-hyperflexion (whiplash) of the cervical spine can occur when the relaxed neck is thrown backward (hyperextension), tearing the anterior longitudinal ligament. Hyperflexion is usually limited when one's chin hits the sternum. Properly adjusted headrests can limit the hyperextension.

5. **B.** Sensation from the skin is mediated by somatic afferents (fibers in the posterior root), and the cell bodies of these sensory neurons (pseudounipolar neurons) associated with the T4 dermatome reside in the T4 spinal ganglion.

6. **D.** Mesoderm derived from the sclerotome normally contributes to the formation of the neural arch (pedicle, lamina, and spinous process), and a folic acid deficiency in the first trimester of pregnancy may contribute to this congenital malformation (spina bifida occulta).

7. **B.** The internal vertebral venous plexus (Batson's plexus) resides in the epidural fat surrounding the meningeal-encased spinal cord. The epidural space lies between the bony vertebral spinal canal and the dura mater surrounding the spinal cord.

8. **E.** The atlantoaxial joint (atlas and axis) functions in the axial rotational movements of the head. The cranium and atlas move as a unit and rotate side to side on the uniaxial synovial pivot joint between the axis (C2) and atlas (C1).

9. **D.** The spinal ganglia between T1 and L2 contain sensory neurons for both somatic and visceral (autonomic) afferent fibers, so both of these modalities would be compromised. Efferent (motor) fibers are not associated with the spinal ganglia.

10. **E.** Of the options, only Schwann cells are derived from the neural crest. While the arachnoid mater and pia mater are derived from neural crest cells (neither of these choices are options), the dura mater is derived from mesoderm.

11. **K.** The only muscle of this group innervated by a cranial nerve is the trapezius muscle by the accessory nerve (CN XI). The other neck muscle innervated by CN XI is the sternocleidomastoid muscle in the lateral neck.

12. **A.** The major extensors along the entire length of the spine, also involved in lateral rotation or bending when unilaterally contracted, are the erector spinae group of muscles (spinalis, longissimus, and iliocostalis muscles).

13. **I.** The only muscles in the list that are associated with the shoulder blade (scapula), attach to the ribs, and elevate them during inspiration are the serratus posterior superior group. These muscles are considered respiratory muscles because they assist in respiratory movements of the ribs.

14. **B.** The latissimus dorsi muscle extends and medially rotates the upper limb at the shoulder and is the only muscle in this list with these combined actions on the upper limb.

15. **E.** The suboccipital nerve (posterior ramus of C1) innervates the suboccipital muscles in the posterior neck, and the rectus posterior major capitis muscle is the only one in the list that extends and rotates the head to the same side.

16. **J.** The splenius capitis muscle is the only epaxial muscle (intrinsic back muscles innervated by posterior rami of the spinal nerves) in this list that has significant attachment to the ligamentum nuchae (origin) and exclusively extends the neck when it contracts bilaterally.

17. **C.** The levator scapulae muscle is innervated by the posterior scapular nerve (C5) and assists the superior portion of the trapezius muscle in shrugging the shoulders.

18. **F.** Hypaxial muscles are innervated by the anterior rami of spinal nerves, and the rhomboid major muscle is a hypaxial muscle that retracts the scapulae.

19. **G.** The rotatores muscles are part of the transversospinales group of muscles that largely fill the spaces between the transverse processes and the spinal processes. Specifically, the rotatores muscles extend between the lamina and transverse processes and stabilize, extend, and rotate the spine.

20. **E.** The vertebral arteries ascend in the neck by passing through the transverse foramina of the C6-C1 vertebrae, then loop medially and superiorly to the posterior arch of the atlas (C1), pass deep (anterior) to the rectus posterior major capitis muscle, and enter the foramen magnum to supply the posterior portion of the brainstem and brain, and the cerebellum by forming the basilar artery and its branches.

21. **C.** Of all the ligaments listed, only the ligamentum flavum is found in the vertebral foramen, where it connects adjacent laminae of two vertebrae.

22. **E.** The thoracodorsal nerve innervates the latissimus dorsi muscle. This muscle can medially rotate, adduct, and extend the humerus; extension of the humerus is its primary action. It is a muscle well developed in competitive swimmers.

23. **C.** Herpes zoster infection affects the sensory distribution of spinal and cranial nerves in a pattern generally following a dermatome. In this instance, it affects the dermatomes associated with the skin overlying the inferior angle of the scapula, or, approximately, the dermatomes of T6-T7. See Clinical Focus 2.10.

24. **E.** As the spinal needle descends in the midline of the back, it would normally encounter the supraspinous ligament and ligament flavum before it enters the vertebral foramen. It would then pierce the dura mater and arachnoid mater before reaching the CSF in the subarachnoid space.

25. **B.** The internal vertebral plexus (of Batson) of veins lies within the vertebral foramen and just outside the dura mater and epidural fat. The other spaces lie beneath the dura mater (subdural or subarachnoid space). The central canal is within the spinal cord itself.

26. **C.** The erector spinae muscles are true intrinsic back muscles innervated by posterior rami of the spinal nerves. They are derived from myotomes (mesoderm) forming the epimeres. Hypomeres give rise to skeletal muscle innervated by the anterior rami of spinal nerves.

27. C. The major anterior segmental medullary artery (of Adamkiewicz) is in the lower thoracic or upper lumbar region. It usually provides the major blood supply to the lower two-thirds of the spinal cord. The other options include arteries that provide blood to more discrete regions of the spinal cord or to the brainstem and cerebellum (the vertebral arteries).

28. A. The spinal cord is anchored cranially by its continuation intracranially as the brainstem and caudally by the terminal filum, which attaches to the coccyx. However, its lateral movement is limited by approximately 21 pairs of triangular-shaped pia mater extensions (denticulate ligaments) that pierce the arachnoid mater and insert into the dura mater. These attachments limit side-to-side movements of the cord.

29. B. The anterior root of a spinal nerve contains only motor (efferent) nerve fibers. The first spinal nerve exits the spinal cord between the C1 vertebra (the atlas) and the skull, and each subsequent spinal nerve exits the vertebral canal above the vertebra of the same number. So the anterior root of the C4 spinal nerve exits between the C3 and C4 vertebrae. However, because there are eight cervical nerves and only seven cervical vertebrae, the C8 spinal nerve exits above the T1 vertebra; hence, all remaining thoracic, lumbar, and sacral nerves exit via the intervertebral foramen below the vertebra of the same number (e.g., the T1 nerve exits the intervertebral foramen between the T1 and T2 vertebrae). See Fig. 2.16.

30. B. See Fig. 2.19.

31. E. The nucleus pulposus lies within the center of the intervertebral disc. See Clinical Focus 2.6.

32. A. The CSF is located in the subarachnoid space, seen here surrounding the cauda equina.

33. G. The spinous process of the L3 vertebra is slanted slightly posteroinferior to the more anterior L3 vertebral body.

34. D. The supraspinous ligament is stretching between adjacent spines of the vertebrae.

35. H. The ligamentum flavum is connecting adjacent laminae of the vertebrae. The ligament also contains some elastic fibers.

Thorax

1. INTRODUCTION

The thorax lies between the neck and abdomen, encasing the great vessels, heart, and lungs, and provides a conduit for structures passing between the head and neck superiorly and the abdomen, pelvis, and lower limbs inferiorly. Functionally, the thorax and its encased visceral structures are involved in the following:

- **Protection:** the thoracic cage and its muscles protect the vital structures in the thorax.
- **Support:** the thoracic cage provides muscular support for the upper limb.
- **Conduit:** the thorax provides for a superior and an inferior thoracic aperture and a central mediastinum.
- **Segmentation:** the thorax provides an excellent example of segmentation, a hallmark of the vertebrate body plan.
- **Breathing:** the movements of the respiratory diaphragm and intercostal muscles are essential for expanding the thoracic cavity to facilitate the entry of air into the lungs in the process of breathing.
- **Pumping blood:** the thorax contains the heart, which pumps blood through the pulmonary and systemic circulations.

The sternum, ribs (12 pairs), and thoracic vertebrae (12 vertebrae) encircle the thoracic contents and provide a stable thoracic cage that both protects the visceral structures of the thorax and offers assistance with breathing. Because of the lower extent of the rib cage, the thorax also offers protection for some of the abdominal viscera, including the liver and gallbladder on the right side, the stomach and spleen on the left side, and the adrenal (suprarenal) glands and upper poles of the kidneys on both sides.

The **superior thoracic aperture** (the anatomical *thoracic inlet*) conveys large vessels, important nerves, the thoracic lymphatic duct, the trachea, and the esophagus between the neck and thorax. Clinicians often refer to "thoracic outlet syndrome," which describes symptoms associated with compression of the brachial plexus as it passes over the first rib (specifically, the T1 anterior ramus). The **inferior thoracic aperture** (the anatomical *thoracic outlet*) conveys the inferior vena cava (IVC), aorta, esophagus, nerves, and thoracic lymphatic duct between the thorax and the abdominal cavity. Additionally, the thorax contains two pleural cavities laterally and a central "middle space" called the **mediastinum,** which is divided as follows (Fig. 3.1):

- **Superior mediastinum:** a midline compartment that lies above an imaginary horizontal transverse thoracic plane that passes through the manubrium of the sternum (sternal angle of Louis) and the intervertebral disc between the T4 and T5 vertebrae
- **Inferior mediastinum:** the midline compartment below this same horizontal plane, which is further subdivided into an anterior, middle (contains the heart), and posterior mediastinum

2. SURFACE ANATOMY

Key Landmarks

Key surface landmarks for thoracic structures include the following (Fig. 3.2):

- **Jugular (suprasternal) notch:** a notch marking the level of the second thoracic vertebra, the top of the manubrium, and the midpoint between the articulation of the two clavicles. The trachea is palpable in the suprasternal notch.
- **Sternal angle (of Louis):** marks the articulation between the manubrium and body of the sternum, the dividing line between the superior and the inferior mediastinum, and the site of articulation of the second ribs (a useful landmark for counting ribs and intercostal spaces).

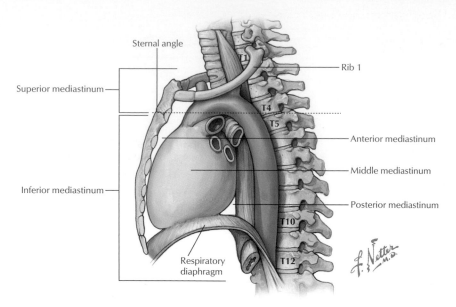

FIGURE 3.1 Subdivisions of the Mediastinum. (From *Netter's atlas of human anatomy,* ed 8, Plate 255; S-411.)

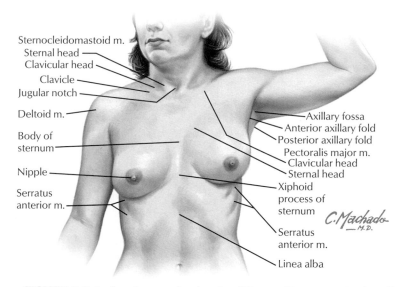

FIGURE 3.2 Surface Anatomy Landmarks of Thorax. (From *Netter's atlas of human anatomy,* ed 8, Plate 202; S-7.)

- **Nipple:** marks the T4 dermatome and approximate level of the dome of the respiratory diaphragm on the right side (variable in the adult female).
- **Xiphoid process:** marks the inferior extent of the sternum and the anterior attachment point of the diaphragm.

Planes of Reference

In addition to the sternal angle of Louis, physicians often use other imaginary planes of reference to assist in locating underlying visceral structures of clinical importance. Important

vertical planes of reference include the following (Fig. 3.3):

- **Midclavicular line:** passing just medial to the nipple.
- **Anterior axillary line:** inferolateral margin of the pectoralis major muscle; demarcates the anterior axillary fold.
- **Midaxillary line:** a descending line from the midpoint of the axilla.
- **Posterior axillary line:** along the margin of the latissimus dorsi and teres major muscles; demarcates the posterior axillary fold.

- **Scapular line**: intersects the inferior angles of the scapula.
- **Midvertebral line** (also called the "posterior median" line): vertically bisects the vertebral column.

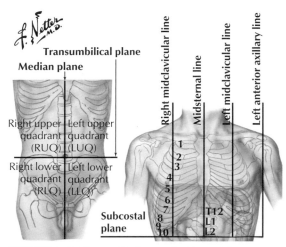

FIGURE 3.3 Planes of Reference for Visceral Structures. (From *Netter's atlas of human anatomy*, ed 8, Plate 269; S-395.)

3. THORACIC WALL

Thoracic Cage

The thoracic cage, which is part of the axial skeleton, includes the thoracic vertebrae, the midline sternum, the 12 pairs of ribs (each with a **head, neck, tubercle,** and **body;** floating ribs 11 and 12 are short and do not have a neck or tubercle), and the costal cartilages (Fig. 3.4). The head of each rib typically articulates with the superior costal facet of the vertebra of the same number, the inferior costal facet of the vertebra above its number, and the intervertebral disc between the two vertebrae (these **costovertebral articulations** are plane synovial joints). The rib's tubercle articulates with the transverse process of the vertebra of the same number. However, ribs 1, 10, 11, and 12 usually articulate only with the vertebra of the same number (Fig. 3.4). This bony framework provides the scaffolding for attachment of the chest wall muscles and the pectoral girdle, which includes the clavicle, scapula, and humerus, and forms the attachment

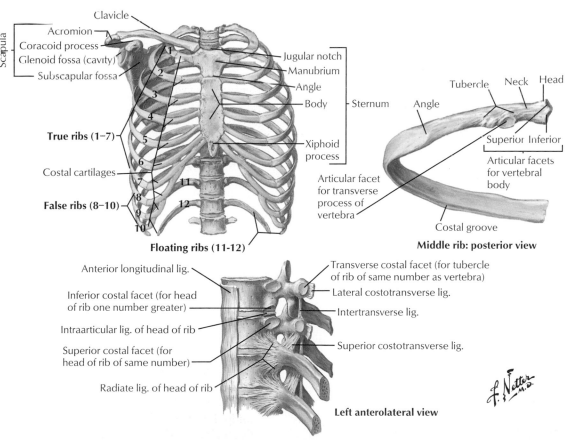

FIGURE 3.4 Thoracic Cage. (From *Netter's atlas of human anatomy*, ed 8, Plates 203 and 204; S-149 and S-150.)

of the upper limb to the thoracic cage at the shoulder joint (Table 3.1).

Rib fractures can be a relatively common and very painful injury (we must continue to breathe) but are less common in children because their thoracic wall is still fairly elastic. The weakest part of the rib is close to the angle (Fig. 3.4).

Joints of Thoracic Cage

Joints of the thoracic cage include articulations between the ribs and the thoracic vertebrae (*discussed in the preceding section*), and between the ribs and the sternum. The clavicle also articulates with the manubrium of the sternum and the first rib. These articulations are summarized in Figure 3.5 and Table 3.2.

Muscles of Anterior Thoracic Wall

The musculature of the anterior thoracic wall includes several muscles that attach to the thoracic cage but that actually are muscles that act on the upper limb (Fig. 3.6). These muscles include the following (for a review, see Chapter 7):

- Pectoralis major.
- Pectoralis minor.
- Serratus anterior.

The *true* anterior thoracic wall muscles fill the intercostal spaces or support the ribs, act on the ribs (elevate or depress the ribs), and keep the intercostal spaces rigid, thereby preventing them from bulging out during expiration and being drawn in during inspiration (Fig. 3.6 and Table 3.3). Note that the external intercostal muscles are replaced by the anterior intercostal membrane at the costochondral junction anteriorly, and that the internal intercostal muscles extend posteriorly to the angle of the ribs and then are replaced by the posterior intercostal membrane. The innermost intercostal

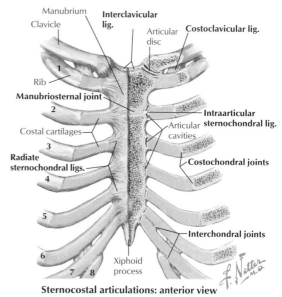

Sternocostal articulations: anterior view

Note: On left side of the rib cage, the sternum and proximal ribs have been shaved down and the ligaments removed to show the bone marrow and articular cavities.

FIGURE 3.5 Sternocostal Articulations of Thoracic Cage (Anterior View). (From *Netter's atlas of human anatomy*, ed 8, Plate 204; S-150.)

TABLE 3.1 Features of the Thoracic Cage

STRUCTURE	CHARACTERISTICS
Sternum	Long, flat bone composed of the manubrium, body, and xiphoid process
True ribs	Ribs 1-7: articulate with the sternum directly
False ribs	Ribs 8-10: articulate to costal cartilages of the ribs above
Floating ribs	Ribs 11 and 12: articulate with vertebrae only

TABLE 3.2 Joints of the Thoracic Cage (Clavicle, Ribs, Sternum)

LIGAMENT	ATTACHMENT	COMMENT
Sternoclavicular (Saddle-Type Synovial) Joint With an Articular Disc		
Capsule	Clavicle and manubrium	Allows elevation, depression, protraction, retraction, circumduction
Sternoclavicular	Clavicle and manubrium	Consists of anterior and posterior ligaments
Interclavicular	Between both clavicles	Connects two sternoclavicular joints
Costoclavicular	Clavicle to first rib	Anchors clavicle to first rib
Sternocostal (Primary Cartilaginous [Synchondroses]) Joints		
First sternocostal	First rib to manubrium	Allows no movement at this joint
Radiate sternochondral	Ribs 2-7 with sternum	Permit some gliding or sliding movement at these synovial plane joints
Costochondral (Primary Cartilaginous) Joints		
Cartilage	Costal cartilage to rib	Normally no movement at these joints
Interchondral (Synovial Plane) Joints		
Interchondral	Between costal cartilages	Allow some gliding movement

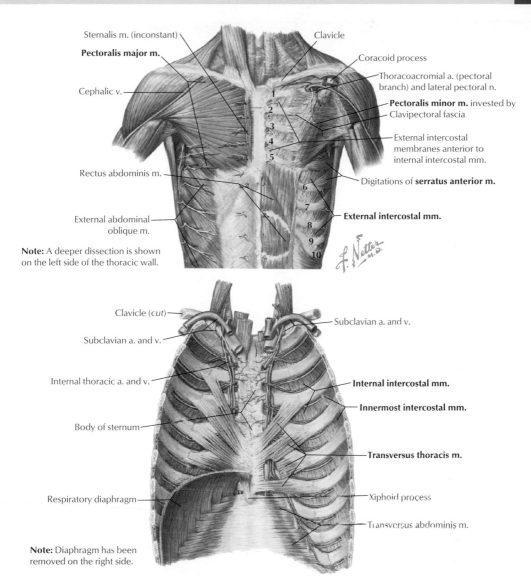

FIGURE 3.6 Muscles of Anterior Thoracic Wall. (From *Netter's atlas of human anatomy,* ed 8, Plates 209 and 211; S-203 and S-205.)

TABLE 3.3 Muscles of the Anterior Thoracic Wall				
MUSCLE	**ORIGIN ATTACHMENT**	**INSERTION ATTACHMENT**	**INNERVATION**	**MAIN ACTIONS**
External intercostal	Inferior border of rib above	Superior border of rib below	Intercostal nerves	Elevate ribs, support intercostal space
Internal intercostal	Inferior border of rib above	Superior border of rib below	Intercostal nerves	Elevate ribs (upper four and five); others depress ribs
Innermost intercostal	Inferior border of rib above	Superior border of rib below	Intercostal nerves	Elevates ribs
Transversus thoracis	Internal surface of costal cartilages 2-6	Posterior surface of lower sternum	Intercostal nerves	Depress ribs and costal cartilages
Subcostal	Internal surface of lower rib near their angles	Superior borders of second or third ribs below	Intercostal nerves	Depress ribs
Levator costarum	Transverse processes of C7 and T1-T11	Subjacent ribs between tubercle and angle	Posterior rami of lower thoracic nerves	Elevate ribs and costal cartilages

Variations in spinal nerve contributions to the innervation of muscles, their attachments, and their actions are common in human anatomy. Therefore, expect differences between texts and realize that anatomical variation is normal.

Clinical Focus 3.1

Thoracic Cage Injuries

Thoracic injuries are responsible for about 25% of trauma deaths. These injuries can involve the heart, great vessels, tracheobronchial tree, and/or thoracic cage. Cage injuries often involve rib fractures (ribs 1 and 2 and 11 and 12 are more protected and often escape being fractured), crush injuries with rib fractures, and penetrating chest wounds such as gunshot and stab wounds. The pain caused by rib fractures can be intense because of the expansion and contraction of the rib cage during respiration; it sometimes requires palliation by anesthetizing the intercostal nerve (nerve block).

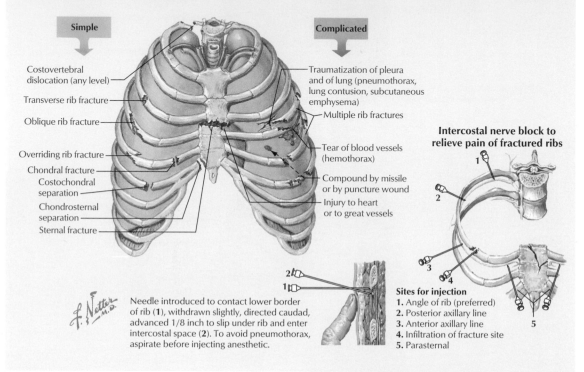

Simple

Costovertebral dislocation (any level)

Transverse rib fracture

Oblique rib fracture

Overriding rib fracture

Chondral fracture

Costochondral separation

Chondrosternal separation

Sternal fracture

Complicated

Traumatization of pleura and of lung (pneumothorax, lung contusion, subcutaneous emphysema)

Multiple rib fractures

Tear of blood vessels (hemothorax)

Compound by missile or by puncture wound

Injury to heart or to great vessels

Needle introduced to contact lower border of rib (**1**), withdrawn slightly, directed caudad, advanced 1/8 inch to slip under rib and enter intercostal space (**2**). To avoid pneumothorax, aspirate before injecting anesthetic.

Intercostal nerve block to relieve pain of fractured ribs

Sites for injection
1. Angle of rib (preferred)
2. Posterior axillary line
3. Anterior axillary line
4. Infiltration of fracture site
5. Parasternal

---

muscles lie deep to the internal intercostals and extend from the midclavicular line to about the angles of the ribs posteriorly (Fig. 3.7).

Intercostal Vessels and Nerves

The **intercostal neurovascular bundles** (vein, artery, and nerve) lie inferior to each rib, running in the costal groove deep to the internal intercostal muscles (Fig. 3.7 and Table 3.4). The veins largely correspond to the arteries and drain into the *azygos system of veins* posteriorly or the *internal thoracic veins* anteriorly. The *intercostal arteries* form an anastomotic loop between the internal thoracic artery (branches of anterior intercostal arteries arise here) and the thoracic aorta posteriorly. Posterior intercostal arteries arise from the aorta, except for the first two, which arise from the supreme intercostal artery, a branch of the costocervical trunk of the subclavian artery.

The **intercostal nerves** are the anterior rami of the first 11 thoracic spinal nerves. The 12th

TABLE 3.4 Arteries of the Internal Thoracic Wall

ARTERY	COURSE
Internal thoracic	Arises from subclavian artery and terminates by dividing into superior epigastric and musculophrenic arteries.
Intercostals	First two posterior branches derived from superior intercostal branch of costocervical trunk and lower nine from thoracic aorta; these anastomose with anterior branches derived from internal thoracic artery (1st-6th spaces) or its musculophrenic branch (7th-9th spaces); the lowest two spaces only have posterior branches.
Subcostal	From aorta, courses inferior to the 12th rib.
Pericardiacophrenic	From internal thoracic artery and accompanies phrenic nerve.

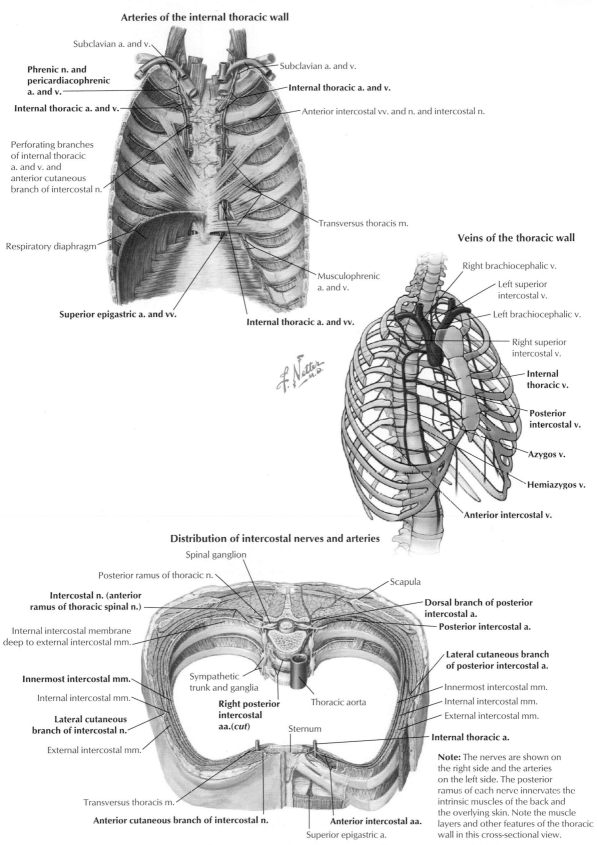

Arteries of the internal thoracic wall

Subclavian a. and v.

Phrenic n. and pericardiacophrenic a. and v.

Internal thoracic a. and v.

Perforating branches of internal thoracic a. and v. and anterior cutaneous branch of intercostal n.

Respiratory diaphragm

Superior epigastric a. and vv.

Subclavian a. and v.

Internal thoracic a. and v.

Anterior intercostal vv. and n. and intercostal n.

Transversus thoracis m.

Musculophrenic a. and v.

Internal thoracic a. and vv.

Veins of the thoracic wall

Right brachiocephalic v.

Left superior intercostal v.

Left brachiocephalic v.

Right superior intercostal v.

Internal thoracic v.

Posterior intercostal v.

Azygos v.

Hemiazygos v.

Anterior intercostal v.

Distribution of intercostal nerves and arteries

Spinal ganglion

Posterior ramus of thoracic n.

Intercostal n. (anterior ramus of thoracic spinal n.)

Internal intercostal membrane deep to external intercostal mm.

Innermost intercostal mm.

Internal intercostal mm.

Lateral cutaneous branch of intercostal n.

External intercostal mm.

Sympathetic trunk and ganglia

Right posterior intercostal aa.(cut)

Transversus thoracis m.

Anterior cutaneous branch of intercostal n.

Scapula

Dorsal branch of posterior intercostal a.

Posterior intercostal a.

Lateral cutaneous branch of posterior intercostal a.

Innermost intercostal mm.

Internal intercostal mm.

External intercostal mm.

Internal thoracic a.

Thoracic aorta

Sternum

Anterior intercostal aa.

Superior epigastric a.

Note: The nerves are shown on the right side and the arteries on the left side. The posterior ramus of each nerve innervates the intrinsic muscles of the back and the overlying skin. Note the muscle layers and other features of the thoracic wall in this cross-sectional view.

FIGURE 3.7 Intercostal Vessels and Nerves. (From *Netter's atlas of human anatomy,* ed 8, Plates 211, 212, 213; S-205, S-206, S-338.)

thoracic nerve gives rise to the subcostal nerve, which courses inferior to the 12th rib. The nerves give rise to lateral and anterior cutaneous branches and branches innervating the intercostal muscles (Fig. 3.7).

Female Breast

The female breast, a modified sweat gland, extends from approximately the second rib to the sixth rib and from the sternum medially to the midaxillary line laterally. Mammary tissue is composed of compound tubuloacinar glands organized into about 15 to 20 lobes, which are supported and separated from each other by fibrous connective tissue septae (the **suspensory retinacula of Cooper**) and fat. Each lobe is divided into lobules of secretory acini and their ducts. Features of the breast include the following (Fig. 3.8):

- **Breast:** fatty tissue containing glands that produce milk; lies in the superficial fascia above the **retromammary space,** which lies above the deep pectoral fascia enveloping the pectoralis major muscle.
- **Areola:** circular pigmented skin surrounding the nipple; it contains modified sebaceous and

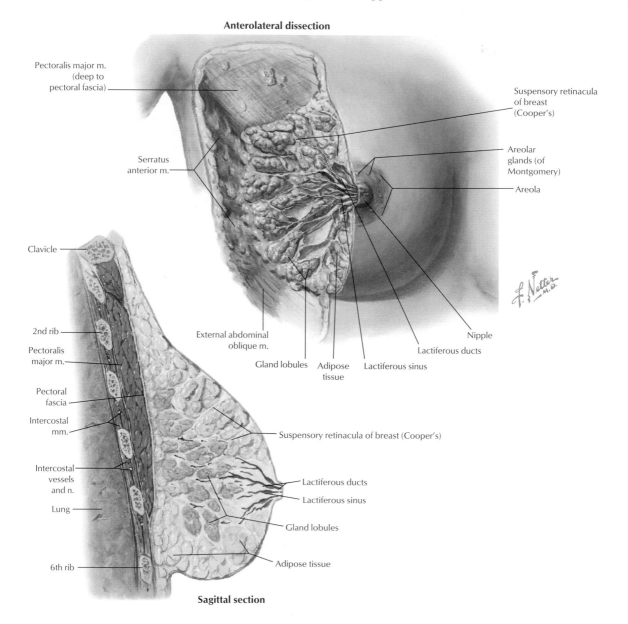

FIGURE 3.8 Anterolateral and Sagittal Views of Female Breast. (From *Netter's atlas of human anatomy,* ed 8, Plate 205; S-473.)

sweat glands **(glands of Montgomery)** that lubricate the nipple and keep it supple.
- **Nipple:** site of opening for the lactiferous ducts, which at their distal ends are dilated into lactiferous sinuses; the nipple usually lies at about the level of the fourth intercostal space.
- **Axillary tail (of Spence):** extension of mammary tissue superolaterally toward the axilla.
- **Lymphatic system:** lymph is drained from breast tissues; about 75% of lymphatic drainage is to the axillary lymph nodes (Fig. 3.9; see also Fig. 7.11), and the remainder drains to parasternal nodes medially or inferiorly to subdiaphragmatic nodes.

The primary **arterial supply** to the breast includes the following:
- Anterior intercostal branches of the internal thoracic (mammary) arteries (from the subclavian artery).

- Lateral mammary branches of the lateral thoracic artery (a branch of the axillary artery).
- Thoracoacromial artery (branch of the axillary artery).

The **venous drainage** (Fig. 3.9) largely parallels the arterial supply, finally draining into the internal thoracic and axillary veins.

4. PLEURA AND LUNGS

Pleural Spaces (Cavities)

The thorax is divided into the following three compartments:
- Right pleural space.
- Left pleural space.
- Mediastinum: a "middle space" lying between the pleural spaces.

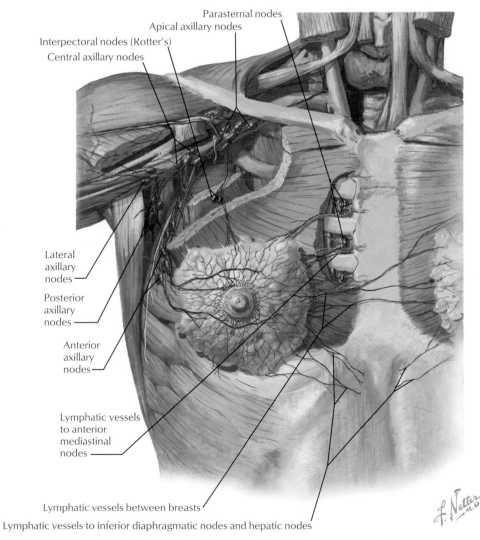

Parasternal nodes
Apical axillary nodes
Interpectoral nodes (Rotter's)
Central axillary nodes
Lateral axillary nodes
Posterior axillary nodes
Anterior axillary nodes
Lymphatic vessels to anterior mediastinal nodes
Lymphatic vessels between breasts
Lymphatic vessels to inferior diaphragmatic nodes and hepatic nodes

FIGURE 3.9 Lymph Vessels and Nodes of Mammary Gland. (From *Netter's atlas of human anatomy,* ed 8, Plate 207; S-348.)

Clinical Focus 3.2

Fibrocystic Breast Disease

Fibrocystic change is a nonspecific term covering a large group of benign conditions occurring in about 80% of women that are often related to cyclic changes in maturation and involution of glandular tissue. **Fibroadenoma,** the second most common form of breast disease and the most common breast mass, has a peak incidence in patients between 20 and 25 years of age, with most below the age of 30 years. The tumors are benign neoplasms of the glandular epithelium and usually are accompanied by a significant increase in periductal connective tissue. They usually present as firm, painless, mobile, solitary palpable masses that may grow rapidly during adolescence and warrant follow-up evaluation.

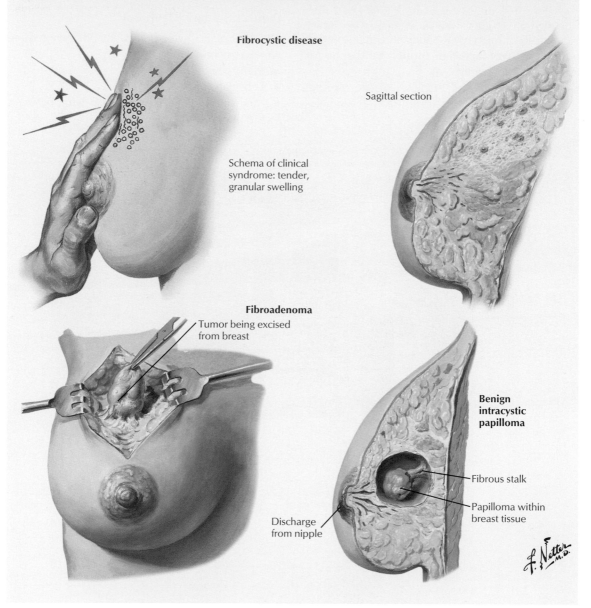

Fibrocystic disease

Sagittal section

Schema of clinical syndrome: tender, granular swelling

Fibroadenoma

Tumor being excised from breast

Benign intracystic papilloma

Fibrous stalk

Papilloma within breast tissue

Discharge from nipple

Clinical Focus 3.3

Breast Cancer

Breast cancer is the most common malignancy in women, and women in the United States have the highest incidence in the world. Well over two-thirds of all cases occur in postmenopausal women. The most common type (occurring in about 75% of cases) is an **infiltrating ductal carcinoma,** which may involve the suspensory retinacula, causing retraction of the ligaments and dimpling of the overlying skin. Invasion and obstruction of the subcutaneous lymphatics can result in dilation and skin edema, creating an "orange peel" appearance (*peau d'orange*). About 60% of the palpable tumors are located in the **upper outer breast quadrant** (the quadrant closest to the axilla, which includes the axillary tail). About 5-10% of breast cancers have a familial or genetic link (mutations of the BRCA1 and 2 tumor suppressor genes). Distant sites of metastasis include the lungs and pleura, liver, bones, and brain.

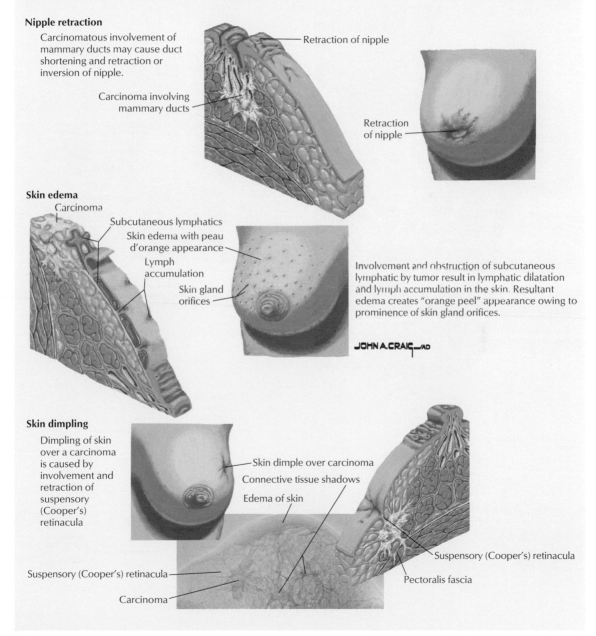

Nipple retraction

Carcinomatous involvement of mammary ducts may cause duct shortening and retraction or inversion of nipple.

Retraction of nipple

Carcinoma involving mammary ducts

Retraction of nipple

Skin edema

Carcinoma

Subcutaneous lymphatics

Skin edema with peau d'orange appearance

Lymph accumulation

Skin gland orifices

Involvement and obstruction of subcutaneous lymphatic by tumor result in lymphatic dilatation and lymph accumulation in the skin. Resultant edema creates "orange peel" appearance owing to prominence of skin gland orifices.

JOHN A.CRAIG—AD

Skin dimpling

Dimpling of skin over a carcinoma is caused by involvement and retraction of suspensory (Cooper's) retinacula

Skin dimple over carcinoma

Connective tissue shadows

Edema of skin

Suspensory (Cooper's) retinacula

Pectoralis fascia

Suspensory (Cooper's) retinacula

Carcinoma

Clinical Focus 3.4

Partial Mastectomy

Several clinical options are available to treat breast cancer, including systemic approaches (chemotherapy, hormonal therapy, immunotherapy) and "local" approaches (radiation therapy, surgery). In a **partial mastectomy,** also called "lumpectomy" or "quadrantectomy," the surgeon performs a breast-conserving surgery that removes the portion of the breast that harbors the tumor along with a surrounding halo of normal breast tissue. Because of the possibility of lymphatic spread, especially to the **axillary nodes,** an incision also may be made for a **sentinel node biopsy** to examine the first axillary node, which is likely to be invaded by metastatic cancer cells from the breast.

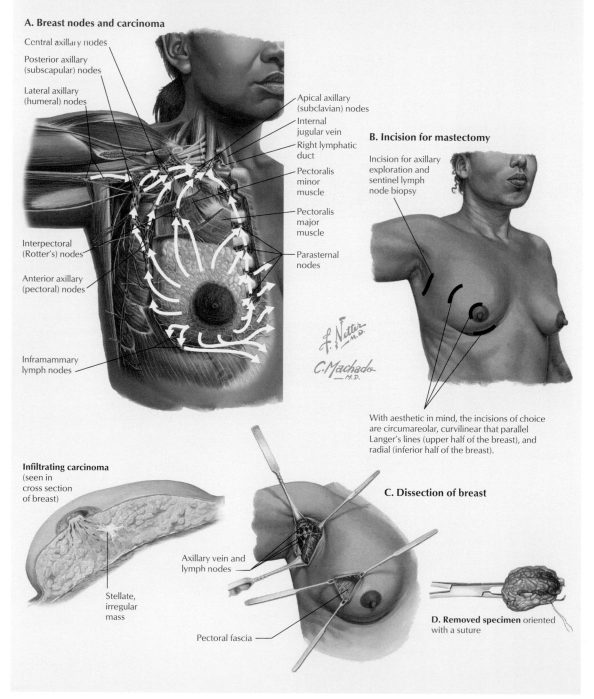

A. Breast nodes and carcinoma

Central axillary nodes
Posterior axillary (subscapular) nodes
Lateral axillary (humeral) nodes
Apical axillary (subclavian) nodes
Internal jugular vein
Right lymphatic duct
Pectoralis minor muscle
Pectoralis major muscle
Interpectoral (Rotter's) nodes
Parasternal nodes
Anterior axillary (pectoral) nodes
Inframammary lymph nodes

B. Incision for mastectomy

Incision for axillary exploration and sentinel lymph node biopsy

With aesthetic in mind, the incisions of choice are circumareolar, curvilinear that parallel Langer's lines (upper half of the breast), and radial (inferior half of the breast).

Infiltrating carcinoma (seen in cross section of breast)

Stellate, irregular mass

C. Dissection of breast

Axillary vein and lymph nodes

Pectoral fascia

D. Removed specimen oriented with a suture

Clinical Focus 3.5

Modified Radical Mastectomy

In addition to breast-conserving surgery, several more invasive mastectomy approaches may be indicated, depending on a variety of factors:

- **Total (simple) mastectomy:** the whole breast is removed, with or without some axillary lymph nodes if indicated, down to the retromammary space.
- **Modified radical mastectomy** (illustrated here): the whole breast is removed along with most of the axillary and pectoral lymph nodes, the axillary fat, and the investing fascia over the chest wall muscles. Care is taken to preserve the pectoralis, serratus anterior, and latissimus dorsi muscles and the long thoracic and thoracodorsal nerves to the latter two muscles, respectively. Damage to the **long thoracic nerve** results in "winging" of the scapula, and damage to the **thoracodorsal nerve** weakens extension at the shoulder.
- **Radical mastectomy:** the whole breast is removed along with the axillary lymph nodes, fat, and chest wall muscles (pectoralis major and minor); use of the radical surgical approach is much less common now.

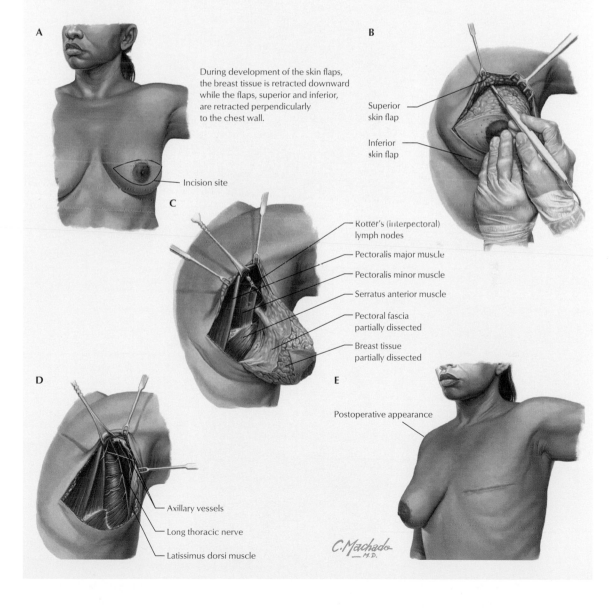

A

During development of the skin flaps, the breast tissue is retracted downward while the flaps, superior and inferior, are retracted perpendicularly to the chest wall.

Incision site

B

Superior skin flap

Inferior skin flap

C

Rotter's (interpectoral) lymph nodes

Pectoralis major muscle

Pectoralis minor muscle

Serratus anterior muscle

Pectoral fascia partially dissected

Breast tissue partially dissected

D

Axillary vessels

Long thoracic nerve

Latissimus dorsi muscle

E

Postoperative appearance

C. Machado
M.D.

The lungs lie within the **pleural cavity** (right and left) (Fig. 3.10). This "potential space" is between the investing **visceral pleura,** which closely envelops each lung, and the **parietal pleura,** which reflects off each lung and lines the inner aspect of the thoracic wall, the superior surface of the diaphragm, and the sides of the pericardial sac (Table 3.5). Normally, the pleural cavity contains a small amount of serous fluid, which lubricates the surfaces and reduces friction during respiration. The parietal pleura is richly innervated with afferent fibers that course in the somatic intercostal nerves. Over most of the surface of the diaphragm and in the parietal pleura facing the mediastinum, the afferent pain fibers course in the **phrenic nerve (C3-C5).** The visceral pleura has few, if any, pain fibers.

Clinically, it is important for physicians to be able to "visualize" the extent of the lungs and pleural cavities topographically on the surface of their patients (Fig. 3.10). The lungs lie adjacent to the

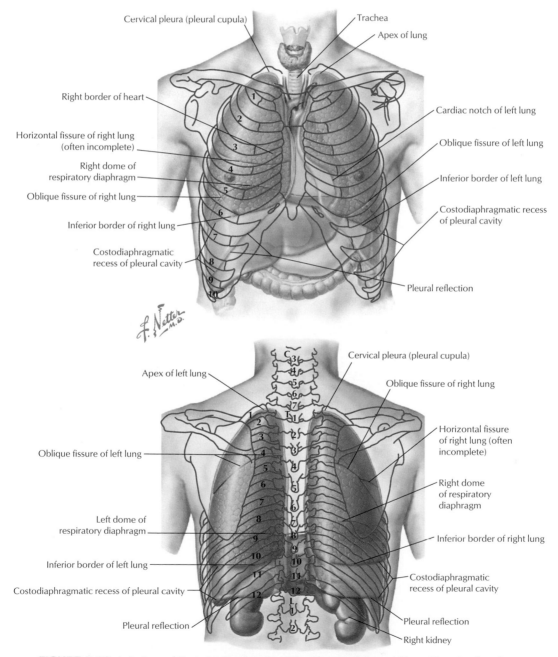

FIGURE 3.10 Anterior and Posterior Topography of the Pleura and Lungs. (From *Netter's atlas of human anatomy*, ed 8, Plates 217 and 218; S-385 and S-386.)

TABLE 3.5 Pleural Features and Recesses

STRUCTURE	DEFINITION
Cupula	Dome of cervical pleura (pleural cupula) extending above the first rib
Parietal pleura	Membrane that in descriptive terms includes costal, mediastinal, diaphragmatic, and cervical (cupula) pleura
Pleural reflections	Points at which parietal pleurae reflect off one surface and extend onto another (e.g., costal to diaphragmatic)
Pleural recesses	Reflection points where the lung does not fully extend into the pleural space (e.g., costodiaphragmatic, costomediastinal)

TABLE 3.6 Surface Landmarks of the Pleura and Lungs

LANDMARK	MARGIN OF LUNG	MARGIN OF PLEURA
Midclavicular line	6th rib	8th rib
Midaxillary line	8th rib	10th rib
Paravertebral line	10th rib	12th rib

parietal pleura inferiorly to the sixth costal cartilage. (Note the presence of the **cardiac notch** on the left side.) Beyond this point, the lungs do not occupy the full extent of the pleural cavity during quiet respiration. These points are important to know if one needs access to the pleural cavity without injuring the lungs, for example, to drain inflammatory exudate **(pleural effusion),** blood **(hemothorax),** or air **(pneumothorax)** that collects in the pleural cavity. In quiet respiration, the lung margins reside two ribs above the extent of the pleural cavity at the midclavicular, midaxillary, and paravertebral lines (Table 3.6).

The Lungs

The paired lungs are invested in the visceral pleura and are attached to mediastinal structures (trachea and heart) at their hilum. Each lung possesses the following surfaces:

- **Apex:** superior part of the upper lobe that extends into the root of the neck (above the clavicles).
- **Hilum:** area located on the medial aspect through which structures enter and leave the lung.
- **Costal:** anterior, lateral, and posterior aspects of the lung in contact with the costal elements of the internal thoracic cage.
- **Diaphragmatic:** inferior part of the lung in contact with the underlying diaphragm.

The right lung has three lobes and is slightly larger than the left lung, which has two lobes. Both lungs are composed of spongy and elastic tissue, which readily expands and contracts to conform to the internal contours of the thoracic cage (Fig. 3.11 and Table 3.7).

The lung's parenchyma is supplied by several small **bronchial arteries** that arise from the proximal portion of the descending thoracic aorta. Usually, one small right bronchial artery and a pair of left bronchial arteries (superior and inferior) can be found on the posterior aspect of the main bronchi. Although much of this blood returns to the heart via the pulmonary veins, some also collects into small **bronchial veins** that drain into the azygos system of veins (see Fig. 3.26).

The lymphatic drainage of both lungs is to **pulmonary** (intrapulmonary) and **bronchopulmonary** (hilar) nodes (i.e., from distal lung tissue sites to the proximal hilum). Lymph then drains into **tracheobronchial** nodes at the tracheal bifurcation and into right and left **paratracheal** nodes (Fig. 3.12). Clinicians often use different names to identify these nodes (intrapulmonary, hilar, carinal, and scalene), so these clinical terms are listed in parentheses after the corresponding anatomical labels in Fig. 3.12.

As visceral structures, the lungs are innervated by the autonomic nervous system. **Sympathetic bronchodilator** fibers relax smooth muscle, vasoconstrict pulmonary vessels, and inhibit the bronchial tree alveolar glands. These fibers arise from upper thoracic spinal cord segments (about T1-T4). **Parasympathetic bronchoconstrictor** fibers contract bronchial smooth muscle, vasodilate pulmonary vessels, and initiate secretion of alveolar glands. They arise from the vagus nerve (CN X).

Visceral afferent fibers that course back to the CNS in the vagus nerve are largely reflexive and convey impulses from the bronchial mucosa, muscles and connective tissue stretch receptors (the Hering-Breuer reflex), pressor receptors on arteries, and chemoreceptors sensitive to blood gas levels and pH. Pain (nociceptive) afferents from the visceral pleura and bronchi pass back via the sympathetic fibers, through the sympathetic trunk, and to the sensory spinal ganglia of the upper thoracic spinal cord levels.

Respiration

During *quiet inspiration* the contraction of the **respiratory diaphragm** alone accounts for most of the decrease in intrapleural pressure, allowing air to expand the lungs. *Active inspiration* occurs when

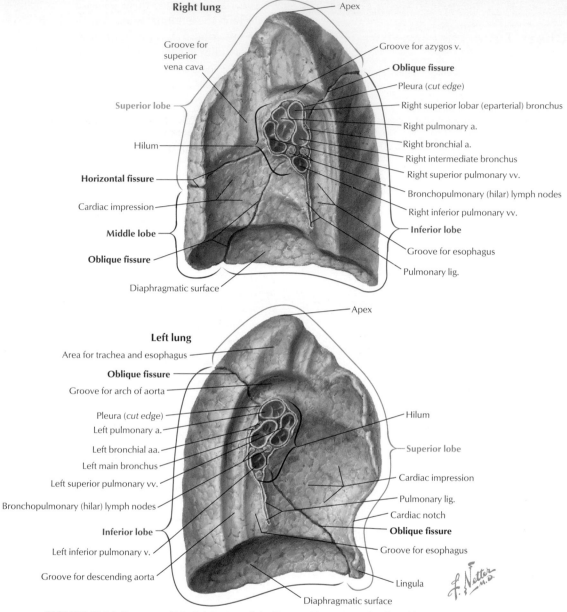

FIGURE 3.11 Features of Medial Aspect of the Lungs. (From *Netter's atlas of human anatomy*, ed 8, Plates 221; S-388.)

TABLE 3.7 External Features of the Lungs

STRUCTURE	CHARACTERISTICS	STRUCTURE	CHARACTERISTICS
Lobes	Three lobes (superior, middle, inferior) in right lung; two in left lung (superior and inferior)	Lingula	Tongue-shaped feature of left lung
Horizontal fissure	Only on right lung, extends along line of fourth rib	Cardiac notch	Indentation for the heart, in left lung
Oblique fissure	On both lungs, extends from T2-T3 vertebra spine to sixth costal cartilage anteriorly	Pulmonary ligament	Double layer of parietal pleura hanging from the hilum that marks reflection of visceral pleura to parietal pleura
Impressions	Made by adjacent structures, in fixed lungs	Bronchopulmonary segment	10 functional segments in each lung supplied by a segmental bronchus and a segmental artery from the pulmonary artery
Hilum	Points at which structures (bronchus, vessels, nerves, lymphatics) enter or leave lungs		

Clinical Focus 3.6

Chest Tube Thoracostomy

1–3. Monitor patient's vital signs. Place patient in supine position. Abduct the patient's arm and flex elbow to position the hand over the patient's head.

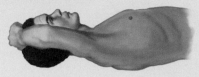

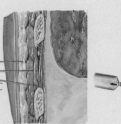

4–7. Use ultrasonography to locate the 4th and 5th intercostal spaces in the anterior axillary line at the level of the nipple. Cleanse the area with antiseptic and drape the patient.

- 4th rib
- 5th rib
- Anterior axillary line

8. Administer anesthetic to a 2- to 3-cm area of the skin and subcutaneous tissue at incision site (A). Continue to anesthetize deeper subcutaneous tissues and intercostal muscles (B).

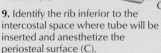

A
B
C

9. Identify the rib inferior to the intercostal space where tube will be inserted and anesthetize the periosteal surface (C).

10. Advance the needle until a flash of pleural fluid or air enters the syringe, confirming entry into the pleural space.

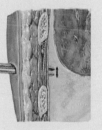

11. Use a scalpel to make a 1- to 2-cm incision parallel to the rib.

12–14. Dissect a tract through subcutaneous tissue and intercostal muscles. Gently enter the pleural space.

Open the clamp while inside the pleural space and then withdraw so that all layers of the dissected tract are enlarged.

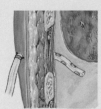

15. Insert a finger into the pleural space and rotate 360 degrees to feel for adhesions.

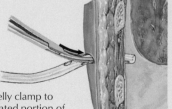

16. Use a Kelly clamp to grab fenestrated portion of the tube and introduce it through the insertion site.

17. Use sutures to close incision. Secure chest tube to chest wall using suture's loose ends to wrap around tube.

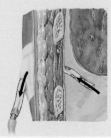

18–20. Wrap petroleum-based gauze around tube and cover with regular gauze. Secure the site with dressings and adhesive tape. Connect chest tube to drainage device. Obtain a chest radiograph to confirm proper tube placement.

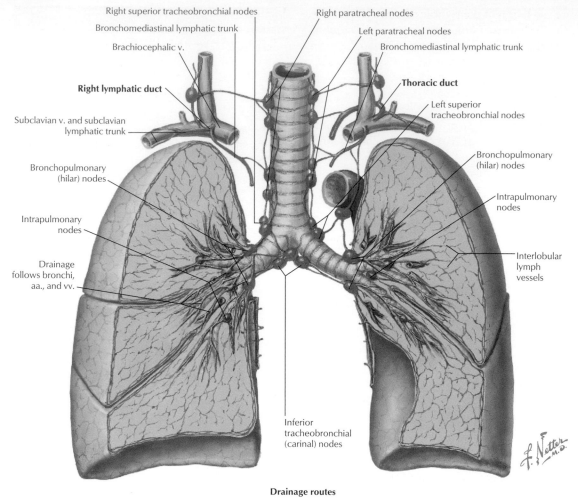

Drainage routes

Right lung: All lobes drain to pulmonary and bronchopulmonary (hilar) nodes, and then to inferior tracheobronchial (carinal) nodes.

Left lung: Superior lobe drains to pulmonary and bronchopulmonary (hilar) nodes and inferior tracheo-bronchial (carinal) nodes. Left inferior lobe drains also to pulmonary and bronchopulmonary (hilar) nodes and to inferior tracheobronchial (carinal) nodes, but then mostly to right superior tracheobronchial nodes, where it follows same route as lymph from right lung.

FIGURE 3.12 Lymphatic Drainage Routes of the Lungs. (From *Netter's atlas of human anatomy*, ed 8, Plates 228; S-350.)

the **diaphragm** and **intercostal muscles** together increase the diameter of the thoracic wall, decreasing intrapleural pressure even more. Although the first rib is stationary, ribs 2 to 6 tend to increase the anteroposterior diameter of the chest wall, and the lower ribs mainly increase the transverse diameter. Accessory muscles of inspiration that attach to the thoracic cage may also assist in very deep inspiration.

During *quiet expiration* the elastic recoil of the lungs, relaxation of the diaphragm, and relaxation of the thoracic cage muscles expel the air. In *forced expiration* the abdominal muscles contract and, by compressing the abdominal viscera superiorly, raise the intraabdominal pressure and force the

diaphragm upward. Having the "wind knocked out of you" shows how forceful this maneuver can be.

Trachea and Bronchi

The **trachea** is a single midline airway that extends from the cricoid cartilage to its bifurcation at the sternal angle of Louis. It lies anterior to the esophagus and is rigidly supported by 16 to 20 C-shaped cartilaginous rings (Fig. 3.13 and Table 3.8). The trachea may be displaced if adjacent structures become enlarged (usually the thyroid gland or aortic arch).

The trachea bifurcates inferiorly into a **right main bronchus** and a **left main bronchus,** which enter the hilum of the right lung and the left lung, respectively, and immediately divide into **lobar (secondary) bronchi** (Fig. 3.13). The right main bronchus often gives rise to the superior lobar (eparterial) bronchus just before entering the hilum of the right lung. Each lobar bronchus then divides again into **tertiary bronchi** supplying the 10 bronchopulmonary segments of each lung (some clinicians identify 8 to 10 segments in the left lung, whereas anatomists identify 10 in each lung) (Fig. 3.13 and Tables 3.7 and 3.8). The **bronchopulmonary segments** are lung segments that are supplied by a tertiary bronchus and a segmental artery of the pulmonary artery that passes to each lung. The tertiary bronchus and artery course together, but the segmental veins draining the segment are at the periphery of each segment. Additionally, each bronchopulmonary segment is surrounded by connective tissue that is continuous with the visceral pleura on the lung's surface, thus forming a functionally independent respiratory unit. The bronchi and respiratory airways continue to divide into smaller and smaller passageways until they terminate in alveolar sacs (about 25 divisional generations from the right and left main bronchi). Gas exchange occurs only in these most distal respiratory regions.

The **right main bronchus** is shorter, more vertical, and wider than the left main bronchus. Therefore, **aspirated objects** often pass more easily into the right main bronchus and right lung.

5. PERICARDIUM AND HEART

The Pericardium

The pericardium and heart lie within the **middle mediastinum.** The heart is enclosed within a fibroserous pericardial pouch that extends and blends into the adventitia of the great vessels that enter or leave the heart. The pericardium has a **fibrous outer layer** that is lined internally by a serous layer, the **parietal serous layer,** which then reflects onto the heart and becomes the **visceral serous layer,** which is the outer covering of the heart itself, also known as the **epicardium** (Fig. 3.14 and Table 3.9). These two serous layers form a potential space known as the **pericardial sac (cavity).**

The Heart

The heart is essentially two muscular pumps in series. The two atria contract in unison, followed by contraction of the two ventricles. The right side of the heart receives the blood from the systemic

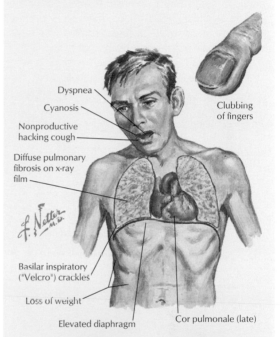
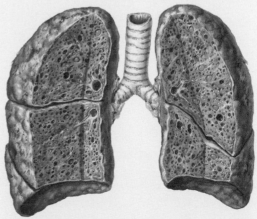

Clinical Focus 3.8

Pulmonary Embolism

The lungs naturally filter **venous clots** larger than circulating blood cells and can usually accommodate small clots because of their fibrinolytic ("clot buster") mechanisms. However, pulmonary embolism (PE) is the cause of death in 10% to 15% of hospitalized patients. **Thromboemboli** originate from deep leg veins in approximately 90% of cases. Major causes are called *Virchow's triad* and include the following:

- Venous stasis (e.g., caused by extended bed rest)
- Trauma (e.g., fracture, tissue injury)
- Coagulation disorders (inherited or acquired)

Other contributors to PE include postoperative and postpartum immobility and some hormone medications that increase the risk of blood clots. Most PEs are "silent" because they are small; larger emboli may obstruct medium-sized vessels and lead to infarction or even obstruction of a vessel as large as the pulmonary trunk (saddle embolus). PE without infarction is common and presents as tachypnea, anxiety, dyspnea, syncope, and vague substernal pressure. Saddle embolus, on the other hand, is an emergency that can precipitate acute cor pulmonale (right-sided heart failure) and circulatory collapse.

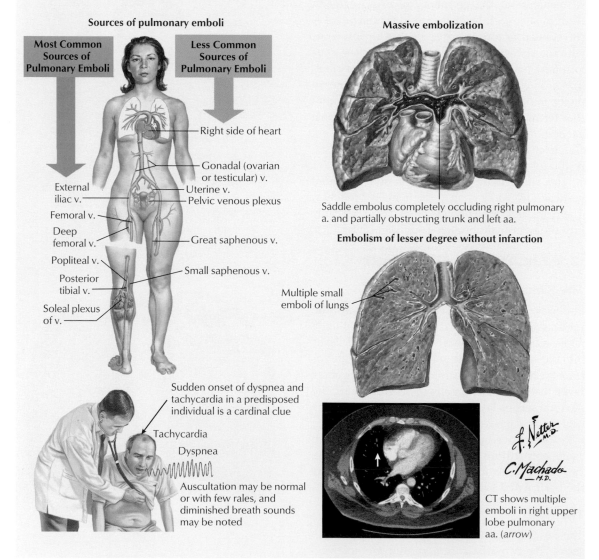

Sources of pulmonary emboli

Most Common Sources of Pulmonary Emboli

Less Common Sources of Pulmonary Emboli

Right side of heart

Gonadal (ovarian or testicular) v.
Uterine v.
Pelvic venous plexus

External iliac v.

Femoral v.

Deep femoral v.

Great saphenous v.

Popliteal v.

Posterior tibial v.

Small saphenous v.

Soleal plexus of v.

Sudden onset of dyspnea and tachycardia in a predisposed individual is a cardinal clue

Tachycardia

Dyspnea

Auscultation may be normal or with few rales, and diminished breath sounds may be noted

Massive embolization

Saddle embolus completely occluding right pulmonary a. and partially obstructing trunk and left aa.

Embolism of lesser degree without infarction

Multiple small emboli of lungs

CT shows multiple emboli in right upper lobe pulmonary aa. (*arrow*)

Clinical Focus 3.9

Lung Cancer

Lung cancer is the leading cause of cancer-related deaths worldwide. Cigarette smoking is the cause in about 85-90% of all cases. Lung cancer arises either from alveolar lining cells of the lung parenchyma or from the epithelium of the tracheobronchial tree. Although there are a number of types, **squamous cell (bronchogenic) carcinoma** (about 20% of lung cancers in the United States) and **adenocarcinoma** (from intrapulmonary bronchi; about 37% of lung cancers in the United States) are the most common types. Bronchiogenic carcinoma may impinge on adjacent anatomical structures. For example, in **Pancoast syndrome,** this apical lung tumor may spread to involve the sympathetic trunk, affect the lower portion of the brachial plexus (C8, T1, and T2), and compromise the sympathetic tone to the head. This may lead to **Horner's syndrome** on the affected side (see Clinical Focus 8.22):

- **Miosis:** constricted pupil
- **Ptosis:** minor drooping of the upper eyelid
- **Anhidrosis:** lack of sweating
- **Flushing:** subcutaneous vasodilation

Additionally, involvement of the neurovascular components passing into the upper limb (trunks of the brachial plexus and subclavian artery) may be affected, resulting in pain and paresthesia in the neck, shoulder, and limb and paresis (incomplete paralysis) of the arm and hand.

Bronchogenic carcinoma: epidermoid (squamous cell) type

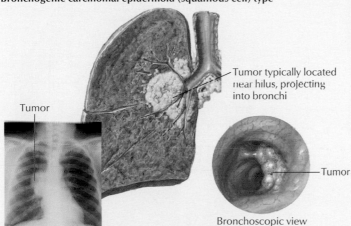

Tumor

Tumor typically located near hilus, projecting into bronchi

Tumor

Bronchoscopic view

Horner's syndrome and wasting, pain, paresthesias, and paresis of arm and hand

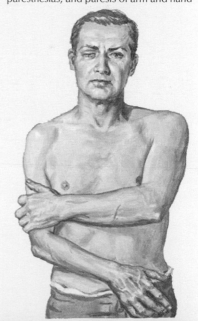

Pancoast syndrome: bronchogenic carcinoma of the apex of the lung

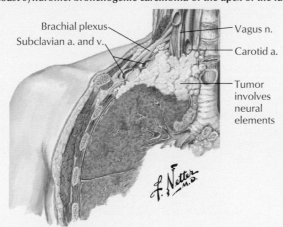

Brachial plexus
Subclavian a. and v.
Vagus n.
Carotid a.
Tumor involves neural elements

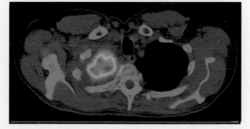

Combined CT/PET images of Pancoast tumor (bright area) seen in axial view

Clinical Focus 3.10

Chronic Obstructive Pulmonary Disease

Chronic obstructive pulmonary disease (COPD) is a broad classification of obstructive lung diseases, the most familiar being **chronic bronchitis, asthma,** and **emphysema.** Emphysema is characterized by permanent enlargement of air spaces at and distal to the respiratory bronchioles, with destruction of the bronchiole walls by chronic inflammation. As a result, lung compliance increases because the elastic recoil of the lung decreases, causing collapse of the airways during expiration. This increases the work of expiration as patients try to force air from their diseased lungs and can lead to a "barrel-chested" appearance caused by hypertrophy of the intercostal muscles. Smoking is a major risk factor for COPD.

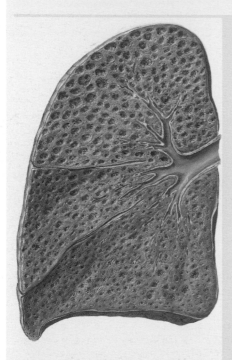

Gross specimen. Involvement tends to be most marked in upper part of lung.

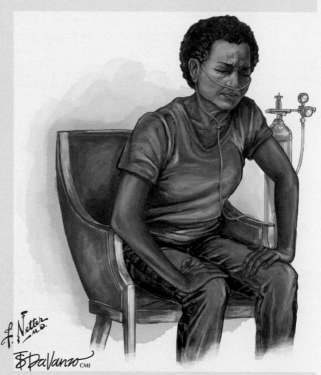

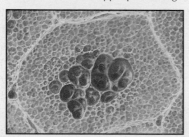

Magnified section. Distended, intercommunicating, saclike spaces in central area of acini.

The typical patient with COPD has clinical, physiological, and radiographic features of both chronic bronchitis and emphysema. She may have chronic cough and sputum production, and need accessory muscles and pursed lips to help her breathe. Pulmonary function testing may reveal variable degrees of airflow limitation, hyperinflation, and reduction in the diffusing capacity, and arterial blood gases may show variable decreases in P_{O_2} and increases in P_{CO_2}. Radiographic imaging often shows components of airway wall thickening, excessive mucus, and emphysema.

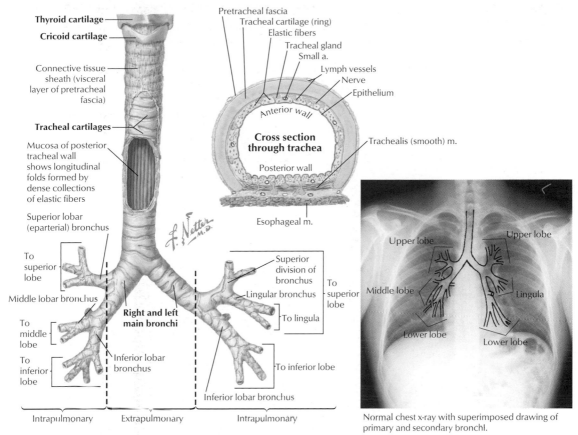

FIGURE 3.13 Trachea and Bronchi. (From *Netter's atlas of human anatomy,* ed 8, Plates 225; S-379; chest radiograph from Major NM: *A practical approach to radiology,* Philadelphia, 2006, Saunders.)

TABLE 3.8 Features of the Trachea and Bronchi	
STRUCTURE	**CHARACTERISTICS**
Trachea	Approximately 5 inches (10 cm) long and 1 inch in diameter; courses inferiorly anterior to esophagus and posterior to aortic arch
Cartilaginous rings	Are 16-20 C-shaped rings
Bronchus	Divides into right and left main (primary) bronchi at level of sternal angle of Louis
Right bronchus	Shorter, wider, and more vertical than left bronchus; aspirated foreign objects more likely to pass into right bronchus
Carina	Internal, keel-like cartilage at bifurcation of trachea
Secondary bronchi	Supply lobes of each lung (three on right, two on left)
Tertiary bronchi	Supply bronchopulmonary segments (10 for each lung)

circulation and pumps it into the pulmonary circulation of the lungs. The left side of the heart receives the blood from the pulmonary circulation and pumps it into the systemic circulation, thus perfusing the organs and tissues of the entire body, including the heart itself. In situ, the heart is oriented in the middle mediastinum and has the following descriptive relationships (Fig. 3.15):

- **Anterior (sternocostal):** the right atrium, right ventricle, and part of the left ventricle.
- **Posterior (base):** the left atrium.
- **Inferior (diaphragmatic):** some of the right ventricle and most of the left ventricle.
- **Acute angle:** the sharp right ventricular margin of the heart, largely the right atrium.
- **Obtuse angle:** the more rounded left margin of the heart, largely the left ventricle.
- **Apex:** the inferolateral part of the left ventricle at the fourth to fifth intercostal space.

The **atrioventricular groove** (coronary sulcus) separates the two atria from the ventricles and marks the locations of the right coronary artery

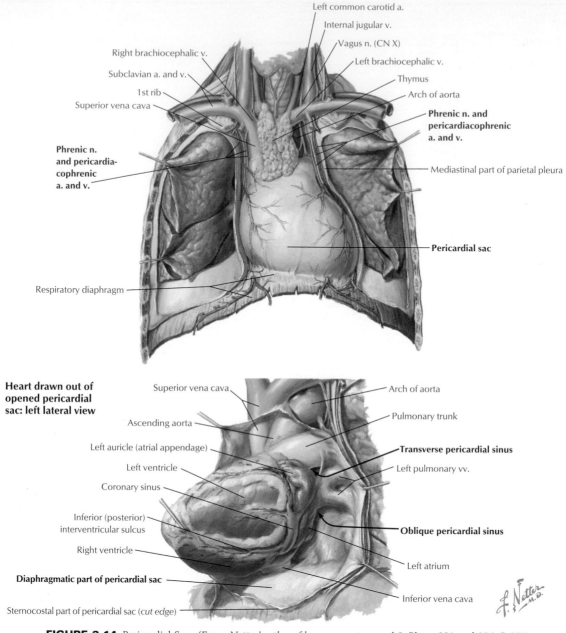

Left common carotid a.

Internal jugular v.

Vagus n. (CN X)

Left brachiocephalic v.

Right brachiocephalic v.

Subclavian a. and v.

1st rib

Superior vena cava

Thymus

Arch of aorta

Phrenic n. and pericardiacophrenic a. and v.

Phrenic n. and pericardia- cophrenic a. and v.

Mediastinal part of parietal pleura

Pericardial sac

Respiratory diaphragm

Heart drawn out of opened pericardial sac: left lateral view

Superior vena cava

Ascending aorta

Left auricle (atrial appendage)

Left ventricle

Coronary sinus

Inferior (posterior) interventricular sulcus

Right ventricle

Diaphragmatic part of pericardial sac

Sternocostal part of pericardial sac (*cut edge*)

Arch of aorta

Pulmonary trunk

Transverse pericardial sinus

Left pulmonary vv.

Oblique pericardial sinus

Left atrium

Inferior vena cava

FIGURE 3.14 Pericardial Sac. (From *Netter's atlas of human anatomy*, ed 8, Plates 231 and 236; S-307 and S-308.)

TABLE 3.9 Features of the Pericardium

STRUCTURE	DEFINITION	STRUCTURE	DEFINITION
Fibrous pericardium	Tough, outer layer that reflects onto great vessels	Transverse sinus	Space posterior to aorta and pulmonary trunk; can clamp vessels with fingers in this sinus and above
Serous pericardium	Layer that lines inner aspect of fibrous pericardium (parietal layer); reflects onto heart as epicardium (visceral layer)	Oblique sinus	Pericardial space posterior to heart
Innervation	Phrenic nerve (C3-C5) for conveying pain; vasomotor innervation via postganglionic sympathetics		

Cardiac Tamponade

Cardiac tamponade can result from fluid accumulation or bleeding into the pericardial sac. Bleeding may be caused by a ruptured aortic aneurysm, a ruptured myocardial infarct, or a penetrating injury (most common cause) that compromises the beating heart and decreases venous return and cardiac output. The fluid can be removed by a **pericardial tap** (i.e., withdrawn by a needle and syringe).

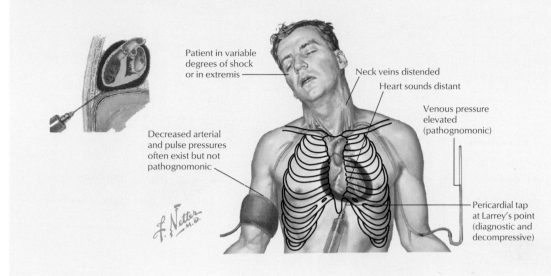

Patient in variable degrees of shock or in extremis

Neck veins distended

Heart sounds distant

Venous pressure elevated (pathognomonic)

Decreased arterial and pulse pressures often exist but not pathognomonic

Pericardial tap at Larrey's point (diagnostic and decompressive)

and the circumflex branch of the left coronary artery. The **anterior** and **posterior interventricular grooves** mark the locations of the left anterior descending (anterior interventricular) branch of the left coronary artery and the inferior (posterior) interventricular branch of right coronary, respectively.

Coronary Arteries and Cardiac Veins

The right and left coronary arteries arise immediately superior to the right and left cusps, respectively, of the **aortic semilunar valve** (Fig. 3.16). The **right coronary artery** courses in the right atrioventricular groove and passes around the acute angle (right side) of the heart. The **left coronary artery** passes between the left auricle and the pulmonary trunk, reaches the left atrioventricular groove, and divides into the **anterior interventricular** (left anterior descending [LAD]) and **circumflex** branches. The LAD descends in the anterior interventricular sulcus between the right and left ventricles, and the circumflex branch courses around the obtuse margin (left side) of the heart. During ventricular diastole, blood enters the coronary arteries to supply the myocardium of each chamber. About 5% of the total cardiac output goes to the heart itself.

Although variations in the coronary artery blood supply to the various chambers of the heart are common, in general, the **right coronary artery** supplies the:

- Right atrium.
- Right ventricle (most of it).
- SA and AV nodes (usually).
- Interatrial septum.
- Left ventricle (a small portion).
- Posteroinferior one-third of the interventricular septum.

In general, the **left coronary artery** supplies:

- Most of the left atrium.
- Most of the left ventricle.
- Most of the interventricular septum.
- Right and left bundle branches (conduction system).
- Small portion of the right ventricle.

The corresponding **great cardiac vein, middle cardiac vein,** and **small cardiac vein** parallel the LAD branch of the left coronary artery, the posterior descending artery (PDA) of the right coronary artery, and the marginal branch of the right coronary artery, respectively. Each of these cardiac veins then empties into the **coronary sinus** on the posterior aspect of the atrioventricular groove

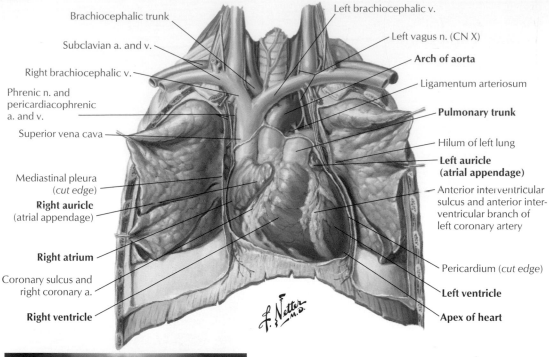

Brachiocephalic trunk

Subclavian a. and v.

Right brachiocephalic v.

Phrenic n. and
pericardiacophrenic
a. and v.

Superior vena cava

Mediastinal pleura
(*cut edge*)

Right auricle
(atrial appendage)

Right atrium

Coronary sulcus and
right coronary a.

Right ventricle

Left brachiocephalic v.

Left vagus n. (CN X)

Arch of aorta

Ligamentum arteriosum

Pulmonary trunk

Hilum of left lung

**Left auricle
(atrial appendage)**

Anterior interventricular
sulcus and anterior interventricular branch of
left coronary artery

Pericardium (*cut edge*)

Left ventricle

Apex of heart

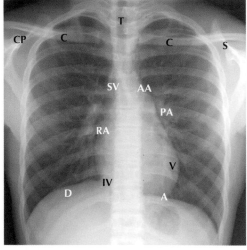

A Apex of heart	**PA** Pulmonary artery (left)
AA Aortic arch	**RA** Right atrium
C Clavicle	**S** Spine of scapula
CP Coracoid process of scapula	**SV** Superior vena cava
D Dome of diaphragm (right)	**T** Trachea (air)
IV Inferior vena cava	**V** Left ventricle

FIGURE 3.15 Anterior In Situ Exposure of the
Heart. (From *Netter's atlas of human anatomy,* ed 8, Plate
232; S-309.)

Clinical Focus 3.12

Dominant Coronary Circulation

About 67% of individuals have a "right dominant"
coronary circulation. This means that the right coronary artery gives rise to the inferior interventricular
branch and the posterolateral artery, as shown in
Fig. 3.16. In about 15% of cases, the left coronary
artery's circumflex branch gives rise to the branch.
In the remaining cases, both the right and the left
coronary arteries may contribute to this branch or
it may be absent and branches from both coronaries
may supply this region.

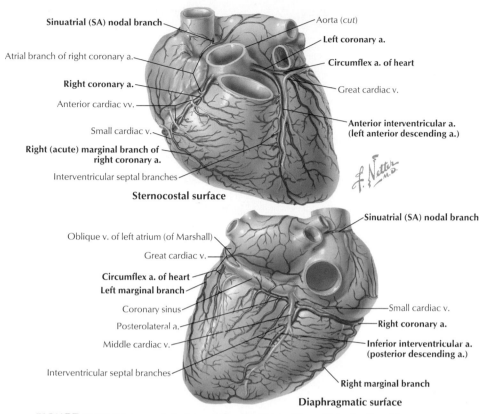

Sinuatrial (SA) nodal branch

Atrial branch of right coronary a.

Right coronary a.

Anterior cardiac vv.

Small cardiac v.

Right (acute) marginal branch of right coronary a.

Interventricular septal branches

Sternocostal surface

Aorta (*cut*)

Left coronary a.

Circumflex a. of heart

Great cardiac v.

Anterior interventricular a. (left anterior descending a.)

Oblique v. of left atrium (of Marshall)

Great cardiac v.

Circumflex a. of heart

Left marginal branch

Coronary sinus

Posterolateral a.

Middle cardiac v.

Interventricular septal branches

Sinuatrial (SA) nodal branch

Small cardiac v.

Right coronary a.

Inferior interventricular a. (posterior descending a.)

Right marginal branch

Diaphragmatic surface

FIGURE 3.16 Coronary Arteries and Cardiac Veins. (From *Netter's atlas of human anatomy,* ed 8, Plate 239; S-317.)

TABLE 3.10 Coronary Arteries and Cardiac Veins

VESSEL	COURSE	VESSEL	COURSE
Right coronary artery	Consists of major branches: sinuatrial (SA) nodal, right marginal, inferior (posterior) interventricular, atrioventricular (AV) nodal	Middle cardiac vein	Parallels inferior (posterior) interventricular branch and drains into coronary sinus
Left coronary artery	Consists of major branches: circumflex, anterior interventricular (left anterior descending [LAD]), left marginal	Small cardiac vein	Parallels right marginal artery and drains into coronary sinus
Great cardiac vein	Parallels LAD artery and drains into coronary sinus	Anterior cardiac veins	Several small veins that drain directly into right atrium
		Smallest cardiac veins	Drain through the cardiac wall directly into all four heart chambers, but mostly the right atrium

(Table 3.10). The coronary sinus empties into the right atrium. Additionally, numerous **smallest cardiac veins** (thebesian veins) empty venous blood into all four chambers of the heart, but mostly into the right atrium.

Chambers of the Heart

The human heart has four chambers, each with unique internal features related to their function (Fig. 3.17 and Table 3.11). The right side of the heart is composed of the **right atrium** and **right ventricle.** These chambers receive blood from the systemic circulation and pump it to the pulmonary circulation for gas exchange.

The **left atrium** and **left ventricle** receive blood from the pulmonary circulation and pump it to the systemic circulation (Fig. 3.18 and Table 3.12).

In both ventricles the **papillary muscles** and their **chordae tendineae** provide a structural mechanism that prevents the **atrioventricular valves** (**tricuspid** and **mitral**) from everting (prolapsing) during ventricular systole. The papillary muscles (actually part of the ventricular muscle) contract as the ventricles contract (ventricular systole) and pull the valve leaflets into alignment. This prevents them from prolapsing into the atrial chamber above as the pressure in the ventricle

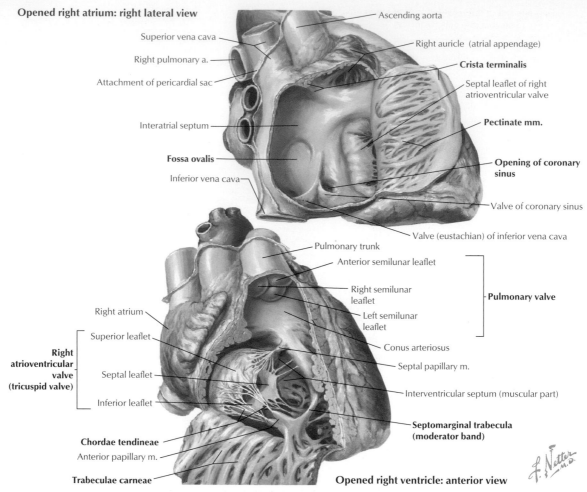

FIGURE 3.17 Right Atrium and Ventricle Opened. (From *Netter's atlas of human anatomy,* ed 8, Plate 241; S-311.)

TABLE 3.11 General Features of Right Atrium and Right Ventricle			
STRUCTURE	**DEFINITION**	**STRUCTURE**	**DEFINITION**
Right Atrium		**Right Ventricle**	
Auricle	Pouchlike appendage of atrium; embryonic heart tube derivative	Trabeculae carneae	Irregular ridges of ventricular myocardium
Pectinate muscles	Ridges of myocardium inside auricle	Papillary muscles	Superoposterior, inferior, and septal projections of myocardium extending into ventricular cavity; prevent valve leaflet prolapse
Crista terminalis	Ridge that runs from inferior vena cava (IVC) to superior vena cava (SVC) openings; its superior extent marks site of SA node and it conveys an internodal conduction pathway to the AV node	Chordae tendineae	Fibrous cords that connect papillary muscles to valve leaflets
		Moderator band	Muscular band that conveys AV bundle from septum to base of ventricle at site of anterior papillary muscle
Fossa ovalis	Depression in interatrial septum; former site of foramen ovale	Ventricular openings	One to pulmonary trunk through pulmonary valve; one to receive blood from right atrium through tricuspid valve
Atrial openings	One each for SVC, IVC, and coronary sinus (venous return from cardiac veins)		

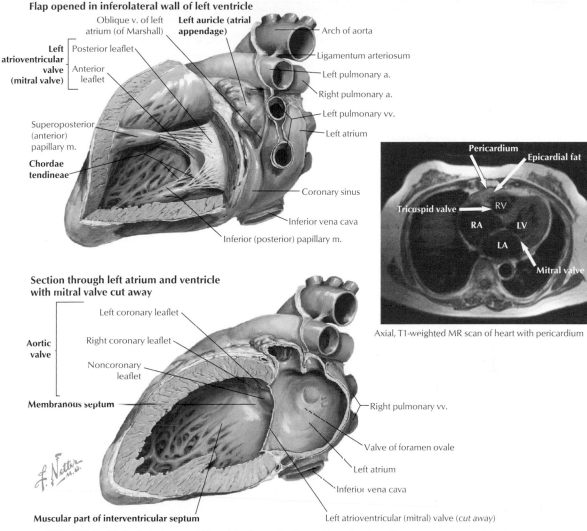

Flap opened in inferolateral wall of left ventricle

Oblique v. of left atrium (of Marshall)

Left auricle (atrial appendage)

Arch of aorta

Ligamentum arteriosum

Left pulmonary a.

Right pulmonary a.

Left pulmonary vv.

Left atrium

Left atrioventricular valve (mitral valve)
Posterior leaflet
Anterior leaflet

Superoposterior (anterior) papillary m.

Chordae tendineae

Coronary sinus

Inferior vena cava

Inferior (posterior) papillary m.

Pericardium
Epicardial fat
Tricuspid valve
RV
RA
LV
LA
Mitral valve

Axial, T1-weighted MR scan of heart with pericardium

Section through left atrium and ventricle with mitral valve cut away

Aortic valve
Left coronary leaflet
Right coronary leaflet
Noncoronary leaflet

Membranous septum

Right pulmonary vv.

Valve of foramen ovale

Left atrium

Inferior vena cava

Muscular part of interventricular septum

Left atrioventricular (mitral) valve (*cut away*)

FIGURE 3.18 Left Atrium and Ventricle Opened. (From *Netter's atlas of human anatomy,* ed 8, Plate 242; S-312; MR image from Kelley LL, Petersen C: *Sectional anatomy for imaging professionals,* St Louis, 2007, Mosby.)

TABLE 3.12 General Features of Left Atrium and Left Ventricle

STRUCTURE	DEFINITION	STRUCTURE	DEFINITION
Left Atrium		Chordae tendineae	Fibrous cords that connect papillary muscles to valve leaflets
Auricle	Small appendage representing primitive embryonic atrium whose wall has pectinate muscle	Ventricular wall	Wall much thicker than that of right ventricle
Atrial wall	Wall slightly thicker than thin-walled right atrium	Membranous septum	Very thin superior portion of IVS and site of most ventricular septal defects (VSDs)
Atrial openings	Usually four openings for four pulmonary veins	Ventricular openings	One to aorta through aortic valve; one to receive blood from left atrium through mitral valve
Left Ventricle			
Papillary muscles	Superoposterior and inferior muscles, larger than those of right ventricle		

Clinical Focus 3.13

Angina Pectoris (the Referred Pain of Myocardial Ischemia)

Angina pectoris ("strangling of the chest") is usually described as pressure, discomfort, or a feeling of choking or breathlessness in the left chest or substernal region that radiates to the left shoulder and arm, as well as the neck, jaw and teeth, abdomen, and back. The discomfort also may radiate to the right arm. This radiating pattern is an example of **referred pain,** in which visceral pain afferents from the heart enter the upper thoracic spinal cord along with somatic afferents, both converging in the spinal cord's posterior horn. The higher brain center's interpretation of this visceral pain may initially be confused with somatic sensations from the same spinal cord levels. Somatic pain is "mapped" on the brain's sensory cortex, but a similar symptomatic mapping of visceral sensations does not occur. This may explain why pain from visceral structures is often mistakenly perceived as somatic pain.

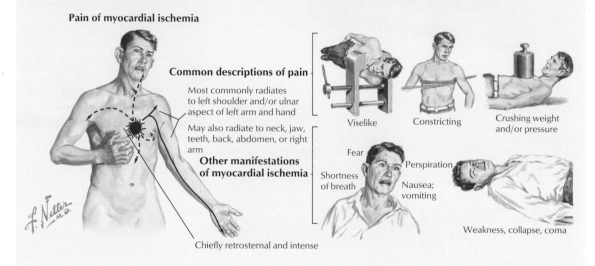

Pain of myocardial ischemia

Common descriptions of pain

Most commonly radiates to left shoulder and/or ulnar aspect of left arm and hand

May also radiate to neck, jaw, teeth, back, abdomen, or right arm

Other manifestations of myocardial ischemia

Chiefly retrosternal and intense

Viselike   Constricting   Crushing weight and/or pressure

Fear   Perspiration

Shortness of breath   Nausea; vomiting

Weakness, collapse, coma

Clinical Focus 3.14

Coronary Bypass

A **coronary artery bypass graft** (CABG), also called "the cabbage procedure," offers a surgical approach for revascularization. Veins or arteries from elsewhere in the patient's body are grafted to the coronary arteries to improve the blood supply. In a *saphenous vein graft* a portion of the great saphenous vein is harvested from the patient's lower limb. Alternatives include internal thoracic artery and radial artery grafts.

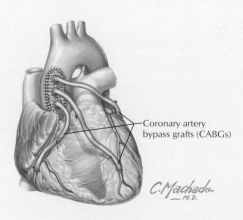

If indicated the physician may prefer to use coronary angioplasty to widen the partially occluded artery, which may include using a stent to keep the artery open.

Coronary artery bypass grafts (CABGs)

Coronary Angiogenesis

Angiogenesis occurs by the budding of new blood vessels from small sprouts of existing vessels, thereby expanding the capillary network. Hypoxia and inflammation are the two major stimuli for new vessel growth. Revascularization of the myocardium after an ischemic episode by angiogenesis, bypass surgery, or percutaneous coronary intervention is vital for establishing blood flow to the ischemic myocardium.

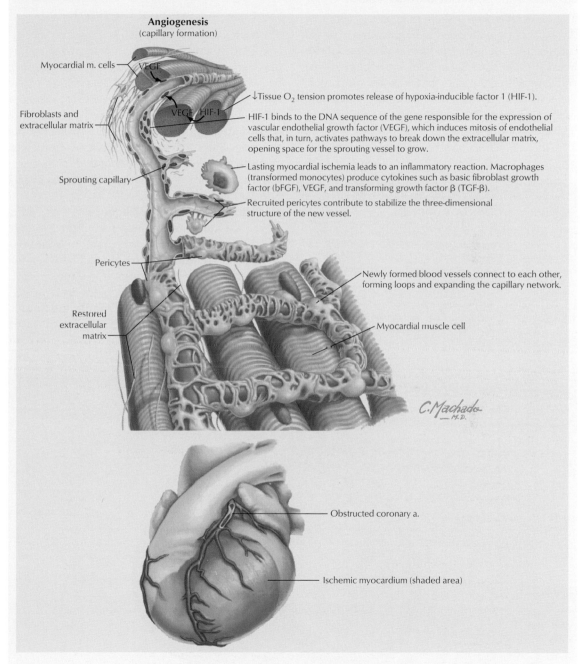

Angiogenesis
(capillary formation)

Myocardial m. cells — VEGF

Fibroblasts and extracellular matrix

VEGF   HIF-1

Sprouting capillary

Pericytes

Restored extracellular matrix

↓Tissue O_2 tension promotes release of hypoxia-inducible factor 1 (HIF-1).

HIF-1 binds to the DNA sequence of the gene responsible for the expression of vascular endothelial growth factor (VEGF), which induces mitosis of endothelial cells that, in turn, activates pathways to break down the extracellular matrix, opening space for the sprouting vessel to grow.

Lasting myocardial ischemia leads to an inflammatory reaction. Macrophages (transformed monocytes) produce cytokines such as basic fibroblast growth factor (bFGF), VEGF, and transforming growth factor β (TGF-β).

Recruited pericytes contribute to stabilize the three-dimensional structure of the new vessel.

Newly formed blood vessels connect to each other, forming loops and expanding the capillary network.

Myocardial muscle cell

C. Machado
— M.D.

Obstructed coronary a.

Ischemic myocardium (shaded area)

increases. During ventricular diastole, the muscle relaxes and the tricuspid and mitral valves open normally to facilitate blood flow into the ventricles. Toward the end of ventricular diastole, the atria contract and "top off" the ventricles, just prior to ventricular systole.

Cardiac Skeleton and Cardiac Valves

The heart has four valves that, along with the myocardium, are attached to fibrous rings of dense collagen that make up the **fibrous skeleton of the heart** (Fig. 3.19 and Table 3.13). In addition to providing attachment points for the valves, the cardiac skeleton separates the atrial myocardium from the ventricular myocardium (which originate from the fibrous skeleton) and electrically isolates the atria from the ventricles. Only the atrioventricular bundle

(of His) conveys electrical impulses between the atria and the ventricles. The following normal heart sounds result from valve closure:

- **First heart sound (S_1):** results from the closing of the mitral and tricuspid valves.
- **Second heart sound (S_2):** results from the closing of the aortic and pulmonary valves.

Conduction System of the Heart

The heart's conduction system is formed by specialized cardiac muscle cells that form nodes and by unidirectional conduction pathways that initiate and coordinate excitation and contraction of the myocardium (Fig 3.20). The system includes the following four elements:

- **Sinuatrial (SA) node:** the "pacemaker" of the heart, where initiation of the action potential occurs; located at the superior end of the crista terminalis near the opening of the superior vena cava (SVC).
- **Atrioventricular (AV) node:** the area of the heart that receives impulses from the SA node and conveys them to the common **atrioventricular bundle (of His)**; located between the opening of the coronary sinus and the origin of the septal cusp of the tricuspid valve.
- **Common atrioventricular bundle and bundle branches:** a collection of specialized heart muscle cells; the AV bundle divides into right

TABLE 3.13 Features of the Heart Valves

VALVE	CHARACTERISTIC
Tricuspid	(Right AV) Between right atrium and right ventricle; has three cusps
Pulmonary	(Semilunar) Between right ventricle and pulmonary trunk; has three semilunar cusps (leaflets)
Mitral	(Bicuspid) Between left atrium and left ventricle; has two cusps
Aortic	(Semilunar) Between left ventricle and aorta; has three semilunar cusps

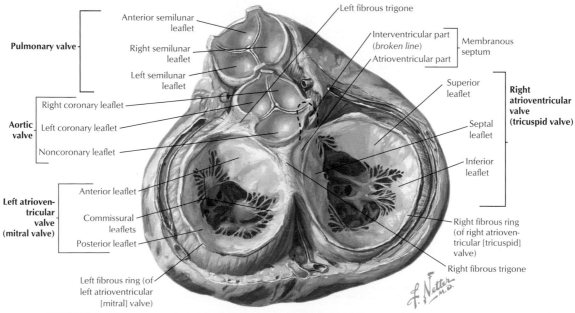

FIGURE 3.19 Heart in Ventricular Diastole Viewed From Above With Atrial Chambers Removed. (From *Netter's atlas of human anatomy*, ed 8, Plate 243; S-314.)

Myocardial Infarction

Myocardial infarction (MI) is a major cause of death. Coronary artery **atherosclerosis** and **thrombosis,** the major causes of MI, precipitate local ischemia and necrosis of a defined myocardial area. Necrosis usually occurs approximately 20 to 30 minutes after coronary artery occlusion. Usually, MI begins in the subendocardium because this region is the most poorly perfused part of the ventricular wall.

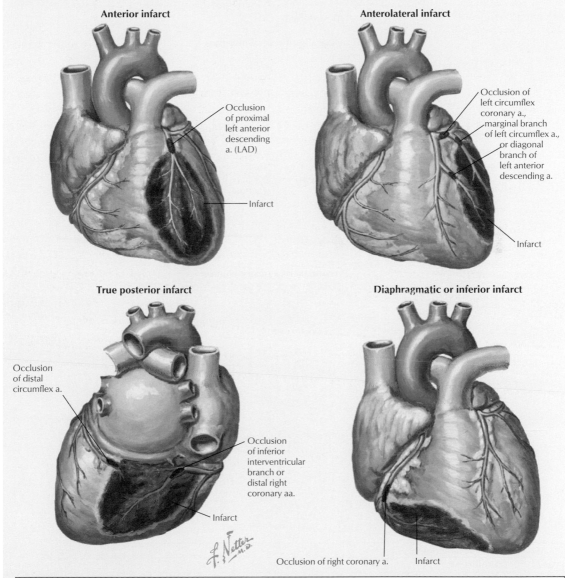

Anterior infarct

Occlusion of proximal left anterior descending a. (LAD)

Infarct

Anterolateral infarct

Occlusion of left circumflex coronary a., marginal branch of left circumflex a., or diagonal branch of left anterior descending a.

Infarct

True posterior infarct

Occlusion of distal circumflex a.

Occlusion of inferior interventricular branch or distal right coronary aa.

Infarct

Diaphragmatic or inferior infarct

Occlusion of right coronary a.   Infarct

Artery and Area Affected by MI	
Artery occluded	Frequency and affected area
LAD	40–50%; affects anterior and apical left ventricle and anterior two-thirds of interventricular septum (IVS)
Right coronary	30–40%; affects posterior wall of left ventricle, posterior one-third of IVS (if right-dominant coronary circulation)
Left circumflex	15–20%; affects lateral wall of left ventricle (can also affect posterior wall if left dominant coronary circulation)

Clinical Focus 3.17

Cardiac Auscultation

Auscultation of the heart requires not only an understanding of normal and abnormal heart sounds but also knowledge of the optimal location to detect the sounds. Sounds are best heard by auscultating the area where **turbulent blood flow radiates** (i.e., distal to the valve through which the blood has just passed). The areas indicated on the image below are approximate, and one must expand the area of auscultation depending on the size of the patient's heart, other normal variations, or pathological conditions that may be present, such as patent ductus arteriosus or ventricular hypertrophy.

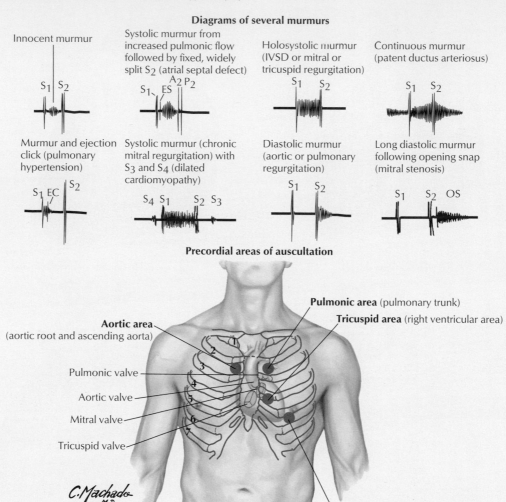

Diagrams of several murmurs

Innocent murmur

S_1 S_2

Systolic murmur from increased pulmonic flow followed by fixed, widely split S_2 (atrial septal defect)

S_1 ES A_2 P_2

Holosystolic murmur (IVSD or mitral or tricuspid regurgitation)

S_1 S_2

Continuous murmur (patent ductus arteriosus)

S_1 S_2

Murmur and ejection click (pulmonary hypertension)

S_1 EC S_2

Systolic murmur (chronic mitral regurgitation) with S_3 and S_4 (dilated cardiomyopathy)

S_4 S_1 S_2 S_3

Diastolic murmur (aortic or pulmonary regurgitation)

S_1 S_2

Long diastolic murmur following opening snap (mitral stenosis)

S_1 S_2 OS

Precordial areas of auscultation

Pulmonic area (pulmonary trunk)

Tricuspid area (right ventricular area)

Aortic area (aortic root and ascending aorta)

Pulmonic valve

Aortic valve

Mitral valve

Tricuspid valve

C. Machado —M.D.

Mitral area (left ventricular area)

Features of Various Heart Sounds	
Area	**Comment**
Aortic	Upper right sternal border; aortic stenosis
Pulmonary	Upper left sternal border to below left clavicle; second heart sound, pulmonary valve murmurs, VSD murmur, continuous murmur of patent ductus arteriosus (PDA)
Tricuspid	Left fourth intercostal space; or sternal border of 5th rib; tricuspid and aortic regurgitation
Mitral	Left fifth intercostal space in midclavicular line; apex; first heart sound, murmurs of mitral or aortic valves, third and fourth heart sounds

Valvular Heart Disease

Although any of the valves may be involved in disease, the mitral and aortic valves are most frequently involved. Major problems include **stenosis** (narrowing) or **insufficiency** (compromised valve function, often leading to regurgitation). Several examples of aortic stenosis are shown (lower right images).

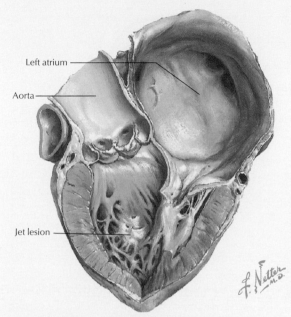

Left atrium

Aorta

Jet lesion

Thickened stenotic mitral valve: aortic leaflet (anterior cusp) has typical convexity; enlarged left atrium, "jet lesion" on left ventricular wall

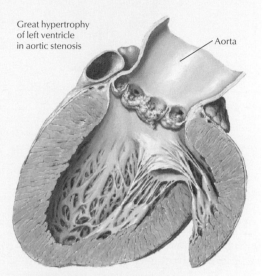

Great hypertrophy of left ventricle in aortic stenosis

Aorta

Elongation of left ventricle with tension on chordae tendineae, which may prevent full closure of mitral valve

Condition	Comment
Aortic stenosis	Leads to left ventricular overload and hypertrophy; caused by rheumatic heart disease (RHD), calcific stenosis, congenital bicuspid valve (1–2%)
Aortic regurgitation (insufficiency)	Caused by congenitally malformed leaflets, RHD, IE, ankylosing spondylitis, Marfan's syndrome, aortic root dilation
Mitral stenosis	Leads to left atrial dilation; usually caused by RHD
Mitral regurgitation (insufficiency)	Caused by abnormalities of valve leaflets, rupture of papillary muscle or chordae tendineae, papillary muscle fibrosis, IE, left ventricular enlargement

IE, infective endocarditis (infection of cardiac valves)

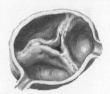

Stenosis and insufficiency (fusion of all commissures)

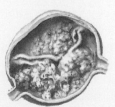

Calcific stenosis

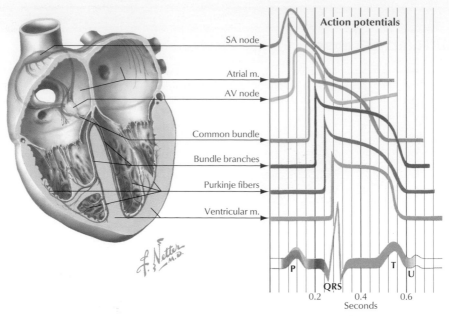

FIGURE 3.20 Conduction System and Electrocardiogram.

and left bundle branches, which course down the interventricular septum.

- **Subendocardial (Purkinje) system**: the ramification of bundle branches in the ventricles of the heart's conduction system; this system includes a subendocardial network of conduction cells that supply the ventricular walls and papillary muscles.

Autonomic Innervation of the Heart

Parasympathetic fibers from the vagus nerve (CN X) course as preganglionic nerves that synapse on postganglionic neurons in the **cardiac plexus** or within the heart wall itself (Fig. 3.21). Parasympathetic stimulation:

- Decreases heart rate.
- Decreases the force of contraction.
- Vasodilates coronary resistance vessels (although most vagal effects are restricted directly to the SA nodal region).

Sympathetic fibers arise from the upper thoracic cord levels (intermediolateral cell column of T1-T4/T5) and enter the sympathetic trunk (Fig. 3.21). These preganglionic fibers synapse in the upper cervical and thoracic sympathetic chain ganglia, and then send postganglionic fibers to the cardiac plexus on and around the aorta and pulmonary trunk. Sympathetic stimulation:

- Increases the heart rate.
- Increases the force of contraction.

- Minimally vasoconstricts the coronary resistance vessels (via alpha adrenoceptors).

This coronary artery vasoconstriction, however, *is masked by a powerful metabolic coronary vasodilation* (mediated by adenosine release from myocytes), which is important because coronary arteries must dilate to supply blood to the heart as it increases its workload.

In the posterior mediastinum, a bilateral thoracic sympathetic chain of ganglia **(sympathetic trunk)** passes across the neck of the upper thoracic ribs and, as it proceeds inferiorly, aligns itself closer to the lateral bodies of the lower thoracic vertebrae (Fig. 3.22). Each of the 11 or 12 pairs of ganglia (number varies) is connected to the anterior ramus of the corresponding spinal nerve by a white ramus communicans (the white ramus conveys preganglionic sympathetic fibers from the spinal nerve). A gray ramus communicans then conveys postganglionic sympathetic fibers back into the spinal nerve and its anterior or posterior rami (see Chapter 1, Nervous System). Additionally, the upper thoracic sympathetic trunk conveys **small thoracic cardiac branches** (postganglionic sympathetic fibers from the upper thoracic ganglia, T1-T4 or T5) to the **cardiac plexus**, where they mix with preganglionic parasympathetic fibers from the vagus nerve (Figs. 3.21 and 3.22). Three other pairs of thoracic splanchnic nerves arise from the lower seven or eight thoracic ganglia and send their preganglionic

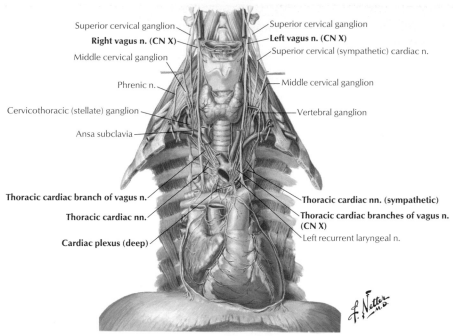

FIGURE 3.21 Autonomic Innervation of the Heart. (From *Netter's atlas of human anatomy*, ed 8, Plate 249; S-99.)

Clinical Focus 3.19

Cardiac Pacemakers

Cardiac pacemakers consist of a pulse generator and one to three endocardial electrode leads. Pacemakers can pace one heart chamber, **dual chambers,** or can provide **biventricular pacing,** with leads in the right atrium and ventricle and one introduced into the coronary sinus and advanced until it is over the surface of the left ventricular wall near the left (obtuse) marginal artery. Depending upon the device, its programming, and its positioning, it can pace the heart chamber (SA node or correct atrial fibrillation), pace the atrium and ventricle sequentially (dual-chamber pacemaker), or provide normal AV pacing and enable pacing of the left ventricular wall (biventricular pacing).

Implantable cardiac pacemaker (dual-chamber cardiac pacing)

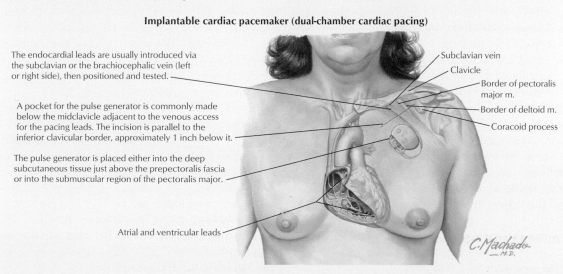

The endocardial leads are usually introduced via the subclavian or the brachiocephalic vein (left or right side), then positioned and tested.

A pocket for the pulse generator is commonly made below the midclavicle adjacent to the venous access for the pacing leads. The incision is parallel to the inferior clavicular border, approximately 1 inch below it.

The pulse generator is placed either into the deep subcutaneous tissue just above the prepectoralis fascia or into the submuscular region of the pectoralis major.

Atrial and ventricular leads

Subclavian vein
Clavicle
Border of pectoralis major m.
Border of deltoid m.
Coracoid process

Clinical Focus 3.20

Cardiac Defibrillators

An implantable cardioverter defibrillator is used for survivors of **sudden cardiac death,** patients with **sustained ventricular tachycardia** (a dysrhythmia originating from a ventricular focus with a heart rate typically greater than 120 beats/min), those at high risk for developing ventricular arrhythmias (ischemic dilated cardiomyopathy), and other indications. In addition to sensing arrhythmias and providing defibrillation to stop them, the device can function as a pacemaker for postdefibrillation bradycardia or atrioventricular dissociation.

Implantable cardiac defibrillator (dual-chamber leads)

In all aspects, the surgical procedure for implantable cardioverter defibrillator (ICD) implantation is very similar to that of cardiac pacemaker implantation.

Due to the number of functions the ICD can perform (cardioverter, defibrillator, and pacemaker), the ICD is usually slightly larger than a pacemaker. The surface of the ICD functions as one of the electrodes of the defibrillation system.

Lead in the right atrium/auricle

Lead with two defibrillation coils. The distal coil is in the right ventricle, and the proximal one is in the superior vena cava/right atrial position.

C. Machado
—M.D.

sympathetic fibers inferiorly to abdominal ganglia. The thoracic splanchnic nerves (spinal levels can vary) (see Chapter 4) contain preganglionic sympathetic fibers and are named as follows:

- **Greater splanchnic nerve:** preganglionic fibers usually arise from the T5-T9 spinal cord levels.
- **Lesser splanchnic nerve:** preganglionic fibers usually arise from the T10-T11 spinal cord levels.
- **Least splanchnic nerve:** preganglionic fibers usually arise from the T12 spinal cord level.

Visceral afferents for **pain or ischemia** from the heart are conveyed back to the upper thoracic spinal cord, usually levels T1-T4 or T5, via the sympathetic fiber pathways (see Clinical Focus 3.13). Visceral afferents mediating **cardiopulmonary reflexes** (stretch receptors, baroreflexes, and chemoreflexes) are conveyed back to the brainstem via the vagus nerve (CN X).

6. MEDIASTINUM

The mediastinum ("middle space") is the middle region of the thoracic cavity and is divided into a superior and an inferior mediastinum by an imaginary horizontal line extending from the sternal angle of Louis to the intervertebral disc between the T4 and T5 vertebrae (Fig. 3.23; see also Fig. 3.1). The superior mediastinum lies behind the manubrium of the sternum, anterior to the first four thoracic vertebrae, and contains the following:

- Thymus gland (largely involuted and replaced by fat in older adults).
- Brachiocephalic veins (right and left).
- Superior vena cava.
- Aortic arch and its three arterial branches (brachiocephalic trunk, left common carotid artery, and left subclavian artery) and pulmonary trunk.
- Trachea.
- Esophagus.
- Phrenic and vagus nerves.
- Thoracic duct and lymphatics.

The inferior mediastinum is further subdivided as follows (Figs. 3.23 and 3.24):

- **Anterior mediastinum:** the region posterior to the body of the sternum and anterior to the

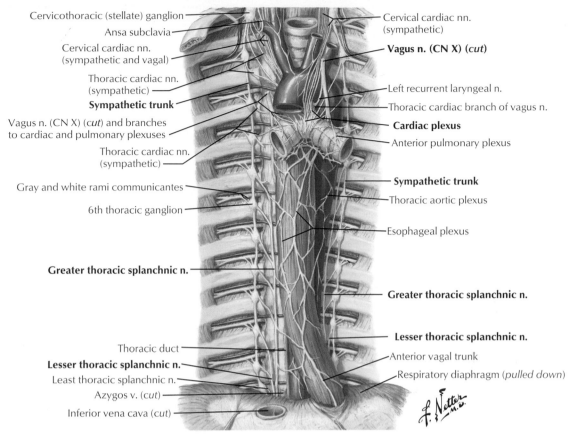

Cervicothoracic (stellate) ganglion

Ansa subclavia

Cervical cardiac nn.
(sympathetic and vagal)

Thoracic cardiac nn.
(sympathetic)

Sympathetic trunk

Vagus n. (CN X) (*cut*) and branches
to cardiac and pulmonary plexuses

Thoracic cardiac nn.
(sympathetic)

Gray and white rami communicantes

6th thoracic ganglion

Greater thoracic splanchnic n.

Thoracic duct

Lesser thoracic splanchnic n.

Least thoracic splanchnic n.

Azygos v. (*cut*)

Inferior vena cava (*cut*)

Cervical cardiac nn.
(sympathetic)

Vagus n. (CN X) (*cut*)

Left recurrent laryngeal n.

Thoracic cardiac branch of vagus n.

Cardiac plexus

Anterior pulmonary plexus

Sympathetic trunk

Thoracic aortic plexus

Esophageal plexus

Greater thoracic splanchnic n.

Lesser thoracic splanchnic n.

Anterior vagal trunk

Respiratory diaphragm (*pulled down*)

FIGURE 3.22 Autonomic Nerves in the Thorax. (From *Netter's atlas of human anatomy,* ed 8, Plate 229; S-101.)

pericardium (substernal region); contains a variable amount of fat.

- **Middle mediastinum:** the region containing the pericardium and heart.
- **Posterior mediastinum:** the region posterior to the heart and anterior to the bodies of the T5-T12 vertebrae; contains the esophagus and its nerve plexus, thoracic aorta, azygos system of veins, sympathetic trunks and thoracic splanchnic nerves, lymphatics, and thoracic duct.

Esophagus and Thoracic Aorta

The **esophagus** extends from the pharynx (throat) to the stomach and enters the thorax posterior to the trachea. As it descends, the esophagus gradually slopes to the left of the median plane, lying anterior to the thoracic aorta (Figs. 3.22–3.25); it pierces the diaphragm at the T10 vertebral level. The esophagus is about 10 cm (4 inches) long and has four points along its course where foreign bodies may become lodged: (1) at its most proximal site at the level of the C6 vertebra (level of the cricoid cartilage), (2) at the point where it is crossed by

the aortic arch, (3) at the point where it is crossed by the left main bronchus, and (4) distally at the point where it passes through the diaphragm at the level of the T10 vertebra. The esophagus receives its blood supply from the inferior thyroid artery, esophageal branches of the thoracic aorta, and branches of the left gastric artery (a branch of the celiac trunk in the abdomen).

The **thoracic aorta** descends alongside and slightly to the left of the esophagus (Fig. 3.25 and see fig. 3.27) and gives rise to the following arteries before piercing the diaphragm at the T12 vertebral level:

- **Pericardial arteries:** small arteries that branch from the thoracic aorta and supply the posterior pericardium; variable in number.
- **Bronchial arteries:** arteries that supply blood to the lungs; usually one artery to the right lung and two to the left lung, but variable in number.
- **Esophageal arteries:** arteries that supply the esophagus; variable in number.
- **Mediastinal arteries:** small branches that supply the lymph nodes, nerves, and connective tissue of the posterior mediastinum.

Superior mediastinum and lungs

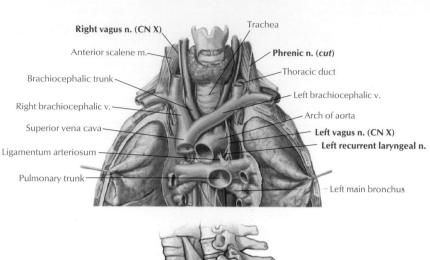

Right vagus n. (CN X)

Anterior scalene m.

Brachiocephalic trunk

Right brachiocephalic v.

Superior vena cava

Ligamentum arteriosum

Pulmonary trunk

Trachea

Phrenic n. (*cut*)

Thoracic duct

Left brachiocephalic v.

Arch of aorta

Left vagus n. (CN X)

Left recurrent laryngeal n.

Left main bronchus

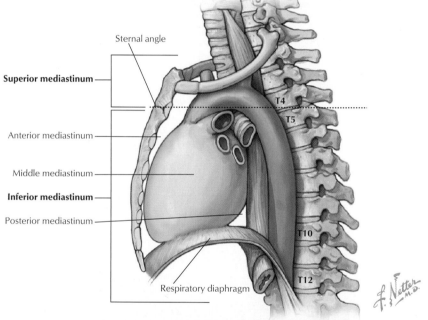

Sternal angle

Superior mediastinum

Anterior mediastinum

Middle mediastinum

Inferior mediastinum

Posterior mediastinum

T4

T5

T10

T12

Respiratory diaphragm

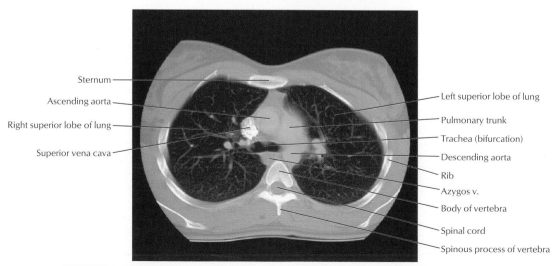

Sternum

Ascending aorta

Right superior lobe of lung

Superior vena cava

Left superior lobe of lung

Pulmonary trunk

Trachea (bifurcation)

Descending aorta

Rib

Azygos v.

Body of vertebra

Spinal cord

Spinous process of vertebra

FIGURE 3.23 Mediastinum. (From *Netter's atlas of human anatomy,* ed 8, Plate 220; S-389.)

Transverse section: level of T7, 3rd interchondral space

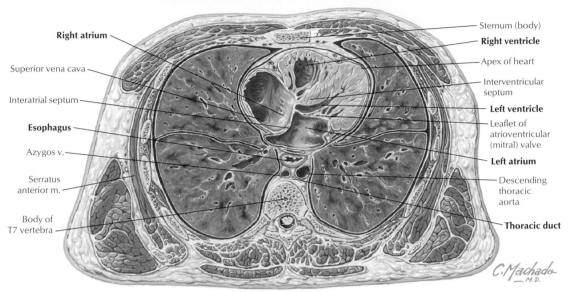

Right atrium

Superior vena cava

Interatrial septum

Esophagus

Azygos v.

Serratus anterior m.

Body of T7 vertebra

Sternum (body)

Right ventricle

Apex of heart

Interventricular septum

Left ventricle

Leaflet of atrioventricular (mitral) valve

Left atrium

Descending thoracic aorta

Thoracic duct

C. Machado M.D.

FIGURE 3.24 Inferior Mediastinum. (From *Netter's atlas of human anatomy,* ed 8, Plate 266; S-538.)

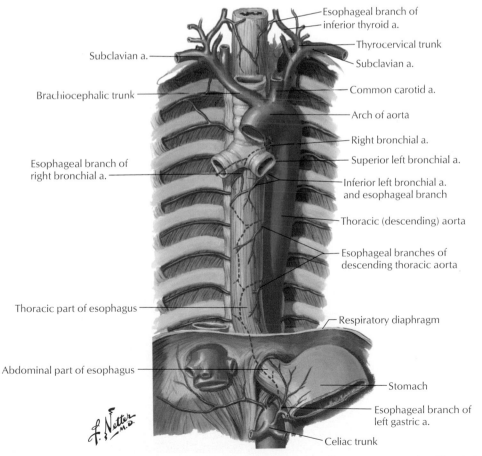

Subclavian a.

Brachiocephalic trunk

Esophageal branch of right bronchial a.

Thoracic part of esophagus

Abdominal part of esophagus

Esophageal branch of inferior thyroid a.

Thyrocervical trunk

Subclavian a.

Common carotid a.

Arch of aorta

Right bronchial a.

Superior left bronchial a.

Inferior left bronchial a. and esophageal branch

Thoracic (descending) aorta

Esophageal branches of descending thoracic aorta

Respiratory diaphragm

Stomach

Esophageal branch of left gastric a.

Celiac trunk

FIGURE 3.25 Esophagus and Thoracic Aorta. (From *Netter's atlas of human anatomy,* ed 8, Plate 258; S-339.)

- **Posterior intercostal arteries:** paired arteries that supply blood to the lower nine intercostal spaces (and their small collateral branches).
- **Superior phrenic arteries:** small arteries to the superior surface of the respiratory diaphragm; anastomose with the musculophrenic and pericardiacophrenic arteries (which arise from the internal thoracic artery).
- **Subcostal arteries:** paired arteries that lie below the inferior margin of the last rib; anastomose with superior epigastric, lower intercostal, and lumbar arteries.

Azygos System of Veins

The azygos venous system drains the posterior thorax and forms an important venous conduit between the **inferior vena cava (IVC)** and **superior vena cava (SVC)** (Fig. 3.26). This system represents the deep venous drainage characteristic of veins throughout the body. Its branches, although variable, largely drain the same regions supplied by the thoracic aorta's branches described earlier. The key veins include the **azygos vein,** with its right ascending lumbar, subcostal, and intercostal tributaries (sometimes the azygos vein also arises from the

IVC before the ascending lumbar and subcostal tributaries join it), the **hemiazygos vein,** and the **accessory hemiazygos vein** (if present, it usually begins at the fourth intercostal space). A small left superior intercostal vein (a tributary of the left brachiocephalic vein) may also connect with the hemiazygos vein. Ultimately, most of the thoracic venous drainage passes into the azygos vein, which ascends right of the midline to empty into the SVC.

Arteriovenous Overview

Arteries of the Thoracic Aorta (Fig. 3.27)

The **heart (1)** gives rise to the **ascending aorta (2),** which receives blood from the left ventricle. The right and left coronary arteries immediately arise from the aorta and supply the heart itself. The **aortic arch (3)** connects the ascending aorta and the **descending aorta (4)** and is found in the superior mediastinum. The descending aorta then continues inferiorly as the **thoracic aorta (5).** The thoracic aorta gives rise to branches to the lungs, esophagus, pericardium, mediastinum, and diaphragm, and also gives rise to posterior intercostal branches to the thoracic wall. The posterior intercostal arteries course along the inferior aspect

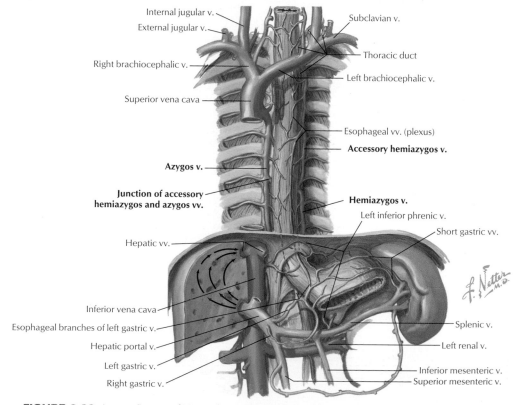

Internal jugular v.
External jugular v.
Right brachiocephalic v.
Superior vena cava
Azygos v.
Junction of accessory hemiazygos and azygos vv.
Hepatic vv.
Inferior vena cava
Esophageal branches of left gastric v.
Hepatic portal v.
Left gastric v.
Right gastric v.

Subclavian v.
Thoracic duct
Left brachiocephalic v.
Esophageal vv. (plexus)
Accessory hemiazygos v.
Hemiazygos v.
Left inferior phrenic v.
Short gastric vv.
Splenic v.
Left renal v.
Inferior mesenteric v.
Superior mesenteric v.

FIGURE 3.26 Azygos System of Veins. (From *Netter's atlas of human anatomy*, ed 8, Plate 259; S-340.)

of each rib (in the costal groove) and supply spinal branches (to the thoracic vertebrae and thoracic spinal cord), small collateral intercostal branches, lateral branches, and branches to the mammary glands. The intercostal arteries anastomose with the anterior intercostal branches from the internal thoracic artery, a branch of the subclavian artery (see Figs. 8.50 and 8.65). The thoracic aorta lies to the left of the thoracic vertebral bodies as it descends

in the thorax, so the left intercostal arteries are shorter than the right intercostal arteries. As it approaches the diaphragm, the aorta shifts closer to the midline of the lower thoracic vertebrae. The lower portion of the esophagus passes anterior to the lower portion of the thoracic aorta **(5)** on its way to the diaphragm and stomach. The thoracic aorta pierces the diaphragm at the level of the T12 vertebra and passes through the aortic hiatus to

Clinical Focus 3.21

Mediastinal Masses

Some of the more common mediastinal masses and their signs and symptoms are noted here.

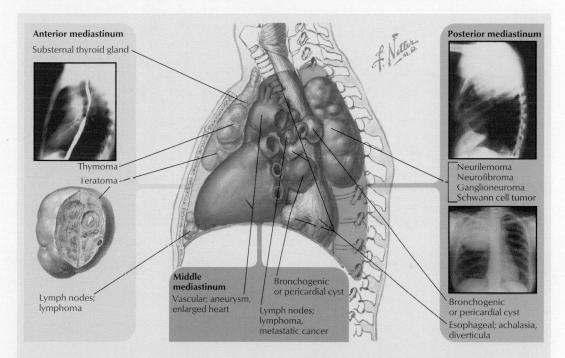

Anterior mediastinum
Substernal thyroid gland
Thymoma
Teratoma
Lymph nodes; lymphoma

Middle mediastinum
Vascular; aneurysm, enlarged heart
Bronchogenic or pericardial cyst
Lymph nodes; lymphoma, metastatic cancer

Posterior mediastinum
Neurilemoma
Neurofibroma
Ganglioneuroma
Schwann cell tumor
Bronchogenic or pericardial cyst
Esophageal; achalasia, diverticula

Types of Mediastinal Masses	
Type of mass	**Comment**
Anterior Mediastinum (retrosternal pain, cough, dyspnea, SVC syndrome, choking sensation)	
Thymoma	Thymus tumors (<50% malignant), often associated with myasthenia gravis
Thyroid mass	Mass that may cause enlarged gland to extend inferiorly and displace trachea
Teratoma	Benign and malignant tumors of totipotent cells, often containing all three germ cell types (ectoderm, mesoderm, and endoderm)
Lymphoma	Hodgkin's, non-Hodgkin's, and primary mediastinal B-cell tumors
Middle Mediastinum (signs and symptoms similar to those of anterior masses)	
Lymph nodes	Enlarged nodes resulting from infections or malignancy
Aortic aneurysm	Aneurysm that is atherosclerotic in origin, may rupture, and can be in any part of the mediastinum
Vascular dilatation	Enlarged pulmonary trunk or cardiomegaly
Cysts	Bronchogenic (at tracheal bifurcation) cysts, pericardial cysts
Posterior Mediastinum (pain, neurologic symptoms, or swallowing difficulty)	
Neurogenic tumors	Tumors of peripheral nerves or sheath cells (e.g., schwannomas)
Esophageal lesions	Diverticula and tumors

1. **Heart (Left Ventricle)***
2. **Ascending Aorta**
3. **Aortic Arch**
4. **Descending Aorta**
5. **Thoracic Aorta**

    Bronchial arteries (branches)

    Esophageal arteries

    Pericardial arteries

    Mediastinal arteries

    Superior phrenic arteries

    Posterior intercostal arteries (lower 9 spaces)

        Dorsal branch

            Medial cutaneous branch

            Lateral cutaneous branch

            Spinal branches

                Postcentral branch

                Prelaminar branch

                Posterior radicular artery

                Anterior radicular artery

                Segmental medullary artery

    Posterior intercostal arteries (cont'd)

        Collateral branch

        Lateral cutaneous branch

        Lateral mammary branches

    Subcostal artery (inferior to rib 12)

        Dorsal branch

        Spinal branch

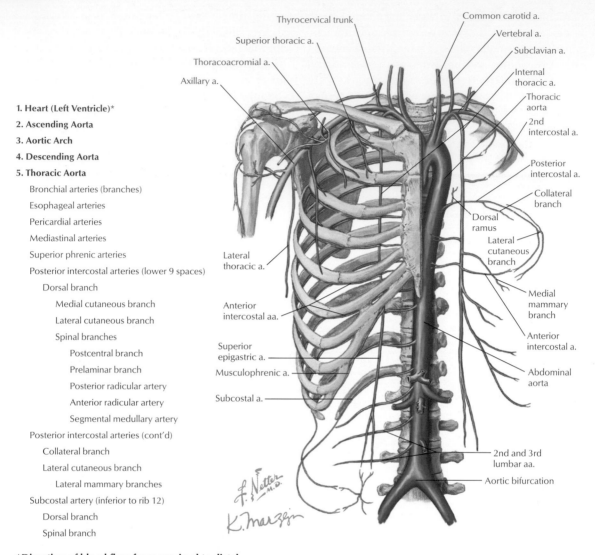

***Direction of blood flow from proximal to distal**

FIGURE 3.27 Arteries of the Thoracic Aorta.

enter the abdominal cavity. The aortic arch gives off very small branches to the aortic body chemoreceptors (not listed in the outline; they function similarly to the carotid body chemoreceptors and are important receptors that monitor blood gas levels and the pH).

Veins of the Thorax (Fig. 3.28)

The venous drainage begins with the **vertebral venous plexus** draining the vertebral column and spinal cord. This plexus includes both an internal and an external vertebral venous plexus. While most of these veins are valveless, recent evidence suggests that some valves do exist in variable numbers in some of these veins. The **posterior intercostal**

veins parallel the posterior intercostal arteries and course in the costal groove at the inferior margin of each rib. The intercostal veins drain largely into **hemiazygos vein (2)** and **azygos vein (3)** in the posterior mediastinum. An **ascending lumbar vein** from the upper abdominal cavity collects venous blood segmentally and often from the left renal vein; it is an important connection between these abdominal caval veins and the azygos system in the thorax. A number of mediastinal veins exist in the posterior mediastinum and drain the diaphragm, pericardium, esophagus, and main bronchi. These veins ultimately drain into the **accessory hemiazygos vein (1)** and **hemiazygos vein (2)** just to the left of the thoracic vertebral bodies or into the **azygos**

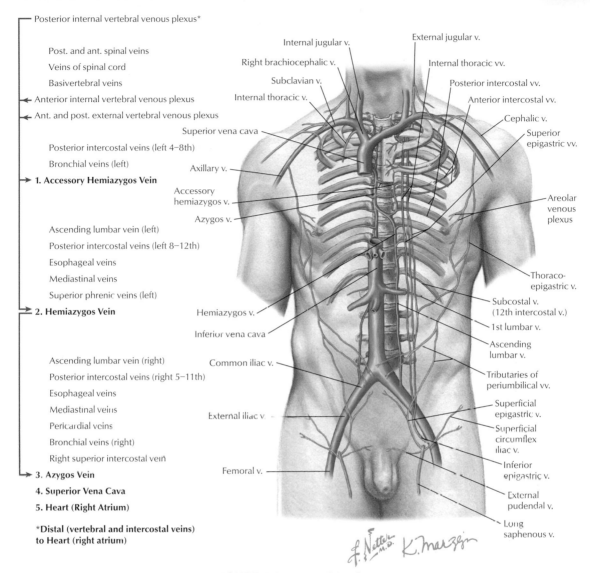

Posterior internal vertebral venous plexus*

Post. and ant. spinal veins
Veins of spinal cord
Basivertebral veins
← Anterior internal vertebral venous plexus
← Ant. and post. external vertebral venous plexus
Superior vena cava
Posterior intercostal veins (left 4–8th)
Bronchial veins (left)
→ **1. Accessory Hemiazygos Vein**

Ascending lumbar vein (left)
Posterior intercostal veins (left 8–12th)
Esophageal veins
Mediastinal veins
Superior phrenic veins (left)
→ **2. Hemiazygos Vein**

Ascending lumbar vein (right)
Posterior intercostal veins (right 5–11th)
Esophageal veins
Mediastinal veins
Pericardial veins
Bronchial veins (right)
Right superior intercostal vein
→ **3. Azygos Vein**
4. Superior Vena Cava
5. Heart (Right Atrium)

*Distal (vertebral and intercostal veins)
to Heart (right atrium)

Internal jugular v.
Right brachiocephalic v.
Subclavian v.
Internal thoracic v.
Axillary v.
Accessory hemiazygos v.
Azygos v.
Hemiazygos v.
Inferior vena cava
Common iliac v.
External iliac v.
Femoral v.

External jugular v.
Internal thoracic vv.
Posterior intercostal vv.
Anterior intercostal vv.
Cephalic v.
Superior epigastric vv.
Areolar venous plexus
Thoraco-epigastric v.
Subcostal v. (12th intercostal v.)
1st lumbar v.
Ascending lumbar v.
Tributaries of periumbilical vv.
Superficial epigastric v.
Superficial circumflex iliac v.
Inferior epigastric v.
External pudendal v.
Long saphenous v.

FIGURE 3.28 Veins of the Thorax.

vein **(3)** just to the right of the vertebral bodies. About midway in the thorax, the hemiazygos vein crosses the midline and drains into the **azygos vein (3),** although the hemiazygos usually maintains its connection with the accessory **hemiazygos vein** as well. Veins tend to connect with one another where possible, and many connections are small, variable, and not readily recognizable. The azygos vein delivers venous blood to the **superior vena cava (4)** just before the SVC enters the **right atrium of the heart (5).** The accessory **hemiazygos vein** also often has connections with the left brachiocephalic vein, providing another venous pathway back to the right side of the heart. Flow in the azygos system of veins is pressure dependent; because the veins are essentially valveless, the flow can go in either direction. As with other regional veins, the number of veins of the azygos system can be variable.

Thoracic Lymphatics

The thoracic lymphatic duct begins in the abdomen at the **cisterna chyli** (found between the abdominal aorta and the right crus of the diaphragm) (Figs. 3.29 and 4.41), ascends through the posterior mediastinum posterior to the esophagus, crosses to the left of the median plane at approximately the T5-T6 vertebral level, and empties into the venous system at the junction of the left internal jugular and left subclavian veins. Lymph from the left hemithorax and left lung generally drains into tributaries that empty into the thoracic duct. Lymph from the right hemithorax and right lung usually

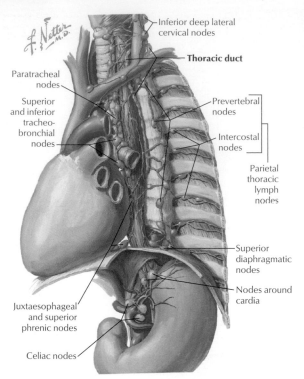

FIGURE 3.29 Mediastinal Lymphatics. (From *Netter's atlas of human anatomy,* ed 8, Plate 260; S-351.)

drains into the right lymphatic duct, which empties into the venous system at the junction of the right subclavian and right internal jugular veins (see Fig. 1.16 and Fig. 3.12.)

7. EMBRYOLOGY

Respiratory System

The airway and lungs begin developing during the fourth week of gestation. Key features of this development include the following (Fig. 3.30):

- Formation of the endodermal **laryngotracheal diverticulum** from the ventral foregut, just inferior to the last pair of pharyngeal pouches
- Division of the laryngotracheal diverticulum into the **left and right lung (bronchial) buds,** each with a primary bronchus
- Division of the lung buds to form the definitive lobes of the lungs (three lobes in the right lung, two lobes in the left lung)
- Formation of segmental bronchi and 10 bronchopulmonary segments in each lung (by weeks 6 to 7)

The airway passages are lined by epithelium derived from the **endoderm of the foregut,** while

mesoderm forms the stroma of each lung. By 6 months of gestation, the alveoli are mature enough for gas exchange, but the production of **surfactant,** which reduces surface tension and helps prevent alveolar collapse, may not be sufficient to support respiration. A premature infant's ability to keep its airways open often is the limiting factor if the premature birth occurs before functional surfactant cells (type II pneumocytes) are present.

Early Embryonic Vasculature

Toward the end of the third week of development, the embryo establishes a primitive vascular system to meet its growing needs for oxygen and nutrients (Fig. 3.31). Blood leaving the embryonic heart enters a series of paired arteries called the **aortic arches,** which are associated with the pharyngeal arches. The blood then flows from these arches into the single midline **aorta** (formed by the fusion of two dorsal aortas), coursing along the length of the embryo. Some of the blood enters the **vitelline arteries** to supply the future bowel (still the yolk sac at this stage), and some passes to the placenta via a pair of **umbilical arteries,** where gases, nutrients, and metabolic wastes are exchanged.

Blood returning from the placenta is oxygenated and carries nutrients back to the heart through the single **umbilical vein.** Blood also returns to the heart through the following veins:

- **Vitelline veins:** drain blood from yolk sac; will become the **portal system** draining the gastrointestinal tract through the liver.
- **Cardinal veins:** form the **superior vena cava** and **inferior vena cava** (and azygos system of veins) and their tributaries; they will become the **caval system** of venous return.

Aortic Arches

Blood pumped from the primitive embryonic heart passes into **aortic arches** that are associated with the pharyngeal arches (Fig. 3.32). The right and left dorsal aortas caudal to the pharyngeal arches fuse to form the single midline aorta, while the aortic arches give rise to the arteries summarized in Table 3.14. Note that the third, fourth, and sixth pairs of embryonic aortic arches are the major contributors to arteries that will persist in the fetus and neonate.

Development of Embryonic Heart Tube and Heart Chambers

The primitive heart begins its development as a single unfolded tube, much like an artery develops

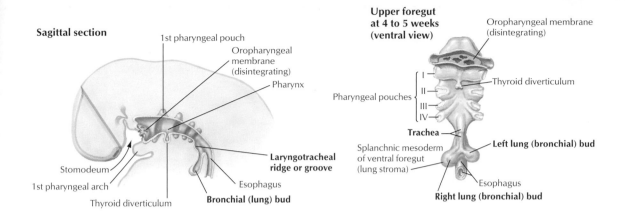

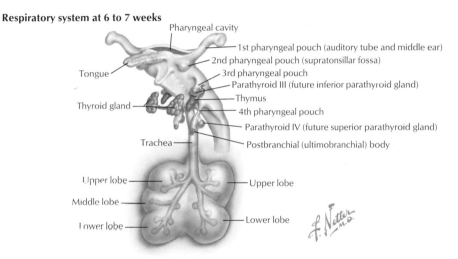

FIGURE 3.30 Embryology of the Respiratory System.

TABLE 3.14 Aortic Arch Derivatives

ARCH	DERIVATIVE
1	Largely disappears (part of maxillary artery in head)
2	Largely disappears (stapedial artery in middle ear)
3	Common carotid and proximal internal carotid arteries
4	Brachiocephalic artery and proximal right subclavian artery and on the left side a small portion of the aortic arch
5	Disappears
6	Ductus arteriosus and proximal portions of both pulmonary arteries

(Fig. 3.33). The **heart tube** receives blood from the embryonic body, which passes through its heart tube segments in the following sequence:

- **Sinus venosus:** receives all the venous return from the embryonic body and placenta.

- **Atrium:** early on it is a single chamber that receives blood from the sinus venosus and passes it to the ventricle.
- **Ventricle:** early on it is a single chamber that receives atrial blood and passes it to the bulbus cordis.
- **Bulbus cordis:** receives ventricular blood and passes it to the truncus arteriosus.
- **Truncus arteriosus:** receives blood from the bulbus cordis and passes it to the aortic arch system for distribution to the lungs and body.

This primitive heart tube soon begins to fold on itself in an "S-bend." The single ventricular chamber folds downward and to the right, and the single atrium and sinus venosus fold upward, posteriorly and to the left, thus forming the definitive positions of the heart's future chambers (atria superior to the ventricles) (Fig. 3.33 and Table 3.15).

The four chambers of the heart (two atria and two ventricles) are formed by the internal septation

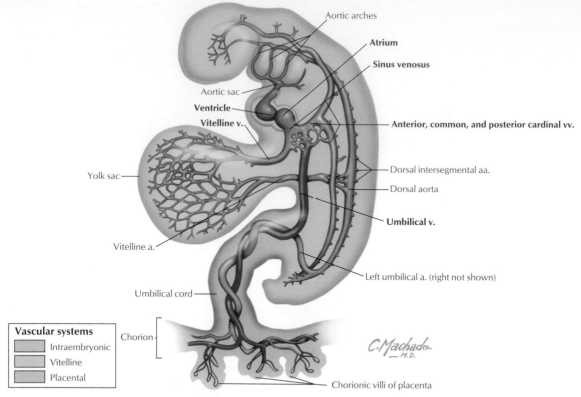

FIGURE 3.31 Early Embryonic Vasculature.

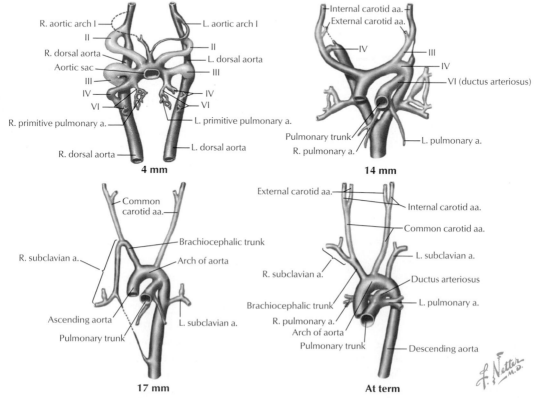

FIGURE 3.32 Sequential Development of Aortic Arch Derivatives (Color-Coded).

Heart tube primordia

Aortic arches (AA)

Truncus arteriosus (TA) — ⎡ Ascending aorta
⎣ Pulmonary trunk

Bulbus cordis (BC) — ⎡ Aortic vestibule of left ventricle
⎣ Conus arteriosus of right ventricle

Ventricle (V) — Trabecular walls of left and right ventricles

Atrium (A) — Auricles/pectinate muscle walls of left
and right atria (smooth wall of left
atrium from pulmonary veins)

Sinus venosus (SV) — ⎡ Coronary sinus
⎣ Smooth wall of right atrium

C. Machado
—M.D.

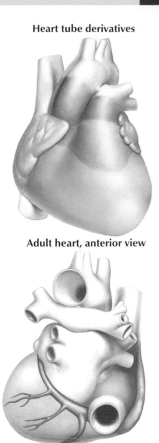

Heart tube derivatives

Adult heart, anterior view

Adult heart, posterior view

FIGURE 3.33 Primitive Heart Tube Formation.

TABLE 3.15 Adult Heart Derivatives of Embryonic Heart Tube

STRUCTURE	DERIVATIVES
Truncus arteriosus	Ascending aorta
	Pulmonary trunk
Bulbus cordis	Smooth part of right ventricle (conus arteriosus)
	Smooth part of left ventricle (aortic vestibule)
Primitive ventricle	Trabeculated part of right ventricle
	Trabeculated part of left ventricle
Primitive atrium	Pectinate wall of right atrium
	Pectinate wall of left atrium
Sinus venosus	Smooth part of right atrium (sinus venarum)*
	Coronary sinus
	Oblique vein of left atrium

From Dudek R: *High-yield embryology: a collaborative project of medical students and faculty*, Philadelphia, 2006, Lippincott Williams & Wilkins.

*The smooth part of the left atrium is formed by incorporation of parts of the pulmonary veins into the atrial wall. The junction of the pectinated and smooth parts of the right atrium is called the *crista terminalis*.

of the single atrium and ventricle of the primitive heart tube. Because most of the blood does not perfuse the lungs *in utero* (the lungs are filled with amniotic fluid and are partially collapsed), most of the blood in the right atrium passes directly to the left atrium via a small opening in the interatrial septum called the **foramen ovale.** The **interatrial septum** is formed by the fusion of a septum primum and a septum secundum (the septum secundum develops on the right atrial side of the septum primum) (Fig. 3.34). Shortly after birth, when the pressure of the left atrium exceeds that of the right atrium (blood now passes into the lungs and returns to the left atrium, raising the pressure on the left side), the two septae are pushed together and fuse, thus forming the **fossa ovalis** of the postnatal heart. While the interatrial septum is forming, the **ventricular septum** forms from the superior growth of the muscular interventricular septum from the base of the heart's common ventricle toward the downward growth of a thin membranous septum from the endocardial cushion (Fig. 3.35).

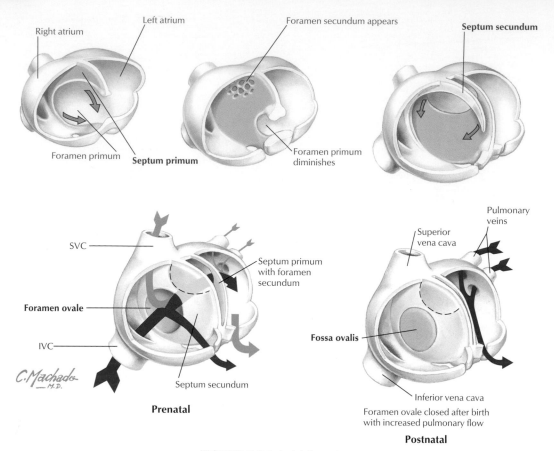

FIGURE 3.34 Atrial Septation.

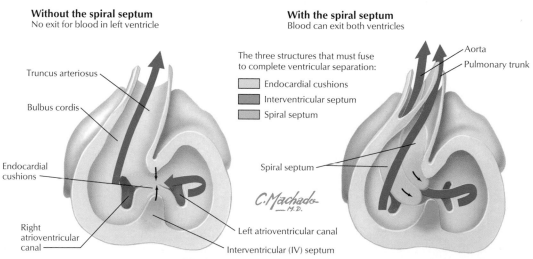

FIGURE 3.35 Ventricular Septation.

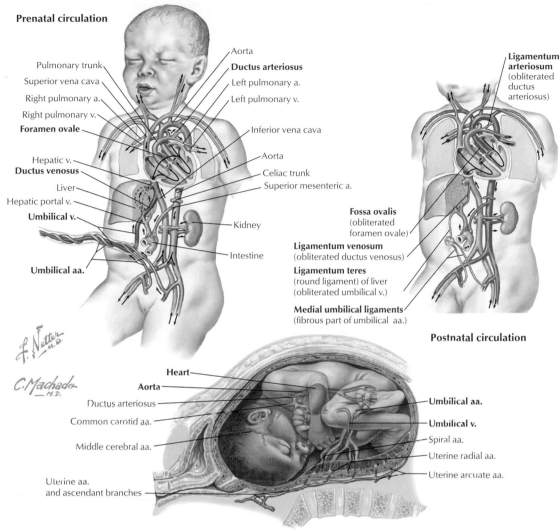

Prenatal circulation

Aorta
Pulmonary trunk
Ductus arteriosus
Superior vena cava
Left pulmonary a.
Right pulmonary a.
Left pulmonary v.
Right pulmonary v.
Foramen ovale
Inferior vena cava
Aorta
Hepatic v.
Celiac trunk
Ductus venosus
Superior mesenteric a.
Liver
Hepatic portal v.
Umbilical v.
Kidney
Intestine
Umbilical aa.

Ligamentum arteriosum
(obliterated ductus arteriosus)

Fossa ovalis
(obliterated foramen ovale)
Ligamentum venosum
(obliterated ductus venosus)
Ligamentum teres
(round ligament) of liver
(obliterated umbilical v.)
Medial umbilical ligaments
(fibrous part of umbilical aa.)

Postnatal circulation

Heart
Aorta
Ductus arteriosus
Common carotid aa.
Middle cerebral aa.
Uterine aa.
and ascendant branches

Umbilical aa.
Umbilical v.
Spiral aa.
Uterine radial aa.
Uterine arcuate aa.

FIGURE 3.36 Fetal Circulation Pattern and Changes at Birth. (From *Netter's atlas of human anatomy*, ed 8, Plate 247; S-305.)

Simultaneously, the **bulbus cordis** and **truncus arteriosus** form the outflow tracts of the ventricles, pulmonary trunk, and aorta. The neural crest plays a key role in the septation and development of the truncus arteriosus as it becomes the pulmonary trunk and ascending aorta.

Fetal Circulation

The pattern of fetal circulation is one of gas exchange and nutrient/metabolic waste exchange across the placenta with the maternal blood (but not the exchange of blood cells), and distribution of oxygen and nutrient-rich blood to the tissues of the fetus

(Fig. 3.36). Various shunts allow fetal blood to largely bypass the liver (not needed for metabolic processing *in utero*) and lungs (not needed for gas exchange *in utero*) so that the blood may gain direct access to the left side of the heart and be pumped into the fetal arterial system. At or shortly after birth, these shunts close, resulting in the normal pattern of pulmonary and systemic circulation observed postnatally. Figure 3.36 highlights these changes and the adult "reminders" that persist in us of our prenatal existence (see the labels associated with **"Postnatal circulation"** in the right image of the figure).

Clinical Focus 3.22

Ventricular Septal Defect

Ventricular septal defect (VSD) is the most common congenital heart defect, representing about 30% of all heart defects. Approximately 80% of cases are **perimembranous** (occur where the muscular septum and membranous septum of the endocardial cushion should fuse). This results in a **left-to-right shunt**, which may precipitate congestive heart failure. The repair illustrated in the figure is through the right atrial approach.

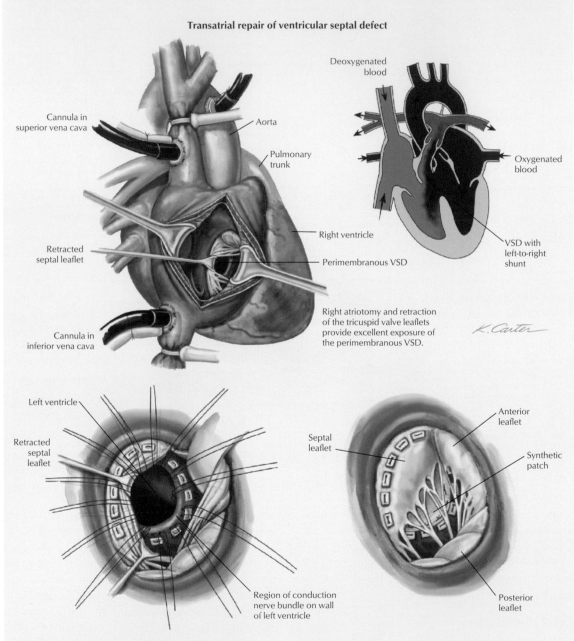

Transatrial repair of ventricular septal defect

Cannula in superior vena cava

Aorta

Pulmonary trunk

Deoxygenated blood

Oxygenated blood

Right ventricle

Perimembranous VSD

VSD with left-to-right shunt

Retracted septal leaflet

Cannula in inferior vena cava

Right atriotomy and retraction of the tricuspid valve leaflets provide excellent exposure of the perimembranous VSD.

K. Carter

Left ventricle

Retracted septal leaflet

Region of conduction nerve bundle on wall of left ventricle

Septal leaflet

Anterior leaflet

Synthetic patch

Posterior leaflet

The septal leaflet of the tricuspid valve may need to be bisected to permit placement of pledgetted sutures at its junction with the VSD. Superficial sutures are placed along the inferior border of the VSD to prevent injury to the conduction system.

The VSD is closed with a synthetic patch and pledgetted sutures. The septal leaflet, if detached, is then repaired with a running suture.

Clinical Focus 3.23

Atrial Septal Defect

Atrial septal defects make up approximately 10% to 15% of congenital cardiac anomalies. Most of these defects are **ostium secundum defects** from incomplete closure of the **foramen ovale**. Larger defects may require a patch that is sutured into place. For smaller atrial septal defects, a percutaneous transcatheter approach using a septal occluder can be deployed and secured. By threading the catheter through the IVC, the catheter is positioned to pass directly into the atrial defect, as shown below, and is then deployed.

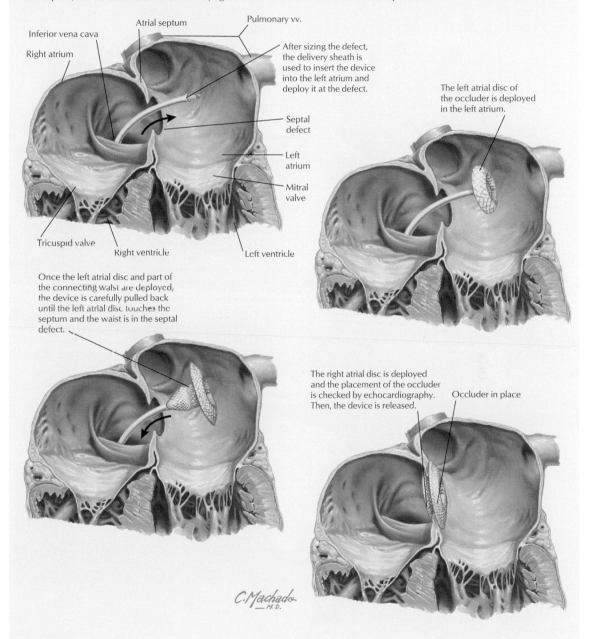

The Amplatzer Septal Occluder is deployed from its delivery sheath, forming two discs, one for either side of the septum, and a central waist available in varying diameters to seat on the rims of the atrial septal defect.

Inferior vena cava

Right atrium

Atrial septum

Pulmonary vv.

After sizing the defect, the delivery sheath is used to insert the device into the left atrium and deploy it at the defect.

Septal defect

Left atrium

Mitral valve

Tricuspid valve

Right ventricle

Left ventricle

The left atrial disc of the occluder is deployed in the left atrium.

Once the left atrial disc and part of the connecting waist are deployed, the device is carefully pulled back until the left atrial disc touches the septum and the waist is in the septal defect.

The right atrial disc is deployed and the placement of the occluder is checked by echocardiography. Then, the device is released.

Occluder in place

C. Machado
_M.D.

Clinical Focus 3.24

Patent Ductus Arteriosus

Patent ductus arteriosus (PDA) is failure of the ductus arteriosus to close shortly after birth. This results in a postnatal shunt of blood from the **aorta into the pulmonary trunk,** which may lead to congestive heart failure. PDA accounts for approximately 10% of congenital heart defects and can be treated medically (or surgically if necessary). Surgical treatment is by direct ligation or a less invasive, catheter-based device that is threaded through the vasculature and positioned to occlude the PDA. Often, children with a PDA may be fine until they become more active and then experience trouble breathing when exercising and demonstrate a failure to thrive. A continuous murmur usually is evident over the left sternal border to just below the clavicle (see Clinical Focus 3.17).

Patent ductus arteriosus

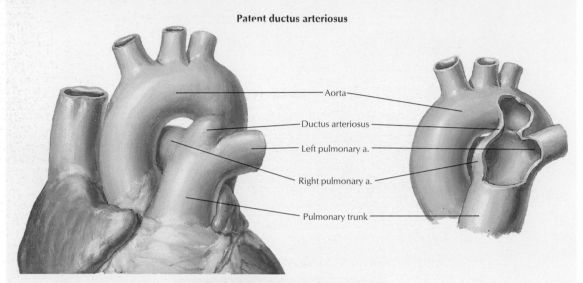

Aorta

Ductus arteriosus

Left pulmonary a.

Right pulmonary a.

Pulmonary trunk

Pathophysiology of patent ductus arteriosus

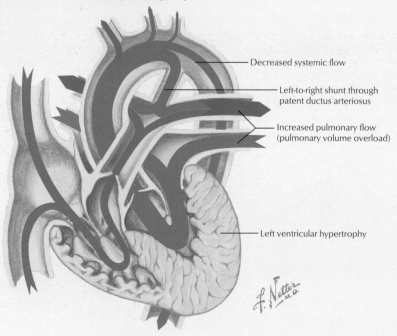

Decreased systemic flow

Left-to-right shunt through patent ductus arteriosus

Increased pulmonary flow (pulmonary volume overload)

Left ventricular hypertrophy

Clinical Focus 3.25

Repair of Tetralogy of Fallot

Tetralogy of Fallot usually results from a maldevelopment of the spiral septum that normally divides the truncus arteriosus into the pulmonary trunk and aorta. This defect involves the following:

- Pulmonary stenosis or narrowing of the right ventricular outflow tract
- Overriding (transposed) aorta
- Right ventricular hypertrophy
- Ventricular septal defect (VSD)

Surgical repair is done on cardiopulmonary bypass to close the VSD and provide unobstructed flow into the pulmonary trunk. The stenotic pulmonary outflow tract is widened by inserting a patch into the wall (pericardial), thus increasing the volume of the subpulmonic stenosis and/or the pulmonary artery stenosis.

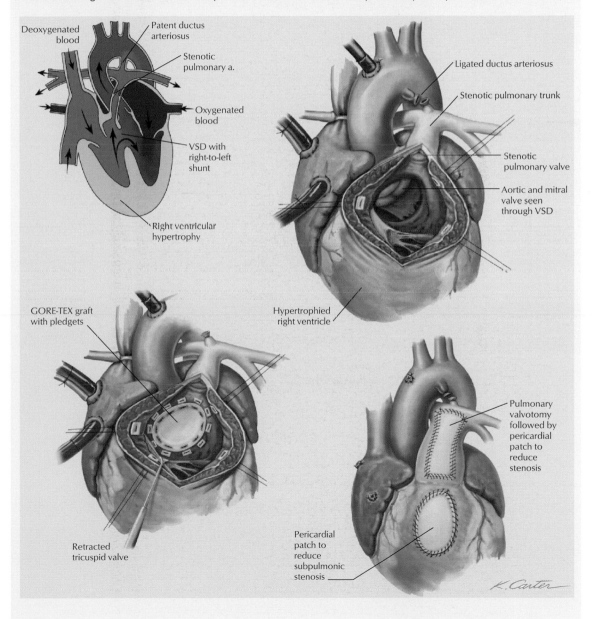

Deoxygenated blood

Patent ductus arteriosus

Stenotic pulmonary a.

Oxygenated blood

VSD with right-to-left shunt

Right ventricular hypertrophy

Ligated ductus arteriosus

Stenotic pulmonary trunk

Stenotic pulmonary valve

Aortic and mitral valve seen through VSD

Hypertrophied right ventricle

GORE-TEX graft with pledgets

Retracted tricuspid valve

Pulmonary valvotomy followed by pericardial patch to reduce stenosis

Pericardial patch to reduce subpulmonic stenosis

K. Carter

Clinical Focus

Available Online

3.26 Hemothorax

3.27 Chronic Cough

3.28 Pneumonia

3.29 Cardiovascular Disease (Elderly and Women)

3.30 Saphenous Vein Graft Disease

3.31 Infective Endocarditis

3.32 Mitral Valve Prolapse

3.33 Ventricular Tachycardia

3.34 Chylothorax

3.35 Coarctation of the Aorta

 Additional figures available online (see inside front cover for details).

Challenge Yourself Questions

1. During open-heart surgery, the pericardial sac is cut open by a longitudinal incision. If a horizontal incision is used, which of the following structures might be transected?

   A. Azygos vein
   B. Inferior vena cava
   C. Internal thoracic artery
   D. Phrenic nerves
   E. Vagus nerves

2. A small, thin, 4-year-old boy presents with an audible continuous murmur that is heard near the left proximal clavicle and is present throughout the cardiac cycle. The murmur is louder in systole than diastole. Which of the following conditions is most likely the cause of this murmur?

   A. Atrial septal defect
   B. Mitral stenosis
   C. Patent ductus arteriosus
   D. Right ventricular hypertrophy
   E. Ventricular septal defect

3. A 61-year-old man presents with severe chest pain and a rhythmic pulsation over the left midclavicular, fifth intercostal space. Which portion of the heart is most likely responsible for this pulsation?

   A. Aortic arch
   B. Apex of the heart
   C. Mitral valve
   D Pulmonary valve
   E. Right atrium

4. After a boating accident, a young child needs a tracheotomy because of injuries to his upper body. Which of the following structures is most at risk for injury during this procedure?

   A. Left brachiocephalic vein
   B. Phrenic nerve
   C. Thoracic duct
   D. Thymus gland
   E. Vagus nerve

5. A coronary artery angiogram for a patient about to undergo coronary bypass surgery shows significant blockage of a vessel that supplies the right and left bundle branches of the heart's conduction system. Which of the following arteries is most likely involved?

   A. Anterior interventricular
   B. Circumflex
   C. Posterior interventricular
   D. Right marginal
   E. Sinuatrial nodal branch

6. An infant presents with left-to-right shunting of blood and evidence of pulmonary hypertension. Which of the following conditions is most likely responsible for this condition?

   A. Atrial septal defect
   B. Mitral stenosis
   C. Patent ductus arteriosus
   D. Patent ductus venosus
   E. Ventricular septal defect

7. An elderly woman presents with valvular stenosis and a particularly loud first heart sound (S_1). Which of the following heart valves are responsible for the S_1 sound?

   A. Aortic and mitral
   B. Aortic and tricuspid
   C. Mitral and tricuspid
   D. Pulmonary and aortic
   E. Tricuspid and pulmonary

8. Endoscopic examination of a 52-year-old man with a history of smoking reveals a malignancy in the right main bronchus. Which of the following lymph structures will most likely be infiltrated first by cancerous cells emanating from this malignancy?

   A. Bronchomediastinal trunk
   B. Bronchopulmonary (hilar) nodes
   C. Inferior tracheobronchial (carinal) nodes
   D. Intrapulmonary nodes
   E. Right paratracheal nodes

 Multiple-choice and short-answer review questions available online; see inside front cover for details.

9. Auscultation of the lungs of a 31-year-old woman reveals crackles heard on the back along the right medial border of the scapula, just above the inferior scapular angle, during late inspiration. Which of the following lobes are most likely involved in this pathology?

   A. Lower lobe of the right lung
   B. Lower lobes of both lungs
   C. Middle lobe of the right lung
   D. Upper lobe of the right lung
   E. Upper lobes of both lungs

10. A penetrating injury in the lower left neck just superior to the medial third of the clavicle results in the collapse of the left lung. Which of the following respiratory structures was most likely injured, resulting in this pneumothorax?

    A. Costal pleura
    B. Cupula
    C. Left main bronchus
    D. Left posterior lobe
    E. Mediastinal parietal pleura

For each condition described below (11-16), select the cardiac feature from the list (A-O) that is most likely responsible.

(A) Aortic valve
(B) Chordae tendineae
(C) Conus arteriosus
(D) Crista terminalis
(E) Fossa ovalis
(F) Membranous ventricular septum
(G) Mitral valve
(H) Moderator band
(I) Opening of coronary sinus
(J) Papillary muscles
(K) Pectinate muscle
(L) Pulmonary valve
(M) Sinuatrial node
(N) Trabeculae carneae
(O) Tricuspid valve

_____ 11. During strenuous exercise, this feature of the right ventricle ensures coordinated contraction of the anterior papillary muscle.

_____ 12. An implantable cardiac defibrillator can function as a pacemaker should this structure be unable to initiate the normal cardiac rhythm.

_____ 13. Most atrial septal defects occur at this site.

_____ 14. Some of the venous blood returning to the right atrium gains access through this feature.

_____ 15. Radiographic contrast imaging of the heart highlights this roughened internal feature of each ventricular wall.

_____ 16. This feature is the postnatal manifestation of the primitive embryonic atrial cardiac muscle.

17. A 67-year-old man experiences chest pain indicative of angina pectoris and myocardial ischemia. The visceral sensory neurons mediating this pain would most likely be found in which of the following locations?

    A. Intermediolateral gray matter of the upper thorax spinal cord
    B. Medial brachial cutaneous nerve
    C. Spinal dorsal root ganglion of T1-T2
    D. Sympathetic chain ganglia
    E. Vagal sensory ganglion

18. Cardiomyopathy results in the enlargement of the left atrium. Which of the following structures is most likely to be compressed by this expansion?

    A. Azygos vein
    B. Esophagus
    C. Left pulmonary artery
    D. Superior vena cava
    E. Sympathetic trunk

19. A woman is diagnosed with metastatic breast cancer with lymph node involvement. Most of the lymphatic drainage of the breast passes to which of the following lymph nodes?

    A. Abdominal
    B. Axillary
    C. Infraclavicular
    D. Parasternal
    E. Pulmonary

20. The sternal angle (of Louis) is an important clinical surface landmark on the anterior chest wall, dividing the thorax into the superior and inferior mediastinum. Which of the following features also is found at the level of the sternal angle?

    A. Articulation of first rib
    B. Azygos vein
    C. Descending aorta
    D. Sinuatrial node
    E. Tracheal bifurcation

21. A 6-year-old boy is diagnosed with decreased blood flow into the proximal descending thoracic aorta. His left brachial arterial pressure is significantly increased and his femoral pressure is decreased. Which of the following embryonic structures has failed to develop normally?

    A. 2nd aortic arch
    B. 3rd aortic arch
    C. 4th aortic arch
    D. 5th aortic arch
    E. 6th aortic arch

22. A 27-year-old comatose anorexic woman is admitted to the emergency department. A nasogastric tube is inserted and passed into her esophagus. What will be the *last* resistance point felt by the physician as the tube passes from the nose into the stomach?

    A. Esophageal hiatus of the diaphragm
    B. Level of the superior thoracic aperture
    C. Posterior to the aortic arch
    D. Posterior to the left atrium
    E. Posterior to the left main bronchus

23. A 68-year-old man is scheduled to have coronary bypass surgery to the inferior (posterior descending) interventricular artery. As this procedure is performed, which of the following vessels is most at risk of injury?

    A. Anterior cardiac vein
    B. Coronary sinus
    C. Great cardiac vein
    D. Middle cardiac vein
    E. Small cardiac vein

24. A 3-year-old girl undergoes corrective surgery to repair a small ventricular septal defect (VSD). To gain access to the site, an incision is made in the anterior surface of the right atrium so instruments may be inserted through the tricuspid valve to repair the VSD. Which of the following structures is the most important to protect as the incision is made in the right atrium?

    A. Anterior papillary muscle
    B. Crista terminalis
    C. Coronary sinus
    D. Pectinate muscles
    E. Valve of the inferior vena cava

25. A 63-year-old man is admitted to the hospital with a myocardial infarction and cardiac tamponade. An emergency pericardiocentesis is ordered to draw off the blood in the pericardial cavity. At which of the following locations will a needle be inserted to perform this procedure?

    A. Left fourth intercostal space in the midaxillary line
    B. Left fifth intercostal space just lateral to the sternum
    C. Just to the right of the xiphoid process
    D. Right third intercostal space 1 inch from the sternum
    E. Right seventh intercostal space 1 inch from the sternum

26. A robbery victim receives a stab injury to the thoracic wall in the area of the right fourth costal cartilage. Which of the following pulmonary structures is present at the site of this injury?

    A. Apex of the lung
    B. Horizontal fissure of the lung
    C. Lingula
    D. Oblique fissure of the lung
    E. Pulmonary ligament

27. A 37-year-old man is admitted to the hospital with a blood pressure measurement of 84/46 mm Hg. A central venous line is placed, and subsequent radiographic imaging detects a chylothorax. Which of the following structures was most likely accidently damaged during this procedure?

    A. Anterior jugular vein
    B. Left proximal external jugular vein
    C. Origin of left brachiocephalic vein
    D. Right external jugular vein
    E. Right subclavian vein

28. A 24-year-old distance runner is admitted to the hospital with severe dyspnea and an acute asthma attack. A bronchodilating drug is administered. Which of the following components of the nervous system must be inhibited by this drug to achieve relaxation of the tracheobronchial smooth muscle?

    A. Postganglionic parasympathetic fibers
    B. Postganglionic sympathetic fibers
    C. Preganglionic sympathetic fibers
    D. Somatic efferent fibers
    E. Visceral afferent fibers

29. A 3-year-old girl aspirates a small peanut and begins coughing and choking. In which component of the tracheobronchial tree is the peanut most likely lodged?

    A. Carina of the trachea
    B. Left main bronchus
    C. Left tertiary bronchus
    D. Proximal trachea
    E. Right main bronchus

30. An examination of a 51-year-old woman shows an orange-peel appearance of her skin on her breast, a tumor in the right upper outer quadrant of her breast, and several deep dimples in the skin over the site of the tumor. Which of the following breast structures is responsible for the deep dimpling of her skin?

    A. Inflammation of her lactiferous ducts
    B. Intraductal obstruction from the cancer
    C. Invasion of the tumor into her retromammary space
    D. Obstruction of her axillary lymphatics
    E. Retraction of her suspensory retinacula

31. A 58-year-old man presents with dyspnea. Examination reveals a mitral valve prolapse. At which of the following locations is auscultation of this valve best performed?

    A. Above the medial third of the left clavicle
    B. Directly over the sternal angle
    C. At the left fifth intercostal space, just below the nipple
    D. At the left second intercostal space, just lateral to the sternum
    E. At the right second intercostal space, just lateral to the sternum

32. A 56-year-old woman undergoes an aortic valve replacement and is connected to a heart-lung machine. The surgeon explores her oblique pericardial sinus and is able to palpate each of the following structures except one. Which structure is not routinely palpable from this perspective?

    A. Inferior left pulmonary vein
    B. Inferior right pulmonary vein
    C. Inferior vena cava
    D. Right atrium
    E. Superior vena cava

For each statement below (33 to 37), select the nerve or nerve fibers that are most likely responsible for the function described or the disorder caused (i.e., the single best answer).

(A) Greater splanchnic nerve
(B) Left recurrent laryngeal nerve
(C) Phrenic nerve
(D) Posterior ramus of a spinal nerve
(E) Postganglionic sympathetic fibers
(F) Right recurrent laryngeal nerve
(G) Somatic afferent fibers
(H) Somatic efferent fibers
(I) Sympathetic trunk
(J) Vagus nerve

_____ 33. Causes contraction of the internal intercostal muscles.

_____ 34. Carries nerve fibers that monitor baroreflexes and chemoreflexes.

_____ 35. Travels to the heart in cervical cardiac nerves.

_____ 36. Consists of a bilateral chain of ganglia.

_____ 37. Carries referred pain from the respiratory diaphragm.

For questions 38 to 40, select the feature shown in the chest radiograph that best satisfies the condition described.

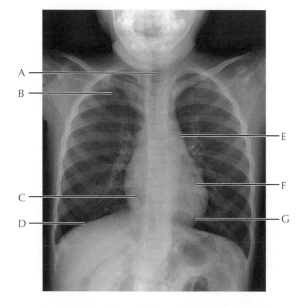

_____ 38. Blood from this heart chamber next passes through the tricuspid valve.

_____ 39. Proximal narrowing of this structure can reduce the blood flow to the left subclavian artery.

_____ 40. The mitral valve can best be auscultated over this structure.

Chapter 3: Thorax

1. **D.** The phrenic nerves course from superior to inferior along the lateral sides of the pericardium, anterior to the root structures entering or leaving the lungs. A longitudinal incision would run parallel to these nerves while a horizontal incision might potentially run across the nerves, unless the surgeon is very careful.

2. **C.** This continuous murmur is caused by the sound of blood rushing through a patent ductus arteriosus from the aorta into the pulmonary trunk (higher-pressure to lower-pressure vessel). This is best heard over the left proximal clavicular area. Normally, the ductus narrows and closes shortly after birth to form the ligamentum arteriosum.

3. **B.** The apex (lower left ventricle) of the heart lies in the left midclavicular line at the fifth intercostal space. Its forceful contraction as it pumps blood into the aorta and systemic circulation is easily heard over this area.

4. **A.** The left brachiocephalic vein passes across the trachea and is very near the sixth cervical vertebra; moreover, in a young child it can lie above the level of the manubrium of the sternum. A tracheotomy is made below the cricoid cartilage and thyroid gland and just superior to this vein at about the level of the C6 vertebra.

5. **A.** The major blood supply to the interventricular septum and the right and left bundle branches is by the left anterior descending (LAD, or anterior interventricular) coronary artery. The posterior interventricular branch supplies the remainder of the interventricular septum.

6. **E.** Ventricular septal defects (VSDs) are the most common congenital heart defect. The shunting of blood from the left to right ventricle results in right ventricular hypertrophy and pulmonary hypertension.

7. **C.** The first heart sound is made by the closing of the two atrioventricular valves (tricuspid and mitral valves). The stenosis (narrowing) most likely involves the mitral valve.

8. **C.** The "carinal" nodes are located at the inferior aspect of the tracheal bifurcation and would be the first nodes involved as lymph moves from the hilar nodes to the carinal nodes.

9. **A.** At this position on the right side of the back, the inferior (lower) lobe of the right lung would be the location of the crackles (see Fig. 3.10). The oblique fissure dividing the right lung into superior and inferior lobes begins posteriorly at the level of the T2-T3 vertebral spine, well above this level.

10. **B.** The cupula is the dome of cervical pleura surrounding the apex of the lung and it extends above the medial portion of the clavicle and the first rib.

11. **H.** The moderator band (septomarginal trabecula) extends from the lower interventricular septum to the base of the anterior papillary muscle in the right ventricle. It conveys the right AV bundle to this distal papillary muscle and probably assists in its coordinated contraction.

12. **M.** The "pacemaker" of the heart is the sinuatrial or SA node. It initiates the action potential that will pass through the atria and down into the AV node and then the ventricles.

13. **E.** Most atrial septal defects (ASDs) occur at the site of the foramen ovale in the fetal heart (fossa ovalis). If the foramen ovale (foramen secundum) remains open after birth, blood can pass from the left atrium into the right atrium.

14. **I.** Venous blood returning from the coronary circulation returns to the right atrium via the coronary sinus. Obviously, the SVC and IVC also return venous blood to the right atrium, but these two vessels are not listed as options.

15. **N.** The roughened appearance of the muscular bundles of the ventricular walls is called the trabeculae carneae (fleshy woody beams).

16. **K.** The roughened muscular walls of the atria (pectinate muscle) represent the "true" embryonic atrium; the smooth portion of each atrium is derived from the embryonic sinus venosus.

17. **C.** Sensory nerve cell bodies conveying somatic or visceral pain are found in the spinal ganglia. Those sensory pain fibers (visceral pain) from myocardial ischemia are conveyed to the upper portion of the sympathetic component of the ANS and reside in the spinal dorsal root ganglia of T1-T2.

18. **B.** The esophagus lies directly posterior to the left atrium and may be compressed by enlargement of this heart chamber.

19. **B.** About three-quarters of all the lymph from the breast passes to the axillary lymph nodes. Lymph can also pass laterally, inferiorly, and superiorly, but most passes to the axilla.

20. **E.** The sternal angle is a good landmark for determining the level of the tracheal bifurcation, the location of the aortic arch, and the articulation of the second ribs with the sternum.

21. **C.** The arch of the aorta develops from the left fourth aortic arch. The second pair of arches largely disappears (it forms the small stapedial artery of the middle ear); the third pair forms the common carotid arteries and a small proximal portion of the internal carotid artery; the right fourth arch forms the brachiocephalic trunk and proximal right subclavian artery; the fifth pair disappears; and the sixth pair forms the proximal pulmonary arteries and, on the left, the ductus arteriosus.

22. **A.** The esophageal hiatus is the last resistance point. It is located at the T10 vertebral level as the esophagus passes through the diaphragm. Other resistance points include the pharyngoesophageal junction, the area posterior to the aortic arch, and the area posterior to the left main bronchus.

23. **D.** The middle cardiac vein parallels the inferior (posterior) interventricular coronary artery and drains into the large coronary sinus, which drains into the right atrium. The great cardiac vein parallels the LAD branch of the left coronary artery.

24. **B.** The crista terminalis, because at its superior margin lies the SA node and beneath its length lies the posterior internodal pathway of conduction fibers between the SA and AV nodes. It also is the site of origin of the atrium's pectinate muscles.

25. **B.** The needle usually is inserted, with ultrasound guidance, in the left fifth intercostal space just to the left of the sternum. In emergencies, if echocardiography is not available, a subxiphoid approach is used just between the xiphisternum and the left costal margin.

26. **B.** The horizontal fissure of the right lung courses along the path of the fourth rib. Both lungs possess an oblique fissure, but only the right lung has a horizontal fissure and three lobes; the left lung has two lobes.

27. **C.** The thoracic lymphatic duct has been damaged, producing a chylothorax. This duct returns lymph from three-quarters of the body to the venous system at the junction of the left internal jugular vein and left subclavian vein where they form the proximal left brachiocephalic vein.

28. **A.** Although sympathetic fibers relax the smooth muscle of the tracheobronchial tree (allowing for increased respiration associated with the fight-or-flight response), postganglionic parasympathetic fibers constrict this smooth muscle and, therefore, must be inhibited.

29. **E.** The right main bronchus is more vertical and shorter and wider than the left main bronchus, so most (but not all!) aspirated objects pass into this bronchus. The tertiary bronchus is usually too small for an object as large as a peanut to be aspirated into it.

30. **E.** Deep dimpling of the skin results from the tension and retraction of the suspensory retinacula of the breast. The peau d'orange (orange peel) appearance of her skin results from obstruction of subcutaneous lymphatics, causing edema and the accumulation of lymph in dilated lymphatics near the surface of the skin.

31. **C.** The mitral valve is heard downstream from the valve as the turbulent flow of blood carries the sound into the left ventricle. The valve is best heard near the apex of the left ventricle, which is at about the fifth intercostal space and to the left of the sternum. In males, this is usually just below the left nipple; in females, the nipple location can vary, depending on the size of the breast.

32. **E.** Although each of the other structures can be palpated by the physician's fingertips, the SVC cannot be felt in the oblique sinus, which is a cul-de-sac lying beneath the atria, IVC, portions of both ventricles, and pulmonary veins.

33. **H.** The intercostal muscles are skeletal muscles and are innervated by anterior rami of the spinal nerves, which contain three types of nerve fibers: somatic efferents, somatic afferents, and postganglionic sympathetics. Only the somatic efferent nerve fibers cause contraction of the skeletal muscle, however.

34. **J.** Baroreceptors and chemoreceptors associated with the heart are found primarily on the aortic arch. Their sensory modalities are conveyed back to the brainstem by the vagus nerve (CN X). Similar receptors also exist at the common carotid bifurcation in the neck, but these afferents are carried by the glossopharyngeal nerve (CN IX). These specialized receptors monitor the blood pressure (baroreceptors), blood pH, and partial pressure of oxygen and carbon dioxide in the blood (chemoreceptors).

35. **E.** Cervical and thoracic cardiac nerves contain postganglionic sympathetic fibers that travel to the heart and increase the heart rate and force of contraction. Their preganglionic sympathetic neurons arise in the upper thoracic (T1-T4) intermediate (intermediolateral) gray matter of the spinal cord, and the postganglionic cell neurons are in the sympathetic trunk ganglia (cervical and upper thoracic regions).

36. **I.** The sympathetic trunk consists of a bilateral chain of ganglia that passes across the neck of the upper thoracic ribs and, as it passes inferiorly, aligns itself closer to the lateral bodies of the lower thoracic vertebrae.

37. **C.** The diaphragm is a skeletal muscle and somatic afferents from it would travel in the phrenic nerve (C3-C5), which innervates the diaphragm. A general answer would be the somatic afferent fibers, but a more specific, and the best, answer is the phrenic nerve. Pain can be referred to the shoulder and lower neck region.

38. **C.** Blood from the right atrium next passes through the tricuspid (right atrioventricular) valve to enter the right ventricle of the heart. Remember, when viewing a radiographic image, that "right" and "left" refer to the patient's right and left, not the right and left side of the image!

39. **E.** Narrowing of the aortic arch (which can happen with coarctation of the proximal aortic arch; see online Clinical Focus 3.35) may reduce blood flow to the left common carotid and subclavian arteries, as well as the descending thoracic aorta.

40. **G.** The mitral valve is best heard over the fifth intercostal space, about 3 inches to the left of the sternum (apex of the heart).

Abdomen

1. INTRODUCTION

The abdomen is the region between the thorax superiorly and the pelvis inferiorly. The abdomen is composed of the following:

- Layers of skeletal muscle that line the abdominal walls and assist in respiration and, by increasing intraabdominal pressure, facilitate micturition (urination), defecation (bowel movement), and childbirth.
- The abdominal cavity is a peritoneal lined cavity that is continuous with the pelvic cavity inferiorly and contains the abdominal viscera (organs).
- Visceral structures that lie within the abdominal peritoneal cavity (intraperitoneal) include the gastrointestinal (GI) tract and its associated organs (the liver, gallbladder, and pancreas), the spleen, and the urinary system (kidneys and ureters), which is located retroperitoneally behind and outside the peritoneal cavity but anterior to the posterior abdominal wall muscles.

In your study of the abdomen, first focus on the abdominal wall and note the continuation of the three muscle layers of the thorax (intercostal muscles) as they blend into the abdominal flank musculature.

Next, note the disposition of the abdominal organs. For example, you should know the region or quadrant of the abdominal cavity in which the organs reside; whether an organ is suspended in a mesentery or lies retroperitoneally (see embryology section in Chapter 1 and Table 4.14 showing the foregut, midgut, and hindgut derivatives); the blood supply and autonomic innervation pattern to the organs; and features of the organs that will allow you to readily identify which organ or part of an organ you are viewing (particularly important in laparoscopic surgery). Also, you should understand the dual venous drainage of the abdomen by the caval and hepatic portal systems and the key anastomoses between these two systems that facilitate venous return to the heart.

Lastly, study the posterior abdominal wall musculature, and identify the components and distribution of the lumbar plexus of somatic nerves.

2. SURFACE ANATOMY

Key Landmarks

Key surface anatomy features of the anterolateral abdominal wall include the following (Fig. 4.1):

- **Rectus sheath:** a fascial sheath containing the rectus abdominis muscle, which runs from the pubic symphysis and crests to the xiphoid process and fifth to seventh costal cartilages.
- **Linea alba:** literally the "white line"; a relatively avascular midline subcutaneous band of fibrous tissue where the fascial aponeuroses of the rectus sheath from each side interdigitate in the midline.
- **Semilunar line:** the lateral border of the rectus abdominis muscle in the rectus sheath.
- **Tendinous intersections:** transverse skin grooves that demarcate transverse fibrous attachment points of the rectus sheath to the underlying rectus abdominis muscle.
- **Umbilicus:** the site that marks the T10 dermatome, lying at the level of the intervertebral disc between L3 and L4; the former attachment site of the umbilical cord.
- **Iliac crest:** the rim of the ilium, which lies at about the level of the L4 vertebra.
- **Inguinal ligament:** a ligament composed of the aponeurotic fibers of the external abdominal oblique muscle, which lies deep to a skin crease that marks the division between the lower abdominal wall and upper thigh of the lower limb.

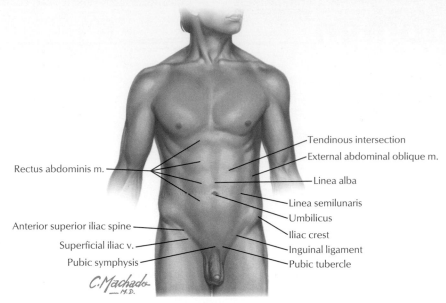

FIGURE 4.1 Key Landmarks in Surface Anatomy of Anterolateral Abdominal Wall. (From *Netter's atlas of human anatomy,* ed 8, Plate 267; S-8.)

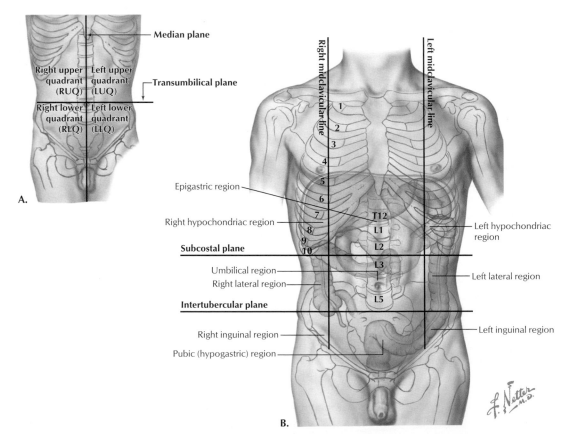

FIGURE 4.2 Four-Quadrant (A) and Nine-Region (B) Abdominal Planes. (From *Netter's atlas of human anatomy,* ed 8, Plate 269; S-395.)

TABLE 4.1 Clinical Planes of Reference for Abdomen

PLANE OF REFERENCE	DEFINITION
Median	Vertical plane from xiphoid process to pubic symphysis
Transumbilical	Horizontal plane across umbilicus at the L4 disc; these planes divide the abdomen into quadrants.
Subcostal	Horizontal plane across inferior margin of 10th costal cartilage
Intertubercular	Horizontal plane across tubercles of ilium.
Midclavicular	Two vertical planes through midpoint of clavicles; these planes divide the abdomen into nine regions.

Surface Topography

Clinically, the abdominal wall is divided descriptively into quadrants or regions so that both the underlying visceral structures and the pain or pathology associated with these structures can be localized and topographically described. Common clinical descriptions use either **quadrants** or the **nine descriptive regions,** demarcated by two vertical midclavicular lines and two horizontal lines: the subcostal and intertubercular planes (Fig. 4.2 and Table 4.1).

3. ANTEROLATERAL ABDOMINAL WALL

Layers

The layers of the abdominal wall include the following:
- **Skin:** epidermis and dermis.
- **Superficial fascia** (subcutaneous tissue): a single, fatty connective tissue layer below the level of the umbilicus that divides into a more superficial fatty layer (Camper's fascia) and a deeper membranous layer (Scarpa's fascia; see Fig. 4.11).
- **Investing fascia:** connective tissue that covers the muscle layers.
- **Abdominal muscles:** three flat layers, similar to the thoracic wall musculature, except in the anterior midregion where the vertically oriented rectus abdominis muscle lies in the rectus sheath.
- **Endoabdominal fascia:** tissue that is unremarkable except for a thicker portion called the **transversalis fascia,** which lines the inner aspect of the transversus abdominis muscle; it is continuous with fascia on the underside of the respiratory diaphragm, fascia of the posterior abdominal muscles, and fascia of the pelvic muscles.

- **Extraperitoneal (fascia) fat:** connective tissue that is variable in thickness and contains a variable amount of fat.
- **Peritoneum:** thin serous membrane that lines the inner aspect of the abdominal wall **(parietal peritoneum)** and occasionally reflects off the walls as a mesentery to invest partially or completely various visceral structures. It then encircles the viscus as **visceral peritoneum.**

Muscles

The muscles of the anterolateral abdominal wall include three flat layers that are continuations of the three layers in the thoracic wall (Fig. 4.3). These include two **abdominal oblique muscles** and the **transversus abdominis muscle** (Table 4.2). In the midregion a vertically oriented pair of **rectus abdominis muscles** lies within the rectus sheath and extends from the pubic symphysis and crest to the xiphoid process and costal cartilages 5 to 7 superiorly. The small pyramidalis muscle just superior to the pubis (Fig. 4.3, *B*) is inconsistent and clinically less significant.

Rectus Sheath

The rectus sheath encloses the vertically running rectus abdominis muscle (and inconsistent pyramidalis), the superior and inferior epigastric vessels, the lymphatics, and the anterior rami of the T7-L1 nerves, which enter the sheath along its lateral margins (Fig. 4.3, *C*). The superior three-quarters of the rectus abdominis is completely enveloped within the rectus sheath, and the inferior one-quarter is supported posteriorly only by the transversalis fascia, extraperitoneal fat, and peritoneum; the site of this transition is called the **arcuate line** (Figs. 4.4, 4.5, and 4.6 and Table 4.3).

Innervation and Blood Supply

The segmental innervation of the anterolateral abdominal skin and muscles is by **anterior rami of T7-L1**. The blood supply includes the following arteries (Figs. 4.3, *C*, and 4.5):
- **Musculophrenic:** a terminal branch of the internal thoracic artery that courses along the costal margin.
- **Superior epigastric:** arises from the terminal end of the internal thoracic artery and anastomoses with the inferior epigastric artery at the level of the umbilicus.
- **Inferior epigastric:** arises from the external iliac artery and anastomoses with the superior epigastric artery.

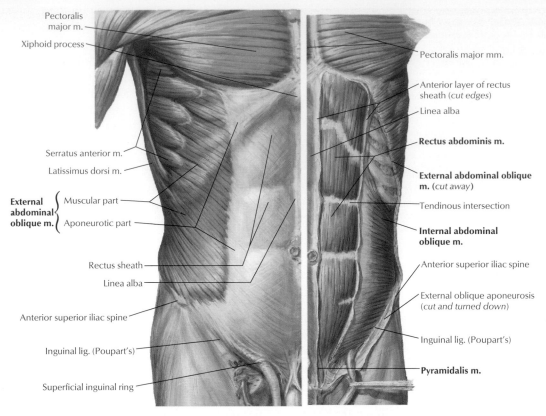

Pectoralis major m.

Xiphoid process

Serratus anterior m.

Latissimus dorsi m.

External abdominal oblique m. { Muscular part
Aponeurotic part

Rectus sheath

Linea alba

Anterior superior iliac spine

Inguinal lig. (Poupart's)

Superficial inguinal ring

Pectoralis major mm.

Anterior layer of rectus sheath (*cut edges*)

Linea alba

Rectus abdominis m.

External abdominal oblique m. (*cut away***)**

Tendinous intersection

Internal abdominal oblique m.

Anterior superior iliac spine

External oblique aponeurosis (*cut and turned down*)

Inguinal lig. (Poupart's)

Pyramidalis m.

A. The external abdominal oblique muscle is shown in this image of the right side of the body.

B. The internal abdominal oblique muscle is shown on the left side of the body and the rectus abdominis muscle is exposed.

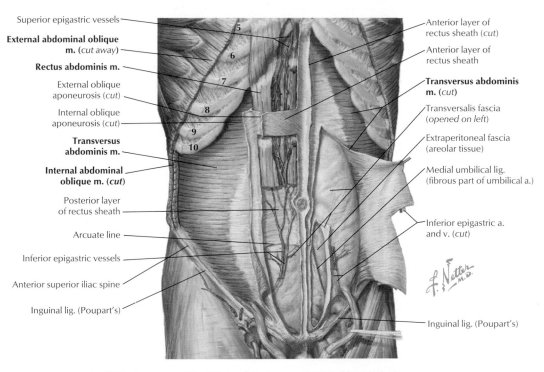

Superior epigastric vessels

External abdominal oblique m. (*cut away***)**

Rectus abdominis m.

External oblique aponeurosis (*cut*)

Internal oblique aponeurosis (*cut*)

Transversus abdominis m.

Internal abdominal oblique m. (*cut*)

Posterior layer of rectus sheath

Arcuate line

Inferior epigastric vessels

Anterior superior iliac spine

Inguinal lig. (Poupart's)

Anterior layer of rectus sheath (*cut*)

Anterior layer of rectus sheath

Transversus abdominis m. (*cut*)

Transversalis fascia (*opened on left*)

Extraperitoneal fascia (areolar tissue)

Medial umbilical lig. (fibrous part of umbilical a.)

Inferior epigastric a. and v. (*cut*)

Inguinal lig. (Poupart's)

C. The transversus abdominis muscle is shown on the right side of the body and is partially reflected on the left side to reveal the underlying transversalis fascia.

FIGURE 4.3 Muscles of Anterolateral Abdominal Wall. (From *Netter's atlas of human anatomy,* ed 8, Plates 270-272; S-211–S-213.)

TABLE 4.2 Principal Muscles of Anterolateral Abdominal Wall

MUSCLE	ORIGIN ATTACHMENT	INSERTION ATTACHMENT	INNERVATION	MAIN ACTIONS
External oblique	External surfaces of 5th to 12th ribs	Linea alba, pubic tubercle, and anterior half of iliac crest	Inferior six thoracic nerves and subcostal nerve	Compresses and supports abdominal viscera; flexes and rotates trunk
Internal oblique	Thoracolumbar fascia, anterior two-thirds of iliac crest, and lateral half of inguinal ligament	Inferior borders of 10th to 12th ribs, linea alba, and pubis via conjoint tendon	Anterior rami of inferior six thoracic nerves and 1st lumbar nerve	Compresses and supports abdominal viscera; flexes and rotates trunk
Transversus abdominis	Internal surfaces of costal cartilages 7-12, thoracolumbar fascia, iliac crest, and lateral third of inguinal ligament	Linea alba with aponeurosis of internal oblique, pubic crest, and pecten pubis via conjoint tendon	Anterior rami of inferior six thoracic nerves and 1st lumbar nerve	Compresses and supports abdominal viscera
Rectus abdominis	Pubic symphysis and pubic crest	Xiphoid process and costal cartilages 5-7	Anterior rami of inferior six thoracic nerves	Compresses abdominal viscera and flexes trunk

Variations in spinal nerve contributions to the innervation of muscles, their attachments, and their actions are common in human anatomy. Therefore, expect differences between texts and realize that anatomical variation is normal.

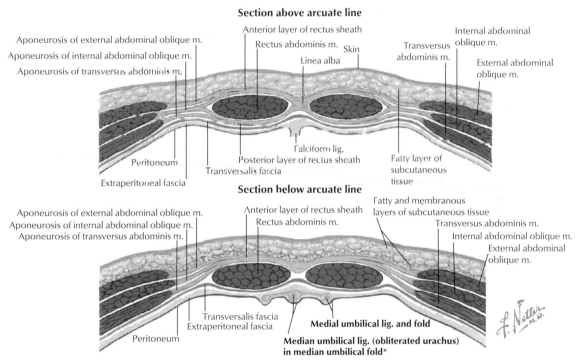

FIGURE 4.4 Features of Rectus Sheath. (From *Netter's atlas of human anatomy*, ed 8, Plate 273; S-214.) (*see Fig. 5.12)

TABLE 4.3 Aponeuroses and Layers Forming Rectus Sheath

LAYER	COMMENT	LAYER	COMMENT
Anterior lamina above arcuate line	Formed by fused aponeuroses of external and internal abdominal oblique muscles	Below arcuate line	All three muscle aponeuroses fuse to form anterior lamina, with rectus abdominis in contact only with transversalis fascia posteriorly
Posterior lamina above arcuate line	Formed by fused aponeuroses of internal abdominal oblique and transversus abdominis muscles		

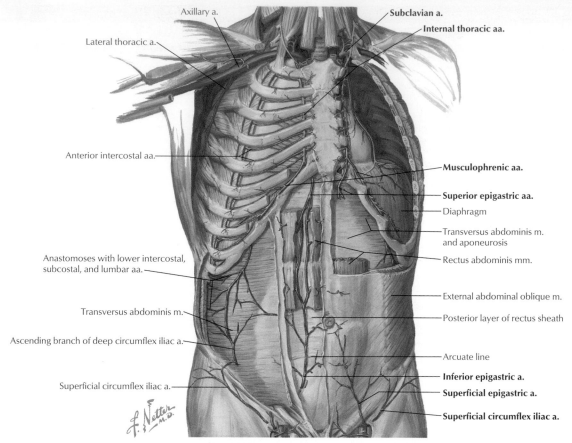

FIGURE 4.5 Arteries of Anterolateral Abdominal Wall. (From *Netter's atlas of human anatomy*, ed 8, Plate 276; S-336.)

- **Superficial circumflex iliac:** arises from the femoral artery and anastomoses with the deep circumflex iliac artery.
- **Superficial epigastric:** arises from the femoral artery and courses toward the umbilicus.
- **External pudendal:** arises from the femoral artery and courses toward the pubis (see Fig. 6.13).

Superficial and deeper veins accompany these arteries, but, as elsewhere in the body, they form extensive anastomoses with each other to facilitate venous return to the heart (Fig. 4.6 and Table 4.4).

Lymphatic drainage of the abdominal wall parallels the venous drainage, with the lymph ultimately coursing to the following lymph node collections: (see Fig. 4.41).

- **Axillary nodes:** superficial drainage above the umbilicus.
- **Superficial inguinal nodes:** superficial drainage below the umbilicus.
- **Parasternal nodes:** deep drainage along the internal thoracic vessels.

- **Lumbar nodes:** deep drainage internally to the nodes along the abdominal aorta.
- **External iliac nodes:** deep drainage along the external iliac vessels.

4. INGUINAL REGION

The inguinal region, or groin, is the transition zone between the lower abdomen and the upper thigh. This region, especially in males, is characterized by a weakened area of the lower abdominal wall that renders this region particularly susceptible to inguinal hernias. Although occurring in either gender, inguinal hernias are much more common in males because of the descent of the testes into the scrotum, which occurs along this boundary region.

The inguinal region is demarcated by the **inguinal ligament,** the inferior border of the external abdominal oblique aponeurosis, which is folded under on itself and attaches to the anterior superior

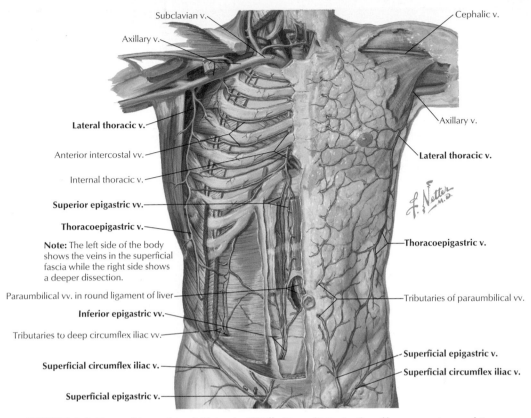

FIGURE 4.6 Veins of Anterolateral Abdominal Wall. (From *Netter's atlas of human anatomy,* ed 8, Plate 277; S-337.)

TABLE 4.4 Principal Veins of Anterolateral Abdominal Wall

VEIN	COURSE
Superficial epigastric	Drains into femoral vein
Superficial circumflex iliac	Drains into femoral vein and parallels inguinal ligament
Inferior epigastric	Drains into external iliac vein
Superior epigastric	Drains into internal thoracic vein
Thoracoepigastric	Anastomoses between superficial epigastric and lateral thoracic
Lateral thoracic	Drains into axillary vein

iliac spine and extends inferomedially to attach to the pubic tubercle (see Figs. 4.1 and 4.3, *B* and *C*). Medially, the inguinal ligament flares into the crescent-shaped **lacunar ligament** that attaches to the pecten pubis of the pubic bone (Fig. 4.7). Fibers from the lacunar ligament also course internally along the pelvic brim as the **pectineal ligament** (see Clinical Focus 4.2). A thickened inferior margin of the transversalis fascia, called the **iliopubic tract,** runs parallel to the inguinal ligament but deep to it and reinforces the medial portion of the inguinal canal.

Inguinal Canal

The gonads in both genders initially develop retroperitoneally from a mass of intermediate mesoderm called the *urogenital ridge.* As the gonads begin to descend toward the pelvis, a peritoneal pouch called the **processus vaginalis** extends through the various layers of the anterior abdominal wall and acquires a covering from each layer, except for the transversus abdominis muscle because the pouch passes beneath this muscle layer. The processus vaginalis and its coverings form the fetal **inguinal canal,** a tunnel or passageway through the anterior abdominal wall. In females the ovaries are attached to the **gubernaculum,** the other end of which terminates in the labioscrotal swellings (which will form the labia majora in females or the scrotum in males). The ovaries descend into the pelvis, where they remain, tethered between the lateral pelvic wall and the uterus medially (by the ovarian ligament, a derivative of the gubernaculum). The gubernaculum then reflects off the uterus

Clinical Focus 4.1

Abdominal Wall Hernias

Abdominal wall hernias often are called **ventral hernias** to distinguish them from inguinal hernias. However, all are technically abdominal wall hernias. Other than inguinal hernias, which are discussed separately, the most common types of abdominal hernias include:

- **Umbilical hernia:** usually seen up to age 3 years and after 40.
- **Linea alba hernia:** often seen in the epigastric region and more common in males; rarely contains visceral structures (e.g., bowel).
- **Linea semilunaris (spigelian) hernia:** usually occurs in midlife and develops slowly.
- **Incisional hernia:** occurs at the site of a previous laparotomy scar.

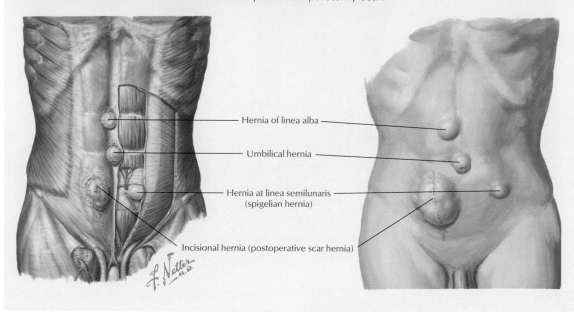

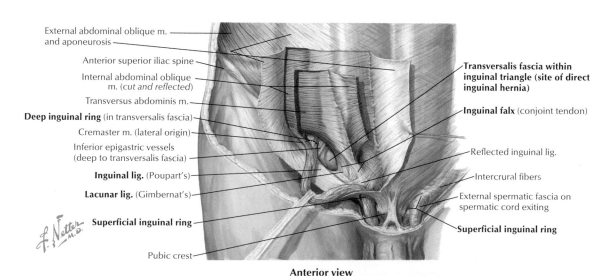

Anterior view

FIGURE 4.7 Adult Inguinal Canal and Retracted Spermatic Cord. (From *Netter's atlas of human anatomy,* ed 8, Plate 280; S-216.)

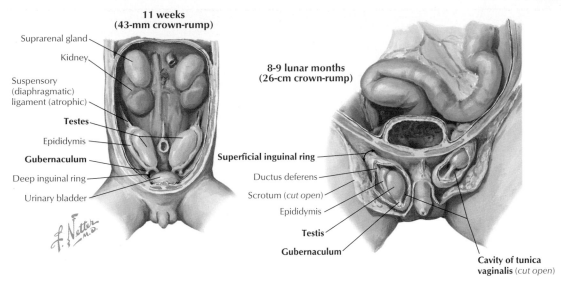

**11 weeks
(43-mm crown-rump)**

Suprarenal gland

Kidney

Suspensory
(diaphragmatic)
ligament (atrophic)

Testes

Epididymis

Gubernaculum

Deep inguinal ring

Urinary bladder

**8-9 lunar months
(26-cm crown-rump)**

Superficial inguinal ring

Ductus deferens

Scrotum (*cut open*)

Epididymis

Testis

Gubernaculum

**Cavity of tunica
vaginalis** (*cut open*)

FIGURE 4.8 Fetal Descent of Testes.

as the **round ligament of the uterus,** passes through the inguinal canal, and ends as a fibrofatty mass in the future labia majora (see Fig. 5.28).

In males the testes descend into the pelvis but then continue their descent through the inguinal canal (formed by the processus vaginalis) and into the **scrotum,** which is the male homologue of the female labia majora (Fig. 4.8). This descent through the inguinal canal occurs around the 26th week of development, usually over several days. The **gubernaculum,** which guides the descent of the testis into the scrotum, terminates in the scrotum and anchors the testis to the floor of the scrotum. A small pouch of the processus vaginalis called the **tunica vaginalis** persists and partially envelops the testis. In both genders the processus vaginalis normally seals itself and is obliterated. Sometimes this fusion does not occur or is incomplete, especially in males, probably caused by descent of the testes through the inguinal canal. Consequently, a weakness may persist in the abdominal wall that can lead to **inguinal hernias** (see Clinical Focus 4.2).

As the testes descend, they bring their accompanying spermatic cord along with them and, as these structures pass through the inguinal canal, they too become ensheathed within the layers of the anterior abdominal wall (Fig. 4.9). The spermatic cord enters the inguinal canal at the **deep inguinal ring** (an outpouching in the transversalis fascia lateral to the inferior epigastric vessels) and exits the 4-cm-long canal via the **superficial inguinal ring** before passing into the scrotum, where it

suspends the testis. In females the only structure in the inguinal canal is the fibrofatty remnant of the round ligament of the uterus, which terminates in the labia majora. The contents in the **spermatic cord** include the following (Fig. 4.9):

- Ductus (vas) deferens.
- Testicular artery, artery of the ductus deferens, and cremasteric artery.
- Pampiniform plexus of veins (testicular veins).
- Autonomic nerve fibers (sympathetic efferents and visceral afferents) coursing on the arteries and ductus deferens.
- Genital branch of the genitofemoral nerve (innervates the cremaster muscle via L1-L2).
- Lymphatics.

Layers of the spermatic cord include the following (see Fig. 4.9):

- **External spermatic fascia:** derived from the external abdominal oblique aponeurosis.
- **Cremasteric (middle spermatic) fascia:** derived from the internal abdominal oblique muscle.
- **Internal spermatic fascia:** derived from the transversalis fascia.

The features of the inguinal canal include its anatomical boundaries, as shown in Fig. 4.10 and summarized in Table 4.5. Note that the **deep inguinal ring** begins internally as an outpouching of the transversalis fascia lateral to the inferior epigastric vessels, and that the **superficial inguinal ring** is the opening in the aponeurosis of the external abdominal oblique muscle. Aponeurotic fibers at the superficial ring envelop the emerging

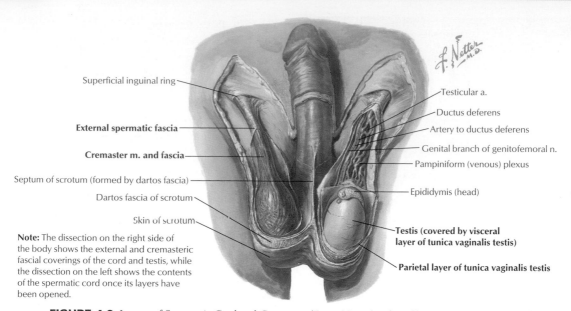

Superficial inguinal ring

External spermatic fascia

Cremaster m. and fascia

Septum of scrotum (formed by dartos fascia)

Dartos fascia of scrotum

Skin of scrotum

Testicular a.

Ductus deferens

Artery to ductus deferens

Genital branch of genitofemoral n.

Pampiniform (venous) plexus

Epididymis (head)

Testis (covered by visceral layer of tunica vaginalis testis)

Parietal layer of tunica vaginalis testis

Note: The dissection on the right side of the body shows the external and cremasteric fascial coverings of the cord and testis, while the dissection on the left shows the contents of the spermatic cord once its layers have been opened.

FIGURE 4.9 Layers of Spermatic Cord and Contents. (From *Netter's atlas of human anatomy,* ed 8, Plate 388; S-497.)

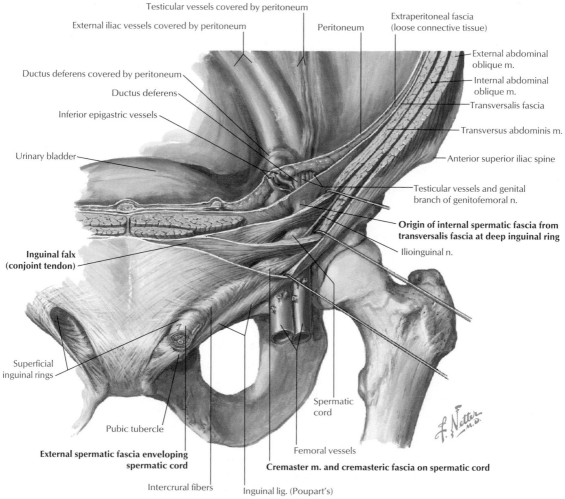

Testicular vessels covered by peritoneum

External iliac vessels covered by peritoneum

Peritoneum

Extraperitoneal fascia (loose connective tissue)

External abdominal oblique m.

Internal abdominal oblique m.

Transversalis fascia

Transversus abdominis m.

Anterior superior iliac spine

Testicular vessels and genital branch of genitofemoral n.

Origin of internal spermatic fascia from transversalis fascia at deep inguinal ring

Ilioinguinal n.

Ductus deferens covered by peritoneum

Ductus deferens

Inferior epigastric vessels

Urinary bladder

Inguinal falx (conjoint tendon)

Superficial inguinal rings

Pubic tubercle

External spermatic fascia enveloping spermatic cord

Intercrural fibers

Inguinal lig. (Poupart's)

Spermatic cord

Femoral vessels

Cremaster m. and cremasteric fascia on spermatic cord

FIGURE 4.10 Features of Male Inguinal Canal. (From *Netter's atlas of human anatomy,* ed 8, Plate 281; S-215.)

TABLE 4.5 Features and Boundaries of Inguinal Canal

FEATURE	COMMENT
Superficial ring	Medial opening in external abdominal oblique aponeurosis
Deep ring	Evagination of transversalis fascia lateral to inferior epigastric vessels, forming internal layer of spermatic fascia
Inguinal canal	Tunnel extending from deep to superficial ring, paralleling inguinal ligament; transmits spermatic cord in males or round ligament of uterus in females
Anterior wall	Aponeuroses of external and internal abdominal oblique muscles
Posterior wall	Transversalis fascia; medially includes conjoint tendon
Roof	Arching muscle fibers of internal abdominal oblique and transversus abdominis muscles
Floor	Medial half of inguinal ligament, and thickened medially by lacunar ligament, an expanded extension of the ligament
Inguinal ligament	Ligament extending between anterior superior iliac spine and pubic tubercle; folded inferior border of external abdominal oblique aponeurosis

spermatic cord medially **(medial crus),** over its top **(intercrural fibers),** and laterally **(lateral crus)** (Fig. 4.10).

The anatomy of the testis is presented in Chapter 5, Pelvis and Perineum.

5. ABDOMINAL VISCERA

Peritoneal Cavity

The abdominal viscera are contained within a serous membrane–lined recess called the **abdominopelvic cavity** (sometimes just "abdominal" or "peritoneal" cavity) or lie in a retroperitoneal position adjacent to this cavity, often with only their anterior surface covered by peritoneum and variable amounts of fat (e.g., the kidneys and ureters). The abdominopelvic cavity extends from the respiratory diaphragm inferiorly to the floor of the pelvis (Fig. 4.11).

The walls of the abdominopelvic cavity are lined by **parietal peritoneum,** which can reflect off the abdominal walls in a double layer of peritoneum called a **mesentery,** which embraces and suspends a visceral structure (e.g., a portion of intestine). As the mesentery wraps around the viscera, it becomes **visceral peritoneum.** Viscera suspended by a mesentery are considered **intraperitoneal,** whereas viscera covered on only one side by peritoneum are considered **retroperitoneal.** Retroperitoneal structures are considered to be either *primarily retroperitoneal* (i.e., those that have never had a mesentery) or *secondarily retroperitoneal* (i.e., those that lost the mesentery during development when they became fused to the abdominal wall). Primarily retroperitoneal structures include the kidneys, ureters, and suprarenal glands; secondarily retroperitoneal structures include most of the duodenum, the pancreas, and the ascending and descending colon.

The parietal peritoneum lines the inner aspect of the abdominal wall and thus is innervated by somatic afferent fibers of the anterior rami of the spinal nerves innervating the abdominal musculature. Therefore, inflammation or trauma to the parietal peritoneum presents as well-localized pain. The visceral peritoneum, on the other hand, is innervated by visceral afferent fibers carried in the sympathetic and parasympathetic nerves (see Innervation section). Pain associated with the visceral peritoneum thus is more poorly localized, giving rise to *referred pain* (see Table 4.12).

Anatomists refer to the peritoneal cavity as a *"potential space"* because it normally contains only a small amount of serous fluid that lubricates its surface. If excessive fluid collects in this space because of edema **(ascites)** or hemorrhage, it becomes a "real space." Many clinicians, however, view the cavity only as a real space because it does contain serous fluid, although they qualify this distinction further when ascites or hemorrhage occurs.

The abdominopelvic cavity is further subdivided into the following (Figs. 4.11 and 4.12):

- **Greater sac:** most of the abdominopelvic cavity.
- **Lesser sac:** also called the **omental bursa;** an irregular part of the peritoneal cavity that forms a cul-de-sac space posterior to the stomach and anterior to the retroperitoneal pancreas; it communicates with the greater sac via the **epiploic foramen** (of Winslow).

In addition to the mesenteries that suspend the bowel, the peritoneal cavity contains a variety of double-layered folds of peritoneum, including the **omenta** (attached to the stomach and duodenum) and **peritoneal ligaments.** These are not "ligaments" in the traditional sense but rather short, distinct mesenteries that connect structures (for

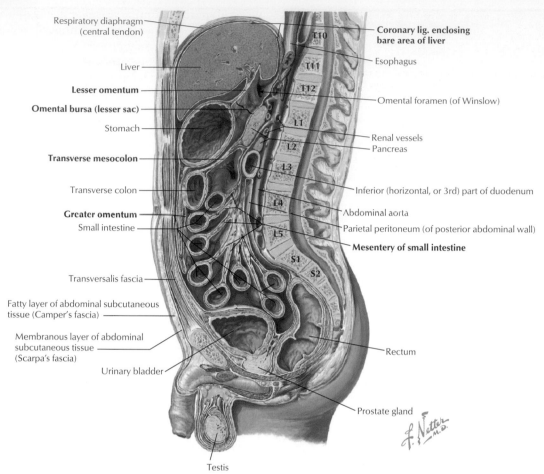

FIGURE 4.11 Parasagittal Section of Peritoneal Cavity. Observe the parietal peritoneum lining the cavity walls, the mesenteries suspending various portions of the viscera, and the lesser and greater sacs. (From *Netter's atlas of human anatomy*, ed 8, Plate 343; S-418.)

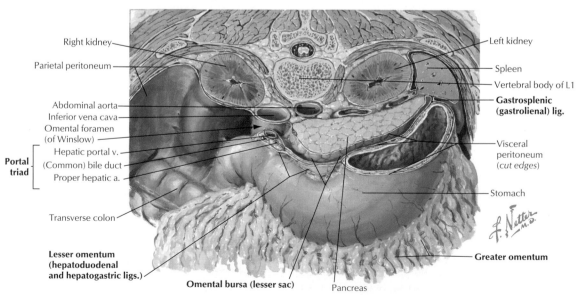

FIGURE 4.12 Lesser Sac of Abdominopelvic Cavity. (From *Netter's atlas of human anatomy*, ed 8, Plate 292; S-417.)

Clinical Focus 4.2

Inguinal Hernias

The protrusion of peritoneal contents (mesentery, fat, and/or a portion of bowel) through the abdominal wall in the groin region is termed an *inguinal hernia.* Inguinal hernias are distinguished by their relationship to the inferior epigastric vessels. There are two types of inguinal hernia:

- **Indirect (congenital) hernia:** represents 75% of inguinal hernias; occurs lateral to the inferior epigastric vessels, passes through the deep inguinal ring and inguinal canal as a protrusion along the spermatic cord, and lies within the internal spermatic fascia.
- **Direct (acquired) hernia:** occurs medial to the inferior epigastric vessels, passes directly through the posterior wall of the inguinal canal, and is separate from the spermatic cord and its fascial coverings derived from the abdominal wall.

Many indirect inguinal hernias arise from incomplete closure or weakness of the processus vaginalis. The herniated peritoneal contents may extend into the scrotum (or labia majora, but much less common in females) if the processus vaginalis is patent along its entire course.

Direct inguinal hernias pass through the **inguinal (Hesselbach's) triangle**, demarcated internally by the inferior epigastric vessels laterally, the rectus abdominis muscle medially, and the inguinal ligament inferiorly. Often, direct hernias are more limited in the extent to which they can protrude through the inferomedial abdominal wall. They occur not because of a patent processus vaginalis but because of an "acquired" weakness in the lower abdominal wall. Direct inguinal hernias can exit at the superficial ring and acquire a layer of external spermatic fascia, with the rare potential to herniate into the scrotum.

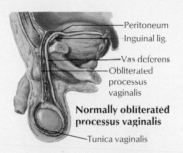

Peritoneum
Inguinal lig.
Vas deferens
Obliterated processus vaginalis

Normally obliterated processus vaginalis

Tunica vaginalis

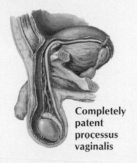

Completely patent processus vaginalis

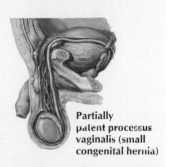

Partially patent processus vaginalis (small congenital hernia)

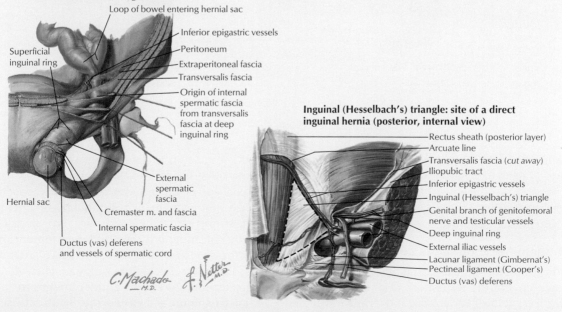

Course of an indirect inguinal hernia

Loop of bowel entering hernial sac

Inferior epigastric vessels
Peritoneum
Extraperitoneal fascia
Transversalis fascia
Origin of internal spermatic fascia from transversalis fascia at deep inguinal ring

Superficial inguinal ring

Hernial sac

External spermatic fascia
Cremaster m. and fascia
Internal spermatic fascia
Ductus (vas) deferens and vessels of spermatic cord

C. Machado M.D.   F. Netter M.D.

Inguinal (Hesselbach's) triangle: site of a direct inguinal hernia (posterior, internal view)

Rectus sheath (posterior layer)
Arcuate line
Transversalis fascia (*cut away*)
Iliopubic tract
Inferior epigastric vessels
Inguinal (Hesselbach's) triangle
Genital branch of genitofemoral nerve and testicular vessels
Deep inguinal ring
External iliac vessels
Lacunar ligament (Gimbernat's)
Pectineal ligament (Cooper's)
Ductus (vas) deferens

Clinical Focus 4.3

Hydrocele and Varicocele

The most common cause of scrotal enlargement is **hydrocele,** an excessive accumulation of serous fluid within the tunica vaginalis (usually a potential space). This small sac of peritoneum is originally from the processus vaginalis that covers about two-thirds of the testis. An infection in the testis or epididymis, trauma, or a tumor may lead to a hydrocele, or it may be idiopathic.

Varicocele is an abnormal dilation and tortuosity of the pampiniform venous plexus within the spermatic cord. Almost all varicoceles are on the left side, perhaps because the left testicular vein drains into the left renal vein rather than the larger inferior vena cava, as the right testicular vein does. A varicocele is evident at physical examination when a patient stands, but it often resolves when the patient is recumbent.

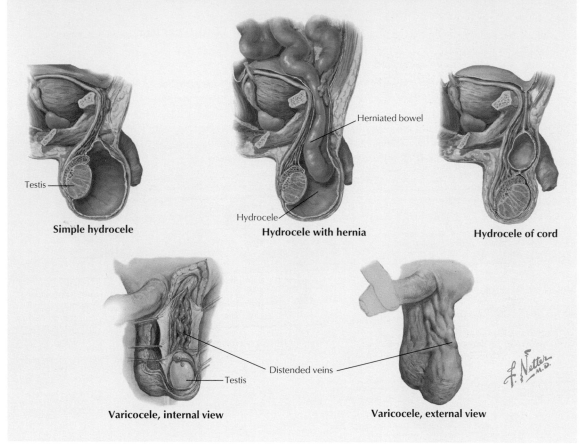

Herniated bowel

Testis

Hydrocele

Simple hydrocele   **Hydrocele with hernia**   **Hydrocele of cord**

Distended veins

Testis

Varicocele, internal view   **Varicocele, external view**

which they are named) together or to the abdominal wall (Table 4.6). Some of these structures are shown in Figs. 4.11, 4.12, and 4.13, and you will encounter the others later in the chapter when the abdominal contents are described.

Abdominal Esophagus and Stomach

The distal end of the esophagus passes through the right crus of the respiratory diaphragm at about the level of the T10 vertebra and terminates in the cardiac portion of the stomach (Fig. 4.13).

The stomach is a dilated, saclike portion of the GI tract that exhibits significant variation in size and configuration. It terminates at the thick, smooth muscle sphincter (**pyloric sphincter**) by joining the first portion of the duodenum. The stomach is tethered superiorly by the **lesser omentum** (hepatogastric ligament portion; Table 4.6) extending from its lesser curvature and is attached along its greater curvature to the **greater omentum** and the **gastrosplenic** and **gastrocolic ligaments** (see Figs. 4.11–4.13). Generally, the J-shaped stomach

TABLE 4.6 Mesenteries, Omenta, and Peritoneal Ligaments

FEATURE	DESCRIPTION	FEATURE	DESCRIPTION
Greater omentum	Double layer of peritoneum comprised of the gastrocolic, gastrosplenic, gastrophrenic, and splenorenal ligaments, and upper anterior part of transverse mesocolon; also includes an apron of mesentery folding upon itself and draped over the bowels	Gastrophrenic ligament	Portion of greater omentum that extends from gastric fundus to diaphragm
		Phrenocolic ligament	Extends from left colic flexure to diaphragm
		Hepatorenal ligament	Connects liver to right kidney
Lesser omentum	Double layer of peritoneum extending from lesser curvature of stomach and proximal duodenum to inferior surface of liver	Hepatogastric ligament	Portion of lesser omentum that extends from liver to lesser curvature of stomach
Mesenteries	Double fold of peritoneum suspending parts of bowel and conveying vessels, lymphatics, and nerves of bowel (mesentery of small bowel, mesoappendix, transverse mesocolon, sigmoid mesocolon)	Hepatoduodenal ligament	Portion of lesser omentum that extends from liver to 1st part of duodenum
		Falciform ligament	Extends from liver to anterior abdominal wall
		Ligamentum teres hepatis	Obliterated left umbilical vein in free margin of falciform ligament
Peritoneal ligaments	Double layer of peritoneum attaching viscera to walls or to other viscera	Coronary ligaments	Reflections of peritoneum from superior aspect of liver to diaphragm
		Ligamentum venosum	Fibrous remnant of obliterated ductus venosus
Gastrocolic ligament	Portion of greater omentum that extends from greater curvature of stomach to transverse colon	Suspensory ligament of ovary*	Extends from lateral pelvic wall to ovary
Gastrosplenic ligament	Left part of greater omentum that extends from hilum of spleen to greater curvature of stomach	Ovarian ligament*	Connects ovary to uterus (part of gubernaculum)
Splenorenal ligament	Connects spleen and left kidney	Round ligament of uterus*	Extends from uterus to deep inguinal ring (part of gubernaculum) and lies within broad ligament of uterus

*See Chapter 5

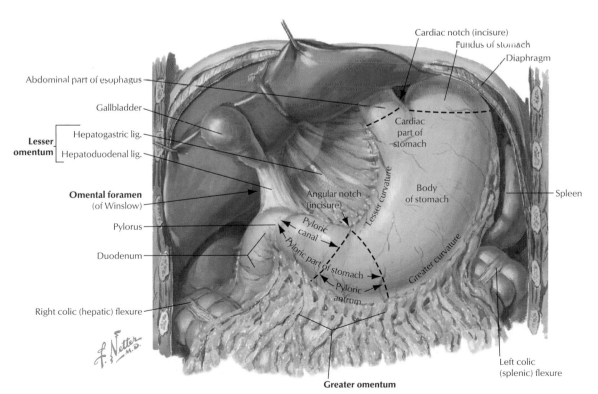

FIGURE 4.13 Abdominal Esophagus and Regions of the Stomach. (From *Netter's atlas of human anatomy*, ed 8, Plate 294; S-415.)

TABLE 4.7 Features of the Stomach

FEATURE	DESCRIPTION
Lesser curvature	Right border of stomach; lesser omentum attaches here and extends to liver as hepatogastric ligament
Greater curvature	Convex inferior border with greater omentum suspended from its margin
Cardiac part	Area of stomach that communicates with esophagus superiorly
Fundus	Superior part just under left dome of diaphragm
Body	Main part between fundus and pyloric antrum
Pyloric part	Portion divided into proximal antrum and distal canal
Pylorus	Site of pyloric sphincter smooth muscle; joins 1st part of duodenum

TABLE 4.8 Features of the Duodenum

PART OF DUODENUM	DESCRIPTION
Superior	First part; attachment site for hepatoduodenal ligament of lesser omentum; technically not retroperitoneal for the first inch (2.5 cm)
Descending	Second part; site where bile and pancreatic ducts empty
Inferior	Third part; crosses inferior vena cava and aorta and is crossed anteriorly by mesenteric vessels
Ascending	Fourth part; tethered by suspensory ligament at duodenojejunal flexure

is divided into the following regions (Fig. 4.13 and Table 4.7):

- **Cardiac region**
- **Fundus**
- **Body**
- **Pyloric region (antrum and canal)**

The interior of the unstretched stomach is lined with prominent longitudinal mucosal gastric folds called **rugae,** which become more evident as they approach the pyloric region. As an embryonic foregut derivative, the stomach's blood supply comes from the **celiac trunk** and its major branches (see Fig. 4.23 and Fig. 4.44 and Embryology section).

Small Intestine

The small intestine measures about 6 meters in length and is divided into the following three parts:

- **Duodenum:** about 25 cm long and largely secondarily retroperitoneal
- **Jejunum:** about 2.5 meters long and suspended by a mesentery
- **Ileum:** about 3.5 meters long and suspended by a mesentery

The **duodenum** is the first portion of the small intestine and descriptively is divided into four parts (Table 4.8). Most of the C-shaped duodenum is retroperitoneal and ends at the duodenojejunal flexure, where it is tethered by a musculoperitoneal fold called the **suspensory muscle of the duodenum** (ligament of Treitz) (Fig. 4.14).

The **jejunum** and **ileum** are both suspended in an elaborate mesentery. The jejunum is recognizable from the ileum because the jejunum (Fig. 4.15):

- Usually occupies the left upper quadrant of the abdomen.
- Is larger in diameter than the ileum.
- Has thicker walls.
- Has mesentery with less fat.
- Has arterial branches with fewer arcades and longer vasa recta (straight arteries).
- Internally has mucosal folds that are higher and more numerous, which increases the surface area for absorption.

The small intestine ends at the **ileocecal junction,** where a smooth muscle sphincter called the **ileocecal valve** controls the passage of ileal contents into the cecum (Fig. 4.16). The valve is actually two internal mucosal folds that cover a thickened smooth muscle sphincter.

The small intestine is a derivative of the embryonic midgut and receives its arterial supply from the **superior mesenteric artery** and its branches (see Fig. 4.24 and Table 4.14). An exception to this generalization is the first part of the duodenum, and sometimes the second part, which receives arterial blood from the gastroduodenal branch (from the common hepatic artery of the celiac trunk). This overlap reflects the embryonic transition from the foregut to the midgut derivatives (stomach to first portions of duodenum).

Large Intestine

The large intestine is about 1.5 meters long, extending from the cecum to the anal canal, and includes the following segments (Figs. 4.16 and 4.17):

- **Cecum:** a pouch that is connected to the ascending colon and the ileum; it extends below the ileocecal junction; it is surrounded by but not suspended by a mesentery.
- **Appendix:** a narrow muscular tube of variable length (usually 6-10 cm) that contains numerous

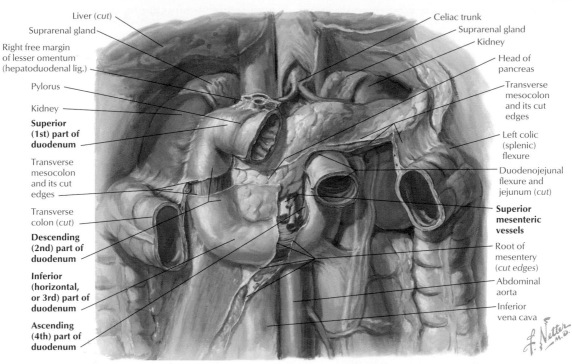

Liver (*cut*)
Suprarenal gland
Right free margin
of lesser omentum
(hepatoduodenal lig.)
Pylorus
Kidney
**Superior
(1st) part of
duodenum**
Transverse
mesocolon
and its cut
edges
Transverse
colon (*cut*)
**Descending
(2nd) part of
duodenum**
**Inferior
(horizontal,
or 3rd) part of
duodenum**
**Ascending
(4th) part of
duodenum**

Celiac trunk
Suprarenal gland
Kidney
Head of
pancreas
Transverse
mesocolon
and its cut
edges
Left colic
(splenic)
flexure
Duodenojejunal
flexure and
jejunum (*cut*)
**Superior
mesenteric
vessels**
Root of
mesentery
(*cut edges*)
Abdominal
aorta
Inferior
vena cava

FIGURE 4.14 Duodenum. (From *Netter's atlas of human anatomy,* ed 8, Plate 296; S-420.)

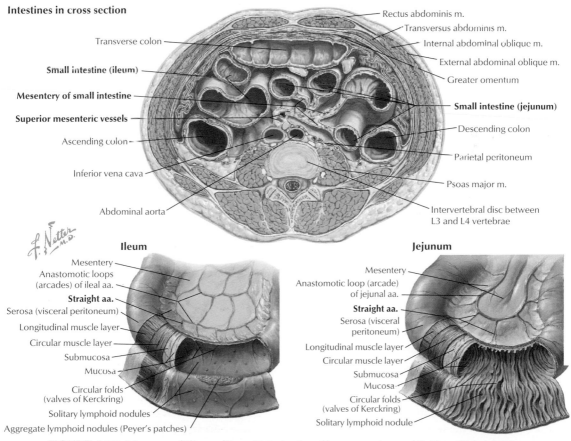

Intestines in cross section

Transverse colon
Small intestine (ileum)
Mesentery of small intestine
Superior mesenteric vessels
Ascending colon
Inferior vena cava
Abdominal aorta

Rectus abdominis m.
Transversus abdominis m.
Internal abdominal oblique m.
External abdominal oblique m.
Greater omentum
Small intestine (jejunum)
Descending colon
Parietal peritoneum
Psoas major m.
Intervertebral disc between
L3 and L4 vertebrae

Ileum
Mesentery
Anastomotic loops
(arcades) of ileal aa.
Straight aa.
Serosa (visceral peritoneum)
Longitudinal muscle layer
Circular muscle layer
Submucosa
Mucosa
Circular folds
(valves of Kerckring)
Solitary lymphoid nodules
Aggregate lymphoid nodules (Peyer's patches)

Jejunum
Mesentery
Anastomotic loop (arcade)
of jejunal aa.
Straight aa.
Serosa (visceral
peritoneum)
Longitudinal muscle layer
Circular muscle layer
Submucosa
Mucosa
Circular folds
(valves of Kerckring)
Solitary lymphoid nodule

FIGURE 4.15 Jejunum and Ileum. (From *Netter's atlas of human anatomy,* ed 8, Plates 297 and 351;
S-421 and S-546.)

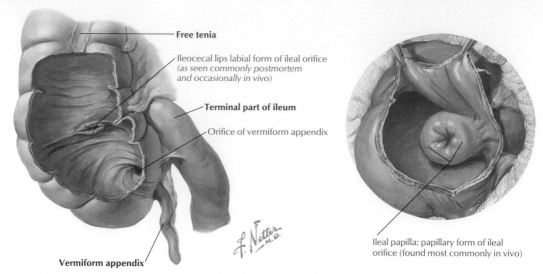

Free tenia

Ileocecal lips labial form of ileal orifice
(*as seen commonly postmortem
and occasionally in vivo*)

Terminal part of ileum

Orifice of vermiform appendix

Vermiform appendix

Ileal papilla: papillary form of ileal
orifice (found most commonly in vivo)

FIGURE 4.16 Ileocecal Junction and Valve. (From *Netter's atlas of human anatomy,* ed 8, Plate 299; S-426.)

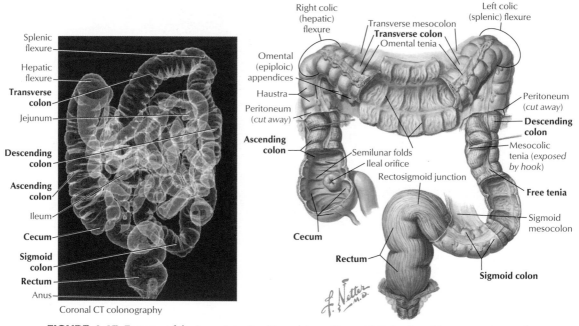

Splenic
flexure

Hepatic
flexure

**Transverse
colon**

Jejunum

**Descending
colon**

**Ascending
colon**

Ileum

Cecum

**Sigmoid
colon**

Rectum

Anus

Coronal CT colonography

Right colic
(hepatic)
flexure

Transverse mesocolon
Transverse colon
Omental tenia

Left colic
(splenic) flexure

Omental
(epiploic)
appendices

Haustra

Peritoneum
(*cut away*)

**Ascending
colon**

Semilunar folds
Ileal orifice

Rectosigmoid junction

Cecum

Rectum

Peritoneum
(*cut away*)

**Descending
colon**

Mesocolic
tenia (*exposed
by hook*)

Free tenia

Sigmoid
mesocolon

Sigmoid colon

FIGURE 4.17 Features of the Large Intestine Musculature. (From *Netter's atlas of human anatomy,* ed
8, Plate 301; S-428. CT image from Kelley LL, Petersen C: *Sectional anatomy for imaging professionals,*
Philadelphia, 2007, Mosby.)

lymphoid nodules and is suspended by a mesentery called the **mesoappendix.**

- **Ascending colon:** is secondarily retroperitoneal and ascends on the right flank to reach the liver, where it bends into the **right colic (hepatic) flexure.**
- **Transverse colon:** is suspended by a mesentery, the **transverse mesocolon,** and runs transversely from the right hypochondrium to the left, where it bends to form the **left colic (splenic) flexure.**

- **Descending colon:** is secondarily retroperitoneal and descends along the left flank to join the sigmoid colon in the left groin region.
- **Sigmoid colon:** is suspended by a mesentery, the **sigmoid mesocolon,** and forms a variable loop of bowel that runs medially to join the midline rectum in the pelvis.
- **Rectum and anal canal:** the superior two-thirds of the rectum is retroperitoneal; the rectum and

anal canal extend from the middle sacrum to the anus (see Chapter 5).

Lateral to the ascending and the descending colon lie the right and the left **paracolic gutters,** respectively. These depressions provide conduits for abdominal fluids to pass from region to region, largely dependent on gravity. Functionally the colon (ascending colon through the sigmoid part) absorbs water and important ions from the feces. It then compacts the feces for delivery to the rectum. Features of the large intestine include the following (Fig. 4.17):

- **Teniae coli:** three longitudinal bands of smooth muscle that are visible on the cecum and colon's surface and assist in peristalsis.
- **Haustra:** sacculations of the colon created by the contracting teniae coli.
- **Omental appendices:** small fat accumulations that are covered by visceral peritoneum and hang from the colon.
- **Greater luminal diameter:** the large intestine has a larger luminal diameter than the small intestine.

The arterial supply to the cecum, ascending colon, appendix, and most of the transverse colon is provided by branches of the **superior mesenteric artery;** these portions of the large intestine are derived from the embryonic midgut (see Fig. 4.36 and Tables 4.11 and 4.14). The embryonic hindgut gives rise to the distal transverse colon, descending colon, sigmoid colon, rectum, and anal canal. These are supplied by branches of the **inferior mesenteric artery** (Table 4.14) and, in the case of the distal rectum and anal canal, rectal branches from the internal iliac and internal pudendal arteries (see Figure 5.14).

Liver

The liver is the largest solid organ in the body and *anatomically* is divided into four lobes (Fig. 4.18):

- **Right lobe:** largest lobe.
- **Left lobe:** lies to the left of the falciform ligament.
- **Quadrate lobe:** lies between the gallbladder and round ligament of the liver.
- **Caudate lobe:** lies between the inferior vena cava (IVC), ligamentum venosum, and porta hepatis.

Surgically the liver is divided into right and left portal lobes and is then further subdivided into eight functional segments based largely on the intrahepatic distribution of vessels and bile ducts; the divisions are useful for partial hepatectomy and/or the excision of metastatic nodules or specific segments. The external demarcation of the two surgical/physiological liver halves runs in an imaginary sagittal plane passing through the gallbladder and the groove for the IVC (Fig. 4.18 and Table 4.9).

Clinical Focus 4.4

Acute Appendicitis

Appendicitis is a fairly common inflammation of the appendix, often caused by bacterial infection. Initially the patient feels diffuse pain in the periumbilical region. However, as the appendix becomes more inflamed and irritates the parietal peritoneum, the pain becomes well localized to the right lower quadrant (circumscribed tenderness to palpation). Surgical resection is the treatment of choice to prevent life-threatening complications such as abscess and peritonitis. Appendicitis is less common in infants and the elderly.

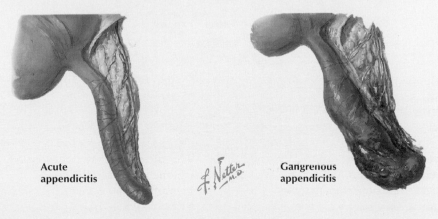

Acute appendicitis

Gangrenous appendicitis

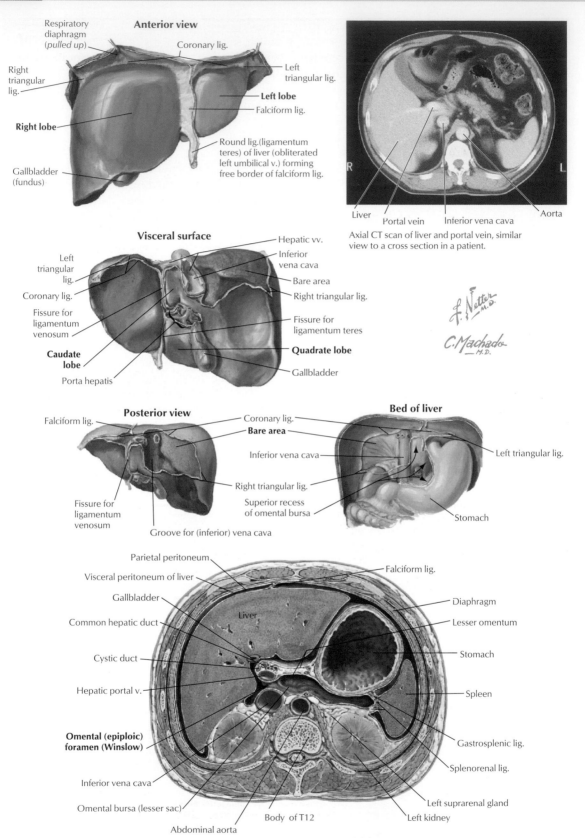

Anterior view

Respiratory diaphragm (*pulled up*)

Coronary lig.

Left triangular lig.

Right triangular lig.

Left lobe

Falciform lig.

Right lobe

Round lig.(ligamentum teres) of liver (obliterated left umbilical v.) forming free border of falciform lig.

Gallbladder (fundus)

Liver

Portal vein

Inferior vena cava

Aorta

R   L

Axial CT scan of liver and portal vein, similar view to a cross section in a patient.

Visceral surface

Hepatic vv.

Left triangular lig.

Inferior vena cava

Bare area

Coronary lig.

Right triangular lig.

Fissure for ligamentum venosum

Fissure for ligamentum teres

Caudate lobe

Quadrate lobe

Porta hepatis

Gallbladder

Posterior view

Bed of liver

Falciform lig.

Coronary lig.

Bare area

Inferior vena cava

Left triangular lig.

Right triangular lig.

Fissure for ligamentum venosum

Superior recess of omental bursa

Stomach

Groove for (inferior) vena cava

Parietal peritoneum

Falciform lig.

Visceral peritoneum of liver

Gallbladder

Diaphragm

Common hepatic duct

Liver

Lesser omentum

Cystic duct

Stomach

Hepatic portal v.

Spleen

Omental (epiploic) foramen (Winslow)

Gastrosplenic lig.

Splenorenal lig.

Inferior vena cava

Left suprarenal gland

Omental bursa (lesser sac)

Left kidney

Body of T12

Abdominal aorta

FIGURE 4.18 Various Views of the Liver and Bed of the Liver. (From *Netter's atlas of human anatomy, ed 8, Plate 302; S-429.* CT image from Kelley LL, Petersen C: *Sectional anatomy for imaging professionals,* Philadelphia, 2007, Mosby.)

Clinical Focus 4.5

Gastroesophageal Reflux Disease (GERD)

The terminal end of the esophagus possesses a **lower esophageal sphincter** (specialized smooth muscle that is physiologically different from the smooth muscle lining the lower esophagus). It prevents the reflux of gastric contents into the lower esophagus. However, it can become compromised, usually by a loss of muscle tone or a sliding hiatal hernia, leading to GERD and inflammation of the esophageal lining. GERD often presents with upper abdominal pain, dyspepsia, gas, heartburn, dysphagia, bronchospasm, or asthma.

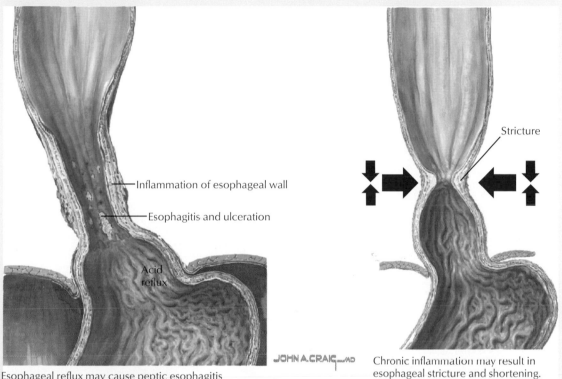

Inflammation of esophageal wall

Esophagitis and ulceration

Acid reflux

Stricture

JOHN A.CRAIG___MD

Esophageal reflux may cause peptic esophagitis and lead to cicatrization and stricture formation.

Chronic inflammation may result in esophageal stricture and shortening.

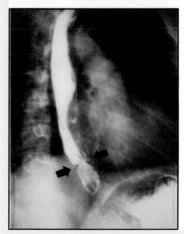

Barium study shows esophageal stricture.

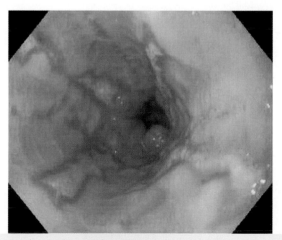

Grade D reflux esophagitis (From Reynolds J. The Netter Collection of Medical Illustrations: Digestive System: Part I - The Upper Digestive Tract, 2016, Elsevier.)

Clinical Focus 4.6

Hiatal Hernia

Herniation of the diaphragm that involves the stomach is referred to as a hiatal hernia. A widening of the space between the muscular right crus forming the esophageal hiatus allows protrusion of part of the stomach superiorly into the posterior mediastinum of the thorax. The two anatomical types are as follows:

- Sliding, rolling, or axial hernia (95% of hiatal hernias): appears as a bell-shaped protrusion
- Paraesophageal, or nonaxial hernia: usually involves the gastric fundus

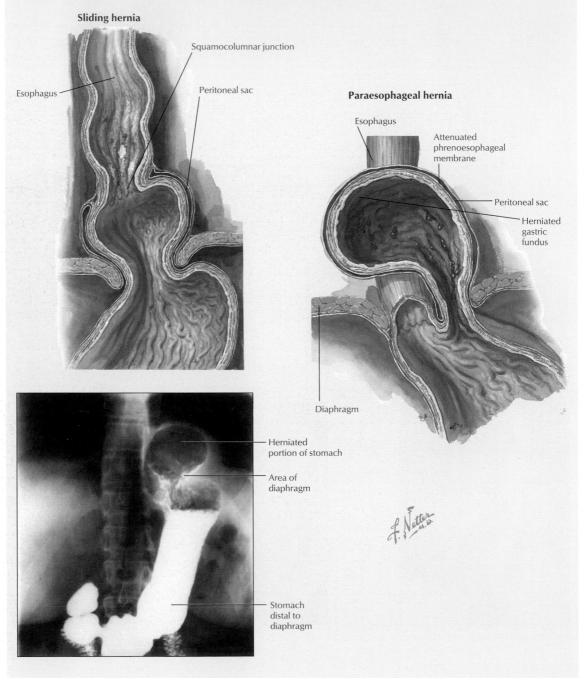

Sliding hernia

Squamocolumnar junction

Esophagus

Peritoneal sac

Paraesophageal hernia

Esophagus

Attenuated
phrenoesophageal
membrane

Peritoneal sac

Herniated
gastric
fundus

Diaphragm

Herniated
portion of stomach

Area of
diaphragm

Stomach
distal to
diaphragm

Clinical Focus 4.7

Peptic Ulcer Disease

Peptic ulcers are GI lesions that extend through the muscularis mucosae and are remitting, relapsing lesions. (*Erosions,* on the other hand, affect only the superficial epithelium.) Acute lesions are small and shallow, whereas chronic ulcers may erode into the muscularis externa or perforate the serosa. Although they may occur in the stomach, most occur in the first part of the duodenum (duodenitis), which is referred to by clinicians as the *duodenal cap* or *bulb.* The two most serious complications of gastric or duodenal peptic ulcers are perforation and hemorrhage.

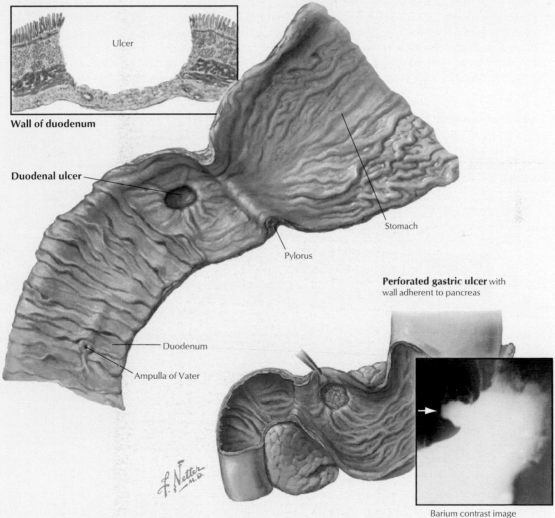

Ulcer

Wall of duodenum

Duodenal ulcer

Stomach

Pylorus

Perforated gastric ulcer with wall adherent to pancreas

Duodenum

Ampulla of Vater

Barium contrast image of perforated ulcer

Characteristics of Peptic Ulcers	
Characteristic	**Description**
Site	98% in first part of duodenum or stomach, in ratio of approximately 4:1
Prevalence	Worldwide approximately 5%; in United States approximately 2% in males and 1.5% in females
Age	Young adults, increasing with age
Aggravating factors	Mucosal exposure to gastric acid and pepsin; *H. pylori* infection (almost 80% of duodenal ulcers and 70% of gastric ulcers); use of nonsteroidal antiinflammatory drugs, aspirin, or alcohol; smoking

Clinical Focus 4.8

Bariatric Surgery

In some cases of morbid obesity, bariatric surgery may offer a viable alternative to failed dieting. The following three approaches may be considered:

- **Gastric stapling** (vertical banded gastroplasty) involves creating a small stomach pouch in conjunction with stomach stapling and banding; this approach is performed less frequently in preference to other options.
- **Sleeve gastrectomy** is becoming a popular option for increased weight loss because of its decreased risk for nutritional deficiencies and the ease with which it can be surgically accomplished.
- **Gastric bypass** (Roux-en-Y) spares a small region of the fundus and attaches it to the proximal jejunum; the main portion of the stomach is stapled off, and the duodenum is reattached to a more distal section of jejunum, allowing for the mixture of digestive juices from the liver and pancreas.
- **Adjustable gastric banding** restricts the size of the proximal stomach, limiting the amount of food that can enter; the band can be tightened or relaxed via a subcutaneous access port if circumstances warrant.

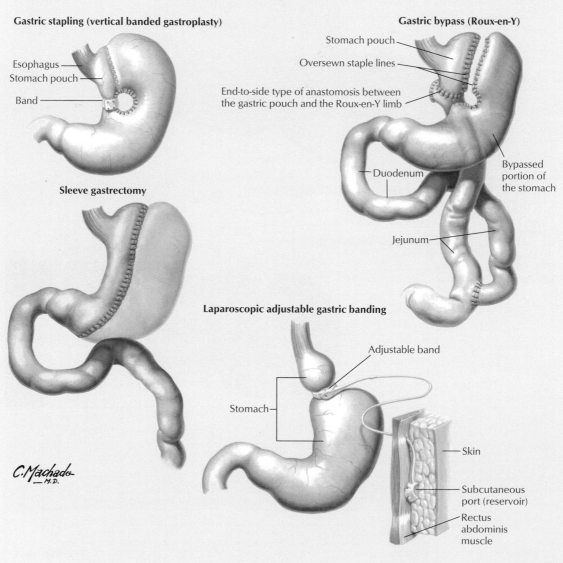

Gastric stapling (vertical banded gastroplasty)

Esophagus
Stomach pouch
Band

Sleeve gastrectomy

Gastric bypass (Roux-en-Y)

Stomach pouch
Oversewn staple lines
End-to-side type of anastomosis between the gastric pouch and the Roux-en-Y limb
Duodenum
Bypassed portion of the stomach
Jejunum

Laparoscopic adjustable gastric banding

Adjustable band
Stomach
Skin
Subcutaneous port (reservoir)
Rectus abdominis muscle

C.Machado
—M.D.

Clinical Focus 4.9

Crohn Disease

Crohn disease is an idiopathic inflammatory bowel disease (affects about 1.5 million people in the United States) that can affect any segment of the GI tract but usually involves the small intestine (terminal ileum) and colon. Young adults of northern European ancestry and/or Jewish descent are more often affected. The incidence in African American and Latino American populations is lower. Transmural edema, follicular lymphocytic infiltrates, epithelioid cell granulomas, and fistulation characterize Crohn disease. Signs and symptoms include the following:

- Diffuse abdominal pain (paraumbilical and right lower quadrant)
- Diarrhea
- Fever, lethargy, malaise
- Dyspareunia (pain during sexual intercourse)
- Urinary tract infection (UTI)
- Malabsorption, unintentional weight loss

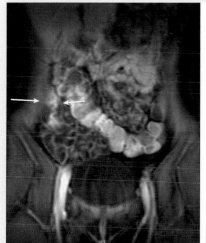

33-year-old woman with Crohn ileitis. MR enterography demonstrates a 5 cm distal terminal ileal stricture.

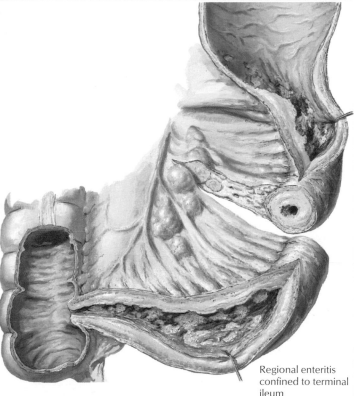

Regional enteritis confined to terminal ileum

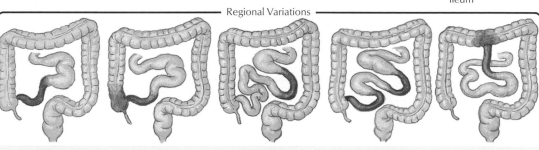

— Regional Variations —

| Terminal ileum | Involving cecum | Upper ileum or jejunum | "Skip" lesions | At ileocolostomy |

Clinical Focus 4.10

Ulcerative Colitis

As with Crohn disease, ulcerative colitis is an idiopathic inflammatory bowel disease that begins in the rectum and extends proximally. Usually the inflammation is limited to the mucosal and submucosal layers of the bowel. Abdominal tenderness in the hypogastrium or left lower quadrant and bloody diarrhea are common.

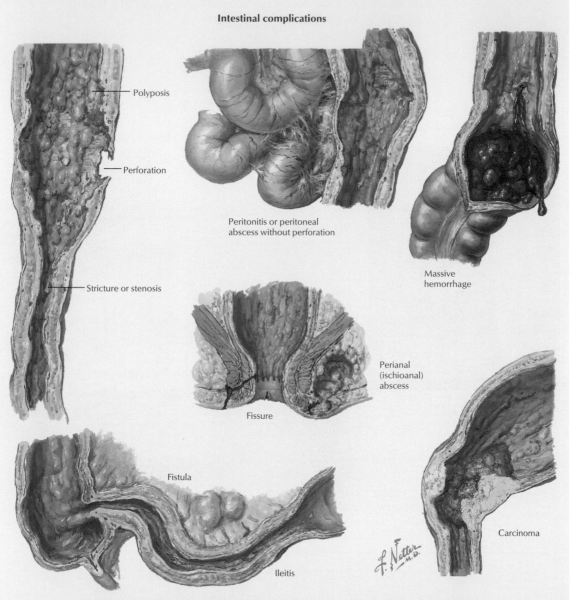

Intestinal complications

Polyposis

Perforation

Stricture or stenosis

Peritonitis or peritoneal abscess without perforation

Massive hemorrhage

Perianal (ischioanal) abscess

Fissure

Fistula

Ileitis

Carcinoma

Characteristic	Description
Prevalence	35-100 cases/100,000 population (80% in rectosigmoid region)
Age	20–50 years; 50% affected are younger than 21 years
Signs and symptoms	Abdominal pain frequently relieved by defecation; diarrhea, fever, arthritis

Diverticulosis

Diverticulosis is a herniation of colonic mucosa and submucosa through the muscular wall, with a diverticular expansion in the adventitia of the bowel visible on its external surface. Common sites of development occur where neurovascular bundles penetrate the muscular wall of the bowel.

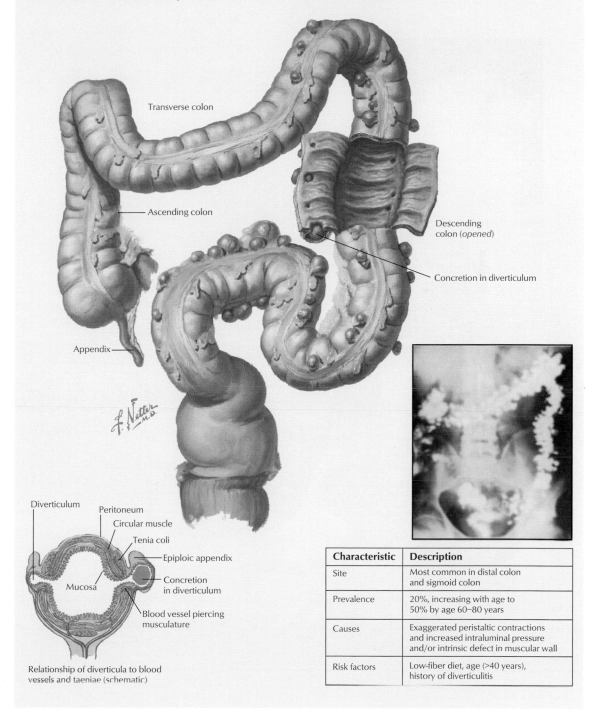

Transverse colon

Ascending colon

Descending colon (*opened*)

Concretion in diverticulum

Appendix

Diverticulum

Peritoneum

Circular muscle

Tenia coli

Epiploic appendix

Concretion in diverticulum

Mucosa

Blood vessel piercing musculature

Relationship of diverticula to blood vessels and taeniae (schematic)

Characteristic	Description
Site	Most common in distal colon and sigmoid colon
Prevalence	20%, increasing with age to 50% by age 60–80 years
Causes	Exaggerated peristaltic contractions and increased intraluminal pressure and/or intrinsic defect in muscular wall
Risk factors	Low-fiber diet, age (>40 years), history of diverticulitis

Clinical Focus 4.12

Colorectal Cancer

Colorectal cancer is the third most common cancer in women and men, accounting for over 50,000 deaths annually in the United States. The cancer appears as polypoid and ulcerating lesions, and spreads by infiltration through the colonic wall, by regional lymph nodes, and to the liver through portal venous tributaries.

Relative regional incidence of carcinoma of large bowel

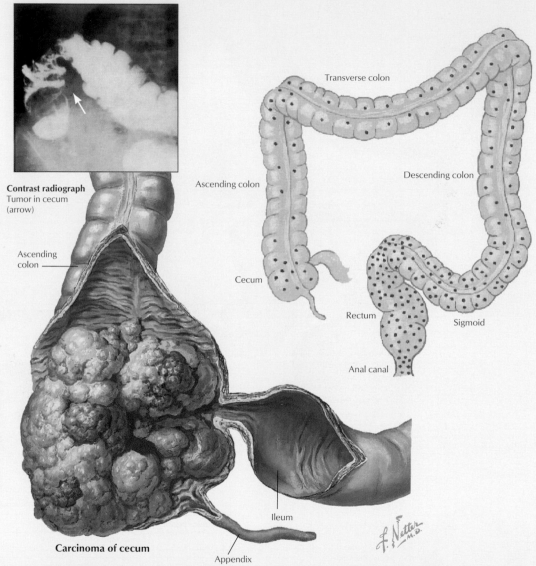

Contrast radiograph
Tumor in cecum
(arrow)

Ascending colon

Transverse colon

Ascending colon

Descending colon

Cecum

Rectum

Sigmoid

Anal canal

Ileum

Carcinoma of cecum

Appendix

Characteristic	Description
Site	98% adenocarcinomas: 25% in cecum and ascending colon, 25% in sigmoid colon, 25% in rectum, 25% elsewhere
Prevalence	Highest in United States, Canada, Australia, New Zealand, Denmark, Sweden; males affected 20% more than females
Age	Peak incidence at 60–70 years
Risk factors	Heredity, high-fat diet, increasing age, inflammatory bowel disease, polyps

Clinical Focus 4.13

Volvulus

Volvulus is the twisting of a bowel loop that may cause bowel obstruction and constriction of its vascular supply, which may lead to infarction. Volvulus affects the small intestine more often than the large intestine. The sigmoid colon is the most common site in the large intestine. The mesenteric mobility of these portions of the bowel accounts for this higher occurrence at these sites. Volvulus is associated with dietary habits, perhaps a bulky vegetable diet that results in an increased fecal load.

Bowel Obstruction Caused by Volvulus

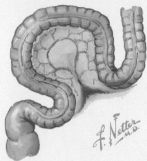 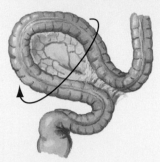 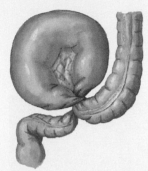

Long sigmoid loop   Contraction of base of mesosigmoid   Torsion, obstruction, strangulation, distention

TABLE 4.9 Features of the Liver and Its Ligaments	
FEATURE	**DESCRIPTION**
Lobes	Divisions, in functional terms, into right and left lobes, with anatomical subdivisions into quadrate and caudate lobes
Round ligament	Ligament that contains obliterated umbilical vein
Falciform ligament	Peritoneal reflection off anterior abdominal wall with round ligament in its margin
Ligamentum venosum	Ligamentous remnant of fetal ductus venosus, allowing fetal blood from placenta to bypass liver
Coronary ligaments	Reflections of peritoneum from liver to diaphragm
Bare area	Area of liver pressed against diaphragm that lacks visceral peritoneum
Porta hepatis	Site at which vessels, ducts, lymphatics, and nerves enter or leave liver

For gross anatomists, the liver has anatomical four lobes: the larger right lobe, the left lobe, the caudate lobe, and the quadrate lobe (Fig. 4.18 and Table 4.9). The liver is important as it receives the venous drainage from the GI tract, its accessory organs, and the spleen via the **portal vein** (see Figs. 4.25

and 4.26). The liver serves the following important functions:

- Storage of energy sources (glycogen, fat, protein, and vitamins).
- Production of cellular fuels (glucose, fatty acids, and ketoacids).
- Production of plasma proteins and clotting factors, and lymph production.
- Metabolism of toxins and drugs.
- Modification of many hormones.
- Production of bile acids.
- Excretion of substances (bilirubin).
- Storage of iron and many vitamins.
- Phagocytosis of foreign materials that enter the portal circulation from the bowel.

The liver is a derivative of the embryonic foregut and receives its arterial supply from branches of the **celiac trunk** (see Fig. 4.23). Its right and left hepatic arteries arise from the **proper hepatic artery,** a branch of the common hepatic artery from the celiac trunk. Variations in the arterial supply to the liver are common, and surgeons operating in this region must remain cognizant of this variability. The **proper hepatic artery** lies in the **hepatoduodenal ligament** with the **common bile duct** and **portal vein** (Figs. 4.18 and 4.19). Deep to the ligament lies the **epiploic foramen** (of Winslow) (Fig. 4.13), which leads

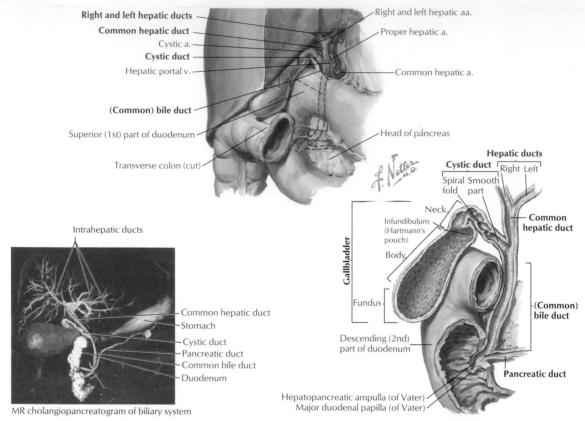

MR cholangiopancreatogram of biliary system

FIGURE 4.19 Gallbladder and Extrahepatic Ducts. (From *Netter's atlas of human anatomy*, ed 8, Plate 305; S-432. MR image from Kelley LL, Petersen C: *Sectional anatomy for imaging professionals*, Philadelphia, 2007, Mosby.)

into the **lesser sac** (also called the omental bursa) posterior to the stomach.

Gallbladder

The gallbladder is composed of a **fundus, body, infundibulum**, and **neck.** Its function is to receive, store, and concentrate bile. Bile secreted by the hepatocytes of the liver passes through the extra-hepatic duct system (Fig. 4.19) as follows:

- Collects in the **right** and **left hepatic ducts** after draining the right and left liver lobes.
- Enters the **common hepatic duct.**
- Enters the **cystic duct** and is stored and con-centrated in the gallbladder.
- On stimulation, largely by vagal efferents and cholecystokinin (CCK), bile leaves the gallbladder and enters the cystic duct.
- Passes inferiorly down the **common bile duct.**
- Enters the **hepatopancreatic ampulla** (of Vater), which is surrounded by a smooth muscle sphincter (of Oddi).

- Empties into the second part of the duodenum (major duodenal papilla).

The liver produces about 900 mL of bile per day. Between meals, most of the bile is stored in the gallbladder, which has a capacity of 30 to 50 mL and where the bile is also concentrated. Consequently, bile that reaches the duodenum is a mixture of the more dilute bile directly flowing from the liver and the concentrated bile from the gallbladder.

As a derivative of the embryonic foregut, the gallbladder is supplied by the **cystic artery,** which is usually a branch of the right hepatic artery, arising from the proper hepatic artery (**celiac trunk dis-tribution,** typical of foregut derivatives). The cystic artery lies in a triangle formed by the liver, cystic duct, and common hepatic duct, clinically referred to as **Calot's cystohepatic triangle** (Figs. 4.19 and 4.23). Variations in the biliary system (ducts and vessels) are common, and surgeons must proceed with caution in this area.

Intussusception

Intussusception is the invagination, or telescoping, of one bowel segment into a contiguous distal segment. In children the cause may be linked to excessive peristalsis. In adults an intraluminal mass such as a tumor may become trapped during a peristaltic wave and pull its attachment site forward into the more distal segment. Intestinal obstruction and infarction may occur.

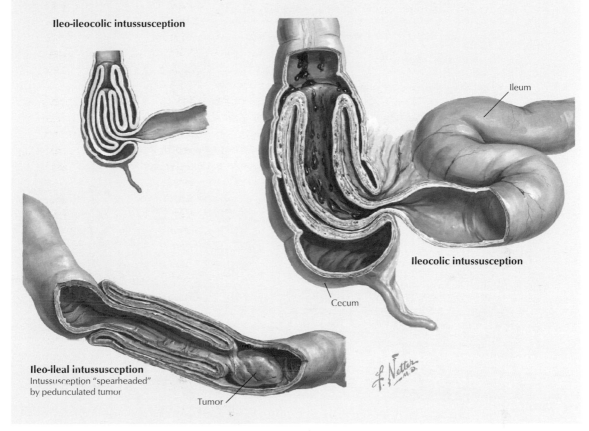

Ileo-ileocolic intussusception

Ileum

Ileocolic intussusception

Cecum

Ileo-ileal intussusception
Intussusception "spearheaded" by pedunculated tumor

Tumor

The gallbladder is innervated by the hepatic plexus of autonomic fibers. *Vagal parasympathetics* cause gallbladder contraction, along with CCK, for bile release. Sympathetic preganglionic efferent fibers from the T6-T9 or T10 levels travel in the greater splanchnic nerve, synapse in the celiac ganglion, and send postganglionic fibers to the liver and gallbladder that travel on the vasculature and inhibit bile secretion.

Pancreas

The pancreas is an exocrine and endocrine organ that lies posterior to the stomach in the posterior wall of the lesser sac (omental bursa). It is a secondarily retroperitoneal organ, except for the distal tail, which is in contact with the spleen (Fig. 4.20).

The anatomical parts of the pancreas include the following:

- **Head:** nestled within the C-shaped curve of the duodenum and overlying the abdominal aorta, the right renal vessels, the left renal vein(s), and the IVC. Its **uncinate process** lies posterior to the superior mesenteric vessels.
- **Neck:** lies anterior to the superior mesenteric vessels, the aorta, and the IVC and deep to the pylorus of the stomach.
- **Body:** extends above the duodenojejunal flexure and across the superior part of the left kidney. The splenic artery courses just superior to the body and tail, and sometimes may be partially surrounded by the parenchyma of the pancreas, as is the splenic vein, which usually courses just inferior to the artery (see Figs. 4.23 and 4.25).

Clinical Focus 4.15

Gallstones (Cholelithiasis)

Cholelithiasis results from stone formation in the gallbladder and extrahepatic ducts. Acute pain (biliary colic) can be referred to several sites. Common sites include the back just below the right scapula (T6-T9 dermatomes) or even the right shoulder region, if an inflamed gallbladder **(cholecystitis)** irritates the diaphragm. Obstruction of bile flow **(bile stasis)** can lead to numerous complications and **jaundice,** a yellow discoloration of the skin and sclera caused by bilirubin accumulation in the blood plasma.

Mechanisms of biliary pain

Sudden obstruction (biliary colic)

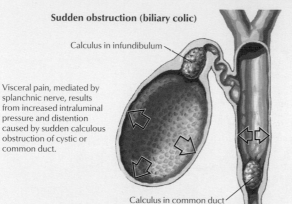

Calculus in infundibulum

Visceral pain, mediated by splanchnic nerve, results from increased intraluminal pressure and distention caused by sudden calculous obstruction of cystic or common duct.

Calculus in common duct

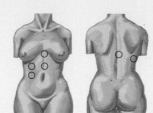

Sites of pain in biliary colic

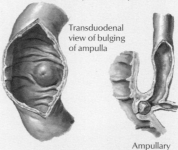

Transduodenal view of bulging of ampulla

Ampullary stone

Persistent obstruction (acute cholecystitis)

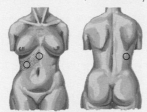

Sites of pain and hyperesthesia in acute cholecystitis

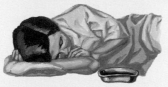

Patient lies motionless because jarring or respiration increases pain. Nausea is common.

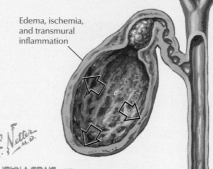

Edema, ischemia, and transmural inflammation

Parietal epigastric or right upper quadrant pain results from ischemia and inflammation of gallbladder wall caused by persistent calculous obstruction of cystic duct.

Features of Cholelithiasis	
Characteristic	**Description**
Prevalence	10–25% of adults in developed countries
Types	Cholesterol stones: (crystalline cholesterol monohydrate); pigment stones (bilirubin calcium salts); mixed stones
Risk factors	Increased age, obesity, female, rapid weight loss, estrogenic factors, gallbladder stasis
Complications	Gallbladder inflammation (cholecystitis), obstructive cholestasis or pancreatitis, empyema

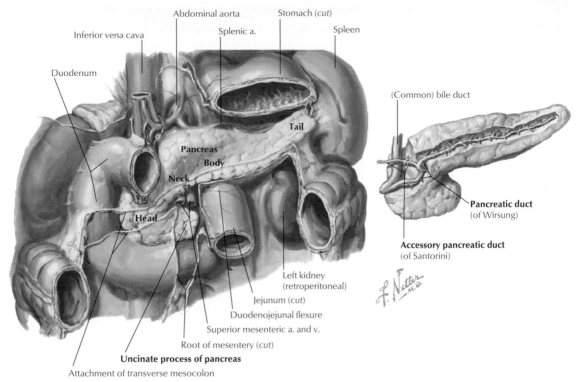

FIGURE 4.20 Pancreas. (From *Netter's atlas of human anatomy*, ed 8, Plate 306; S-433.)

- **Tail:** extends from the left kidney, which it crosses, and terminates at the hilum of the spleen in the splenorenal ligament (Fig. 4.21).

The acinar cells of the exocrine pancreas secrete a number of enzymes necessary for digestion of proteins, starches, and fats. The pancreatic ductal cells secrete fluid with a high bicarbonate content that serves to neutralize the acid entering the duodenum from the stomach. Pancreatic secretion is under neural (vagus nerve) and hormonal (secretin and CCK) control, and the exocrine secretions (a variety of proteases, amylase, lipases, and nucleases) empty primarily into the **main pancreatic duct** (of Wirsung), which joins the common bile duct at the hepatopancreatic ampulla (of Vater). A smaller, and variable, **accessory pancreatic duct** (of Santorini) also empties into the second part of the duodenum about 2 cm above the major duodenal papilla (Fig. 4.20).

The endocrine pancreas includes clusters of islet cells (of Langerhans) and a heterogeneous population of cells responsible for the elaboration and secretion primarily of insulin, glucagon, somatostatin, pancreatic polypeptide, and several lesser hormones (see Table 1.5).

The pancreas is a derivative of the embryonic foregut. It receives its arterial supply primarily from the **celiac trunk** (splenic artery and gastroduodenal branch from the common hepatic branch of the celiac artery) and also from branches of the **superior mesenteric artery** (inferior pancreaticoduodenal branches; see Fig. 4.23). The pancreas is innervated by parasympathetics from the vagus nerve (CN X) and by preganglionic sympathetics that run in the greater splanchnic nerve, synapse in the celiac and superior mesenteric ganglia, and distribute as perivascular postganglionic fibers to the organ (the sympathetics to the pancreas are largely vasomotor fibers).

Spleen

The spleen normally is slightly larger than a clenched fist and weighs about 180 to 250 grams. It lies in the left upper quadrant (hypochondriac region) of the abdomen and is tucked posterolateral to the stomach under the protection of the lower-left rib cage and diaphragm (Figs. 4.12, 4.20, and 4.21). Simplistically, the spleen is a large lymph node, becoming larger during infections, although it is also involved in the following very important functions:

- Lymphocyte proliferation (B and T cells).
- Immune surveillance and response.
- Blood filtration.

Clinical Focus 4.16

Pancreatic Cancer

Carcinoma of the pancreas is the fifth leading cause of cancer death in the United States. Pancreatic carcinomas, which are mostly adenocarcinomas, arise from the exocrine part of the organ (cells of the duct system); 60% of cancers are found in the pancreatic head and often cause **obstructive jaundice.** Islet tumors of the endocrine pancreas are less common. Because of the anatomical position of the pancreas, adjacent sites may be directly involved (duodenum, stomach, liver, colon, spleen), and pancreatic metastases via the lymphatic network are common and extensive.

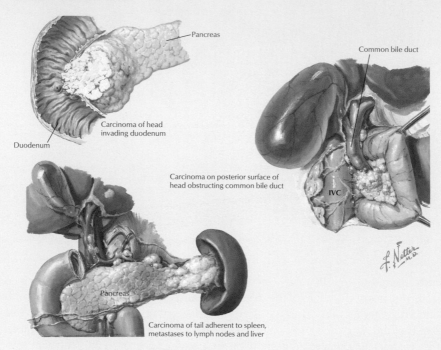

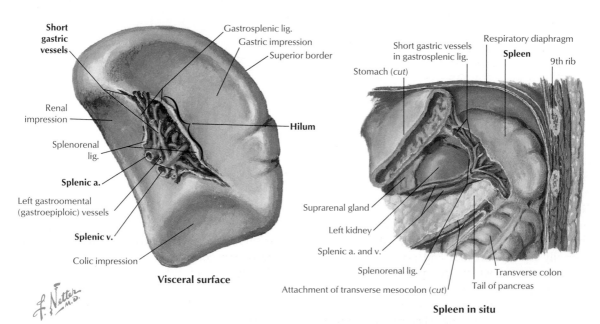

FIGURE 4.21 Spleen. (From *Netter's atlas of human anatomy,* ed 8, Plate 307; S-434.)

Clinical Focus 4.17

Rupture of the Spleen

Trauma to the left upper quadrant can lead to splenic rupture. The adventitial capsule of the spleen is very thin, making traumatic rupture a medical emergency, as the spleen receives a rich vascular supply and can bleed profusely.

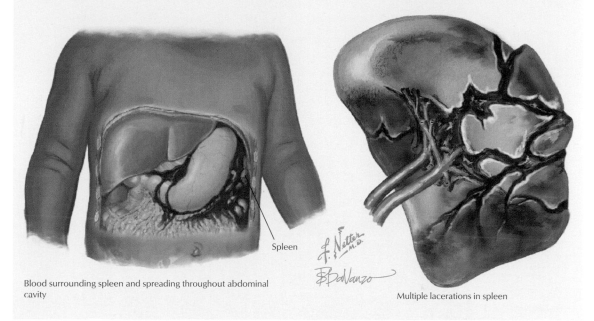

Blood surrounding spleen and spreading throughout abdominal cavity

Spleen

Multiple lacerations in spleen

- Destruction of old or damaged red blood cells (RBCs).
- Destruction of damaged platelets.
- Recycling iron and globin.
- Providing a reservoir for blood.
- Providing a source of RBCs in early fetal life.

The spleen is tethered to the stomach by the **gastrosplenic ligament** and to the left kidney by the **splenorenal ligament.** Vessels, nerves, and lymphatics enter or leave the spleen at the hilum (Fig. 4.21). The **splenorenal ligament** contains the splenic artery and vein, and the **gastrosplenic ligament** contains the short gastric arteries, which are branches of the splenic artery that supply the fundus of the stomach (see Fig. 4.23 and Table 4.6). The spleen also is tethered by the **splenocolic ligament** (between the spleen and the left colic flexure) and **phrenicosplenic ligament** (between the spleen and the diaphragm). The splenic artery typically is very tortuous and can accommodate those occasions when the spleen may become enlarged (from infections, such as infectious mononucleosis). The primary arterial supply is via the splenic artery from the celiac trunk. Although supplied by the **celiac trunk,** the spleen is not a foregut embryonic derivative (see the next section). The spleen is derived from mesoderm, unlike the ductal and epithelial linings of the abdominal GI tract and its accessory organs (liver, gallbladder, and pancreas).

Arterial Supply to the Abdominal Viscera

The arterial supply and the innervation pattern of the abdominopelvic viscera are directly reflected in the embryology of the GI tract, which is discussed later at the end of the chapter. The GI tract is derived from the following three embryonic gut regions:

- **Foregut**: gives rise to the abdominal esophagus, stomach, proximal half of the duodenum, liver, gallbladder, and pancreas.
- **Midgut**: gives rise to the distal half of the duodenum, jejunum, ileum, cecum, appendix, ascending colon, and proximal two-thirds of the transverse colon.
- **Hindgut**: gives rise to the distal third of the transverse colon, descending colon, sigmoid colon, rectum, and proximal anal canal.

The following three unpaired large arteries arise from the anterior aspect of the **abdominal aorta;**

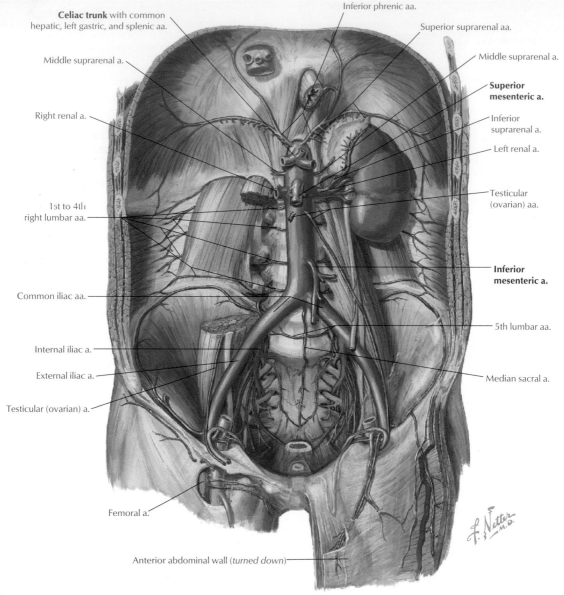

FIGURE 4.22 Abdominal Aorta and Branches. (From *Netter's atlas of human anatomy*, ed 8, Plate 284; S-341.)

each artery supplies the derivatives of the three embryonic gut regions (Fig. 4.22):
- **Celiac trunk** (artery): foregut derivatives and the spleen.
- **Superior mesenteric artery (SMA):** midgut derivatives.
- **Inferior mesenteric artery (IMA):** hindgut derivatives.

The **celiac trunk** arises from the aorta immediately inferior to the respiratory diaphragm, at the T12-L1 vertebral level, and divides into the following three main branches (Fig. 4.23):

- **Common hepatic artery:** supplies the liver, gallbladder, stomach, duodenum, and pancreas (its head and neck).
- **Left gastric artery:** the smallest branch; supplies the stomach and esophagus.
- **Splenic artery:** the largest branch; takes a tortuous course along the superior margin of the pancreas and supplies the spleen, stomach, and pancreas (its neck, body, and tail).

The **SMA** arises from the aorta about one finger's breadth inferior to the celiac trunk, at about the L1 vertebral level. It then passes posterior to the

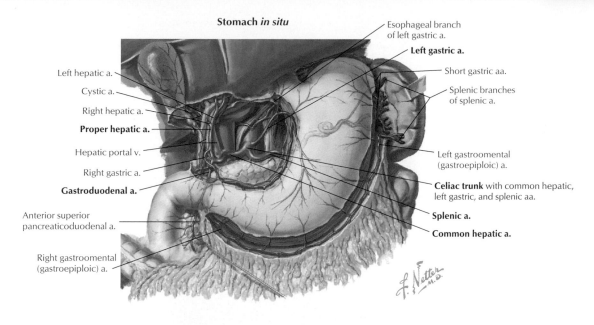

Stomach in situ

Esophageal branch
of left gastric a.

Left gastric a.

Left hepatic a.

Cystic a.

Right hepatic a.

Proper hepatic a.

Hepatic portal v.

Right gastric a.

Gastroduodenal a.

Anterior superior
pancreaticoduodenal a.

Right gastroomental
(gastroepiploic) a.

Short gastric aa.

Splenic branches
of splenic a.

Left gastroomental
(gastroepiploic) a.

Celiac trunk with common hepatic,
left gastric, and splenic aa.

Splenic a.

Common hepatic a.

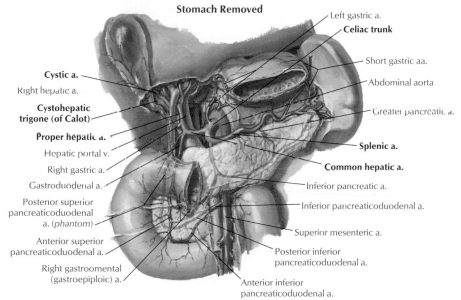

Stomach Removed

Left gastric a.

Celiac trunk

Cystic a.

Right hepatic a.

**Cystohepatic
trigone (of Calot)**

Proper hepatic a.

Hepatic portal v.

Right gastric a.

Gastroduodenal a.

Posterior superior
pancreaticoduodenal
a. (phantom)

Anterior superior
pancreaticoduodenal a.

Right gastroomental
(gastroepiploic) a.

Short gastric aa.

Abdominal aorta

Greater pancreatic a.

Splenic a.

Common hepatic a.

Inferior pancreatic a.

Inferior pancreaticoduodenal a.

Superior mesenteric a.

Posterior inferior
pancreaticoduodenal a.

Anterior inferior
pancreaticoduodenal a.

FIGURE 4.23 Celiac Trunk, With Major and Secondary Branches. (From *Netter's atlas of human anatomy*, ed 8, Plate 308; S-435.)

neck of the pancreas and anterior to the distal duodenum (the inferior, or third, part of the duodenum). Its major branches include the following (Fig. 4.24):

- **Inferior pancreaticoduodenal artery:** supplies the head of the pancreas and duodenum.
- **Jejunal and ileal branches:** give rise to 15 to 18 intestinal branches; they run in the mesentery tethering the jejunum and ileum.
- **Middle colic artery:** runs in the transverse mesocolon; supplies the transverse colon.

- **Right colic artery:** courses retroperitoneally to the right side; supplies the ascending colon; is variable in location.
- **Ileocolic artery:** passes to the right iliac fossa and supplies the ileum, cecum, appendix, and proximal ascending colon; terminal branch of the SMA.

The **IMA**, the smallest of these three unpaired arteries, arises from the anterior aorta at about the level of the L3 vertebra (the aorta divides anterior to the L4 vertebra), angles to the

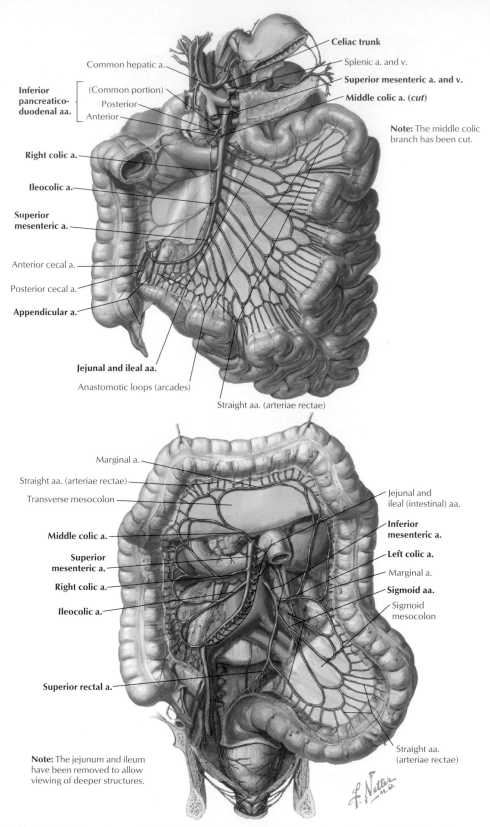

Celiac trunk

Common hepatic a.

Splenic a. and v.

Superior mesenteric a. and v.

Middle colic a. (*cut*)

Inferior pancreatico-duodenal aa.

(Common portion)

Posterior

Anterior

Note: The middle colic branch has been cut.

Right colic a.

Ileocolic a.

Superior mesenteric a.

Anterior cecal a.

Posterior cecal a.

Appendicular a.

Jejunal and ileal aa.

Anastomotic loops (arcades)

Straight aa. (arteriae rectae)

Marginal a.

Straight aa. (arteriae rectae)

Transverse mesocolon

Jejunal and ileal (intestinal) aa.

Inferior mesenteric a.

Middle colic a.

Superior mesenteric a.

Right colic a.

Ileocolic a.

Left colic a.

Marginal a.

Sigmoid aa.

Sigmoid mesocolon

Superior rectal a.

Straight aa. (arteriae rectae)

Note: The jejunum and ileum have been removed to allow viewing of deeper structures.

FIGURE 4.24 Superior and Inferior Mesenteric Arteries and Branches. (From *Netter's atlas of human anatomy,* ed 8, Plates 313 and 314; S-439 and S-440.)

left, and gives rise to the following branches (Fig. 4.24):

- **Left colic artery:** courses to the left and ascends retroperitoneally to supply the distal transverse colon (by an ascending branch that enters the transverse mesocolon) and the descending colon.
- **Sigmoid arteries:** a variable number of arteries (two to four) that enter the sigmoid mesocolon to supply the sigmoid colon.
- **Superior rectal artery:** a small terminal branch that supplies the distal sigmoid colon and proximal rectum.

Along the extent of the abdominal GI tract, the branches of each of these arteries *anastomose* with each other, providing alternative routes of arterial supply. The celiac artery and the SMA anastomose via their branches in the head, body, and tail of the pancreas. The SMA and IMA anastomose along the transverse colon by the **marginal artery** (of Drummond) (Fig. 4.24), which is a large, usually continuous branch that interconnects the right, middle, and left colic branches supplying the large intestine. The IMA forms anastomoses with the arteries of the rectum via its superior rectal artery (Fig. 4.24). All of these arteries are sequentially listed and illustrated in Fig. 4.38.

Venous Drainage

The **hepatic portal system** drains the abdominal GI tract, pancreas, gallbladder, and spleen and ultimately drains into the liver and its sinusoids (Fig. 4.25). By definition, a *portal system* implies that arterial blood flows into a capillary system (in this case the bowel and its accessory organs), then into larger veins (portal tributaries), and then again into another capillary sinusoidal system (liver sinusoids), before ultimately being collected into larger veins (hepatic veins, IVC) that return the blood to the heart.

The **portal vein** ascends from behind the pancreas and courses superiorly in the **hepatoduodenal ligament** (which also contains the *common bile duct* and *proper hepatic artery)* to the hilum of the liver; it is formed by the following veins (Figs. 4.25 and 4.26):

- **Superior mesenteric vein (SMV):** large vein that lies to the right of the SMA and drains portions of the foregut and all of the midgut derivatives.

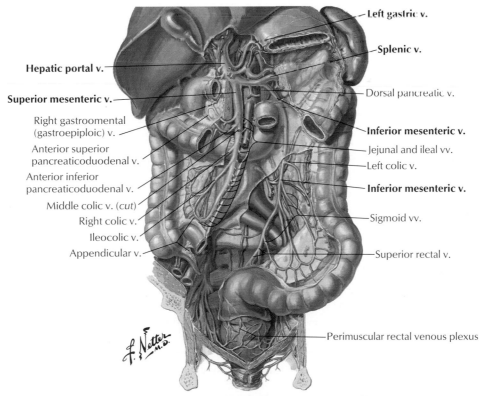

Left gastric v.
Splenic v.
Hepatic portal v.
Superior mesenteric v.
Dorsal pancreatic v.
Right gastroomental (gastroepiploic) v.
Inferior mesenteric v.
Jejunal and ileal vv.
Anterior superior pancreaticoduodenal v.
Left colic v.
Anterior inferior pancreaticoduodenal v.
Inferior mesenteric v.
Middle colic v. (cut)
Sigmoid vv.
Right colic v.
Ileocolic v.
Appendicular v.
Superior rectal v.
Perimuscular rectal venous plexus

FIGURE 4.25 Venous Tributaries of Hepatic Portal System. (From *Netter's atlas of human anatomy,* ed 8, Plate 317; S-444.)

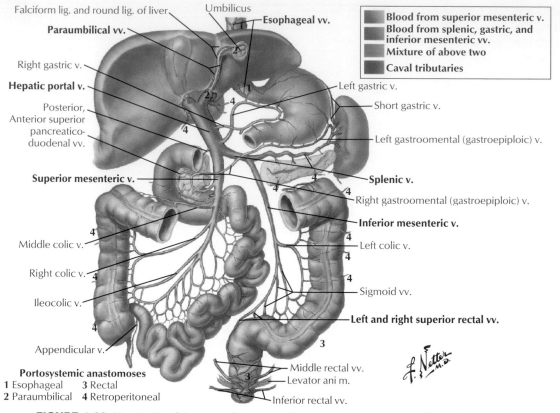

Falciform lig. and round lig. of liver

Paraumbilical vv.

Umbilicus

Esophageal vv.

Blood from superior mesenteric v.
Blood from splenic, gastric, and inferior mesenteric vv.
Mixture of above two
Caval tributaries

Right gastric v.

Hepatic portal v.

Posterior, Anterior superior pancreatico- duodenal vv.

Superior mesenteric v.

Middle colic v.

Right colic v.

Ileocolic v.

Appendicular v.

Left gastric v.

Short gastric v.

Left gastroomental (gastroepiploic) v.

Splenic v.

Right gastroomental (gastroepiploic) v.

Inferior mesenteric v.

Left colic v.

Sigmoid vv.

Left and right superior rectal vv.

Middle rectal vv.
Levator ani m.
Inferior rectal vv.

Portosystemic anastomoses
1 Esophageal   3 Rectal
2 Paraumbilical 4 Retroperitoneal

FIGURE 4.26 Hepatic Portal System and Important Portosystemic Anastomoses. (From *Netter's atlas of human anatomy,* ed 8, Plate 318; S-446.)

- **Splenic vein:** large vein that lies inferior to the splenic artery, parallels its course, and drains the spleen, pancreas, foregut, and, usually, hindgut derivatives (via the **inferior mesenteric vein**).

The **inferior mesenteric vein (IMV)** drains much of the hindgut and then usually drains into the splenic vein (see Figs. 4.25 and 4.26). The IMV also may drain into the junction of the SMV and splenic vein, or drain directly into the SMV (remember, veins are variable).

Typical of most veins in the body, the portal system has *numerous anastomoses* with other veins, specifically in this case with the tributaries of the caval system (IVC and azygos system of veins; Fig. 4.26). These anastomoses allow for the rerouting of venous return to the heart (these veins do not possess valves) should a major vein become occluded. The most important portosystemic anastomoses are around the lower esophagus (these esophageal veins can enlarge and form varices; Clinical Focus 4.19), around the rectum and anal canal (these engorged veins present as hemorrhoids; see Clinical Focus 5.19), and in the paraumbilical

region (these subcutaneous engorged veins present clinically as a caput medusae, resembling the tortuous snakes on the head of Medusa; Clinical Focus 4.18).

Lymphatics

Lymphatic drainage from the stomach, portions of the duodenum, liver, gallbladder, pancreas, and spleen is largely from regional nodes associated with those organs to a central collection of lymph nodes around the celiac trunk (Fig. 4.27). Lymphatic drainage from the midgut derivatives is largely to superior mesenteric nodes adjacent to the superior mesenteric artery, and hindgut derivatives (from the distal transverse colon to the proximal rectum) drain to inferior mesenteric nodes adjacent to the artery of the same name (Fig. 4.28). These nodal collections often are referred to as the **preaortic** and **paraaortic nodes** and ultimately drain to the **cisterna chyli** (dilated proximal end of the thoracic duct), which is located adjacent to the celiac trunk, just to the right of the T12 vertebral body. Lateral aortic lymph nodes lie adjacent to the abdominal aorta, especially between the SMA and the

Clinical Focus 4.18

Portal Hypertension

If the portal vein becomes occluded or its blood cannot pass through the hepatic sinusoids, a significant increase in portal venous pressure will ensue, resulting in portal hypertension. Normal portal venous pressure is 3 to 6 mm Hg but can exceed 12 mm Hg (portal hypertension), resulting in dilated, tortuous veins (varices) and variceal rupture. Three major mechanisms are defined as follows:

- **Prehepatic:** obstructed blood flow to the liver
- **Posthepatic:** obstructed blood flow from the liver to the heart
- **Intrahepatic:** cirrhosis or another liver disease, affecting hepatic sinusoidal blood flow

Clinical consequences of portal hypertension include the following:

- Ascites, usually detectable when 500 mL of fluid accumulates in the abdomen
- Formation of portosystemic shunts via anastomotic channels (see Fig. 4.26)
- Congestive splenomegaly (becomes engorged with venous blood backing up from the splenic vein)
- Hepatic encephalopathy (neurologic problems caused by inadequate removal of toxins in the blood by the diseased liver)

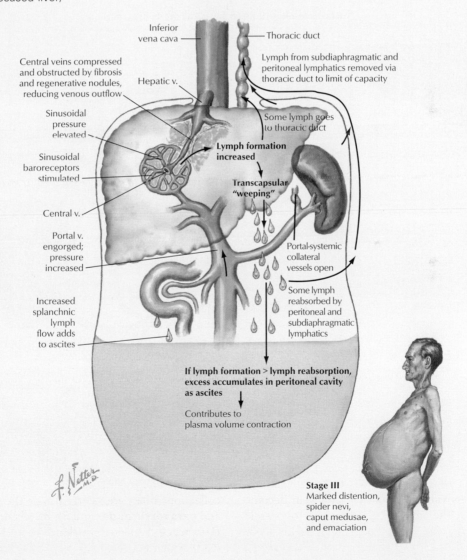

Inferior vena cava

Thoracic duct

Central veins compressed and obstructed by fibrosis and regenerative nodules, reducing venous outflow

Lymph from subdiaphragmatic and peritoneal lymphatics removed via thoracic duct to limit of capacity

Hepatic v.

Sinusoidal pressure elevated

Some lymph goes to thoracic duct

Lymph formation increased

Sinusoidal baroreceptors stimulated

Transcapsular "weeping"

Central v.

Portal v. engorged; pressure increased

Portal-systemic collateral vessels open

Some lymph reabsorbed by peritoneal and subdiaphragmatic lymphatics

Increased splanchnic lymph flow adds to ascites

If lymph formation > lymph reabsorption, excess accumulates in peritoneal cavity as ascites

Contributes to plasma volume contraction

Stage III
Marked distention, spider nevi, caput medusae, and emaciation

Clinical Focus 4.19

Cirrhosis of the Liver

Cirrhosis is a largely irreversible disease characterized by diffuse fibrosis, parenchymal nodular regeneration, and disturbed hepatic architecture. Progressive fibrosis disrupts the portal blood flow, leading to portal hypertension. Major causes of cirrhosis include the following:

- Alcoholic liver disease (60% to 70%)
- Viral hepatitis (10%)
- Biliary diseases (5% to 10%)
- Genetic hemochromatosis (5%)
- Cryptogenic cirrhosis (10% to 15%)

Portal hypertension can lead to **esophageal** and **rectal varices** (tortuous enlargement of the esophageal and rectal veins) as the portal venous blood is shunted into the caval system using portosystemic anastomoses (see Fig. 4.26). Additionally, the engorgement of the superficial venous channels in the subcutaneous tissues of the abdominal wall (see Fig. 4.6, via the paraumbilical portosystemic route) can appear as a **caput medusae** (tortuous subcutaneous varices that resemble the snakes of Medusa's head).

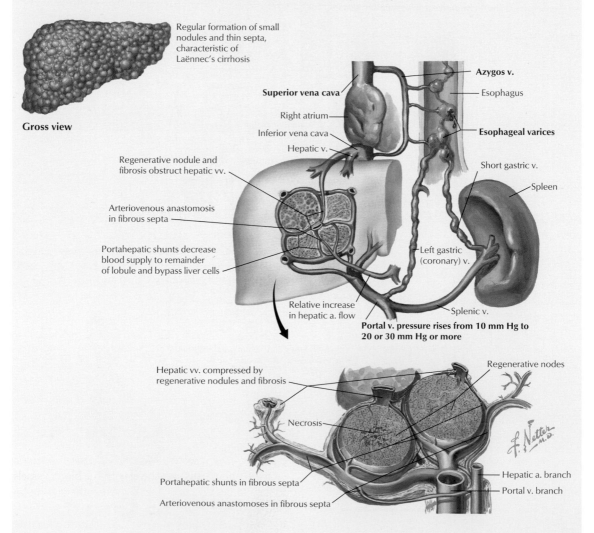

Changes resulting from cirrhosis and portal hypertension

Regular formation of small nodules and thin septa, characteristic of Laënnec's cirrhosis

Gross view

Azygos v.

Superior vena cava

Esophagus

Right atrium

Inferior vena cava

Esophageal varices

Hepatic v.

Regenerative nodule and fibrosis obstruct hepatic vv.

Short gastric v.

Spleen

Arteriovenous anastomosis in fibrous septa

Portahepatic shunts decrease blood supply to remainder of lobule and bypass liver cells

Left gastric (coronary) v.

Relative increase in hepatic a. flow

Splenic v.

Portal v. pressure rises from 10 mm Hg to 20 or 30 mm Hg or more

Hepatic vv. compressed by regenerative nodules and fibrosis

Regenerative nodes

Necrosis

Hepatic a. branch

Portal v. branch

Portahepatic shunts in fibrous septa

Arteriovenous anastomoses in fibrous septa

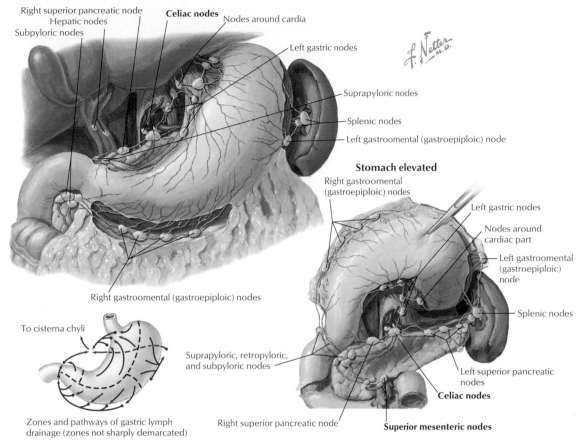

Right superior pancreatic node
Hepatic nodes
Subpyloric nodes
Celiac nodes Nodes around cardia
Left gastric nodes
Suprapyloric nodes
Splenic nodes
Left gastroomental (gastroepiploic) node

Stomach elevated
Right gastroomental (gastroepiploic) nodes
Left gastric nodes
Nodes around cardiac part
Left gastroomental (gastroepiploic) node
Right gastroomental (gastroepiploic) nodes
Splenic nodes

To cisterna chyli
Suprapyloric, retropyloric, and subpyloric nodes
Left superior pancreatic nodes
Celiac nodes

Zones and pathways of gastric lymph drainage (zones not sharply demarcated)
Right superior pancreatic node
Superior mesenteric nodes

FIGURE 4.27 Lymphatics of Epigastric Region.

bifurcation of the aorta at the level of the L4 vertebral body.

Innervation

The abdominal viscera are innervated by the **autonomic nervous system (ANS),** and the pattern of innervation closely parallels the arterial supply to the various embryonic gut regions (see Table 4.14). Additionally, the **enteric nervous system** provides an "intrinsic" network of ganglia with connections to the ANS, which helps coordinate peristalsis and secretion (see Chapter 1). The enteric ganglia and nerve plexuses include the **myenteric plexus** and **submucosal plexus** within the layers of the bowel wall (see Fig. 1.27).

The **sympathetic innervation** of the viscera is derived from the following nerves (Figs. 4.29 and 4.30):

- **Thoracic splanchnic nerves:** greater (T5-T9 or T10), lesser (T10-T11), and least (T12) splanchnic nerves (the spinal cord levels contributing these nerve fibers may vary) will arise from the associated **thoracic sympathetic**

chain, convey preganglionic axons to **abdominal prevertebral ganglia** (celiac and superior mesenteric ganglia), and synapse in these ganglia. Postganglionic sympathetic nerve fibers will innervate the embryonic foregut and midgut visceral derivatives.

- **Lumbar splanchnic nerves:** several pairs of lumbar splanchnic nerves (L1-L2 or L3) that convey sympathetic preganglionic axons to the **inferior mesenteric ganglion** and plexus to innervate the embryonic hindgut visceral derivatives (see Figs. 1.24, 1.26, and 4.29 and Table 4.14).

Postganglionic sympathetic axons arise from the postganglionic neurons in the prevertebral ganglia (*celiac, superior mesenteric, and inferior mesenteric ganglia*) and plexus and travel with the blood vessels to their target viscera. Generally, sympathetic stimulation of the GI tract leads to the following:

- Vasoconstriction to shunt blood to other parts of the body, thus inhibiting digestion.
- Reduced bowel motility.
- Reduced bowel secretion.

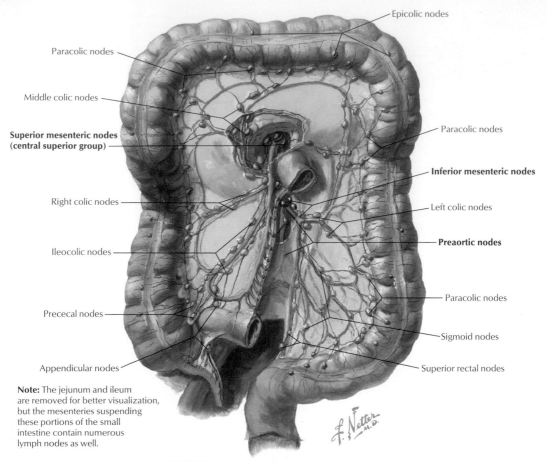

FIGURE 4.28 Lymphatics of the Intestines.

The **parasympathetic innervation** of the viscera is derived from the following nerves (see Table 4.14 and Fig. 4.30):

- **Vagus nerves:** anterior and posterior vagal trunks enter the abdomen on the esophagus and send *preganglionic axons* directly to postganglionic neurons in or near the walls of the viscera derived from the embryonic foregut and midgut (distal esophagus to the proximal two-thirds of the transverse colon).
- **Pelvic splanchnic nerves:** *preganglionic axons* from S2-S4 travel via these splanchnic nerves to the prevertebral plexus (inferior hypogastric plexus) and distribute to the postganglionic neurons of the embryonic hindgut derivatives. (**Note:** pelvic splanchnic nerves are *not* part of the sympathetic trunk; only sympathetic neurons and axons reside in the sympathetic trunk and chain ganglia.)

Many postganglionic parasympathetic neurons are in the **myenteric** and **submucosal ganglia** and plexuses that compose the *enteric nervous system*

(see Chapter 1), Fig. 1.27. Generally, parasympathetic stimulation leads to the following:

- Increased bowel motility
- Increased secretion
- Increased blood flow

Visceral afferent fibers travel with the ANS components and can be summarized as follows:

- **Pain afferents:** include the pain modalities of distention/compression, inflammation, and ischemia, which are conveyed to the central nervous system (CNS) largely by the sympathetic components to the spinal ganglia (DRG) associated with the *T5-L2 spinal cord levels.* These visceral pain fibers travel back in the sympathetic nerves until they reach the spinal nerve and then pass to the respective spinal ganglion and into the spinal cord. Thus, GI pain may be perceived over the body regions represented by the T5-L2 dermatomes. Pain afferents for the distal hindgut also pass to spinal ganglia via pelvic splanchnics (S2-S4). These pain signals then

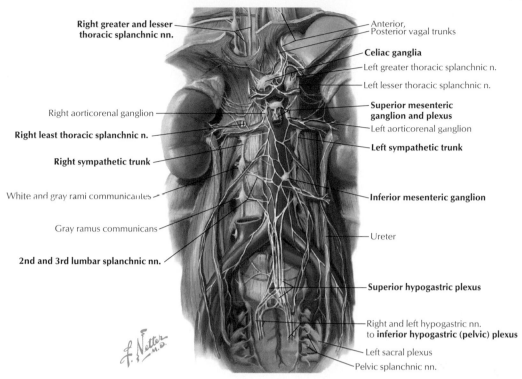

Right greater and lesser thoracic splanchnic nn.

Anterior, Posterior vagal trunks

Celiac ganglia

Left greater thoracic splanchnic n.

Left lesser thoracic splanchnic n.

Right aorticorenal ganglion

Superior mesenteric ganglion and plexus

Left aorticorenal ganglion

Right least thoracic splanchnic n.

Left sympathetic trunk

Right sympathetic trunk

White and gray rami communicantes

Inferior mesenteric ganglion

Gray ramus communicans

Ureter

2nd and 3rd lumbar splanchnic nn.

Superior hypogastric plexus

Right and left hypogastric nn. to **inferior hypogastric (pelvic) plexus**

Left sacral plexus

Pelvic splanchnic nn.

FIGURE 4.29 Abdominal Autonomic Nerves. (From *Netter's atlas of human anatomy*, ed 8, Plate 319; S-105.)

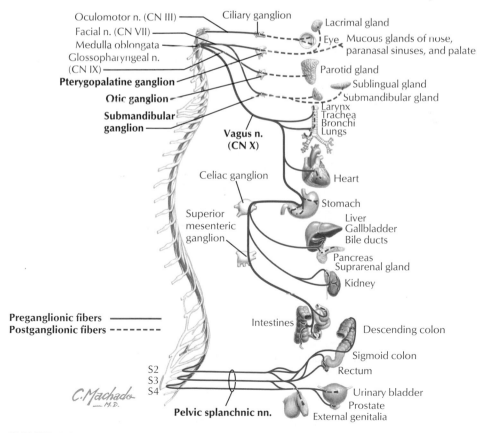

Oculomotor n. (CN III)

Ciliary ganglion

Lacrimal gland

Facial n. (CN VII)

Eye   Mucous glands of nose, paranasal sinuses, and palate

Medulla oblongata

Glossopharyngeal n. (CN IX)

Parotid gland

Pterygopalatine ganglion

Sublingual gland

Otic ganglion

Submandibular gland

Submandibular ganglion

Larynx
Trachea
Bronchi
Lungs

Vagus n. (CN X)

Celiac ganglion

Heart

Stomach

Superior mesenteric ganglion

Liver
Gallbladder
Bile ducts

Pancreas
Suprarenal gland

Kidney

Preganglionic fibers ——————
Postganglionic fibers – – – – – –

Intestines

Descending colon

Sigmoid colon

Rectum

S2
S3
S4

Urinary bladder
Prostate
External genitalia

Pelvic splanchnic nn.

FIGURE 4.30 Parasympathetic Innervation of Abdominal Viscera. (From *Netter's atlas of human anatomy*, ed 8, Plate 7; S-21.)

ascend through the spinal cord to the brainstem and brain.

- **Reflex afferents:** include information from *chemoreceptors, osmoreceptors, and mechanoreceptors,* which are conveyed to autonomic centers in the medulla oblongata of the brainstem via the **vagus nerves** from the embryonic foregut and midgut derivatives of the GI tract. Reflex afferents from the embryonic hindgut derivatives of the GI tract course back to the spinal cord via the **pelvic splanchnic nerves** to the spinal ganglia associated with the S2-S4 spinal cord levels.

Gastrointestinal function is a coordinated effort not only by the "hard-wired" components of the ANS and enteric nervous system, as described earlier, but also by the *immune and endocrine systems.* In fact, many view the GI tract as the largest endocrine organ in the body, secreting and responding to dozens of GI hormones and other neuroeffector substances.

6. POSTERIOR ABDOMINAL WALL AND VISCERA

Posterior Abdominal Wall

The posterior abdominal wall and its visceral structures lie deep to the parietal peritoneum **(retroperitoneal)** lining the posterior abdominal cavity. This region contains skeletal structures, muscles, major vascular channels, the kidneys and suprarenal (adrenal) glands, nerves, and lymphatics.

Fascia and Muscles

Deep to the parietal peritoneum, the muscles of the posterior abdominal wall are enveloped in a layer of investing fascia called the *endoabdominal fascia,* which is continuous laterally with the *transversalis fascia* of the transversus abdominis muscle. For identification, the fascia is named according to the structures it covers and includes the following layers (Figs. 4.31 and 4.32):

- **Psoas fascia:** covers the psoas major muscle and is thickened superiorly, forming the medial arcuate ligament.
- **Thoracolumbar fascia:** anterior layer covers the quadratus lumborum muscle and is thickened superiorly, forming the lateral arcuate ligament; middle and posterior layers of the thoracolumbar fascia envelop the erector spinae muscles of the back.

The muscles of the posterior abdominal wall have attachments to the lower rib cage, the T12-L5 vertebrae, and bones of the pelvic girdle (Table 4.10 and Fig. 4.32). Note that the **diaphragm** has a central tendinous portion and is attached to the lumbar vertebrae by a right crus and a left crus (leg), which are joined centrally by the median arcuate ligament that passes over the emerging abdominal aorta. The **inferior vena cava** passes through the diaphragm at the T8 vertebral level to enter the right atrium of the heart. The right phrenic nerve may accompany the IVC as it passes through

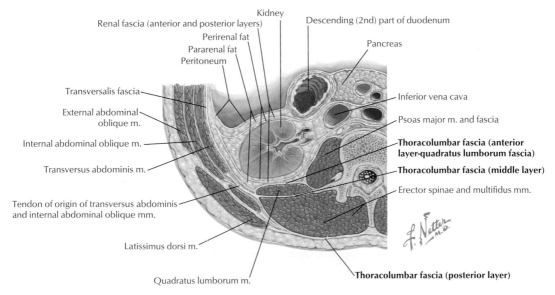

FIGURE 4.31 Transverse Section Through L2 Vertebra. (From *Netter's atlas of human anatomy,* ed 8, Plate 200; S-545.)

TABLE 4.10 Muscles of Posterior Abdominal Wall

MUSCLE	ORIGIN ATTACHMENT	INSERTION ATTACHMENT	INNERVATION	ACTIONS
Psoas major	Transverse processes of lumbar vertebrae; sides of bodies of T12-L5 vertebrae, and intervening intervertebral discs	Lesser trochanter of femur	Lumbar plexus via anterior branches of L1-L3 nerves	Acting superiorly with iliacus, flexes hip; acting inferiorly, flexes vertebral column laterally; used to balance trunk in sitting position; acting inferiorly with iliacus, flexes trunk
Iliacus	Superior two-thirds of iliac fossa, ala of sacrum, and anterior sacroiliac ligaments	Lesser trochanter of femur and shaft inferior to it and to psoas major tendon	Femoral nerve (L2-L4)	Flexes thigh at hip and stabilizes hip joint; acts with psoas major
Quadratus lumborum	Medial half of inferior border of 12th rib and tips of lumbar transverse processes	Iliolumbar ligament and internal lip of iliac crest	Anterior rami of T12 and L1-L4 nerves	Extends and laterally flexes vertebral column; fixes 12th rib during inspiration
Respiratory diaphragm	Thoracic outlet: xiphoid, lower six costal cartilages, L1-L3 vertebrae	Converges into central tendon	Phrenic nerve (C3-C5)	Draws central tendon down and forward during inspiration

Variations in spinal nerve contributions to the innervation of muscles, their attachments, and their actions are common in human anatomy. Therefore, expect differences between texts and realize that anatomical variation is normal.

the diaphragm, which it innervates. The **esophagus** passes through the diaphragm at the T10 vertebral level, along with the anterior and posterior vagal trunks esophageal branches of the left gastric artery. The **aorta** passes through the diaphragm at the T12 vertebral level and is accompanied by the thoracic duct and often the azygos vein as they course superiorly.

Kidneys and Adrenal (Suprarenal) Glands

The kidneys and adrenal glands are retroperitoneal organs that receive a rich arterial supply (Fig. 4.33). The right kidney usually lies somewhat lower than the left kidney because of the presence of the liver.

Each **kidney** is enclosed in the following layers of fascia and fat (Figs. 4.31 and 4.34):

- **Renal capsule:** covers each kidney and forms a thick fibroconnective tissue capsule.
- **Perirenal (perinephric) fat:** directly surrounds the kidney (and adrenal glands) and cushions it.
- **Renal (Gerota's) fascia:** surrounds the kidney (and adrenal glands), the ureter, the renal vessels, and the perirenal fat; superiorly it is continuous with the fascia covering the diaphragm; inferiorly it may blend with the transversalis fascia; medially the anterior layer blends with the vessels in the renal hilum and the connective tissue of the aorta and IVC. A thin renal capsule intimately invests each kidney and lies deep to the renal fat.

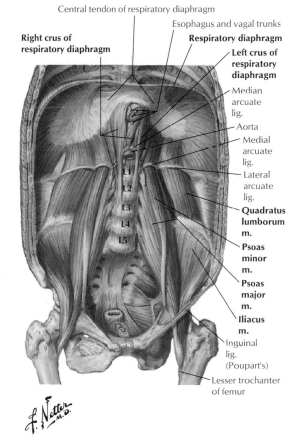

Central tendon of respiratory diaphragm

Esophagus and vagal trunks

Right crus of respiratory diaphragm

Respiratory diaphragm

Left crus of respiratory diaphragm

Median arcuate lig.

Aorta

Medial arcuate lig.

Lateral arcuate lig.

Quadratus lumborum m.

Psoas minor m.

Psoas major m.

Iliacus m.

Inguinal lig. (Poupart's)

Lesser trochanter of femur

L1
L2
L3
L4
L5

FIGURE 4.32 Muscles of Posterior Abdominal Wall. (From *Netter's atlas of human anatomy*, ed 8, Plate 283; S-219.)

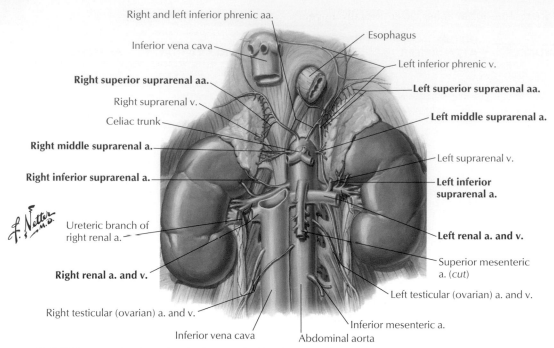

Right and left inferior phrenic aa.

Esophagus

Inferior vena cava

Left inferior phrenic v.

Right superior suprarenal aa.

Left superior suprarenal aa.

Right suprarenal v.

Left middle suprarenal a.

Celiac trunk

Right middle suprarenal a.

Left suprarenal v.

Right inferior suprarenal a.

**Left inferior
suprarenal a.**

Ureteric branch of
right renal a.

Left renal a. and v.

Right renal a. and v.

Superior mesenteric
a. (*cut*)

Left testicular (ovarian) a. and v.

Right testicular (ovarian) a. and v.

Inferior mesenteric a.

Inferior vena cava   Abdominal aorta

FIGURE 4.33 Blood Supply of Kidneys and Adrenal Glands. (From *Netter's atlas of human anatomy*,
ed 8, Plate 332; S-531.)

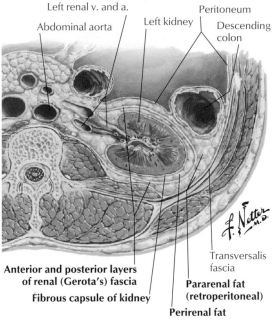

Left renal v. and a.

Abdominal aorta

Left kidney

Peritoneum

Descending
colon

Transversalis
fascia

**Anterior and posterior layers
of renal (Gerota's) fascia**

**Pararenal fat
(retroperitoneal)**

Fibrous capsule of kidney

Perirenal fat

FIGURE 4.34 Renal Fascia and Fat. (From *Netter's atlas
of human anatomy*, ed 8, Plate 337; S-461.)

- **Pararenal (paranephric) fat:** an outer layer of
  fat outside of the renal fascia that is variable in
  thickness and is continuous with the extraperitoneal (retroperitoneal) fat.

The kidneys are related posteriorly to the respiratory diaphragm and muscles of the posterior
abdominal wall, as well as the 11th and 12th (floating)
ribs. They move with respiration, and anteriorly are
in relation to the abdominal viscera and mesenteries
shown in Figs. 4.14 and 4.18. For the right kidney,
this includes the liver, second part of the duodenum,
ascending colon, and/or right colic flexure. For the left
kidney, this includes the pancreas, spleen, descending
colon, and/or left colic flexure. Each kidney also is
"capped" by the **adrenal (suprarenal) glands**. Variability in these relationships is common because the
size of the kidneys can be quite variable, as can the
size of the adjacent viscera, disposition of mobile
portions of the bowel, and extent of the mesenteries.

Structurally, each kidney has the following gross
features (Fig. 4.35):

- **Renal capsule:** a thin fibroconnective tissue
  capsule that surrounds the renal cortex.
- **Renal cortex:** outer layer that surrounds the
  renal medulla and contains nephrons (units of
  filtration numbering about a million in each
  kidney) and renal tubules.

- **Renal medulla:** inner layer (usually appears darker) that contains renal tubules and collecting ducts that convey the filtrate to minor calyces; the renal cortex extends as renal columns between the medulla, demarcating the distinctive medullary **renal pyramids** whose apex **(renal papilla)** terminates with a minor calyx.
- **Minor calyx:** structure that receives urine from the collecting ducts of the renal pyramids.
- **Major calyx:** site at which several minor calyces drain.
- **Renal pelvis:** point at which several major calyces unite; conveys urine to the proximal **ureter.**
- **Hilum:** medial aspect of each kidney, where the renal pelvis emerges from the kidney and where vessels, nerves, and lymphatics enter or leave the kidney.

The kidneys filter about 180 liters of fluid each day, as about 20% of the cardiac output each minute passes through the kidneys. The kidneys function to:

- Filter plasma and begin the process of urine formation.
- Reabsorb important electrolytes, organic molecules, vitamins, and water from the filtrate.
- Excrete metabolic wastes, metabolites, and foreign chemicals (e.g., drugs).
- Regulate fluid volume, composition, and pH.
- Secrete hormones that regulate the blood pressure, erythropoiesis, and calcium metabolism.
- Convey urine to the ureters, which then pass the urine to the bladder.

The **ureters** are 25-30 cm long, extend from the renal pelvis to the urinary bladder, are composed of a thick layer of smooth muscle, and lie in a retroperitoneal position.

The **right adrenal (suprarenal) gland** often is pyramidal in shape, whereas the left gland is often semilunar in shape (see Fig. 4.33). Each adrenal gland "caps" the superior pole of the kidney and is surrounded by perirenal fat and renal fascia. The right adrenal gland is close to the IVC and liver, whereas the stomach, pancreas, and even the spleen can lie anterior to the left adrenal gland.

As endocrine organs, the adrenal glands have a rich vascular supply from **superior suprarenal arteries** (branches of the inferior phrenic arteries), **middle suprarenal arteries** directly from the aorta, and **inferior suprarenal arteries** from the renal arteries (see Figs. 4.33 and 4.36). The kidneys and adrenal glands are innervated by the ANS.

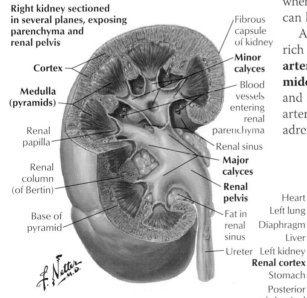

Right kidney sectioned in several planes, exposing parenchyma and renal pelvis

- Cortex
- Medulla (pyramids)
- Renal papilla
- Renal column (of Bertin)
- Base of pyramid
- Fibrous capsule of kidney
- Minor calyces
- Blood vessels entering renal parenchyma
- Renal sinus
- Major calyces
- Renal pelvis
- Fat in renal sinus
- Ureter

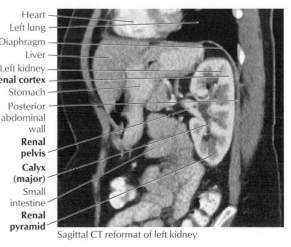

- Heart
- Left lung
- Diaphragm
- Liver
- Left kidney
- Renal cortex
- Stomach
- Posterior abdominal wall
- Renal pelvis
- Calyx (major)
- Small intestine
- Renal pyramid

Sagittal CT reformat of left kidney

FIGURE 4.35 Features of Right Kidney Sectioned in Several Planes. (From *Netter's atlas of human anatomy*, ed 8, Plate 333; S-462; CT image from Kelley LL, Petersen C: *Sectional anatomy for imaging professionals*, Philadelphia, 2007, Mosby.)

Clinical Focus 4.20

Renal Stones (Calculi)

Renal stones may form in the kidney and remain there or more often pass down the ureters to the bladder. When they traverse the ureter, the stones cause significant pain **(renal colic)** that typically distributes on the side of the insult radiating from "loin to groin." The ureters narrow at three points along their course to the bladder. This is a common location for renal stones to become lodged and cause pain. This pain distribution reflects the pathway of visceral pain afferents (pain is from distention of the ureter) that course to the spinal cord levels T11-L2 via the sympathetic splanchnic nerves. Complications of renal stones include obstruction to the flow of urine, infection, and destruction of the renal parenchyma.

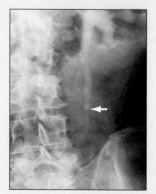

Midureteral obstruction

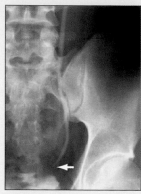

Distal ureteral obstruction

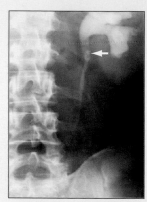

Ureteropelvic obstruction

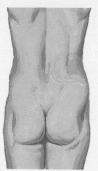

Distribution of pain in renal colic

JOHN A. CRAIG—AD

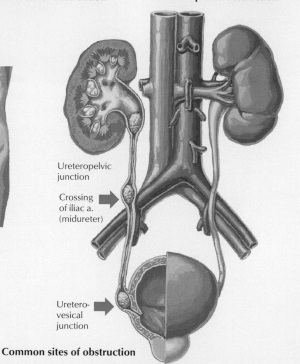

Ureteropelvic junction

Crossing of iliac a. (midureter)

Uretero-vesical junction

Common sites of obstruction

Features of Urinary Tract Calculi	
Characteristic	Description
Type	75% calcium oxalate (phosphate), 15% magnesium ammonium phosphate, 10% uric acid or cystine
Prevalence	Approximately 15% in the United States, highest in Southeast; 2-3 times more common in men than in women; uncommon in African-Americans and Asians
Risk factors	Concentrated urine, heredity, diet, associated diseases (sarcoidosis, inflammatory bowel disease, cancer)

Clinical Focus 4.21

Obstructive Uropathy

Obstruction to the normal flow of urine, which may occur anywhere from the level of the renal nephrons to the urethral opening, can precipitate pathologic changes that with infection can lead to serious uropathies. This composite figure shows a number of obstructive possibilities and highlights important aspects of the adjacent anatomy one sees along the extent of the urinary tract.

Possible obstructive entities along the urinary tract

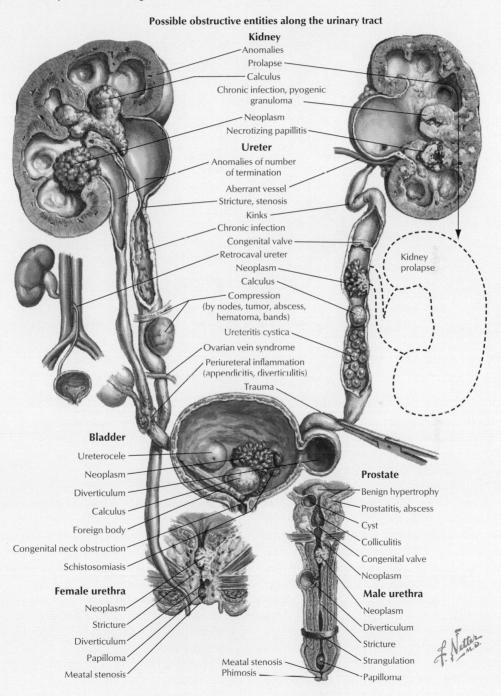

Kidney
Anomalies
Prolapse
Calculus
Chronic infection, pyogenic granuloma
Neoplasm
Necrotizing papillitis

Ureter
Anomalies of number of termination
Aberrant vessel
Stricture, stenosis
Kinks
Chronic infection
Congenital valve
Retrocaval ureter
Neoplasm
Calculus
Compression (by nodes, tumor, abscess, hematoma, bands)
Ureteritis cystica
Ovarian vein syndrome
Periureteral inflammation (appendicitis, diverticulitis)
Trauma

Kidney prolapse

Bladder
Ureterocele
Neoplasm
Diverticulum
Calculus
Foreign body
Congenital neck obstruction
Schistosomiasis

Female urethra
Neoplasm
Stricture
Diverticulum
Papilloma
Meatal stenosis

Prostate
Benign hypertrophy
Prostatitis, abscess
Cyst
Colliculitis
Congenital valve
Neoplasm

Male urethra
Neoplasm
Diverticulum
Stricture
Strangulation
Papilloma

Meatal stenosis
Phimosis

Clinical Focus 4.22

Malignant Tumors of the Kidney

Of the malignant kidney tumors, 80% to 90% are *adenocarcinomas* that arise from the tubular epithelium. They account for about 2% of all adult cancers, often occur after age 50, and occur twice as often in men as in women. **Wilms tumor** accounts for about 7% of all malignancies in children and is associated with congenital malformations related to chromosome 11.

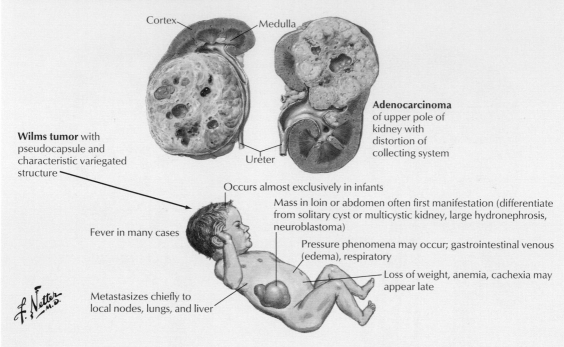

Cortex

Medulla

Adenocarcinoma of upper pole of kidney with distortion of collecting system

Ureter

Wilms tumor with pseudocapsule and characteristic variegated structure

Occurs almost exclusively in infants

Mass in loin or abdomen often first manifestation (differentiate from solitary cyst or multicystic kidney, large hydronephrosis, neuroblastoma)

Fever in many cases

Pressure phenomena may occur; gastrointestinal venous (edema), respiratory

Loss of weight, anemia, cachexia may appear late

Metastasizes chiefly to local nodes, lungs, and liver

Sympathetic nerves arise from the T10-L2 spinal levels; they synapse in the superior mesenteric ganglia and superior hypogastric plexuses and send postganglionic fibers to the kidney and adrenal glands. In the adrenal glands, these sympathetic postganglionic fibers are vasomotor in function. Additionally, *preganglionic fibers* from the lower thoracic levels travel directly to the medulla of each adrenal gland and synapse on the **medullary cells** (the neuroendocrine [chromaffin] cells of the medulla are the postganglionic cells of the sympathetic system). These neuroendocrine cells secrete primarily epinephrine and, to a lesser extent, norepinephrine into the bloodstream. These catecholamines increase the heart rate and blood flow to essential tissues, increase the blood pressure, and increase the rate of respiration. **Parasympathetic nerves** to the kidneys and adrenal glands travel with the **vagus nerves** and synapse on postganglionic neurons within the kidney and

adrenal cortex (see Figs. 4.29 and 4.30). The adrenal cortex secretes cortisol, aldosterone, and adrenal androgens.

Abdominal Vessels

The **abdominal aorta** extends from the aortic hiatus (T12) to the lower level of the L4 vertebra, where it divides into the right and left common iliac arteries (Figs. 4.22, 4.36, and 4.38). The abdominal aorta gives rise to the following three groups of arteries (Table 4.11):

- **Unpaired visceral arteries** to the GI tract, spleen, pancreas, gallbladder, and liver.
- **Paired visceral arteries** to the kidneys, adrenal glands, and gonads.
- **Parietal arteries** to musculoskeletal structures of the abdominal wall.

The **inferior vena cava** (IVC) (Fig. 4.37) drains abdominal structures other than the GI tract, pancreas, and the spleen, which are drained by the

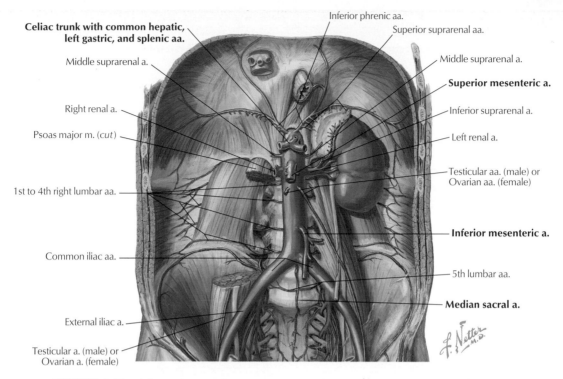

FIGURE 4.36 Abdominal Aorta. (From *Netter's atlas of human anatomy*, ed 8, Plate 284; S-341.)

TABLE 4.11 Branches of Abdominal Aorta

ARTERIAL BRANCH	STRUCTURES SUPPLIED
Unpaired Visceral	
Celiac trunk	Embryonic foregut derivatives and spleen*
SMA	Embryonic midgut derivatives*
IMA	Embryonic hindgut derivatives*
Paired Visceral	
Middle suprarenals	Adrenal (suprarenal) glands
Renals	Kidneys
Gonadal	Ovarian or testicular branches to gonad
Parietal Branches	
Inferior phrenics	Paired arteries to diaphragm
Lumbars	Usually four pairs to posterior abdominal wall and spine
Median sacral	Unpaired artery to sacrum (caudal artery)

SMA, Superior mesenteric artery; *IMA*, inferior mesenteric artery.

*See Table 4.14 for list of derivatives

hepatic portal system (Figs. 4.25, 4.26, and 4.40). The IVC begins by the union of the two common iliac veins just to the right and slightly inferior of the midline bifurcation of the distal abdominal aorta, at about the level of the L5 vertebra (Fig. 4.37). The IVC ascends to pierce the diaphragm at the level of the T8 vertebral level, where it empties into the right atrium. Most of the IVC tributaries parallel the arterial branches of the aorta, but two or three hepatic veins also enter the IVC just inferior to the diaphragm (Fig. 4.37). It is important to note that the ascending lumbar veins connect adjacent lumbar veins and drain superiorly into the **azygos venous system** (see Chapter 3, Figs. 3.26 and 3.28). This venous anastomosis is a very important route of *collateral circulation* should the IVC should become obstructed.

Arteries of the Abdominal Aorta

The **abdominal aorta (1)** is a continuation of the thoracic aorta beginning at about the level of the T12 vertebra, where the aorta passes through the aortic hiatus of the diaphragm. It gives off three sets of **parietal arteries** that supply the diaphragm **(inferior phrenic artery [2]),** usually four pairs of **lumbar arteries (3),** and an unpaired **median sacral artery (4),** our equivalent of the "caudal artery" (for the tail) in most other mammals. These arteries arise from the posterolateral aspect of the aorta (Fig. 4.38).

The **abdominal aorta (1)** also gives rise to three **unpaired visceral arteries** that arise from the anterior aspect of the aorta. The **celiac trunk (5)** supplies the embryonic foregut derivatives of

Clinical Focus 4.23

Surgical Management of Abdominal Aortic Aneurysm

Aneurysms (bulges in the arterial wall) usually involve the large arteries. The multifactorial etiology includes family history, hypertension, breakdown of collagen and elastin within the vessel wall (which leads to inflammation and weakening of the arterial wall), and atherosclerosis. The abdominal aorta (*infrarenal segment*) and iliac arteries are most often involved, but the thoracic aorta and the femoral and popliteal arteries can also have aneurysms. Symptoms include abdominal and back pain, nausea, and early satiety, but up to 75% of patients may be asymptomatic. If surgical repair is warranted, an open procedure may be done using durable synthetic grafts (illustrated) or an endovascular repair, in which a new synthetic lining is inserted using hooks or stents to hold the lining in place.

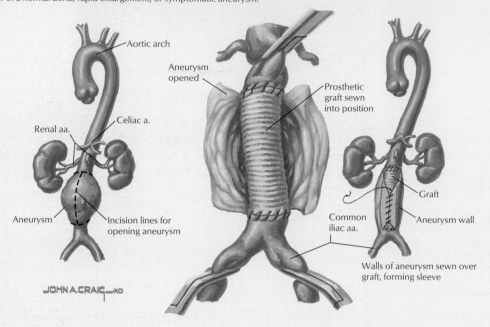

Indications for surgery include an aneurysm diameter that is twice the diameter of a normal aorta, rapid enlargement, or symptomatic aneurysm.

Aortic arch

Aneurysm opened

Prosthetic graft sewn into position

Celiac a.

Renal aa.

Aneurysm

Incision lines for opening aneurysm

Graft

Common iliac aa.

Aneurysm wall

Walls of aneurysm sewn over graft, forming sleeve

JOHN A. CRAIG—MD

the gastrointestinal tract and its accessory organs, the gallbladder, liver, and pancreas. It also supplies the spleen, an organ of the immune system. The **superior mesenteric artery (6)** supplies the embryonic midgut derivatives (distal half of the duodenum, small intestine, cecum, appendix, ascending colon, and proximal two-thirds of the transverse colon) and also portions of the pancreas. The **inferior mesenteric artery (7)** supplies the embryonic hindgut derivatives (distal transverse colon, descending colon, sigmoid colon, and proximal rectum).

The **abdominal aorta (1)** finally gives rise to three **paired visceral arteries** that supply the adrenal (suprarenal) glands via the paired **middle suprarenal arteries (8),** the kidneys via the paired **renal arteries (9),** and the gonads via

the paired **ovarian or testicular arteries (10).** The paired visceral branches arise from the lateral aspect of the **abdominal aorta (1).** The aorta then divides into the right and left **common iliac arteries.**

A rich blood supply is common around the stomach, duodenum, and pancreas. The adrenal glands also receive a rich vascular supply (superior, middle, and inferior suprarenal arteries). The small bowel has a collateral circulation via its *arcades* and the colon via its *marginal artery*, although the pattern and supply by these arteries is variable.

In the outline of the arteries (Fig. 4.38), major vessels often dissected in anatomy courses include the first-order arteries (in bold and numbered) and their second-order major branches. In more detailed dissection courses, some or all of the third- and/or fourth-order arteries may also be dissected.

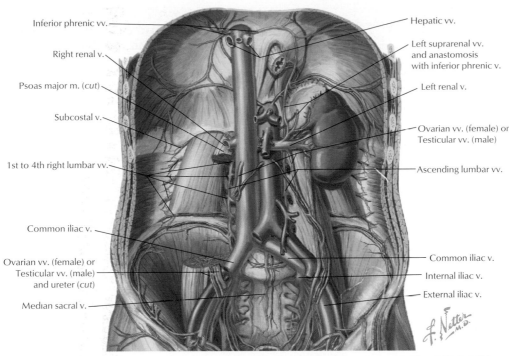

Inferior phrenic vv.

Right renal v.

Psoas major m. (cut)

Subcostal v.

1st to 4th right lumbar vv.

Common iliac v.

Ovarian vv. (female) or
Testicular vv. (male)
and ureter (cut)

Median sacral v.

Hepatic vv.

Left suprarenal vv.
and anastomosis
with inferior phrenic v.

Left renal v.

Ovarian vv. (female) or
Testicular vv. (male)

Ascending lumbar vv.

Common iliac v.

Internal iliac v.

External iliac v.

FIGURE 4.37 Inferior Vena Cava. (From *Netter's atlas of human anatomy*, ed 8, Plate 285; S-342.)

Thoracic Aorta*
1. Abdominal Aorta
2. Inferior Phrenic Arteries
   Superior suprarenal arteries
3. Lumbar Arteries (usually 4 pairs)
   Dorsal branch
   Spinal branch
     Segmental medullary artery
4. Median Sacral Artery
5. Celiac Trunk
   Left gastric artery
     Esophageal branches
   Common hepatic artery
     Gastroduodenal artery
       Post. sup. pancreaticoduodenal artery
       Retroduodenal arteries
       Right gastroepiploic artery
       Ant. sup. pancreaticoduodenal artery
     Right gastric artery
     Proper hepatic artery
       Right branch
         Cystic artery
         Artery to caudate lobe/segmental aa.
       Left branch
         Artery to caudate lobe/segmental aa.
   Splenic artery
     Pancreatic aa. (various small branches)
     Left gastroepiploic artery
     Short gastric arteries
     Splenic branches
     Post. gastric artery
6. Superior Mesenteric Artery
   Inferior pancreaticoduodenal artery
   Jejunal and ileal branches
   Middle colic artery
   Right colic artery
   Ileocolic artery
     Appendicular artery
   Marginal artery (arcade)
7. Inferior Mesenteric Artery
   Left colic artery (ascending/descending br.)
   Sigmoid arteries (2–4 branches)
   Superior rectal artery
8. Middle Suprarenal Artery
9. Renal Artery (variable number)
   Inferior suprarenal artery
   Ant. and post. branches
   Ureteric branch
10. Ovarian Artery (female) or Testicular Artery (male)
   Ureteric branches
   Tubal (epididymal) branches
Right and Left Common Iliac Arteries

*Proximal (thoracic aorta) to Distal (aortic bifurcation)

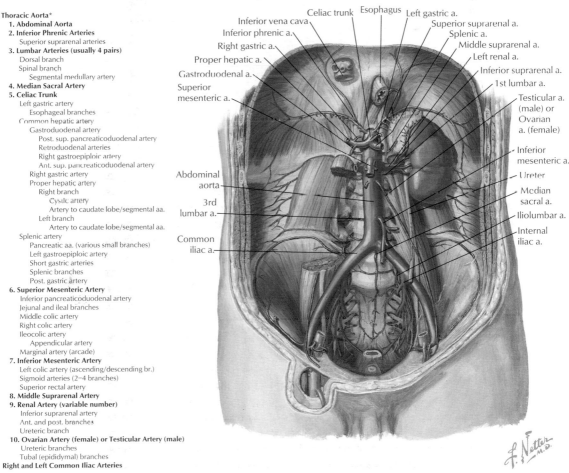

Inferior vena cava
Inferior phrenic a.
Right gastric a.
Proper hepatic a.
Gastroduodenal a.
Superior mesenteric a.

Celiac trunk   Esophagus   Left gastric a.
Superior suprarenal a.
Splenic a.
Middle suprarenal a.
Left renal a.
Inferior suprarenal a.
1st lumbar a.
Testicular a. (male) or Ovarian a. (female)
Inferior mesenteric a.
Ureter
Median sacral a.
Iliolumbar a.
Internal iliac a.

Abdominal aorta

3rd lumbar a.

Common iliac a.

FIGURE 4.38 Arteries of the Abdominal Aorta.

Veins of the Abdomen (Caval System)

As elsewhere in the body, the veins of the abdomen include a deep group and a superficial group. The *deep veins* drain essentially the areas supplied by the "parietal and paired visceral" branches of the abdominal aorta (Fig. 4.39). (Note that the "unpaired visceral" branches of the abdominal aorta supplying the GI tract, its accessory organs, and the spleen are drained by the **hepatic portal system of veins**.)

Beginning at the level of the pelvic brim, the **common iliac vein (1)** is formed by the internal and external iliac veins. The two **common iliac veins (1)** join to form the **inferior vena cava (2)**, which receives venous drainage from the gonads, kidneys, posterior abdominal wall (lumbar veins), liver, and diaphragm. The IVC then drains into the **right atrium of the heart (3).**

The superficial set of veins drain the anterolateral abdominal wall, the superficial inguinal region, rectus sheath, and lateral thoracic wall (Fig. 4.6).

Most of its connections ultimately drain into the **axillary vein (4),** then into the **subclavian vein** and the two **brachiocephalic veins**, which unite to form the **superior vena cava**, and then into the **heart (3).** The inferior epigastric veins (from the external iliac veins) enter the posterior rectus sheath, course cranially above the umbilicus as the superior epigastric veins, and then anastomose with the internal thoracic veins that drain into the subclavian veins (see Figs. 3.28, 4.3, and 4.6).

The superficial veins can become enlarged during *portal hypertension*, when the venous flow through the liver is compromised. Important **portosystemic anastomoses** between the portal system and caval system can allow venous blood to gain access to the caval veins (both deep and superficial veins) to assist in returning blood to the heart (see Figs. 4.25 and 4.26).

Variations in the venous pattern and in the number of veins and their sizes are common, so it is best to understand the major venous channels

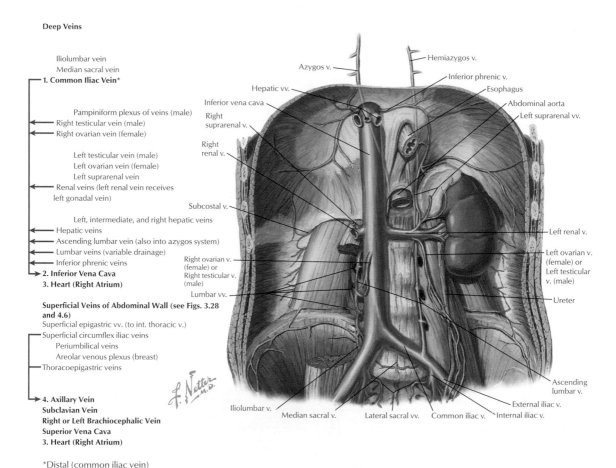

Deep Veins

Iliolumbar vein
Median sacral vein
1. Common Iliac Vein*

Pampiniform plexus of veins (male)
Right testicular vein (male)
Right ovarian vein (female)

Left testicular vein (male)
Left ovarian vein (female)
Left suprarenal vein
Renal veins (left renal vein receives left gonadal vein)

Left, intermediate, and right hepatic veins
Hepatic veins
Ascending lumbar vein (also into azygos system)
Lumbar veins (variable drainage)
Inferior phrenic veins
2. Inferior Vena Cava
3. Heart (Right Atrium)

Superficial Veins of Abdominal Wall (see Figs. 3.28 and 4.6)
Superficial epigastric vv. (to int. thoracic v.)
Superficial circumflex iliac veins
Periumbilical veins
Areolar venous plexus (breast)
Thoracoepigastric veins

4. Axillary Vein
Subclavian Vein
Right or Left Brachiocephalic Vein
Superior Vena Cava
3. Heart (Right Atrium)

*Distal (common iliac vein)
to Heart (right atrium)

Azygos v.
Hemiazygos v.
Inferior phrenic v.
Hepatic vv.
Esophagus
Inferior vena cava
Abdominal aorta
Right suprarenal v.
Left suprarenal vv.
Right renal v.
Subcostal v.
Left renal v.
Right ovarian v. (female) or Right testicular v. (male)
Left ovarian v. (female) or Left testicular v. (male)
Lumbar vv.
Ureter
Ascending lumbar v.
Iliolumbar v.
External iliac v.
Median sacral v.
Lateral sacral vv.
Common iliac v.
Internal iliac v.

FIGURE 4.39 Veins of the Abdomen.

and realize that smaller veins often are more variable.

Hepatic Portal System of Veins

The hepatic portal system of veins drains the abdominal GI tract and two of its accessory organs (pancreas and gallbladder) and the spleen (immune system organ) (Fig. 4.40). This blood then collects largely in the liver, where processing of absorbed GI contents takes place. (However, most fats are absorbed by the lymphatics and returned via the **thoracic duct** to the venous system in the neck (Fig. 1.16), at the junction of the left internal jugular and left subclavian veins.) Venous blood in the liver collects in the **right, intermediate, and left hepatic veins (5)** and is drained into the **inferior vena cava (6)** and then the **right atrium of the heart (7)**.

The **inferior mesenteric vein (1)** essentially drains the area supplied by the inferior mesenteric

artery (embryonic hindgut derivatives) and then drains into the **splenic vein (2).** (Sometimes it also drains into the junction between the splenic and superior mesenteric vein [SMV] or into the SMV directly.) The **splenic vein (2)** drains the spleen and portions of the stomach and pancreas. The **superior mesenteric vein (3)** essentially drains the same region as that supplied by the superior mesenteric artery (embryonic midgut derivatives), as well as portions of the pancreas and stomach.

The **splenic vein (2)** and **superior mesenteric vein (3)** unite to form the **portal vein (4)**. The **portal vein (4)** is about 8-10 cm long and receives not only venous blood from the **splenic vein (2)** and **SMV (3)** but also smaller tributaries that drain from the stomach, paraumbilical region, and cystic duct (of the gallbladder). Just before entering the liver, the **portal vein (4)** divides into its right and left branches, one to each of the two major lobes of the liver (with

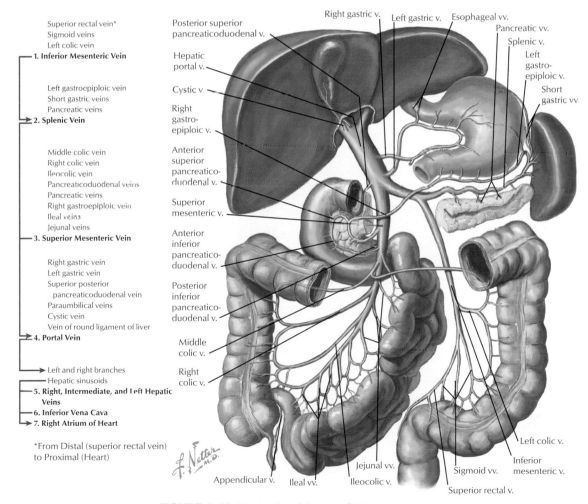

FIGURE 4.40 Hepatic Portal System of Veins.

intrahepatic veins passing to each of the eight physiological intrahepatic segments). Blood leaving the liver collects into **hepatic veins (5)** and drains into the **IVC (6)** and then the **heart (7).**

If blood cannot traverse the hepatic sinusoids (because of liver disease), it backs up in the portal system and causes **portal hypertension**. The large amount of venous blood in the portal system then must find its way back to the heart and does so by important portosystemic anastomotic connections that utilize the inferior and superior venae cavae as alternate routes to the heart. Important **portosystemic anastomoses** occur in the following regions (see Fig. 4.26):

- **Esophageal veins** from the portal vein that connect with the azygos system of veins draining into the SVC (see Fig. 3.26).
- **Rectal veins** (superior rectal vein of portal system to middle and inferior rectal veins) that ultimately drain into the IVC (Fig. 4.26).
- **Paraumbilical veins** of the superficial abdominal wall that can drain into the tributaries of either the SVC or the IVC (Figs. 4.6 and 4.26).
- **Retroperitoneal (colic) venous connections** wherever the bowel is up against the abdominal wall (secondarily retroperitoneal) and is drained by small parietal venous tributaries.

As with all veins, these veins can be *variable* in number and size, but the major venous channels are relatively constant anatomically.

Lymphatic Drainage

Lymph from the posterior abdominal wall and retroperitoneal viscera drains medially, following the arterial supply back to lumbar and visceral preaortic and lateral aortic lymph nodes (Fig. 4.41). Ultimately, the lymph is collected into the **cisterna chyli** and conveyed to the venous system by the **thoracic duct** (Figs. 3.29 and Fig. 4.41).

Innervation

Retroperitoneal visceral structures of the posterior abdominal wall (adrenal glands, kidneys, and ureters) are supplied by *parasympathetic fibers* from the **vagus nerve** and by the **pelvic splanchnic nerves** (S2-S4) to the distal ureters (pelvic ureters) (see Fig. 4.30). *Sympathetic nerves (secretomotor fibers)* to the adrenal medulla come from the **lesser** and **least splanchnic nerves,** and sympathetic nerves to the kidneys and proximal ureters come from the **lesser** and **least splanchnic nerves** (T10-T12) and the **lumbar splanchnic nerves** (L1-L2) (see Figs. 3.22 and 4.29). They synapse in the superior mesenteric ganglion and the

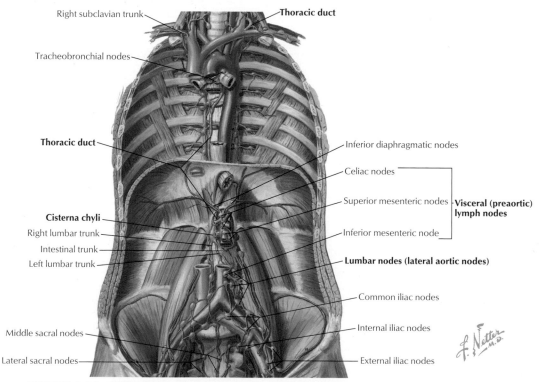

FIGURE 4.41 Abdominal Lymphatics. (From *Netter's atlas of human anatomy*, ed 8, Plate 286; S-352.)

superior mesenteric hypogastric plexus, and send postganglionic sympathetic perivascular fibers to the kidneys.

Pain afferents from all the abdominal viscera pass retrogradely back to the spinal cord by coursing in the **thoracic and lumbar splanchnic sympathetic nerves** (T5-L2). The neuronal cell bodies of these afferent fibers reside in the respective spinal ganglia of spinal cord segments T5-L2. Thus, visceral pain may be perceived as somatic pain over these dermatome regions, a phenomenon known clinically as **referred pain.** Pain afferents from pelvic viscera largely follow **pelvic splanchnic parasympathetic nerves** (S2-S4) into the cord, and the pain is largely confined to the pelvic region. Common sites of referred visceral

pain are shown in Fig. 4.42 and summarized in Table 4.12.

Somatic nerves of the posterior abdominal wall are derived from the **lumbar plexus**, which is composed of the anterior rami of L1-L4 (often with a small contribution from T12) (Fig. 4.43). The branches of the lumbar plexus innervate the posterior abdominal wall muscles (Fig. 4.32 and Table 4.10), as well as some pelvic and thigh muscles, and are summarized in Table 4.13.

7. EMBRYOLOGY

Summary of Gut Development

The embryonic gut begins as a midline endoderm-lined tube that is divided into **foregut, midgut,**

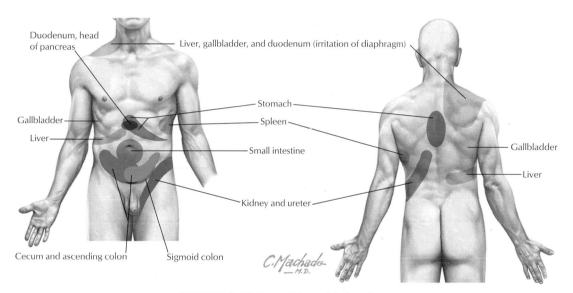

FIGURE 4.42 Sites of Visceral Referred Pain.

TABLE 4.12 Spinal Cord Levels for Visceral Referred Pain*

ORGAN	SPINAL CORD LEVEL	ANTERIOR ABDOMINAL REGION OR QUADRANT
Stomach	T5-T9	Epigastric or left hypochondrium
Spleen	T6-T8	Left hypochondrium
Duodenum**	T5-T8	Epigastric or right hypochondrium
Pancreas	T7-T9	Inferior part of epigastric
Liver or gallbladder**	T6-T9	Epigastric or right hypochondrium
Jejunum	T6-T10	Umbilical
Ileum	T7-T10	Umbilical
Cecum	T10-T11	Umbilical or right lumbar or right lower quadrant
Appendix	T10-T11	Umbilical or right inguinal or right lower quadrant
Ascending colon	T10-T12	Umbilical or right lumbar
Sigmoid colon	L1-L2	Left lumbar or left lower quadrant
Kidney	T10-L2	Lower hypochondrium or lumbar
Ureter	T11-L2	Lumbar to inguinal (loin to groin)

*These spinal cord levels are approximate. Although normal variations are common from individual to individual, these levels do show the approximate contributions.
**Irritation of the diaphragm can lead to pain referred to the back (inferior scapular region) and shoulder region when these organs are inflamed.

TABLE 4.13 Branches of Lumbar Plexus

NERVE	FUNCTION AND INNERVATION
Subcostal (T12)	Last thoracic nerve; courses inferior to 12th rib
Iliohypogastric (L1)	Motor and sensory; above pubis and posterolateral buttocks
Ilioinguinal (L1)	Motor and sensory; sensory to inguinal region
Genitofemoral (L1-L2)	Genital branch to cremaster muscle; femoral branch to femoral triangle
Lateral cutaneous nerve of thigh (L2-L3)	Sensory to anterolateral thigh
Femoral (L2-L4)	Motor in pelvis (to iliacus) and anterior thigh muscles; sensory to thigh and medial leg
Obturator (L2-L4)	Motor to adductor muscles in thigh; sensory to medial thigh
Accessory obturator	Inconstant (10%); motor to pectineus muscle

and **hindgut** regions, each giving rise to adult visceral structures with a segmental vascular supply and autonomic innervation (Fig. 4.44 and Table 4.14). Knowing this pattern of distribution related to the three embryonic gut regions will help you better organize your thinking about the abdominal viscera and their neurovascular supply.

The gut undergoes a series of rotations and differential growth that ultimately contributes to the postnatal disposition of the abdominal GI tract (see Fig. 4.44). This sequence of events can be summarized as follows:

- The **stomach** rotates 90 degrees clockwise (from the embryo's perspective) on its longitudinal axis so that the left side of the gut tube faces anteriorly and the right side posteriorly.
- As the stomach rotates, the **duodenum** swings to the right into its familiar C-shaped configuration and becomes largely secondarily retroperitoneal.

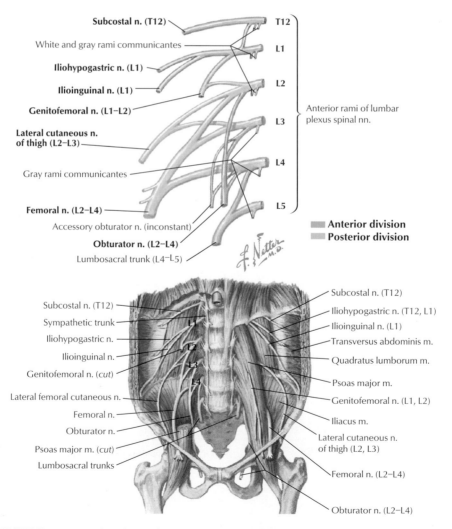

FIGURE 4.43 Lumbar Plexus. (From *Netter's atlas of human anatomy*, ed 8, Plate 507; S-113.)

Congenital Megacolon

Congenital megacolon results from the failure of **neural crest cells** to migrate distally along the colon (usually the sigmoid colon and rectum). The incidence of megacolon is about 1 in 5000 live births. It is more common in boys. The condition leads to an aganglionic segment that lacks both the **Meissner's submucosal plexus** and the **Auerbach's myenteric plexus** (see Fig. 1.27). Distention proximal to the aganglionic region may occur shortly after birth or may cause symptoms in early childhood. Surgical repair involves prolapse and eversion of the segment.

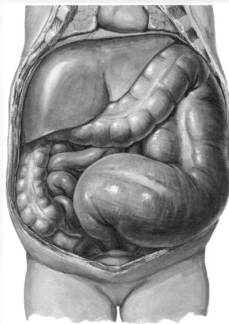

Tremendous distention and hypertrophy of sigmoid and descending colon; moderate involvement of transverse colon; distal constricted segment

Bowel "freed up" transperitoneally

Rectum prolapsed and divided circumferentially exposing underlying everted bowel

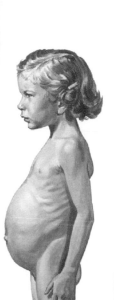

Typical abdominal distention

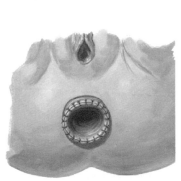

Rectal and colonic mucosa approximated

Colon further everted, sutured to rectal stump, and divided

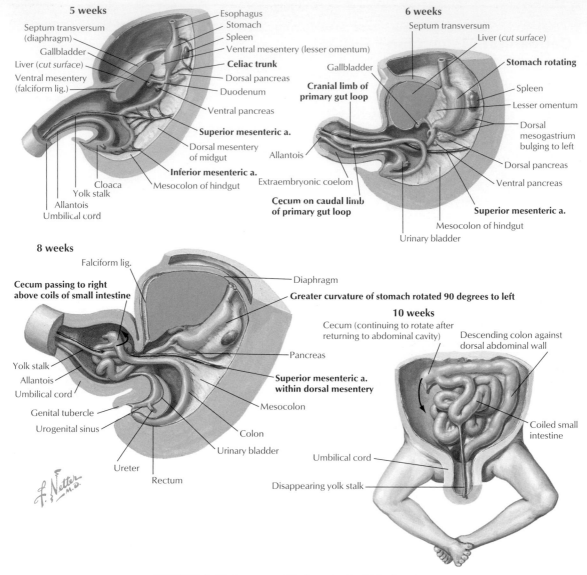

FIGURE 4.44 Sequence of Embryonic Gut Tube Rotations.

- The **midgut** forms an initial primary intestinal loop by rotating 180 degrees clockwise around the axis of the **SMA** (which supplies blood to the midgut) and, because of its fast growth, herniates out into the umbilical cord (6-8 weeks).
- By the 10th week, the gut loop returns into the abdominal cavity and completes its rotation with a 90-degree clockwise swing to the right lower abdominal quadrant (see Clinical Focus 4.25).
- Thus, the midgut loop completes a *270-degree rotation* about the axis of the **SMA** and undergoes significant differential growth to form the

small intestine and proximal portions of the large intestine.
- The **hindgut** then develops into the remainder of the large intestine and proximal rectum, supplied by the **IMA**, and ending in the cloaca (Latin for "sewer").

The embryonic pattern of development from the three gut regions helps one understand how the various derivatives of each gut region are supplied by major branches of the abdominal aorta and how they are innervated by the autonomic nervous system (Table 4.14).

TABLE 4.14 Summary of Embryonic Gut Development

	FOREGUT	MIDGUT	HINDGUT
Organs	Stomach Liver Gallbladder Pancreas Spleen 1st half of duodenum	2nd half of duodenum Jejunum Ileum Cecum Ascending colon Two-thirds of transverse colon	Left one-third of transverse colon Descending colon Sigmoid colon Rectum
Arteries	Celiac trunk: Splenic Left gastric Common hepatic	Superior mesenteric: Ileocolic Right colic Middle colic	Inferior mesenteric: Left colic Sigmoid branches Superior rectal
Ventral mesentery	Lesser omentum Falciform ligament Coronary/triangular ligaments of liver	None	None
Dorsal mesentery	Gastrosplenic ligament Splenorenal ligament Gastrocolic ligament Greater omentum and omental apron	Mesointestine Mesoappendix Transverse mesocolon	Sigmoid mesocolon
Nerve Supply			
Parasympathetic	Vagus	Vagus	Pelvic splanchnics (S2-S4)
Sympathetic	Thoracic splanchnics (T5-T11)	Thoracic splanchnics (T11-T12)	Lumbar splanchnics (L1-L2)

Liver, Gallbladder, and Pancreas Development

During the third week of development, an endodermal outpocketing of the foregut gives rise to the **hepatic diverticulum** (Fig. 4.45). The hepatic diverticulum gives rise to the liver, which grows into the primitive diaphragm (called the *septum transversum* at this early stage of development), which is derived from mesoderm. The liver hepatocytes are endodermal derivatives, and the Kupffer cells, hematopoietic cells, fibroblasts, and endothelium of the liver sinusoids are derived from mesoderm. Further development of the original diverticulum gives rise to the **biliary duct system** and the **gallbladder**. A short time later, two **pancreatic buds** (ventral and dorsal buds) originate as endodermal outgrowths of the developing duodenum. As the duodenum swings to the right during rotation of the stomach, the ventral pancreatic bud (which will form part of the pancreatic head and the uncinate process) swings around posteriorly and fuses with the dorsal bud to form the union of the two pancreatic ducts (main and accessory ducts) and buds. This fused pancreas embraces the **SMV** and **SMA**, which are in relationship to these developing embryonic buds (see Figs. 4.20 and 4.45). The endoderm of the pancreas gives rise to the exocrine and endocrine cells of the organ, whereas the connective tissue stroma and vasculature are formed by mesoderm.

Urinary System Development

Initially, retroperitoneal intermediate mesoderm differentiates into the nephrogenic (kidney) tissue and forms the following (Fig. 4.46):
- **Pronephros**, a primary kidney that *degenerates*.
- **Mesonephros** with its mesonephric duct, which *functions briefly before degenerating*.
- **Metanephros,** the *definitive kidney tissue* (nephrons and loop of Henle) into which the **ureteric bud** (an outgrowth of the mesonephric duct) grows and differentiates into the ureter, renal pelvis, major and minor calyces, and collecting ducts; the metanephric mesoderm gives rise to the renal nephrons and their loops of Henle, as well as the connecting tubules.

By differential growth and some migration, the kidney "ascends" from the pelvic region, first with its hilum directed anteriorly and then medially, until it reaches its adult location (Fig. 4.47). Around the 12th week, the kidney becomes functional as the fetus swallows amniotic fluid, urinates into the amniotic cavity, and continually recycles fluid in this manner. Toxic fetal wastes, however, are removed through the placenta into the maternal circulation.

Clinical Focus 4.25

Meckel's Diverticulum

Meckel's diverticulum is the most common developmental anomaly of the bowel. It results from failure of the vitelline (yolk stalk) duct to involute once the gut loop has reentered the abdominal cavity. It is often referred to as the "syndrome of twos" for the following reasons:

- It occurs in approximately 2% of the population.
- It is about 2 inches (5 cm) long.
- It is located about 2 feet from the ileocecal junction.
- It often contains at least two types of mucosa.

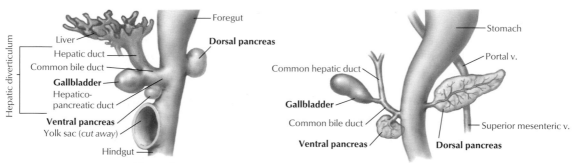

Ileum

Meckel's
diverticulum

Meckel's diverticulum with fibrous
cord extending to umbilicus

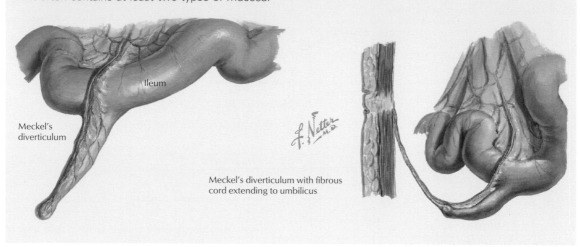

Hepatic diverticulum

1. Bud formation

2. Beginning rotation of common duct and of ventral pancreas

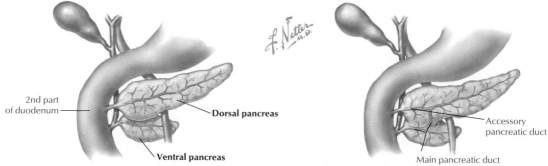

3. Rotation completed but fusion has not yet taken place

**4. Fusion of ventral and dorsal pancreas
and union of ducts**

FIGURE 4.45 Development of Hepatic Diverticulum and Pancreas.

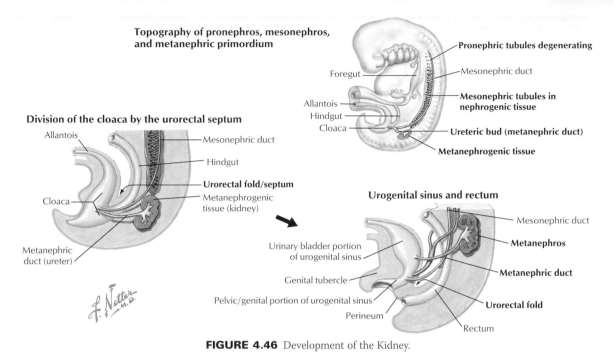

Topography of pronephros, mesonephros, and metanephric primordium

Pronephric tubules degenerating

Foregut

Mesonephric duct

Allantois

Hindgut

Cloaca

Mesonephric tubules in nephrogenic tissue

Ureteric bud (metanephric duct)

Metanephrogenic tissue

Division of the cloaca by the urorectal septum

Allantois

Mesonephric duct

Hindgut

Urorectal fold/septum

Metanephrogenic tissue (kidney)

Cloaca

Metanephric duct (ureter)

Urogenital sinus and rectum

Mesonephric duct

Metanephros

Urinary bladder portion of urogenital sinus

Genital tubercle

Metanephric duct

Pelvic/genital portion of urogenital sinus

Perineum

Urorectal fold

Rectum

FIGURE 4.46 Development of the Kidney.

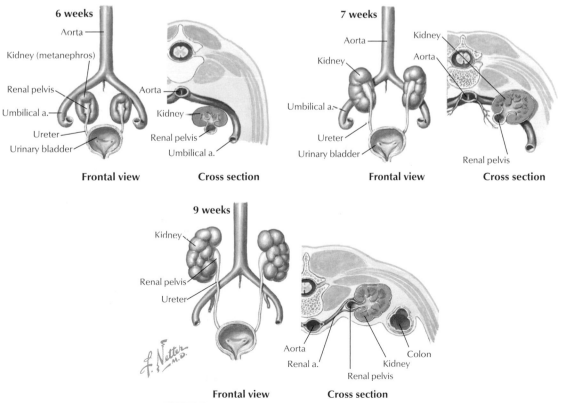

Apparent "ascent and rotation" of the kidneys in embryologic development

6 weeks

Aorta

Kidney (metanephros)

Renal pelvis

Aorta

Umbilical a.

Kidney

Ureter

Renal pelvis

Urinary bladder

Umbilical a.

Frontal view   **Cross section**

7 weeks

Aorta

Kidney

Aorta

Kidney

Umbilical a.

Ureter

Urinary bladder

Renal pelvis

Frontal view   **Cross section**

9 weeks

Kidney

Renal pelvis

Ureter

Aorta

Renal a.

Renal pelvis

Kidney

Colon

Frontal view   **Cross section**

FIGURE 4.47 Ascent and Rotation of the Kidney.

Clinical Focus 4.26

Congenital Malrotation of the Colon

Many congenital lesions of the GI tract cause intestinal obstruction, which commonly results from malrotation of the midgut, atresia, volvulus, meconium ileus, or imperforate anus. Vomiting, absence of stool, and abdominal distention characterize the clinical picture. Intestinal obstruction can be life threatening, requiring surgical intervention. The corrective procedure for congenital malrotation with volvulus of the midgut is illustrated.

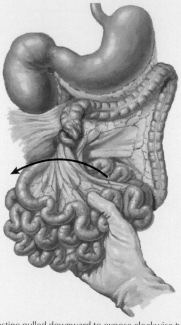

1. Small intestine pulled downward to expose clockwise twist and strangulation at apex of incompletely anchored mesentery; unwinding is done in counterclockwise direction (arrow)

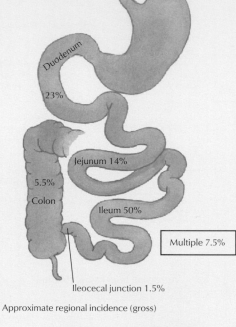

Duodenum 23%

Jejunum 14%

5.5% Colon

Ileum 50%

Multiple 7.5%

Ileocecal junction 1.5%

Approximate regional incidence (gross)

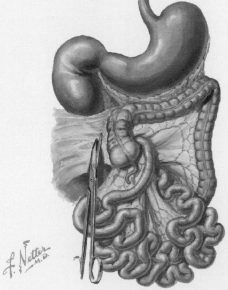

2. Volvulus unwound; peritoneal band compressing duodenum is being divided

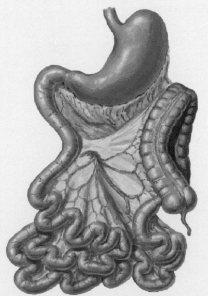

3. Complete release of obstruction; duodenum descends toward root of superior mesenteric artery; cecum drops away to left

Clinical Focus 4.27

Pheochromocytoma

Although pheochromocytomas are relatively rare neoplasms composed largely of adrenal medullary cells, which secrete excessive amounts of catecholamines, they can occur elsewhere throughout the body and are associated with the sympathetic chain or at other sites where **neural crest cells** typically migrate (remember that the neural crest cells contribute to a wide variety of cells; see Fig. 2.24). Common clinical features of pheochromocytoma include the following:

- Vasoconstriction and elevated blood pressure
- Headache, sweating, and flushing
- Anxiety, nausea, tremor, and palpitations or chest pain

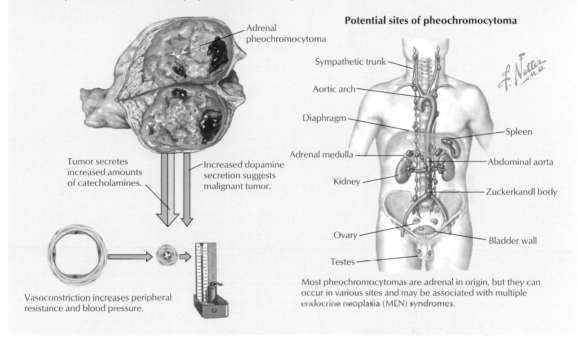

Adrenal pheochromocytoma

Tumor secretes increased amounts of catecholamines.

Increased dopamine secretion suggests malignant tumor.

Vasoconstriction increases peripheral resistance and blood pressure.

Potential sites of pheochromocytoma

Sympathetic trunk

Aortic arch

Diaphragm

Spleen

Adrenal medulla

Abdominal aorta

Kidney

Zuckerkandl body

Ovary

Bladder wall

Testes

Most pheochromocytomas are adrenal in origin, but they can occur in various sites and may be associated with multiple endocrine neoplasia (MEN) syndromes.

Adrenal (Suprarenal) Gland Development

The adrenal cortex develops from mesoderm, whereas the adrenal medulla forms from **neural crest cells,** which migrate into the cortex and aggregate in the center of the gland (see Clinical Focus 4.27). The neuroendocrine chromaffin cells of the medulla are essentially the postganglionic neurons of the sympathetic division of the ANS, but they secrete their catecholamines into the bloodstream rather than as neurotransmitters at synapses. This unique feature means that instead of having a limited effect at one target site, the catecholamines can quickly circulate throughout the body and have a *mass-action effect* that mobilizes the "fight, fright, or flight" response.

Clinical Focus 4.28

Renal Fusion

The term *renal fusion* refers to various common defects in which the two kidneys fuse to become one. The **horseshoe kidney**, in which developing kidneys fuse (usually the lower lobes) anterior to the aorta, often lies low in the abdomen and is the most common kind of fusion. Fused kidneys are close to the midline, have multiple renal arteries, and are malrotated. Obstruction, stone formation, and infection are potential complications.

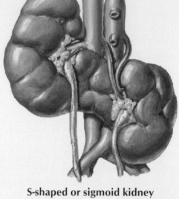

S-shaped or sigmoid kidney

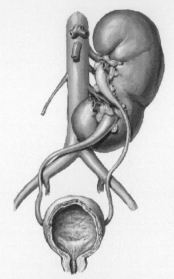

Simple crossed ectopia with fusion

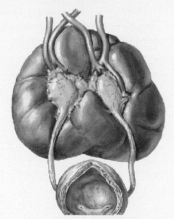

Pelvic cake or lump kidney

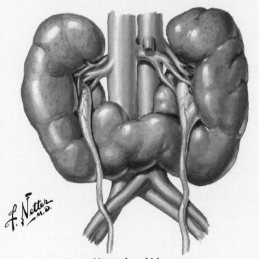

Horseshoe kidney

Clinical Focus

Available Online

4.29 Acute Abdomen: Visceral Etiology

4.30 Irritable Bowel Syndrome

4.31 Acute Pyelonephritis

4.32 Causes and Consequences of Portal Hypertension

Additional figures available online (see inside front cover for details).

Challenge Yourself Questions

1. Which of the descriptive levels accurately describes why the umbilicus can be an important clinical landmark?
   - **A.** Level of celiac trunk
   - **B.** Level of L3 vertebra
   - **C.** Level of transverse colon
   - **D.** Level of T10 dermatome
   - **E.** Level of third part of duodenum

2. Clinically, which of the following statements regarding an indirect inguinal hernia is false?
   - **A.** Can be a congenital hernia.
   - **B.** Enters the deep inguinal ring.
   - **C.** Herniates lateral to the inferior epigastric vessels.
   - **D.** Lies within the internal spermatic fascia.
   - **E.** Passes through the inguinal triangle.

3. A 42-year-old obese woman comes to the clinic with episodes of severe right hypochondrial pain, usually associated with eating a fatty meal. A history of gallstones suggests that she is experiencing cholecystitis (gallbladder inflammation). Which of the following nerves carries the visceral pain associated with this condition?
   - **A.** Greater splanchnic
   - **B.** Intercostal
   - **C.** Phrenic
   - **D.** Pelvic splanchnic
   - **E.** Vagus

4. The metastatic spread of stomach (gastric) cancer through lymphatics would most likely travel first to which of the following lymph nodes?
   - **A.** Celiac
   - **B.** Inferior mesenteric
   - **C.** Inferior phrenic
   - **D.** Lumbar
   - **E.** Superior mesenteric

5. A 51-year-old woman with a history of alcohol abuse is diagnosed with cirrhosis of the liver and portal hypertension. In addition to esophageal varices, she presents with rectal varices. Which of the following portosystemic anastomoses is most likely responsible for these rectal varices?
   - **A.** Inferior mesenteric vein to inferior rectal veins
   - **B.** Left gastric veins to inferior rectal veins
   - **C.** Portal vein to the middle and inferior rectal veins
   - **D.** Superior mesenteric vein to superior rectal veins
   - **E.** Superior rectal vein to the middle and inferior rectal veins

6. A patient presents with acute abdominal pain and fever. Examination of her abdomen reveals fluid (ascites) within the lesser sac, which is now draining into the greater peritoneal sac. Which of the following pathways accounts for the seepage of fluid from the lesser to the greater sac?
   - **A.** Epiploic foramen
   - **B.** Left paracolic gutter
   - **C.** Posterior fornix
   - **D.** Right paracolic gutter
   - **E.** Vesicouterine pouch

7. A 59-year-old man presents with deep epigastric pain. A CT scan of the abdomen reveals a pancreatic tumor that partially envelops a large artery. Which of the following arteries is most likely involved?
   - **A.** Common hepatic
   - **B.** Gastroduodenal
   - **C.** Left gastric
   - **D.** Middle colic
   - **E.** Superior mesenteric

 Multiple-choice and short-answer review questions available online; see inside front cover for details.

8. A kidney stone (calculus) passing from the kidney to the urinary bladder can become lodged at several sites along its pathway to the bladder, leading to "loin-to-groin" pain. One common site of obstruction can occur about halfway down the pathway of the ureter where it crosses which of the following structures?

   A. Common iliac vessels
   B. Lumbosacral trunk
   C. Major renal calyx
   D. Renal pelvis
   E. Sacroiliac joint

9. An obese 46-year-old woman presents in the clinic with right upper quadrant pain for the past 48 hours, jaundice for the last 24 hours, nausea, and acute bouts of severe pain (biliary colic) after she tries to eat a meal. A diagnosis of cholelithiasis (gallstones) is made. Which of the following structures is most likely obstructed by the stone?

   A. Common bile duct
   B. Cystic duct
   C. Main pancreatic duct
   D. Right hepatic duct
   E. Thoracic duct

10. A gunshot wound to the spine of a 29-year-old man damages the lower portion of his spinal canal at about the L3-L4 level, resulting in loss of some of the central parasympathetic control of his bowel. Which of the following portions of the gastrointestinal tract is most likely affected?

    A. Ascending colon
    B. Descending colon
    C. Ileum
    D. Jejunum
    E. Transverse colon

11. If access to several arterial arcades supplying the distal ileum is required, which of the following layers of peritoneum would a surgeon need to enter to reach these vessels?

    A. Greater omentum and lesser omentum
    B. Greater omentum and mesentery
    C. Greater omentum and transverse mesocolon
    D. Parietal peritoneum and greater omentum
    E. Parietal peritoneum and mesentery
    F. Parietal peritoneum and transverse mesocolon

12. Clinically, inflammation in which of the following organs is *least* likely to present as periumbilical pain?

    A. Ascending colon
    B. Descending colon
    C. Ileum
    D. Jejunum
    E. Proximal duodenum

13. During abdominal surgery, resection of a portion of the descending colon necessitates the sacrifice of a nerve lying on the surface of the psoas major muscle. Which of the following nerves would *most* likely be sacrificed?

    A. Femoral
    B. Genitofemoral
    C. Ilioinguinal
    D. Lateral cutaneous nerve of thigh
    E. Subcostal

14. At autopsy it is discovered that the deceased had three ureters, one on the left side and two on the right. The condition was apparently asymptomatic. Which of the following embryonic events might account for the presence of two ureters on one side?

    A. Duplication of the mesonephric duct
    B. Early splitting of the ureteric bud
    C. Failure of the mesonephros to form
    D. Failure of the urorectal septum to form
    E. Persistent allantois

For each of the clinical descriptions below (15-20), select the organ from the list (A-P) that is most likely responsible.

(A)	Adrenal gland	(I)	Kidney
(B)	Appendix	(J)	Liver
(C)	Ascending colon	(K)	Pancreas
(D)	Descending colon	(L)	Rectum
(E)	Duodenum	(M)	Sigmoid colon
(F)	Gallbladder	(N)	Spleen
(G)	Ileum	(O)	Stomach
(H)	Jejunum	(P)	Transverse colon

_____ 15. This retroperitoneal structure is often a site of ulceration.

_____ 16. Volvulus in this segment of the bowel may also constrict its vascular supply by the inferior mesenteric artery.

_____ 17. Inflammation of this structure may begin as diffuse periumbilical pain, but as the affected structure contacts the parietal peritoneum, the pain becomes acute and well localized to the right lower quadrant, often necessitating surgical resection.

_____ 18. A sliding or axial hernia is the most common type of hiatal hernia and involves this structure.

_____ 19. The failure of the vitelline duct to involute (occurs in about 2% of the population) during embryonic development leads to a persistent diverticulum on this structure.

_____ 20. During embryonic development, this structure forms from both a dorsal and a ventral bud, which then fuse into a single structure.

21. You, as a resident, are assisting the chief surgeon during abdominal surgery and mistakenly clamp the hepatoduodenal ligament! Which of the following vessels would most likely be occluded as a result?

    A. Common hepatic artery
    B. Hepatic vein
    C. Inferior vena cava
    D. Proper hepatic artery
    E. Superior mesenteric artery

22. A 3-year-old child presents with severe vomiting. Radiographic examination reveals the presence of an anular pancreas. Which one of the following portions of the gastrointestinal system is most likely obstructed by this developmental condition?

    A. Antrum of the stomach
    B. 1st part of the duodenum
    C. Jejunum
    D. Proximal transverse colon
    E. 2nd part of the duodenum

23. A 41-year-old woman has a history of acute pain while she eats and for a period of time after she eats; the pain then subsides. Her pain is in the epigastric region and radiates to her back just inferior to her scapula. A CT scan reveals that she has gallstones. Which of the following nerves possess the afferent fibers that convey the referred pain she is experiencing?

    A. Greater thoracic splanchnic nerves
    B. Phrenic nerves
    C. Posterior rami of the midintercostal nerves
    D. Thoracodorsal nerves
    E. Vagus nerves

24. During an open surgical approach to repair an indirect inguinal hernia, the spermatic cord, internal abdominal oblique muscle, and transversus abdominis fascia are identified. Which layer of the spermatic cord is derived from the internal abdominal oblique muscle?

    A. Cremasteric fascia
    B. External spermatic fascia
    C. Internal spermatic fascia
    D. Membranous (Scarpa's) fascia
    E. Tunica vaginalis

25. A 67-year-old man with a history of alcoholism is brought into the emergency department because he is vomiting blood. It is determined that his bleeding is from esophageal varices. These varices are most likely the result of an anastomosis between the left gastric vein and which of the following vessels?

    A. Azygos system
    B. Hepatic veins
    C. Inferior vena cava
    D. Portal vein
    E. Subcostal veins

26. How might a surgeon differentiate between the jejunum and the ileum when she is performing exploratory laparotomy?

    A. Jejunum has fewer villi
    B. Jejunum has less mesenteric fat
    C. Jejunum has more vascular arcades
    D. Jejunum has more lymphatic follicles
    E. Jejunum has a smaller diameter

27. A 52-year-old gentleman presents with excruciating pain that radiates from his left back around to just above his pubic symphysis. Further imaging reveals a kidney stone lodged in his renal pelvis at the point where the pelvis narrows into the proximal ureter. Which of the following nerves conveys the pain fibers associated with this condition?

    A. Femoral nerve
    B. Iliohypogastric nerve
    C. Lateral femoral cutaneous nerve
    D. Lumbar splanchnics
    E. Sympathetic trunk

28. A 33-year-old woman presents with a 4-month history of elevated blood pressure, headaches, episodes of flushing and sweating, anxiety, a slight tremor, and palpitations in her chest. A CT scan reveals a 4-cm mass just to the left of the abdominal aorta at about the level of the celiac trunk. Which of the following organs is most likely to harbor this mass?

A. Appendix
B. Gallbladder
C. Jejunum
D. Spleen
E. Suprarenal gland

29. A 51-year-old man presents in the emergency department with a complaint of sharp pain and cramping. Follow-up imaging reveals a tumor in the head and uncinate process of the pancreas. Which of the following vessels is most immediately at risk for occlusion if this tumor enlarges?

A. Common hepatic artery
B. Left renal artery
C. Portal vein
D. Splenic artery
E. Superior mesenteric artery

For questions 30 to 35, select the one blood vessel from the list (A to L) that best fits the structure described.

(A) Common hepatic artery
(B) Inferior mesenteric artery
(C) Inferior suprarenal artery
(D) Inferior vena cava
(E) Left gastric vein
(F) Left renal vein
(G) Portal vein
(H) Splenic artery
(I) Splenic vein
(J) Superior mesenteric artery
(K) Superior mesenteric vein
(L) Superior rectal vein

_____ 30. This vessel forms an important portosystemic anastomosis with esophageal vessels and the azygos system.

_____ 31. The branches of this vessel provide the blood supply to the appendix.

_____ 32. This vessel drains the ascending colon into the portal vein.

_____ 33. This vessel crosses directly anterior to the abdominal aorta and drains an organ

that normally receives about 10% of the blood flow each minute.

_____ 34. This vessel specifically drains the pancreas, stomach, and spleen.

_____ 35. This vessel contributes to the portosystemic anastomosis found deep within the pelvis.

For questions 36 to 40, select the label (A to L) shown in the abdominal image that best fits the structure described.

_____ 36. This structure receives its major blood supply from both the superior and inferior mesenteric arteries.

_____ 37. When this structure is obstructed and inflamed, a patient will initially present with periumbilical pain that radiates to the lower right quadrant.

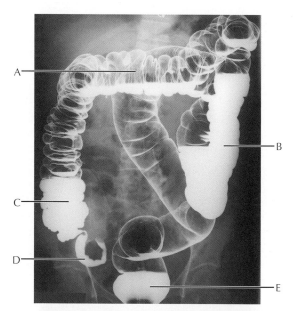

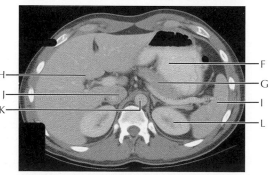

Reused with permission from Major NM: *A practical approach to radiology,* St Louis, 2006, Elsevier.

_____ 38. This structure is a paired retroperitoneal organ.

_____ 39. This important organ lies deep to the omental bursa.

_____ 40. This structure has a direct connection to the right atrium.

Answers to Challenge Yourself Questions

1. **D.** The umbilicus denotes the T10 dermatome, just one of several key dermatome points. The shoulder is C5, the middle finger C7, the nipple T4, the inguinal region L1, the knee L4, and the second toe L5. The S1-S2 dermatomes then run up the back side of the leg and thigh.

2. **E.** The inguinal (Hesselbach's) triangle is demarcated medially by the rectus sheath, superolaterally by the inferior epigastric vessels, and inferomedially by the inguinal ligament. A hernia that does not pass down the inguinal canal but rather herniates through this triangle is considered a direct inguinal hernia. Direct inguinal hernias also are referred to as acquired hernias.

3. **A.** General visceral pain, in this case from the gallbladder, travels back to the CNS via the sympathetic pathway and the greater splanchnic nerve (T5-T9). The sensory neuronal cell bodies reside in the spinal ganglia associated with these spinal cord levels. If the gallbladder expands and contacts the diaphragm, the pain may be felt over the right C3-C5 region of the back and shoulder, because the pain is referred by the phrenic nerve to these dermatomes.

4. **A.** The lymphatic drainage will parallel the venous drainage and/or arterial supply. The celiac nodes, therefore, will receive the bulk of the lymphatic drainage from the stomach. Other adjacent nodes may also be involved, but not to the same degree as the celiac nodes.

5. **E.** The superior rectal veins (portal drainage) of the inferior mesenteric vein would communicate with the middle rectal veins, which drain into the internal iliac veins (systemic circulation into the IVC via the common iliac veins). The middle rectal and inferior rectal veins (drain into the pudendal veins, a systemic route ultimately to the IVC) also communicate and can form rectal varices in portal hypertension. Thus, venous blood flow would go from portal tributaries (superior rectal veins) into the caval (systemic) tributaries (middle and inferior rectal veins) in an effort to return blood back to the heart.

6. **A.** The epiploic foramen (of Winslow) connects the lesser sac (omental bursa), a cul-de-sac space posterior to the stomach, with the greater sac (remainder of the abdominopelvic cavity).

7. **E.** The superior mesenteric artery passes between the neck and the uncinate process of the pancreas and then anterior to the third portion of the duodenum.

8. **A.** The ureter crosses the common iliac vessels about halfway on its journey to the urinary bladder. It is slightly stretched and its lumen narrowed as it crosses these vessels, so a calculus can become lodged at this point. This site also is close to the pelvic brim.

9. **A.** The common bile duct is probably obstructed, causing the pain and jaundice. Blockage of the cystic duct may not be associated with jaundice, and obstruction of the main pancreatic duct would probably cause pancreatitis.

10. **B.** All the other portions of his bowel that are listed are innervated by the vagus nerve and its parasympathetic nerve fibers (innervates the foregut and midgut embryonic derivatives of the bowel). Only the descending colon is a hindgut embryonic derivative and it receives parasympathetic efferents from the S2-S4 pelvic splanchnic nerves.

11. **E.** The surgeon would need to incise the parietal peritoneum to enter the abdominal cavity, move the apron of the greater omentum aside, and then incise the mesentery of the small bowel to access the arterial arcades.

12. **E.** The duodenum, especially its proximal portion, would present largely as epigastric pain. The other portions of the bowel would be more likely to present with periumbilical pain.

13. **B.** The genitofemoral nerve is almost always found lying on the anterior surface of the psoas major muscle.

14. **B.** Most likely this is the result of an early division of the ureteric bud, which ultimately gives rise to the ureters, renal pelvis, calyces, and collecting ducts.

15. **E.** The first part of the duodenum is prone to ulcers (peptic ulcers) and is largely retroperitoneal. Ulcerative colitis may also occur in some portions of the retroperitoneal large bowel but not as commonly as duodenal peptic ulcers.

16. **M.** Volvulus, or a twisting, of the bowel is most common in the small bowel (supplied by the superior mesenteric artery). However, when volvulus occurs in the large bowel, it is most common in the sigmoid colon, which can be

quite mobile because it is tethered by a mesentery. The inferior mesenteric artery supplies the distal portion of the transverse, descending, and sigmoid colon and the proximal rectum.

17. **B.** This is the "classic" presentation of appendicitis. The pain localizes to the lower left quadrant once the somatic pain fibers of the peritoneal wall are stimulated. This point is called "McBurney's point" and is about two-thirds the distance from the umbilicus to the right anterior superior iliac spine.

18. **O.** A hiatal hernia is a herniation of a portion of the stomach through a widened space between the muscular right crus of the diaphragm that forms the esophageal hiatus. Sliding (also called axial or rolling) hernias account for the vast majority of hiatal hernias.

19. **G.** This diverticulum is called a "Meckel's diverticulum" and is the most common developmental anomaly of the bowel. It occurs about 2 feet from the ileocecal junction and is a diverticulum of the distal ileum (midgut derivative).

20. **K.** The pancreas develops as a fusion of a ventral and a dorsal bud. With the rotation of the duodenum, the ventral bud "flips" over and fuses with the larger dorsal bud, forming part of the head and uncinate process of the pancreas.

21. **D.** The hepatoduodenal ligament, a portion of the lesser omentum, contains the proper hepatic artery (which supplies blood to the gallbladder and liver), the common bile duct, and the portal vein.

22. **E.** The pancreas develops from a dorsal bud and a ventral bud that are endodermal outgrowths of the future duodenum. As the primitive gut tube begins to rotate, the future duodenum swings right and the ventral pancreatic bud (which forms the head and uncinate process of the pancreas) swings posteriorly and fuses with the dorsal pancreatic bud. During this rotation, a portion of the ventral pancreatic bud may swing anterior to the duodenum and entrap the duodenum by forming an anular pancreas.

23. **A.** This referred pain from the gallbladder is conveyed back to the spinal ganglia of the midthoracic spinal cord via the greater thoracic splanchnic nerve (T5-T9), which provides sympathetic fibers to the foregut derivatives and conveys visceral pain afferents back to the spinal cord via its splanchnic nerves. This visceral pain is perceived as somatic pain at the dermatome levels of the thoracic spinal cord segments associated with that sympathetic outflow.

24. **A.** The internal abdominal oblique muscle gives rise to the cremasteric (middle spermatic) fascia. The external spermatic fascia is derived from the external abdominal oblique aponeurosis, and the internal spermatic fascia is derived from the transversalis fascia.

25. **D.** These varices arise from engorged esophageal veins. They drain into the azygos system of veins. This portosystemic anastomosis provides an alternative route for portal venous blood to bypass the obstructed liver and reach the right atrium of the heart (see Clinical Focus 4.18).

26. **B.** The jejunum exhibits less fat in its mesentery. It also usually occupies the left upper quadrant, usually has a larger diameter, and has fewer arcades, but it has longer vasa rectae. The other features (villi, follicles) are internal features, not routinely visible to a surgeon.

27. **D.** This visceral pain from the ureter is conveyed by sympathetic fibers from the T11-L2 splanchnic nerves to the corresponding dorsal root ganglion at those spinal cord levels. The referred pain from the most proximal portion of the ureter (L1) is perceived somatically along this dermatome, but the visceral pain afferents are carried back to the spinal cord via the lesser thoracic splanchnic (T12) and L1 lumbar splanchnic nerves. The other choices are somatic nerves which do not convey visceral pain.

28. **E.** Each of these findings suggests a hyperactive suprarenal (adrenal) gland, which is releasing epinephrine and norepinephrine into the bloodstream. The location of the tumor just superior to the left kidney and to the left of the aorta is consistent with this diagnosis (see Clinical Focus 4.27, Pheochromocytoma).

29. **E.** The superior mesenteric artery passes between the dorsal and ventral pancreatic buds of the embryonic pancreas, and postnatally is usually found crossing the uncinate process of the embryonic ventral pancreatic bud, just to the left of the pancreatic head and anterior to the third part of the duodenum. None of the other vessels are as closely related to the pancreatic head and uncinate process as this artery.

30. **E.** Portal venous blood that is unable to pass through the diseased liver will pass into the left gastric veins, the esophageal veins (causing esophageal varices), and the azygos system of veins that return to the heart. This is the most proximal and most common portosystemic anastomotic option.

31. **J.** The appendicular artery is a branch of the ileocolic artery from the superior mesenteric artery, which supplies blood to the embryonic midgut derivatives.

32. **K.** Blood from the ascending colon, an embryonic midgut derivative, is drained by the superior mesenteric vein, which then is joined by the splenic vein to form the portal vein.

33. **F.** The left renal vein passes anterior to the abdominal aorta before emptying into the inferior vena cava. Each kidney normally receives about 10% of the cardiac output each minute (both kidneys combined receive about 20%; see Fig. 1.12).

34. **I.** The best answer is the splenic vein (see Fig. 4.26). This vein often also receives venous blood from the inferior mesenteric vein before emptying into the portal vein.

35. **L.** The superior rectal veins possess portosystemic connections with the middle and inferior rectal veins (these veins ultimately connect with the inferior vena cava). The superior rectal veins drain into the inferior mesenteric vein (part of the portal venous drainage to the liver).

36. **A.** The transverse colon is derived from both the embryonic midgut and the hindgut. Its proximal portion receives blood from the SMA and its distal portion is supplied by the IMA. In this air contrast barium enema, the transverse colon is clearly visible crossing horizontally from right to left.

37. **D.** This is the classic referred pain pattern of appendicitis. The appendix is clearly seen filled with barium and hanging off of the cecum.

38. **L.** The two kidneys are retroperitoneal structures and are clearly visible in this normal axial CT image.

39. **G.** The omental bursa (lesser sac) is the space that lies posterior to the stomach and anterior to the largely retroperitoneal pancreas (the tip of the pancreatic tail is not retroperitoneal and terminates at the hilum of the spleen in the splenorenal ligament). The pancreas is visible posterior to the stomach; the stomach (F) in this image is largely obliterating a view of the omental bursa.

40. **J.** The inferior vena cava is seen in the CT image just to the right (i.e., the patient's right) of the abdominal aorta (K), which lies almost in contact with the vertebral body.

Pelvis and Perineum

1. INTRODUCTION

The bowl-shaped pelvic cavity is continuous superiorly with the abdomen and bounded inferiorly by the perineum, the region between the proximal thighs. The bones of the pelvic girdle demarcate the following two regions:

- **Greater or false pelvis:** the lower portion of the abdomen that lies between the flared iliac crests.
- **Lesser or true pelvis:** demarcated by the pelvic brim, sacrum, and coccyx, and contains the pelvic viscera. The **pelvic inlet** is the upper border of the true pelvis (the pelvic brim) and the **pelvic outlet** is the lower border of the true pelvis.

The pelvis contains the terminal gastrointestinal tract and urinary system and the internal reproductive organs. The perineum lies below the "pelvic diaphragm," or muscles that form the pelvic floor, and contains the external genitalia. Our review of the pelvis and perineum focuses on the musculoskeletal structures that support the pelvis and then examines the viscera, blood supply, and innervation of these two regions.

2. SURFACE ANATOMY

Key landmarks of the surface anatomy of the pelvis and perineum include the following (Fig. 5.1):

- **Umbilicus:** site that marks the T10 dermatome, that lies at the level of the intervertebral disc between the L3 and L4 vertebral bodies; can lie slightly lower in infants or morbidly obese individuals and higher in late pregnancy.
- **Iliac crest:** rim of the ilium that lies at approximately the L4 vertebral level; also the approximate level of the bifurcation of the abdominal aorta into its two common iliac branches.
- **Anterior superior iliac spine:** superior attachment point for the inguinal ligament.
- **Inguinal ligament:** ligament formed by the aponeurosis of the external abdominal oblique muscle; forms a line of demarcation separating the lower abdominopelvic region from the thighs.
- **Pubic tubercle:** the inferior attachment point of the inguinal ligament.
- **Posterior superior iliac spine:** often seen as a "dimpling" of the skin just above the intergluteal (natal) cleft; often more obvious in females.

The surface anatomy of the perineum is reviewed later in this chapter.

3. MUSCULOSKELETAL ELEMENTS

Bony Pelvic Girdle

The pelvic girdle is the attachment point of the lower limb to the body's trunk. (The pectoral girdle is its counterpart for the attachment of the upper limb.) The bones of the pelvis include the following (Fig. 5.2):

- **Right and left pelvic bones (coxal or hip bones):** fusion of three separate bones—the **ilium, ischium,** and **pubis**—that join in the **acetabulum** (cup-shaped surface where the pelvis articulates with the head of the femur).
- **Sacrum:** fusion of the five sacral vertebrae; the two pelvic bones, at the medial aspect of the ilium on each side, articulate with the sacrum posteriorly (**sacroiliac joint**). Superiorly, the sacrum articulates with the fifth lumbar vertebra (**lumbosacral joint**) (Table 5.1).
- **Coccyx:** terminal end of the vertebral column; a remnant of our embryonic tail; articulates with the last fused sacral vertebra at the sacrococcygeal joint (see Tables 5.1 and 2.2).

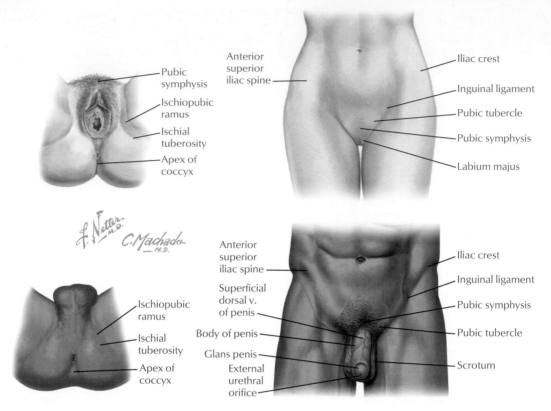

FIGURE 5.1 Key Landmarks in Surface Anatomy of Male Pelvis and Perineum. (From *Netter's atlas of human anatomy*, ed 8, Plate 352; S-9.)

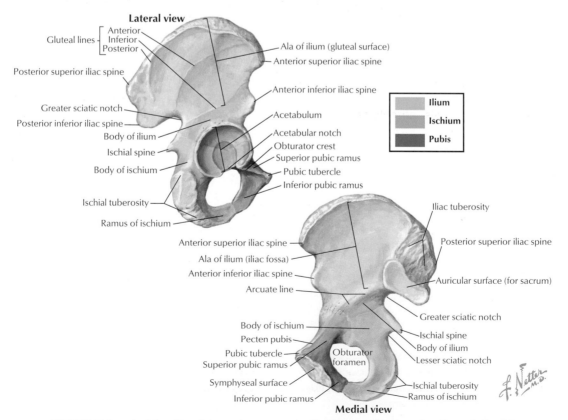

FIGURE 5.2 Right Pelvic (Coxal) Bone. (From *Netter's atlas of human anatomy*, ed 8, Plate 496; S-170.)

Pelvic Fractures

Clinically, the term *pelvic fractures* is used to describe fractures of the pelvic ring and does not typically include *acetabular fractures,* which are a separate type of fracture, usually from high-impact falls or automobile crashes. Pelvic fractures may be high or low impact; high-impact fractures often involve significant bleeding and may be life threatening. Pelvic ring fractures are classified as *stable,* involving only one side of the ring, or *unstable,* involving both parts of the pelvic ring.

Stable pelvic ring fractures

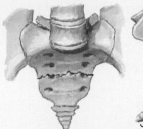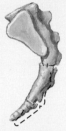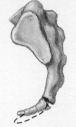

Fracture usually requires no treatment other than care in sitting; inflatable ring helpful.

Transverse fracture of the sacrum that is minimally displaced

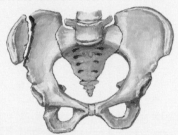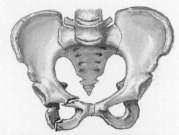

Fracture of iliac wing from direct blow

Fracture of ipsilateral pubic and ischial ramus requires only symptomatic treatment with short-term bed rest and limited activity with walker- or crutch-assisted ambulation for 4 to 6 weeks.

Unstable pelvic fractures

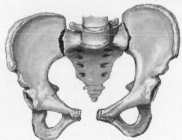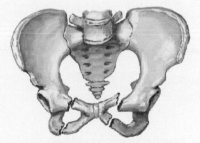

Open book fracture. Disruption of symphysis pubis with wide anterior separation of pelvic ring. Anterior sacroiliac ligaments are torn, with slight opening of sacroiliac joints. Intact posterior sacroiliac ligaments prevent vertical migration of the pelvis.

Straddle fracture. Double break in continuity of anterior pelvic ring causes instability but usually little displacement. Visceral (especially genito-urinary) injury likely.

Vertical shear fracture. Upward and posterior dislocation of sacroiliac joint and fracture of both pubic rami on same side result in upward shift of hemipelvis. Note also fracture of transverse process of L5 vertebra, avulsion of ischial spine, and stretching of sacral nerves.

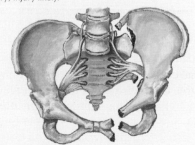

TABLE 5.1 Joints and Ligaments of the Pelvis

LIGAMENT	ATTACHMENT	COMMENT
Lumbosacral Joint*		
Intervertebral disc	Between L5 and sacrum	Allows little movement
Iliolumbar	Transverse process of L5 to crest of ilium	Can be involved in avulsion fracture
Sacroiliac (Plane Synovial) Joint		
Sacroiliac	Sacrum to ilium	Allows little movement; consists of **posterior** (strong), **anterior** (provides rotational stability), and **interosseous** (strongest) ligaments
Sacrococcygeal (Symphysis) Joint		
Sacrococcygeal	Between coccyx and sacrum	Allows some movement; consists of anterior, posterior, and lateral ligaments; contains intervertebral disc between S5 and Co1
Pubic Symphysis		
Pubic	Between pubic bones	Allows some movement, fibrocartilage disc
Accessory Ligaments		
Sacrotuberous	Iliac spines and sacrum to ischial tuberosity	Provides vertical stability
Sacrospinous	Ischial spine to sacrum and coccyx	Divides sciatic notch into greater and lesser sciatic foramina

*Other ligaments include those binding any two vertebrae and facet joints.

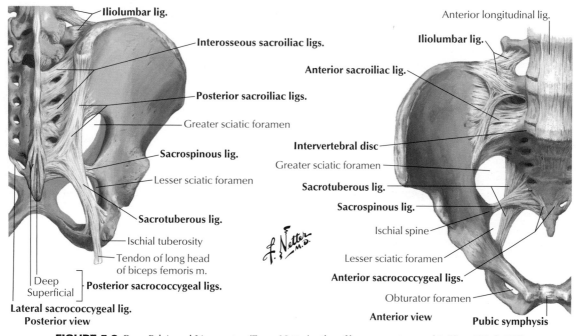

FIGURE 5.3 Bony Pelvis and Ligaments. (From *Netter's atlas of human anatomy,* ed 8, Plate 397; S-224.)

The pelvis protects the pelvic viscera, supports the weight of the body, aids in ambulation by swinging side to side in a rotary movement at the lumbosacral articulation, provides for muscle attachments, and provides a bony support for the lower birth canal. The **pelvic inlet** is the circular opening where the lower abdominal cavity is continuous with the pelvic cavity; the promontory of the sacrum protrudes into this opening and represents its posterior midline boundary (Fig. 5.3). The **pelvic outlet** is diamond shaped and bounded by the pubic symphysis anteriorly, the pubic arches, the inferior pubic rami and ischial rami, the sacrotuberous ligament, and the coccyx. The perineum is enclosed by these boundaries and lies below the pelvic floor (see Fig. 5.18).

The pelvic girdle forms a stable articulation to support the transfer of weight from the trunk to the lower limb. Weight is transferred from the lumbar vertebral column to the sacrum, across the sacroiliac joints to the coxal (pelvic or hip) bones, and then to the femur (thigh bone). The joints and ligaments reflect this stability (Fig. 5.3 and Table 5.1). The **sacroiliac ligaments** are strong, especially posteriorly, as they support the weight of the upper body.

Anatomical differences in the **female bony pelvis** reflect the adaptations for childbirth. The differences from the male pelvis include the following:

- The bones of the female pelvis usually are smaller, lighter, and thinner.
- The pelvic inlet is **oval** in the female and **heart shaped** in the male.
- The female pelvic outlet is larger because of everted ischial tuberosities.
- The female pelvic cavity is **wider** and **shallower**.
- The female pubic arch is larger and wider.
- The greater sciatic notch is wider in females.
- The female sacrum is **shorter** and **wider**.
- The obturator foramen is oval or triangular in females and round in males.

The female pelvis may assume variable shapes, as follows:

- **Gynecoid:** normal, and most suitable shape for childbirth.
- **Android:** a masculine pelvic type, with a heart-shaped inlet, prominent ischial spines, and a narrower pelvic outlet.
- **Platypelloid:** foreshortened in the anteroposterior dimension of the pelvic inlet and wider in the transverse dimension.

- **Anthropoid:** resembling the pelvis of an anthropoid ape, with an oval-shaped inlet with a greatly elongated anteroposterior dimension and a shortened transverse dimension. It possesses a larger outlet.

Various asymmetric shapes may also result from scoliosis, poliomyelitis, fractures, and other pathologies. The characteristic shapes of the female pelvic inlet and outlet are important from the gynecological point of view.

Muscles of the Pelvis

The muscles of the true pelvis line its lateral wall and form a floor over the pelvic outlet. (The pelvic inlet is demarcated by the pelvic brim.) Two muscles line the lateral wall (**obturator internus** and **piriformis muscles**) and attach to the femur (see Table 6.5), and two muscles form the floor, or **pelvic diaphragm** (levator ani and coccygeus muscles) (Fig. 5.4 and Table 5.2). The **levator ani muscle** consists of three muscle groups intermingled to form a single sheet of muscle (*iliococcygeus, pubococcygeus, and puborectalis muscles*). The levator ani muscle is an important support structure for the pelvic viscera in bipeds (upright-walking humans) and helps maintain closure of the vagina and rectum. Bipedalism places greater pressure on the lower pelvic floor, and the coccygeus and levator ani muscles have been "co-opted" for a different use than originally intended in most land-dwelling quadruped mammals. Thus, the muscles once used to tuck the tail between the hind legs (coccygeus) and wag the tail (levator ani) now subserve an important support function during our evolution as bipeds.

TABLE 5.2 Muscles of the Pelvis

MUSCLE	ORIGIN ATTACHMENT	INSERTION ATTACHMENT	INNERVATION	MAIN ACTIONS
Obturator internus	Pelvic aspect of obturator membrane and pelvic bones	Medial surface of greater trochanter of femur	Nerve to obturator internus (L5.S1)	Rotates extended thigh laterally; abducts flexed thigh at hip
Piriformis	Anterior surface of 2nd to 4th sacral segments and sacrotuberous ligament	Superior border of greater trochanter of femur	Anterior rami of L5, S1-S2	Rotates extended thigh laterally; abducts flexed thigh; stabilizes hip joint
Levator ani	Body of pubis, tendinous arch of obturator fascia, and ischial spine	Perineal body, coccyx, anococcygeal raphe, walls of prostate gland or vagina, rectum, and anal canal	Anterior rami of S3-S4, perineal nerve	Supports pelvic viscera; raises pelvic floor
Coccygeus (ischiococcygeus)	Ischial spine and sacrospinous ligament	Inferior sacrum and coccyx	Anterior rami of S4-S5	Supports pelvic viscera; draws coccyx forward

Variations in spinal nerve contributions to the innervation of muscles, their attachments, and their actions are common in human anatomy. Therefore, expect differences between texts and realize that anatomical variation is normal.

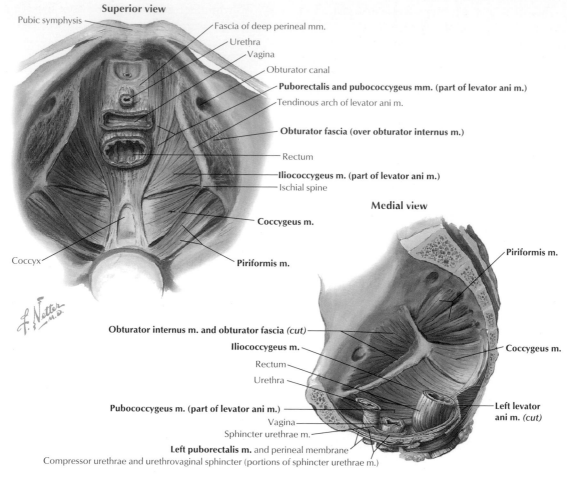

Superior view

Pubic symphysis

Fascia of deep perineal mm.

Urethra

Vagina

Obturator canal

Puborectalis and pubococcygeus mm. (part of levator ani m.)

Tendinous arch of levator ani m.

Obturator fascia (over obturator internus m.)

Rectum

Iliococcygeus m. (part of levator ani m.)

Ischial spine

Medial view

Coccygeus m.

Piriformis m.

Coccyx

Piriformis m.

Obturator internus m. and obturator fascia *(cut)*

Iliococcygeus m.

Coccygeus m.

Rectum

Urethra

Pubococcygeus m. (part of levator ani m.)

Left levator ani m. *(cut)*

Vagina

Sphincter urethrae m.

Left puborectalis m. and perineal membrane

Compressor urethrae and urethrovaginal sphincter (portions of sphincter urethrae m.)

FIGURE 5.4 Muscles of the Female Pelvis. (From *Netter's atlas of human anatomy*, ed 8, Plate 359; S-479.)

4. VISCERA

Distal Gastrointestinal Tract

In both genders the distal gastrointestinal tract passes into the pelvis as the **rectum** and **anal canal**. The rectosigmoid junction superiorly lies at about the level of the S3 vertebra, and the rectum extends inferiorly to become the anal canal just below the coccyx (Fig. 5.5). As the rectum passes through the pelvic diaphragm, it bends posteriorly at the **anorectal flexure** and becomes the anal canal. The anorectal flexure helps maintain fecal continence through the muscle tone maintained by the puborectalis portion of the levator ani muscle. During defecation this muscle relaxes, the anorectal flexure straightens, and fecal matter can then move into the anal canal. Superiorly, the rectum is covered on its anterolateral surface with peritoneum, which gradually covers only the anterior surface, while

the distal portion of the rectum descends below the peritoneal cavity (subperitoneal) to form the **anorectal flexure.** Features of the rectum and anal canal are summarized in Table 5.3.

Pelvic Fascia

The pelvic fascia forms a connective tissue layer between the skeletal muscles forming the lateral walls and floor of the pelvis and the pelvic viscera itself. Two types of pelvic fascia are recognized:

- **Membranous fascia**: one very thin layer of this fascia (termed the **parietal pelvic fascia**) lines the walls and floor of the pelvic cavity muscles; a second thin layer (termed the **visceral pelvic fascia**) lines visceral structures and, where visceral peritoneum covers the viscera, lies just beneath this peritoneum (it is difficult to distinguish between these layers).
- **Endopelvic fascia**: a loose connective tissue layer that permits expansion of the visceral

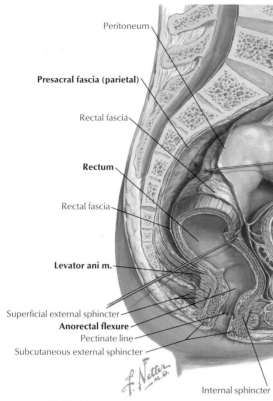

Peritoneum

Presacral fascia (parietal)

Rectal fascia

Rectum

Rectal fascia

Levator ani m.

Superficial external sphincter

Anorectal flexure

Pectinate line

Subcutaneous external sphincter

Internal sphincter

FIGURE 5.5 Rectum and Anal Canal.

TABLE 5.3 Features of the Rectum and Anal Canal	
STRUCTURE	**CHARACTERISTICS**
Pelvic diaphragm	Consists of levator ani and coccygeus muscles; supports pelvic viscera
Internal sphincter	Smooth muscle anal sphincter
Pectinate line	Demarcates visceral (above) from somatic (below) portions of anal canal by type of epithelium, innervation, and embryology
External sphincter	Skeletal muscle anal sphincter (subcutaneous, superficial, and deep)

structures and fills the subperitoneal space between the parietal and visceral membranous fascia. This fascia also contributes to stronger condensations that support the rectum and urinary bladder in men and women and, in women, the uterus (see Figs. 5.5, 5.6, and 5.12).

Distal Urinary Tract

The distal elements of the urinary tract lie within the pelvis and include the following (Fig. 5.6):

- **Distal ureters:** they pass *retroperitoneally* into the pelvic inlet, passing over and near the bifurcation of the common iliac artery; they are crossed anteriorly by the *uterine artery* in females (see Fig. 5.13) and the *ductus deferens* in males (see Fig. 5.11) before terminating in the posterolateral wall of the urinary bladder. As the ureter enters the urinary bladder it passes obliquely through the smooth muscle wall of the bladder, and this arrangement provides for a sphincter-like action.
- **Urinary bladder:** lies behind the pubic symphysis in a subperitoneal position; holds about 500 mL of urine (less in women and even less during pregnancy). Internally, the bladder contains a smooth triangular area between the

openings of the two ureters and the single urethral opening inferiorly that is referred to as the **trigone of the bladder** (see Clinical Focus 5-2). The smooth muscle of the bladder wall is the **detrusor muscle.**

- **Urethra:** short in the female (3-4 cm) and contains two small **paraurethral mucous glands** (Skene's glands) at its aperture; longer in the male (18-20 cm) and divided into the prostatic, membranous, and spongy portions. The **prostatic** portion (about 3 cm) traverses the prostate gland, the **membranous** portion (2-2.5 cm) traverses the external urethral sphincter (skeletal muscle), and the **spongy** portion traverses the corpus spongiosum on the ventral aspect of the penis.

Females have an **external urethral sphincter** composed of skeletal muscle under voluntary control and innervated by the somatic nerve fibers in the **pudendal nerve** (S2-S4). Males have the following urethral sphincters:

- **Internal sphincter:** smooth-muscle involuntary sphincter at the neck of the bladder and innervated by *sympathetic fibers from L1 to L2;* during ejaculation, it contracts and prevents semen from entering the urinary bladder.
- **External sphincter:** skeletal muscle voluntary sphincter surrounding the membranous urethra and innervated by the somatic nerve fibers in the **pudendal nerve** (S2-S4).

Micturition (urination/voiding) occurs by the following sequence of events:

- Normally, the *sympathetic fibers* relax the bladder wall and constrict the internal urethral sphincter (smooth muscle around the bladder neck, present only in males), thus inhibiting emptying.
- Micturition is initiated by the stimulation of *stretch receptors* (afferents enter the spinal cord

Female: Median (sagittal) section

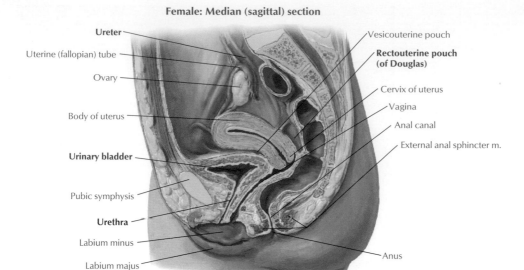

Ureter
Uterine (fallopian) tube
Ovary
Body of uterus
Urinary bladder
Pubic symphysis
Urethra
Labium minus
Labium majus

Vesicouterine pouch
Rectouterine pouch (of Douglas)
Cervix of uterus
Vagina
Anal canal
External anal sphincter m.
Anus

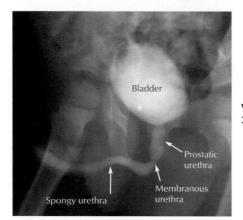

Bladder

Voiding cystourethrogram, 2-year-old male

Prostatic urethra
Membranous urethra
Spongy urethra

Male: Median (sagittal) section

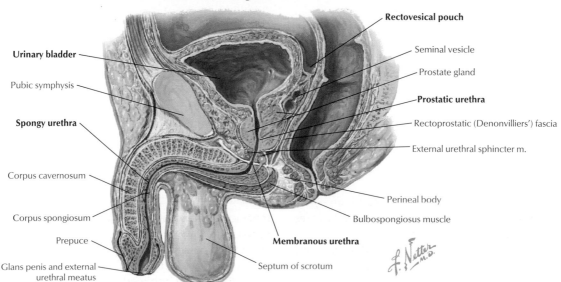

Urinary bladder
Pubic symphysis
Spongy urethra
Corpus cavernosum
Corpus spongiosum
Prepuce
Glans penis and external urethral meatus

Rectovesical pouch
Seminal vesicle
Prostate gland
Prostatic urethra
Rectoprostatic (Denonvilliers') fascia
External urethral sphincter m.
Perineal body
Bulbospongiosus muscle
Membranous urethra
Septum of scrotum

FIGURE 5.6 Distal Urinary Tract. (From *Netter's atlas of human anatomy,* ed 8, Plates 364 and 368; S-485 and S-495.)

Clinical Focus 5.2

Urinary Tract Infections

Urinary tract infection (UTI) is more common in females, likely directly related to their shorter urethra, urinary tract trauma, and exposure to pathogens in an environment conducive for growth and propagation. As illustrated, a number of other risk factors also may precipitate infections in either gender. *Escherichia coli* is the usual pathogen involved. UTI may lead to urethritis, cystitis (bladder inflammation), and pyelonephritis. Symptoms of cystitis include the following:

- Dysuria
- Frequency of urination
- Urgency of urination

- Suprapubic discomfort and tenderness
- Hematuria (less common)

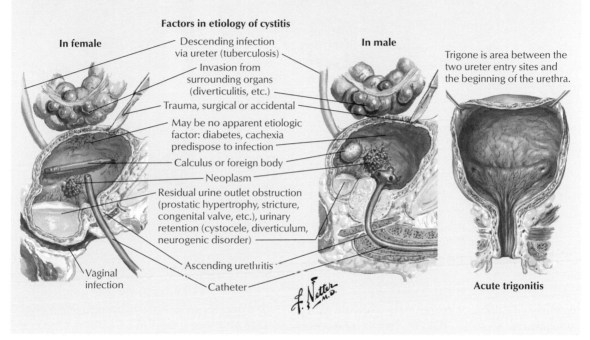

Factors in etiology of cystitis

In female

Descending infection via ureter (tuberculosis)

Invasion from surrounding organs (diverticulitis, etc.)

Trauma, surgical or accidental

May be no apparent etiologic factor: diabetes, cachexia predispose to infection

Calculus or foreign body

Neoplasm

Residual urine outlet obstruction (prostatic hypertrophy, stricture, congenital valve, etc.), urinary retention (cystocele, diverticulum, neurogenic disorder)

Ascending urethritis

Vaginal infection

Catheter

In male

Trigone is area between the two ureter entry sites and the beginning of the urethra.

Acute trigonitis

via the *pelvic splanchnic nerves, S2-S4*) located in the detrusor (smooth) muscle of the bladder when it begins to fill.

- *Parasympathetic efferents (pelvic splanchnics)* induce a reflex contraction of the detrusor muscle and relaxation of the internal sphincter (males only), enhancing the urge to void.
- When appropriate to void (and sometimes not!), *somatic efferents via the pudendal nerve* (S2-S4) cause a voluntary relaxation of the external urethral sphincter, and the bladder begins to empty. In both sexes, the external urethral sphincter (skeletal muscle under voluntary control) relaxes so the passage of urine may occur.
- When voiding is complete, the *external urethral sphincter* contracts (in males the bulbospongiosus muscle contracts as well to expel the last few drops of urine from the spongy urethra), and

the detrusor muscle relaxes under *sympathetic control.*

Female Pelvic Reproductive Viscera

The female pelvic reproductive viscera include the midline **uterus** and **vagina** and the adnexa (paired **ovaries** and **uterine tubes**), which are positioned between the urinary bladder anteriorly and the rectum posteriorly (Fig. 5.6).

The **uterus** is pear shaped, about 7 to 8 cm long, and exhibits a *body* (fundus and isthmus) and *cervix* (neck). The cervix has an internal os (opening), a cervical canal, and an external os that opens into the vagina. While the uterine cavity looks triangular in coronal section (see Fig. 5.8), in sagittal section it appears only as a narrow space (Fig. 5.6, *top*). The usual position of the uterus is in an anteflexed (anteverted) position and lies almost in

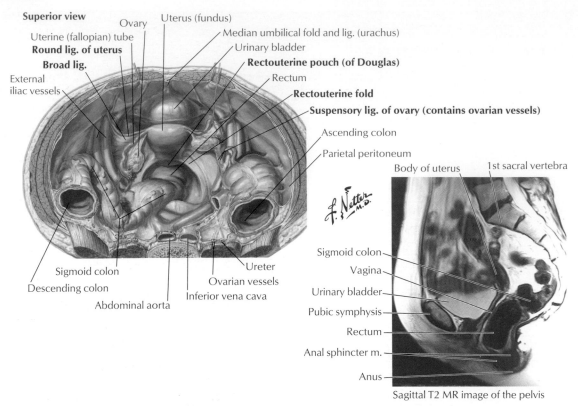

FIGURE 5.7 Peritoneal Relationships of the Female Pelvic Viscera. (From *Netter's atlas of human anatomy,* ed 8, Plate 367; S-484; MR image from Kelley LL, Petersen C: *Sectional anatomy for imaging professionals,* Philadelphia, 2007, Mosby.)

the horizontal plane. A double sheet of peritoneum (actually a mesentery) called the **broad ligament** envelops the ovaries, uterine tubes, and uterus (Figs. 5.7 and 5.8). During embryonic development the ovaries are pulled into the pelvis by a fibromuscular band (homologue of the male gubernaculum). This **ovarian ligament** attaches the inferomedial pole of the ovary to the uterus, then reflects anterolaterally off the uterus as the **round ligament of the uterus,** enters the deep inguinal ring, courses down the inguinal canal, and ends in the **labium majus of the perineum** as a fibrofatty mass. Features of the female pelvic reproductive viscera are summarized in Table 5.4.

The **vagina,** about 8 to 9 cm long, is a fibromuscular tube that surrounds the uterine cervix and passes inferiorly through the pelvic floor to open in the **vestibule** (area enclosed by the **labium minus**). Because the uterine cervix projects into the superoanterior aspect of the vagina, a continuous gutter surrounds the cervical opening, shallower anteriorly and deeper posteriorly, forming the anterior, lateral, and posterior fornices.

The **ovaries** are almond-shaped female gonads 3 to 4 cm long (but smaller in older women) attached to the broad ligament by its mesovarium portion. The ovary is suspended between two attachments: laterally to the pelvic wall by the **suspensory ligament of the ovary** (contains the ovarian vessels, lymphatics, and autonomic nerve fibers) and medially to the uterus by the **ovarian ligament.** The ovary is covered by its own epithelium and has no peritoneal covering.

The **uterine tubes** (fallopian tubes), about 8-10 cm long, are suspended in the mesosalpinx portion of the broad ligament and are subdivided into four parts:

- **Infundibulum:** fimbriated, expanded distal portion that opens at the ostium into the peritoneal cavity and lies close to the ovary.
- **Ampulla:** wide portion of the tube lying between the infundibulum and the isthmus; the usual site of fertilization.
- **Isthmus:** proximal, narrow, straight, and thickened portion of the tube that joins the body of the uterus.
- **Intramural portion:** traverses the uterine wall to open into the uterine cavity.

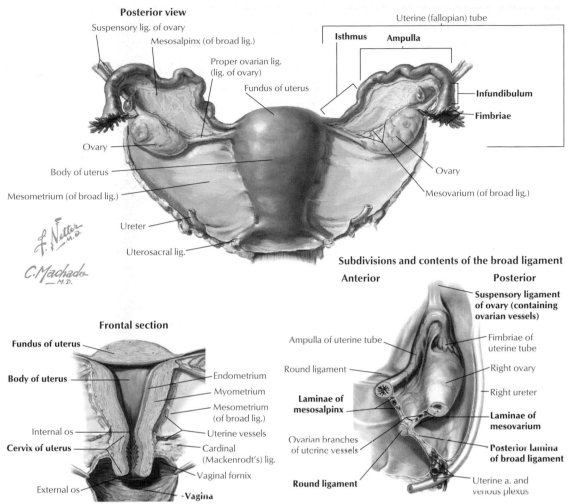

Posterior view

Suspensory lig. of ovary
Mesosalpinx (of broad lig.)
Proper ovarian lig. (lig. of ovary)
Fundus of uterus
Ovary
Body of uterus
Mesometrium (of broad lig.)
Ureter
Uterosacral lig.

Uterine (fallopian) tube
Isthmus Ampulla
Infundibulum
Fimbriae
Ovary
Mesovarium (of broad lig.)

Frontal section

Fundus of uterus
Body of uterus
Endometrium
Myometrium
Mesometrium (of broad lig.)
Internal os
Uterine vessels
Cervix of uterus
Cardinal (Mackenrodt's) lig.
Vaginal fornix
External os
Vagina

Subdivisions and contents of the broad ligament

Anterior Posterior

Suspensory ligament of ovary (containing ovarian vessels)
Ampulla of uterine tube
Fimbriae of uterine tube
Round ligament
Right ovary
Laminae of mesosalpinx
Right ureter
Ovarian branches of uterine vessels
Laminae of mesovarium
Round ligament
Posterior lamina of broad ligament
Uterine a. and venous plexus

FIGURE 5.8 Uterus and Adnexa. (From *Netter's atlas of human anatomy,* ed 8, Plates 374 and 376; S-487 and S-489.)

TABLE 5.4 Features of the Female Pelvic Viscera

STRUCTURE	CHARACTERISTICS
Urinary bladder	Covered by peritoneum
Uterus	Consists of a body (fundus and isthmus) and cervix; supported by pelvic diaphragm and ligaments; enveloped in broad ligament
Ovaries	Suspended between suspensory ligament of ovary (contains ovarian vessels, nerves, and lymphatics) and ovarian ligament (tethered to uterus)
Uterine tubes (fallopian tubes)	Courses in mesosalpinx of broad ligament and consists of fimbriated end (collects ovulated ova), infundibulum, ampulla, isthmus, and intrauterine portions
Vagina	Fibromuscular tube that includes the fornix, a superior recess around protruding uterine cervix
Rectum	Distal retroperitoneal portion of large intestine
Vesicouterine pouch	Peritoneal recess between bladder and uterus
Rectouterine pouch (of Douglas)	Peritoneal recess between rectum and uterus and lowest point in female pelvis
Broad ligament	Peritoneal fold that suspends uterus and uterine tubes; includes mesovarium (enfolds ovary), mesosalpinx (enfolds uterine tube), and mesometrium (remainder of ligament)
Round ligament of uterus	Reflects off uterus and keeps uterus anteverted and anteflexed; passes into inguinal canal and ends as fibrofatty mass in labia majus
Transverse cervical (cardinal or Mackenrodt's) ligaments	Fibrous condensations of subperitoneal pelvic fascia that support uterus
Uterosacral ligaments	Extend from sides of cervix to sacrum, support uterus, and lie beneath peritoneum (form uterosacral fold)

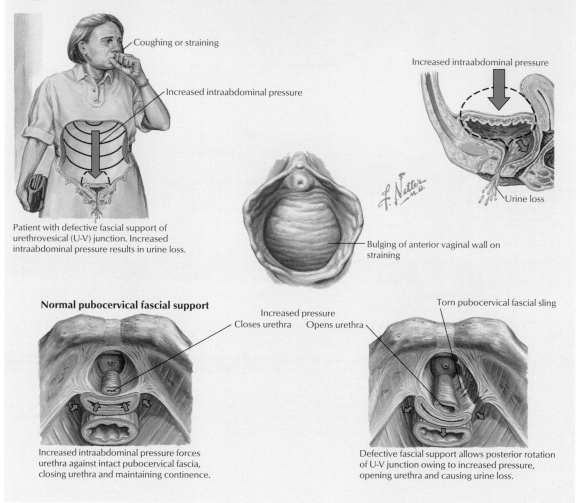

Clinical Focus 5.3
Stress Incontinence in Women

Involuntary loss of urine after an increase in intraabdominal pressure is often associated with a weakening of the support structures of the pelvic floor, including the following:

- Medial and lateral pubovesical ligaments
- Pubovesical fascia at the urethrovesical junction (blends with the perineal membrane and body)
- Levator ani (provides support at the urethrovesical junction)
- Functional integrity of the urethral sphincter

Common predisposing factors for stress incontinence include multiparity, obesity, chronic cough, and heavy lifting.

Coughing or straining

Increased intraabdominal pressure

Increased intraabdominal pressure

Urine loss

Patient with defective fascial support of urethrovesical (U-V) junction. Increased intraabdominal pressure results in urine loss.

Bulging of anterior vaginal wall on straining

Normal pubocervical fascial support

Increased pressure
Closes urethra   Opens urethra

Torn pubocervical fascial sling

Increased intraabdominal pressure forces urethra against intact pubocervical fascia, closing urethra and maintaining continence.

Defective fascial support allows posterior rotation of U-V junction owing to increased pressure, opening urethra and causing urine loss.

Male Pelvic Reproductive Viscera

The male pelvic reproductive viscera include the **prostate gland** and paired **seminal vesicles.** These structures lie in a subperitoneal position and are in close association with the urethra (Figs. 5.6 and 5.9). The testes descend into the scrotum late in human prenatal development and are connected to the seminal vesicles by the **ductus (vas) deferens,** which passes in the spermatic cord, ascends in the scrotum, passes through the inguinal canal, and then courses retroperitoneally to join the duct of the seminal vesicles **(ejaculatory ducts)** (Table 5.5 and Figs. 5.9 and 5.10).

Text continued on p. 249.

Uterine Prolapse

Uterine prolapse may occur when the support structures of the uterus, especially the **cardinal ligaments, uterosacral ligaments,** and **levator ani muscle,** are weakened.

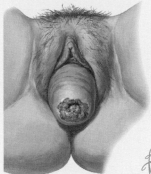

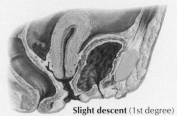

Slight descent (1st degree)

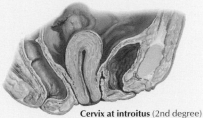

Cervix at introitus (2nd degree)

Procidentia clinical appearance

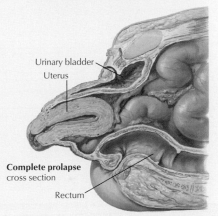

Urinary bladder

Uterus

Complete prolapse
cross section

Rectum

Characteristic	Description
Prevalence	Some descent common in parous women
Age	Late reproductive and older age groups
Risk factors	Birth trauma, obesity, chronic cough, lifting, weak ligaments

Cervical Carcinoma

Approximately 85% to 90% of cervical carcinomas are squamous cell carcinomas, whereas 10% to 15% are adenocarcinomas. Most carcinomas occur near the *external cervical os*, where the cervical epithelium changes from simple columnar to stratified squamous epithelium (the transformation zone). The most common cause of cervical carcinoma is contraction of human papillomavirus (HPV) during sexual intercourse.

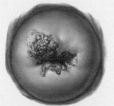

Adenocarcinoma

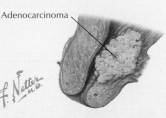

Uterus

Cancer of the cervix with
direct extension to vaginal
wall, bladder, and rectum

Early carcinoma

Rectum

Characteristic	Description
Risk factors	Early sexual activity, multiple sex partners, human papillomavirus (HPV) infection, African-American, smoking
Prevalence	10,000 cases/year, with 4,000 deaths/year
Age	40–60 years

Clinical Focus 5.6

Uterine Leiomyomas (Fibroids)

Leiomyomas are benign tumors of smooth muscle and connective tissue cells of the myometrium of the uterus. These "fibroids" are firm and can range in size from 1 to 20 cm. The composite drawing shows various sizes and sites of potential leiomyomas.

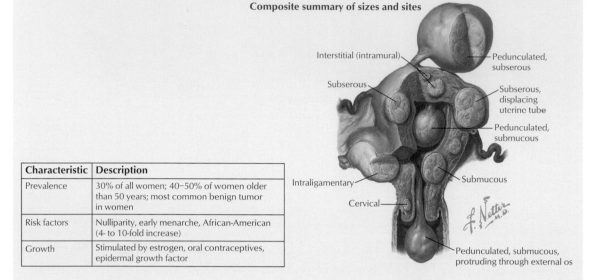

Composite summary of sizes and sites

Characteristic	Description
Prevalence	30% of all women; 40–50% of women older than 50 years; most common benign tumor in women
Risk factors	Nulliparity, early menarche, African-American (4- to 10-fold increase)
Growth	Stimulated by estrogen, oral contraceptives, epidermal growth factor

Clinical Focus 5.7

Endometriosis

Endometriosis is a progressive benign condition characterized by ectopic foci of endometrial tissue, called *implants,* that grow in the pelvis—on the ovaries and in the rectouterine pouch, uterine ligaments, and uterine tubes—or in the peritoneal cavity. As with the uterine lining, these estrogen-sensitive ectopic implants can grow and then break down and bleed in cycle with the woman's normal menstrual cycle.

Characteristic	Description
Prevalence	5–10% of all women; 30–50% of infertility patients
Age	25–45 years
Causes	Genetic, menstrual backflow through tubes, lymphatic or vascular spread, metaplasia of coelomic epithelium
Risk factors	Obstructive anomalies (cervical or vaginal outflow pathway)

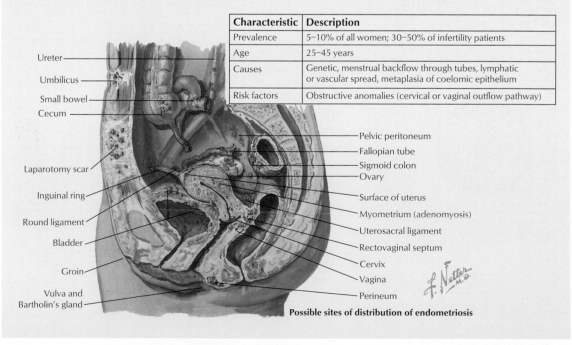

Possible sites of distribution of endometriosis

Uterine Endometrial Carcinoma

Endometrial carcinoma is the most common malignancy of the female reproductive tract. It often occurs between the ages of 55 and 65 years, and risk factors include the following:

- Obesity (increased estrogen synthesis from fat cells without concomitant progesterone synthesis)
- Estrogen replacement therapy without concomitant progestin
- Breast or colon cancer
- Early menarche or late menopause (prolonged estrogen stimulation)
- Chronic anovulation
- No prior pregnancies or periods of breastfeeding
- Diabetes

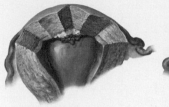

Early carcinoma
involving only endometrium

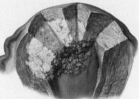

More extensive carcinoma
deeply involving muscle

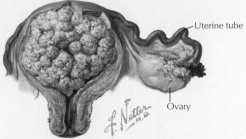

Uterine tube

Ovary

Extensive carcinoma invading full thickness of myometrium and escaping through tube to implant on ovary

Chronic Pelvic Inflammatory Disease

Recurrent or chronic infections of the *uterine tubes or other adnexa (uterine appendages)* result in cystic dilation (hydrosalpinx) and can account for approximately 40% of female infertility cases. Chronic pelvic inflammatory disease (PID) can cause scarring, causing problems with fertility, pelvic pain, or tubal (ectopic) pregnancy. The most affected age group is 15 to 25 years of age, and risk factors include the following:

- Early sexual activity
- Failure to use condoms
- Multiple sexual partners
- Sexually transmitted diseases (STDs)

Unilateral or bilateral adnexal masses are usually sausage shaped and may be palpable.

Examples of adnexal masses resulting from PID
Fully developed abscess

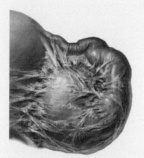

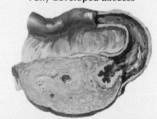

PID: hydrosalpinx (dilation of uterine tube)

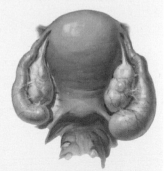

Pathogenesis of tuboovarian abscess
Adherence of tube and infection of ruptured follicle (corpus luteum)

Small and moderate-sized hydrosalpinx

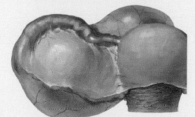

Large tuboovarian cyst

Clinical Focus 5.10

Dysfunctional Uterine Bleeding

Dysfunctional uterine bleeding (DUB) involves an irregular cycle or intermenstrual bleeding (painless) with no clinically identifiable cause. The etiology and pathogenesis are extensive and include local uterine, ovarian, or adnexal disorders, as well as systemic and pregnancy-related disorders. Hormonal imbalance is a common cause.

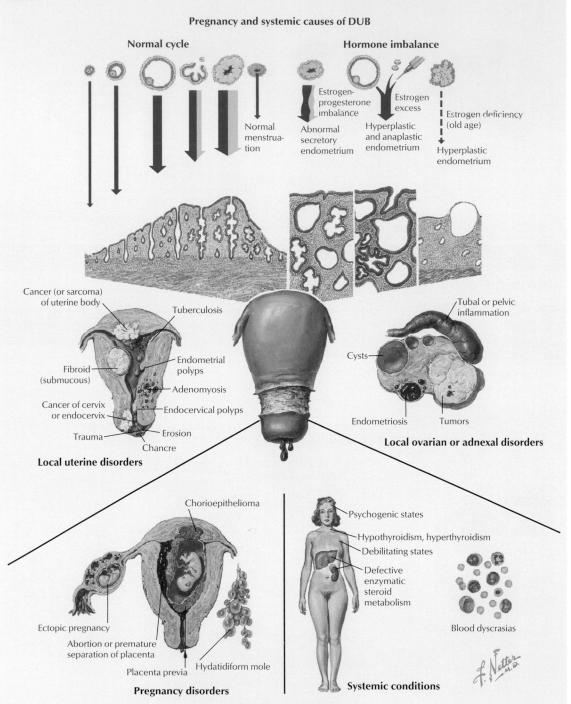

Pregnancy and systemic causes of DUB

Normal cycle

Hormone imbalance

Estrogen-progesterone imbalance

Estrogen excess

Estrogen deficiency (old age)

Normal menstruation

Abnormal secretory endometrium

Hyperplastic and anaplastic endometrium

Hyperplastic endometrium

Cancer (or sarcoma) of uterine body

Tuberculosis

Fibroid (submucous)

Endometrial polyps

Adenomyosis

Cancer of cervix or endocervix

Endocervical polyps

Trauma

Erosion

Chancre

Local uterine disorders

Tubal or pelvic inflammation

Cysts

Endometriosis

Tumors

Local ovarian or adnexal disorders

Chorioepithelioma

Ectopic pregnancy

Abortion or premature separation of placenta

Placenta previa

Hydatidiform mole

Pregnancy disorders

Psychogenic states

Hypothyroidism, hyperthyroidism

Debilitating states

Defective enzymatic steroid metabolism

Blood dyscrasias

Systemic conditions

Ectopic Pregnancy

Ectopic pregnancy involves implantation of a **blastocyst** outside the uterine cavity, most often in the **fallopian tube.** Because of the potential medical danger of an ectopic pregnancy, the pregnancy is usually terminated medically (if detected early enough) or surgically (often laparoscopically).

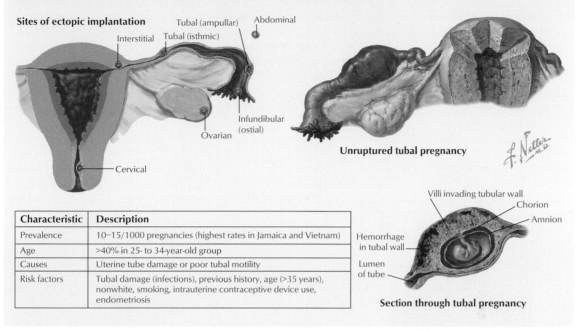

Sites of ectopic implantation

Interstitial · Tubal (isthmic) · Tubal (ampullar) · Abdominal · Infundibular (ostial) · Ovarian · Cervical

Unruptured tubal pregnancy

Villi invading tubular wall · Chorion · Amnion · Hemorrhage in tubal wall · Lumen of tube

Section through tubal pregnancy

Characteristic	Description
Prevalence	10–15/1000 pregnancies (highest rates in Jamaica and Vietnam)
Age	>40% in 25- to 34-year-old group
Causes	Uterine tube damage or poor tubal motility
Risk factors	Tubal damage (infections), previous history, age (>35 years), nonwhite, smoking, intrauterine contraceptive device use, endometriosis

Assisted Reproduction

Approximately 10% to 15% of infertile couples may benefit from various assisted reproductive strategies.

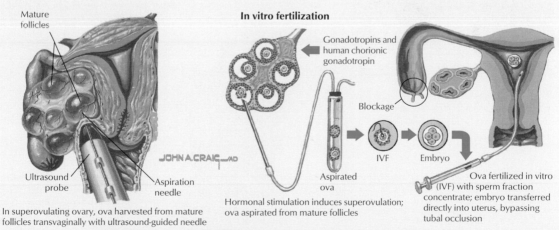

In vitro fertilization

Mature follicles

Gonadotropins and human chorionic gonadotropin

Blockage

IVF · Embryo

Ultrasound probe · Aspiration needle

JOHN A.CRAIG—MD

Aspirated ova

In superovulating ovary, ova harvested from mature follicles transvaginally with ultrasound-guided needle

Hormonal stimulation induces superovulation; ova aspirated from mature follicles

Ova fertilized in vitro (IVF) with sperm fraction concentrate; embryo transferred directly into uterus, bypassing tubal occlusion

Technique	Definition
Artificial insemination	Use of donor sperm
GIFT	Gamete intrafallopian transfer
IUI	Intrauterine insemination (partner's or donor's sperm)
IVF/ET	In vitro fertilization with embryo transfer to uterine cavity (illustrated)
ZIFT	In vitro fertilization with zygote transfer to fallopian tube

Clinical Focus 5.13

Ovarian Cancer

Ovarian cancer is the *most lethal cancer* of the female reproductive tract. From 85% to 90% of all malignancies occur from the surface epithelium, with cancerous cells often breaking through the capsule and **seeding the peritoneal surface,** invading the adjacent pelvic organs, or seeding the omentum, mesentery, and intestines. Additionally, the cancer cells may spread via the **venous system** to the lungs (by the ovarian vein and inferior vena cava) and liver (by the portal system) and via **lymphatics**. Risk factors include the following:

- Family history of ovarian cancer
- High-fat diet
- Age
- Nulliparity
- Early menarche or late menopause (prolonged estrogen stimulation)
- White race
- Higher socioeconomic status

Routes of metastases

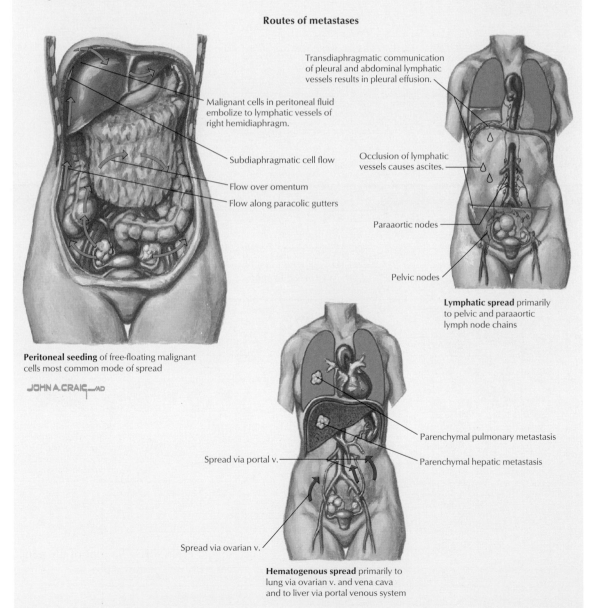

Transdiaphragmatic communication of pleural and abdominal lymphatic vessels results in pleural effusion.

Malignant cells in peritoneal fluid embolize to lymphatic vessels of right hemidiaphragm.

Subdiaphragmatic cell flow

Occlusion of lymphatic vessels causes ascites.

Flow over omentum

Flow along paracolic gutters

Paraaortic nodes

Pelvic nodes

Lymphatic spread primarily to pelvic and paraaortic lymph node chains

Peritoneal seeding of free-floating malignant cells most common mode of spread

JOHN A. CRAIG—MD

Parenchymal pulmonary metastasis

Spread via portal v.

Parenchymal hepatic metastasis

Spread via ovarian v.

Hematogenous spread primarily to lung via ovarian v. and vena cava and to liver via portal venous system

The **testes** are paired gonads about the size of a chestnut with the following features (Fig. 5.10):

- During descent of the testes into the scrotum, a pouch of abdominopelvic peritoneum called the **tunica vaginalis** attaches to the anterior and lateral aspect of the testes (has visceral and parietal layers).
- Testes are encased within a thick capsule, the **tunica albuginea.**
- Testes are divided into lobules that contain **seminiferous tubules.**
- The seminiferous tubules are lined with germinal epithelium that gives rise to **spermatozoa**.
- Testes drain spermatozoa into the **rete testes** (straight tubules) and **efferent ductules** of the epididymis.
- Sperm mature and are stored in the **epididymis,** a long coiled tube about 6 meters in length if uncoiled.

It is within the **seminiferous tubules** that spermatogenesis occurs. The testis is divided into about 250 lobules, each containing one to four seminiferous tubules of the testes and each about 50 cm (20 inches) long on average at full length. The complete cycle of spermatogenesis takes about 74 days and 12 more days for the sperm to mature and pass through the epididymis. About 300 million sperm cells are produced daily in the human testis.

The **ductus deferens** is 40 to 45 cm long and joins the ducts of the **seminal vesicles** to form the **ejaculatory ducts,** which empty into the **prostatic urethra,** the first portion of the male urethra leaving the urinary bladder (Fig. 5.11; see Fig. 5.9 and Table 5.5). The **seminal vesicles** have the following features:

- Contribute fluid to the ejaculate and account for about 70% of the ejaculate volume.

TABLE 5.5 Features of the Male Pelvic Viscera

STRUCTURE	CHARACTERISTICS
Urinary bladder	Lies retroperitoneal and has detrusor muscle (smooth muscle) lining its walls
Prostate gland	Walnut-sized gland with five lobes (anterior, middle, posterior, right lateral, left lateral); middle lobe prone to benign hypertrophy and surrounds prostatic urethra
Seminal vesicles	Lobulated glands whose ducts join ductus deferens to form ejaculatory duct; secretes alkaline seminal fluid
Bulbourethral (Cowper's) glands	Pea-sized glands located posterolateral to the membranous urethra that secrete a mucus-like lubrication into the urethra
Rectum	Distal portion of large intestine that is retroperitoneal
Rectovesical pouch	Recess between bladder and rectum
Testes	Develop in retroperitoneal abdominal wall and descend into scrotum
Epididymis	Consists of head, body, and tail and functions in maturation and storage of sperm
Ductus (vas) deferens	Passes in spermatic cord through inguinal canal to join duct of seminal vesicles (ejaculatory duct)

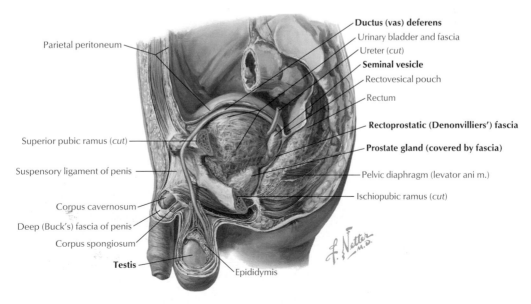

FIGURE 5.9 Male Reproductive Viscera. (From *Netter's atlas of human anatomy,* ed 8, Plate 368; S-495.)

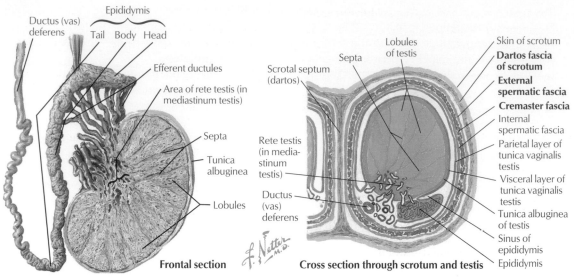

FIGURE 5.10 Testis, Epididymis, and Ductus Deferens. (From *Netter's atlas of human anatomy*, ed 8, Plate 392; S-498.)

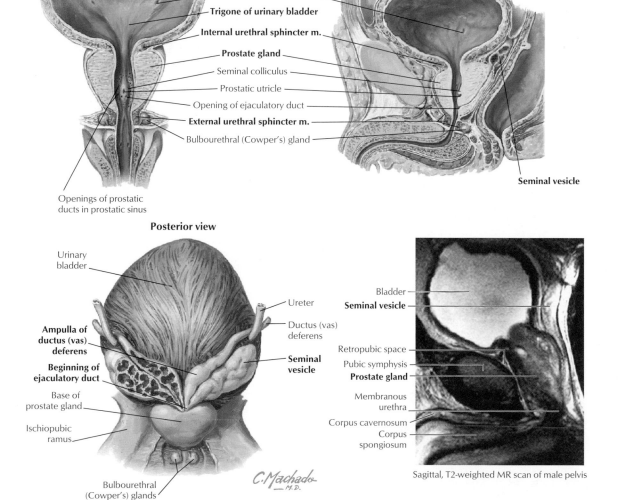

FIGURE 5.11 Bladder, Prostate, Seminal Vesicles, and Proximal Urethra. (From *Netter's atlas of human anatomy*, ed 8, Plate 385; S-496; MR image from Weber E, Vilensky J, Carmichael M: *Netter's concise radiologic anatomy*, Philadelphia, 2009, Saunders.)

- Produce a viscous and alkaline fluid that *nourishes* the spermatozoa and *protects* them from the acidic environment of the female vagina.

The **prostate** is a walnut-sized gland that surrounds the proximal urethra and has the following features:

- Contributes fluid to the ejaculate and accounts for about 20% of the ejaculate volume.
- Produces a thin, milky, slightly alkaline fluid that helps to liquefy coagulated semen after it is deposited in the vagina; this fluid contains citric acid, proteolytic enzymes, sugars, phosphate, and various ions.

About 3 to 5 mL of **semen** and 100 million sperm/mL are present in each ejaculation. The pH of the ejaculate is between 7 and 8.

Pelvic Peritoneum

In both sexes, the peritoneum on the lower internal aspect of the anterior abdominal wall reflects off the midline from the urinary bladder as the **median umbilical ligament** (a remnant of the embryonic urachus). The **medial umbilical ligaments** pass superiorly about 2 cm laterally on each side; they contain the inferior epigastric vessels, which will course superiorly in the posterior lamina of the rectus sheath (Figs. 4.3, 4.4, and 5.12).

In *females,* the peritoneum reflects onto the superior aspect of the urinary bladder, over the body of the uterus, as the **broad ligament,** and onto the anterolateral aspect of the rectum (Fig. 5.6). In *males,* the peritoneum reflects off of the urinary bladder and directly onto the anterolateral aspect of the

---

Clinical Focus 5.14

Vasectomy

Vasectomy offers *birth control* with a failure rate below that of the pill, condom, intrauterine device, and tubal ligation. It can be performed as an office procedure with a local anesthetic. (Approximately 500,000 are performed each year in the United States.) One approach uses a small incision on each side of the scrotum to isolate the vas deferens; another uses a small puncture (no incision) in the scrotal skin to isolate both the right vas and left vas. The muscular vas is identified, and a small segment is isolated between two small metal clips or sutures. The isolated segment is resected, the clipped ends of the vas are cauterized, and the incision is closed (or, in the nonincisional approach, the puncture wound is left unsutured).

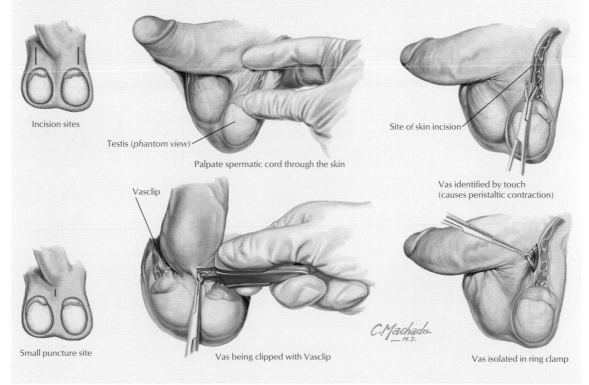

Incision sites

Testis (*phantom view*)

Palpate spermatic cord through the skin

Site of skin incision

Vas identified by touch (causes peristaltic contraction)

Vasclip

Small puncture site

Vas being clipped with Vasclip

Vas isolated in ring clamp

Testicular Cancer

Testicular tumors are heterogeneous neoplasms, with 95% arising from **germ cells** and almost all malignant. Of the germ cell tumors, 60% show mixed histologic features, and 40% show a single histologic pattern. Surgical resection usually is performed using an inguinal approach (radical inguinal orchiectomy) to avoid spread of the cancer to the adjacent scrotal tissues. Testicular cancer is the *most common cancer* in men 15 to 35 years old. It has a high incidence among Caucasians, with the highest prevalence rates in Scandinavia, Germany, and New Zealand.

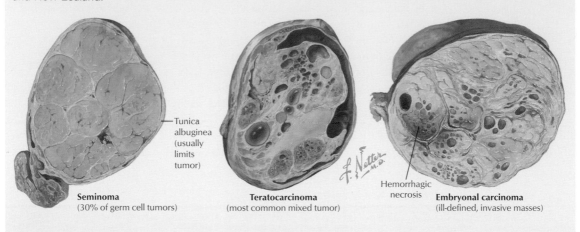

Seminoma
(30% of germ cell tumors)

Teratocarcinoma
(most common mixed tumor)

Embryonal carcinoma
(ill-defined, invasive masses)

Hydrocele and Varicocele

The most common cause of scrotal enlargement is *hydrocele,* an excessive accumulation of serous fluid within the **tunica vaginalis** (usually a potential space). An infection in the testis or epididymis, trauma, or a tumor may lead to hydrocele, or it may be idiopathic.

Varicocele is an abnormal dilation and tortuosity of the **pampiniform venous plexus.** Almost all varicoceles are on the left side (90%), perhaps because the left testicular vein drains into the left renal vein, which has a slightly higher pressure, rather than into the larger inferior vena cava, as the right testicular vein does. A varicocele is evident at physical examination when a patient stands, but it usually resolves when the patient is recumbent.

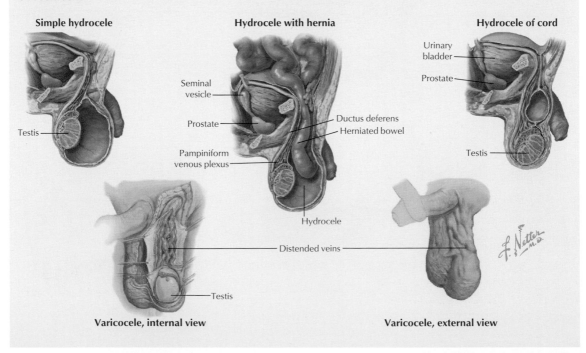

Simple hydrocele

Hydrocele with hernia

Hydrocele of cord

Varicocele, internal view

Varicocele, external view

Clinical Focus 5.17

Transurethral Resection of the Prostate

Benign prostatic hypertrophy (BPH) occurs in about 20% of men by age 40, increasing with age to 90% of males older than 80. BPH is really a nodular *hyperplasia,* not hypertrophy, and results from proliferation of epithelial and stromal tissues, often in the periurethral area. This growth can lead to urinary urgency, decreased stream force, frequency, and nocturia. Symptoms may necessitate transurethral resection of the prostate (TURP), in which the obstructing periurethral part of the gland is removed using a resectoscope.

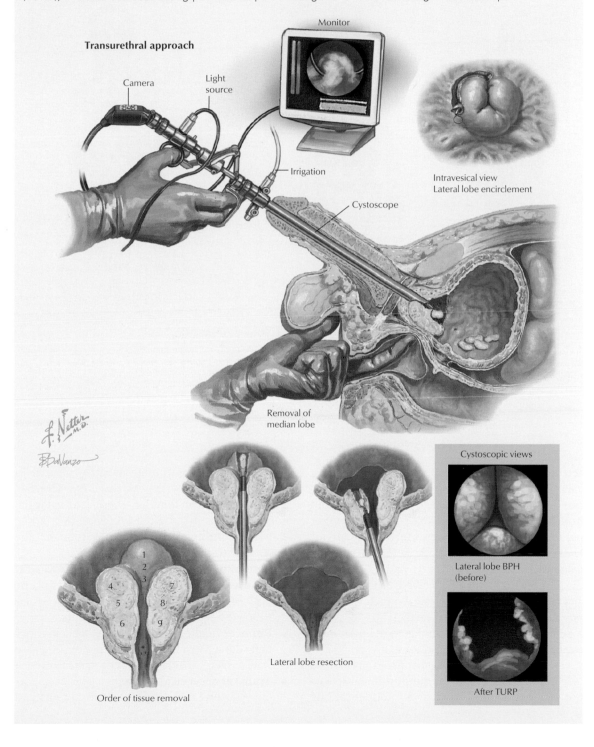

Transurethral approach

Monitor

Camera

Light source

Irrigation

Cystoscope

Intravesical view
Lateral lobe encirclement

Removal of median lobe

Order of tissue removal

Lateral lobe resection

Cystoscopic views

Lateral lobe BPH (before)

After TURP

Clinical Focus 5.18

Prostatic Carcinoma

Prostatic carcinoma is the *most common visceral cancer* in males and the second leading cause of death in men older than 50, after lung cancer. Primary lesions invade the prostatic capsule and then spread along the ejaculatory ducts into the space between the seminal vesicles and bladder. The pelvic lymphatics and rich venous drainage of the prostate (prostatic venous plexus) facilitate metastatic spread to distant sites.

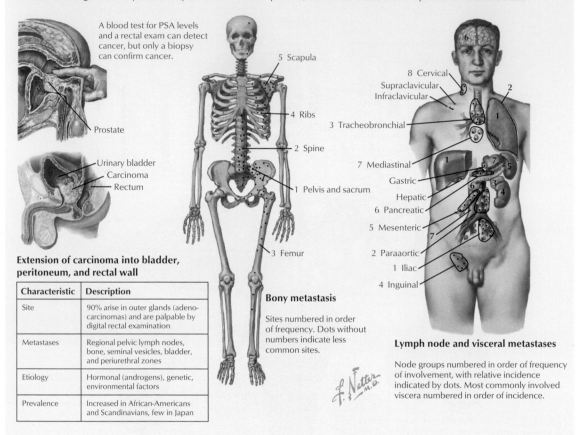

A blood test for PSA levels and a rectal exam can detect cancer, but only a biopsy can confirm cancer.

Prostate

Urinary bladder
Carcinoma
Rectum

Extension of carcinoma into bladder, peritoneum, and rectal wall

Characteristic	Description
Site	90% arise in outer glands (adenocarcinomas) and are palpable by digital rectal examination
Metastases	Regional pelvic lymph nodes, bone, seminal vesicles, bladder, and periurethral zones
Etiology	Hormonal (androgens), genetic, environmental factors
Prevalence	Increased in African-Americans and Scandinavians, few in Japan

5 Scapula
4 Ribs
3 Tracheobronchial
2 Spine
1 Pelvis and sacrum
3 Femur

Bony metastasis

Sites numbered in order of frequency. Dots without numbers indicate less common sites.

8 Cervical
Supraclavicular
Infraclavicular
7 Mediastinal
Gastric
Hepatic
6 Pancreatic
5 Mesenteric
2 Paraaortic
1 Iliac
4 Inguinal

Lymph node and visceral metastases

Node groups numbered in order of frequency of involvement, with relative incidence indicated by dots. Most commonly involved viscera numbered in order of incidence.

---

rectum. Reflection of the peritoneum in females causes a trough or pouch to form between the bladder and the uterus, called the **vesicouterine pouch**. Between the uterus and the rectum, the peritoneum forms the **rectouterine pouch** (of Douglas), which represents the *lowest point* in the female peritoneal cavity (Figs. 5.6 and 5.7). In males, the peritoneum forms a pouch between the bladder and rectum called the **rectovesical pouch**, the *lowest point* in the male peritoneal cavity (Fig. 5.6). When a person is upright, excess fluids in the peritoneal cavity (ascites) may collect in these low points.

The **endopelvic fascia,** discussed previously (see Pelvic Fascia), fills the subperitoneal spaces but also contributes to stronger condensations

that support the rectum and urinary bladder in both sexes and the uterus in females (see Figs. 5.5, 5.6, and 5.12). In females, these major fascial condensations include the following (Fig. 5.12):

- **Medial pubovesical ligament:** connects the bladder to the pubis in both genders.
- **Lateral ligament of the bladder (pubovesical ligament):** provides lateral support for the bladder and conveys the superior vesical vessels supplying the bladder in both genders.
- **Pubocervical ligaments:** fascial condensations that course from the cervix to the anterior pelvic wall, passing on either side of the female bladder.
- **Transverse cervical ligaments:** provide important posterolateral support of the uterus and

Female: superior view (peritoneum and loose areolar tissue removed)

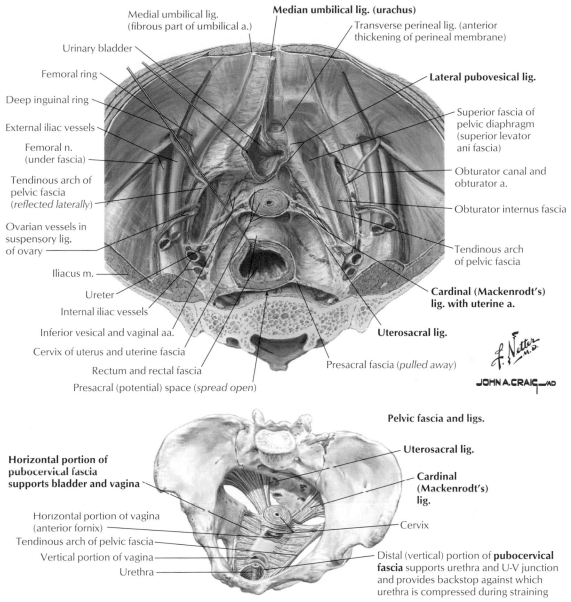

FIGURE 5.12 Endopelvic Fascia in the Female. (From *Netter's atlas of human anatomy,* ed 8, Plate 266 and 373; S-490 and S-478)

upper vagina and convey the uterine vessels; also called **cardinal,** lateral cervical, or **Mackenrodt's ligaments.**

- **Uterosacral ligaments:** fascial condensations that course from the cervix posteriorly to the pelvic walls.
- **Rectovaginal septum:** fascial condensations between the rectum and vagina.

The same ligaments that support the female urinary bladder also support the male bladder. Males have a condensation called the **prostatic fascia** that surrounds the anterolateral aspect of the prostate gland, envelops the prostatic venous plexus, and extends posteriorly to envelop the prostatic arteries and nerve plexus (**rectoprostatic fascia** or Denonvilliers' fascia; see Fig. 5.9).

5. BLOOD SUPPLY

The arterial supply to the pelvis arises from the paired **internal iliac arteries,** which not only supply the pelvis but also send branches into the perineum, the gluteal region, and the medial thigh. The arteries in the female pelvis are shown in Fig. 5.13 and summarized in Table 5.6.

The arteries in the male are similar, except that the uterine, vaginal, and ovarian branches are replaced by arteries to the ductus deferens (from a vesical branch), the prostatic artery (from the inferior vesical artery), and the testicular arteries (from the abdominal aorta). Significant variability exists for these pelvic arteries, so they are best identified and named for the structure they supply (Figs. 5.14 and 5.15). Corresponding veins, *usually multiple in number,* course with each of these arterial branches and drain into the **internal iliac veins** directly or into other larger veins. (*Multiple connections among veins are common.*) Extensive venous plexuses are associated with the bladder, rectum, vagina, uterus, and prostate, and are referred to as the **pelvis plexus of veins.** Fig. 5.15 shows this extensive arterial and venous drainage in the male pelvis. This extensive venous plexus in both sexes facilitates the metastatic spread of cancer (see Clinical Focus 5.13 and 5.18). The veins surrounding the rectum form an important **portosystemic anastomosis** via the superior rectal vein (*portal system*) and the middle and inferior rectal veins (*cava system*) (see Figs. 4.26 and 5.20). Likewise, the **right gonadal vein** (ovarian or testicular) drains into the inferior vena cava (IVC), and the **left gonadal vein** drains into the left renal vein. The **superior rectal vein** drains into the inferior mesenteric vein of the hepatic portal system, and the **vertebral venous plexus** drains superiorly into the azygos venous system, although several smaller veins may drain directly into lumbar veins and the IVC (see Fig. 4.39).

Overview of Pelvic and Perineal Arteries

The aorta bifurcates at about the L4 vertebral level into the **common iliac artery (1)** (right and left branches), which then bifurcates into the **internal iliac artery (2)** and the **external iliac artery (3)** at about the L5-S1 intervertebral level. The external iliac artery passes inferiorly to the thigh, where it becomes the femoral artery after passing deep to the inguinal ligament (Figs. 5.14 and 5.15).

The **internal iliac artery (2)** provides branches to the sacrum, the obturator artery to the medial compartment of the thigh (adductor muscles of hip), the gluteal arteries to the gluteal muscles, and a partially patent umbilical artery (becomes the medial umbilical ligament as it approaches the anterior abdominal wall). The internal iliac artery also gives rise to arteries to the urinary bladder (the vesical artery, usually from the umbilical artery), to the uterus and vagina in females, and middle rectal artery to the rectum (with vaginal and prostatic branches, depending on the sex).

The **internal pudendal artery** passes out the greater sciatic foramen and around the sacrospinous ligament and enters the pudendal canal through the lesser sciatic foramen to pass forward and inferiorly to the perineum. The internal pudendal artery supplies the skin, external genitalia, and muscles of the perineum (anal and urogenital triangle).

Some anatomists divide the branches of the internal iliac artery into anterior and posterior trunks for descriptive purposes. The posterior branches are the iliolumbar, lateral sacral, and superior gluteal arteries; all the other major arteries are from the anterior trunk (Table 5.6).

The veins of the pelvis and perineum course with the arteries and generally have the same names. They drain largely back into the **internal iliac vein,** common iliac vein, inferior vena cava, and then to the heart. Important **portosystemic anastomoses** occur between the superior rectal vein (drains into the inferior mesenteric vein of the portal system) and the middle **(internal iliac vein)** and inferior (internal pudendal vein) rectal veins of the caval system (see Fig. 5.20).

6. LYMPHATICS

Much of the lymphatic drainage of the pelvis parallels the venous drainage and drains into lymph nodes along the **internal iliac vessels** (Fig. 5.16 and Table 5.7). The major exception is the drainage from the ovaries and the adjacent uterine tubes and upper uterus, and from the testes and scrotal structures, which flows directly back to the **aortic (lumbar) nodes** of the midabdomen. Because some lymph from the uterus may drain along the round ligament of the uterus to the **inguinal nodes**, physicians must be aware that uterine cancer could spread to these nodes as well as the external iliac nodes.

Lymph from the deep structures of the perineum drains primarily into the internal iliac lymph nodes, as described above. However, lymph from the more superficial structures of the perineum drains into the **superfical** and **deep inguinal lymph nodes**.

Right paramedian section: lateral view

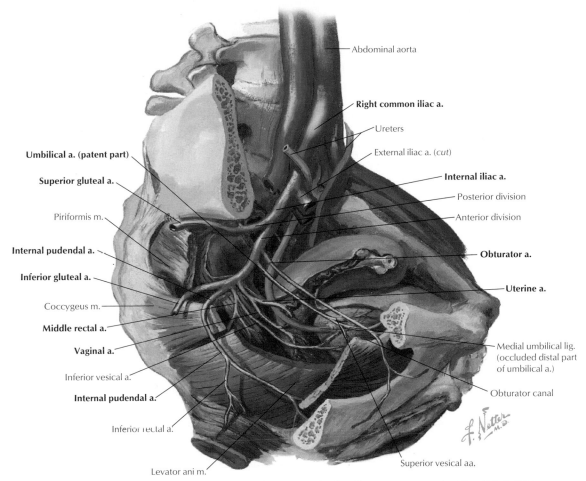

FIGURE 5.13 Pelvic Arteries in the Female. (From *Netter's atlas of human anatomy*, ed 8, Plate 404; S-507.)

TABLE 5.6 Branches (Divisions) of the Female Pelvic Arteries

ARTERIAL BRANCH*	COURSE AND STRUCTURES SUPPLIED
Common iliac	Divides into external (to thigh) and internal (to pelvis) iliac
Internal iliac	Divides into posterior division (P) and anterior division (A)
Iliolumbar (P)	To iliacus muscle (iliac artery), psoas, quadratus lumborum, and spine (lumbar artery)
Lateral sacral (P)	To piriformis muscle and sacrum (meninges and nerves)
Superior gluteal (P)	Between lumbosacral trunk and S1 nerves, through greater sciatic foramen and to gluteal region
Inferior gluteal (A)	Between S1 or S2 and S2 or S3 nerves to gluteal region
Internal pudendal (A)	To perineal structures through greater sciatic foramen and into lesser sciatic foramen to perineum
Umbilical (A)	Gives rise to superior vesical artery to bladder and becomes medial umbilical ligament when it reaches anterior abdominal wall
Obturator (A)	Passes into medial thigh via obturator foramen (with obturator nerve)
Uterine (A)	Runs over levator ani muscle and ureter to reach uterus (may give rise to vesical arteries supplying the bladder)
Vaginal (A)	From internal iliac or uterine, passes to vagina
Middle rectal (A)	To lower rectum and superior part of anal canal
Ovarian	From abdominal aorta, runs in suspensory ligament of ovary
Superior rectal	Continuation of inferior mesenteric artery to rectum
Median sacral	From aortic bifurcation, unpaired artery to sacrum and coccyx (caudal artery)

*A, Branch of anterior trunk; P, branch of posterior trunk.

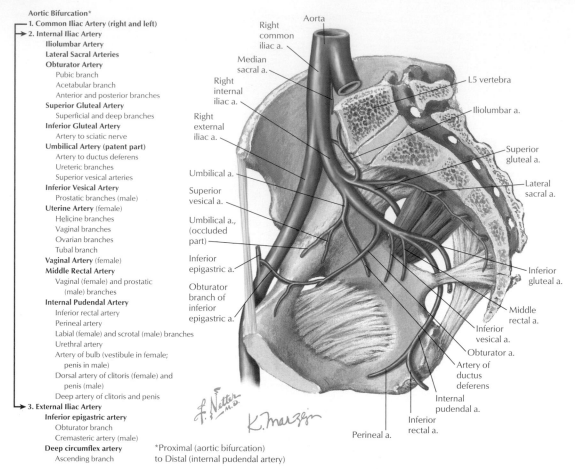

Aortic Bifurcation*
- 1. **Common Iliac Artery (right and left)**
- 2. **Internal Iliac Artery**
  - **Iliolumbar Artery**
  - **Lateral Sacral Arteries**
  - **Obturator Artery**
    - Pubic branch
    - Acetabular branch
    - Anterior and posterior branches
  - **Superior Gluteal Artery**
    - Superficial and deep branches
  - **Inferior Gluteal Artery**
    - Artery to sciatic nerve
  - **Umbilical Artery (patent part)**
    - Artery to ductus deferens
    - Ureteric branches
    - Superior vesical arteries
  - **Inferior Vesical Artery**
    - Prostatic branches (male)
  - **Uterine Artery (female)**
    - Helicine branches
    - Vaginal branches
    - Ovarian branches
    - Tubal branch
  - **Vaginal Artery (female)**
  - **Middle Rectal Artery**
    - Vaginal (female) and prostatic
      (male) branches
  - **Internal Pudendal Artery**
    - Inferior rectal artery
    - Perineal artery
    - Labial (female) and scrotal (male) branches
    - Urethral artery
    - Artery of bulb (vestibule in female;
      penis in male)
    - Dorsal artery of clitoris (female) and
      penis (male)
    - Deep artery of clitoris and penis
- 3. **External Iliac Artery**
  - **Inferior epigastric artery**
    - Obturator branch
    - Cremasteric artery (male)
  - **Deep circumflex artery**
    - Ascending branch

*Proximal (aortic bifurcation)
to Distal (internal pudendal artery)

FIGURE 5.14 Arteries of Pelvis and Perineum in the Male. (From *Netter's atlas of human anatomy,* ed 8, Plate 406; S-511.)

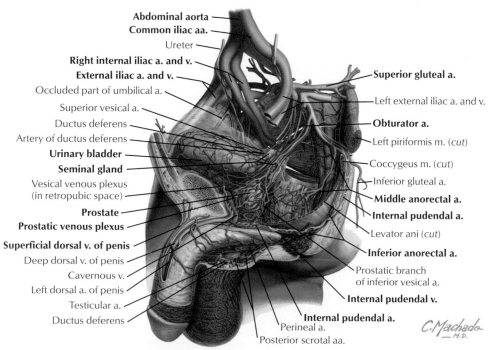

FIGURE 5.15 Arteries and Veins of Pelvis: Male. (From *Netter's atlas of human anatomy*, ed 8, Plate 405; S-509.)

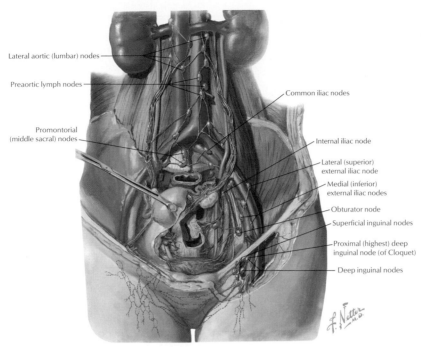

FIGURE 5.16 Lymphatics of the Female Pelvis. (From *Netter's atlas of human anatomy*, ed 8, Plate 408; S-355.)

As noted previously, lymph from the testes drains upward in the spermatic cord and follows the testicular veins to the **aortic (lumbar) lymph nodes** in the midabdomen (Table 5.7).

7. INNERVATION

The skin and skeletal muscle of the pelvis are innervated by the somatic division of the peripheral nervous system. The muscle innervation is summarized in Table 5.2 and is derived from the anterior rami of the **sacral** (L4-S4) and **coccygeal plexus.** Although most of the sacral plexus is involved in innervation of the gluteal muscles and muscles of the lower limb, several small twigs innervate the pelvic musculature (nerve to the obturator internus muscle and nerves to the pelvic diaphragm) and the perineum, which is supplied by the **pudendal nerve** (S2-S4). **Somatic afferent fibers** convey pain, touch, and temperature from the skin, skeletal muscle, and joints via nerves from these plexuses to the same relative spinal cord levels.

The smooth muscle and glands of the pelvis are innervated by the autonomic division of the peripheral nervous system via the **pelvic splanchnics** (S2-S4; parasympathetic) and the **lumbar and sacral splanchnics** (L1-L2; sympathetic) (Fig. 5.17 and Table 5.8).

The **parasympathetic efferent fibers** generally mediate the following functions:
- Vasodilate.
- Contract the bladder's detrusor smooth muscle.
- Stimulate engorgement of the erectile tissues in both sexes.
- Modulate the enteric nervous system's control of the distal bowel (from splenic flexure to rectum).
- Inhibit contraction of both the male internal urethral sphincter for urination and the internal anal sphincter for defecation in both genders.

TABLE 5.7 Pelvic Lymphatics

LYMPH NODES	DRAINAGE
Superficial inguinal	Receive lymph from perineum (and lower limb and lower abdomen) and deep pelvic viscera (part of uterus) and drain lymph to external iliac nodes
Deep inguinal	Receive lymph from perineum (and lower limb) and drain lymph to external iliac nodes
Internal iliac	Receive lymph from pelvic viscera and drain lymph along iliac nodes, ultimately to reach aortic (lumbar) nodes
External iliac	Convey lymph along iliac nodes to reach aortic (lumbar) nodes
Gonadal lymphatics	Drain lymph from gonads directly to aortic (lumbar) nodes

TABLE 5.8 Summary of Pelvic Nerves	
NERVE	**INNERVATION**
Lumbar splanchnics	From T10 to L2 or L3: sympathetics to hypogastric plexus (superior and inferior) to innervate hindgut derivatives and pelvic reproductive viscera
Sacral splanchnics	From L1 to L2 or L3: sympathetics to inferior hypogastric plexus that first travel down sympathetic chain before synapsing in the plexus
Pelvic splanchnics	From S2 to S4: parasympathetics to inferior hypogastric plexus to innervate hindgut derivatives and pelvic reproductive viscera
Inferior hypogastric plexus	Plexus of nerves (splanchnics) and ganglia where sympathetic and parasympathetic preganglionic fibers synapse
Pudendal nerve	From anterior rami of S2 to S4: somatic nerve that innervates skin and skeletal muscle of pelvic diaphragm and perineum (from sacral plexus)

The **sympathetic efferent fibers** generally mediate the following functions:

- Vasoconstrict and/or maintain vasomotor tone.
- Increase secretion from the skin's sweat glands and sebaceous glands.
- Contract the male internal urethral sphincter and the internal anal sphincters in both genders.
- Through smooth muscle contraction, move the sperm along the male reproductive tract and stimulate secretion from the seminal vesicles and prostate.
- Stimulate secretion from the greater vestibular (Bartholin's) glands in females and the bulbourethral (Cowper's) glands in males, along with minor lubricating glands associated with the reproductive tract in both genders.

Visceral afferent fibers convey pelvic sensory information (largely pain) via both the *sympathetic fibers* (to the upper lumbar spinal cord [L1-L2] or lower thoracic levels [T11-T12]) and *parasympathetic fibers* (to the S2-S4 levels of the spinal cord).

8. FEMALE PERINEUM

The perineum is a diamond-shaped region between the proximal thighs and is divided descriptively into an anterior **urogenital triangle** and a posterior **anal triangle** (Fig. 5.18). The boundaries of the perineum include the following:

- Pubic symphysis anteriorly.

- Ischial tuberosities laterally (lateral margins are demarcated by the ischiopubic rami anteriorly and the sacrotuberous ligaments posteriorly; see Fig. 5.3.).
- Coccyx posteriorly.
- Roof formed largely by levator ani muscle.

Anal Triangle (Both Genders)

The key feature of the anal triangle is the anal opening and the **external anal sphincter,** which has the following attachments (Fig. 5.19):

- Subcutaneous part: located just beneath the skin.
- Superficial part: attaches to the perineal body and coccyx.
- Deep part: surrounds the anal canal.

Similar to the skin and all the skeletal muscles of the perineum, the external anal sphincter is innervated by the **pudendal nerve** (S2-S4) (via the nerve's inferior rectal branches; see Fig. 5.24) from the sacral plexus. This region is supplied by the **internal pudendal artery** (via its rectal branches). The internal pudendal artery is a branch of the internal iliac artery in the pelvis (see Figs. 5.13 and 5.14). The venous drainage of the lower rectum and anal canal provides an important **portosystemic anastomosis** between the superior rectal vein (portal system) and the median sacral vein and middle and inferior rectal branches (all draining into the caval system) (Fig. 5.20 and Table 5.9).

The anal canal and external anal sphincter are flanked on either side by a wedge-shaped fat-filled space called the **ischioanal** (ischiorectal) **fossa** (Fig. 5.21). This space allows for the expansion of the anal canal during defecation and accommodates the fetus during childbirth. The ischioanal fossa can become infected (e.g., glandular, abrasive lesions, boils), and because the two fossae communicate posterior to the anal canal, the infection can easily spread from side to side or spread anteriorly into the *urogenital triangle* superior to the perineal membrane (Fig. 5.19).

Deep to the external anal sphincter there is a smooth muscle **internal anal sphincter,** a thickened continuation of the smooth muscle lining the anal canal (Fig. 5.21). It is an involuntary sphincter and is innervated by the autonomic nervous system. *Sympathetic innervation* maintains a tonic contraction of this smooth muscle, except when feces expand the rectal ampulla; then the *parasympathetic stimulation* relaxes this sphincter to allow for defecation. Internally, the anal canal exhibits anal columns (vertical mucosal ridges) that lie above the **pectinate (dentate) line** (Fig. 5.21). This line demarcates the dual embryology of the anal canal;

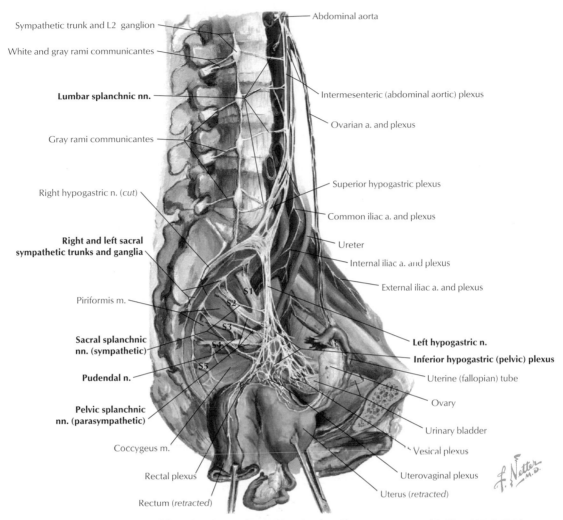

Sympathetic trunk and L2 ganglion
White and gray rami communicantes
Lumbar splanchnic nn.
Gray rami communicantes
Right hypogastric n. (*cut*)
Right and left sacral sympathetic trunks and ganglia
Piriformis m.
Sacral splanchnic nn. (sympathetic)
Pudendal n.
Pelvic splanchnic nn. (parasympathetic)
Coccygeus m.
Rectal plexus
Rectum (*retracted*)

Abdominal aorta
Intermesenteric (abdominal aortic) plexus
Ovarian a. and plexus
Superior hypogastric plexus
Common iliac a. and plexus
Ureter
Internal iliac a. and plexus
External iliac a. and plexus
Left hypogastric n.
Inferior hypogastric (pelvic) plexus
Uterine (fallopian) tube
Ovary
Urinary bladder
Vesical plexus
Uterovaginal plexus
Uterus (*retracted*)

S1
S2
S3
S4
S5

FIGURE 5.17 Nerves of the Pelvic Cavity. (From *Netter's atlas of human anatomy,* ed 8, Plate 414; S-513.)

Regions (triangles) of perineum: surface topography

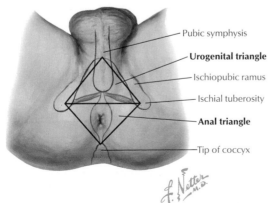

Pubic symphysis
Urogenital triangle
Ischiopubic ramus
Ischial tuberosity
Anal triangle
Tip of coccyx

FIGURE 5.18 Subdivisions of the Perineum. (From *Netter's atlas of human anatomy,* ed 8, Plate 381; S-500.)

above this line the canal and rectum are derived from the *hindgut endoderm,* and below this line the distal anal canal is derived from the *ectoderm.*

Urogenital Triangle

The female urogenital triangle is divided into a **superficial pouch and deep pouch. The superficial pouch** contains the external genitalia and associated skeletal muscles, including the **bulbospongiosus, ischiocavernosus,** and **superficial transverse perineal muscles** (Figs. 5.19, 5.22, and 5.23). The bulbospongiosus skeletal muscle, which envelops the **bulb of the vestibule,** lies deep to the labium (lip) majora and is split by the vaginal opening. Laterally along both pubic rami, the paired ischiocavernosus muscles cover the **corpora cavernosa** (crura), which form the body and glans of the clitoris (Figs. 5.22

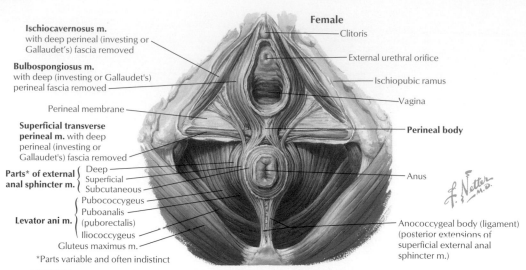

Female

Ischiocavernosus m.
with deep perineal (investing or
Gallaudet's) fascia removed

Bulbospongiosus m.
with deep (investing or Gallaudet's)
perineal fascia removed

Perineal membrane

Superficial transverse
perineal m. with deep
perineal (investing or
Gallaudet's) fascia removed

Parts* of external
anal sphincter m. { Deep
Superficial
Subcutaneous

Levator ani m. { Pubococcygeus
Puboanalis
(puborectalis)
Iliococcygeus

Gluteus maximus m.

*Parts variable and often indistinct

Clitoris

External urethral orifice

Ischiopubic ramus

Vagina

Perineal body

Anus

Anococcygeal body (ligament)
(posterior extensions of
superficial external anal
sphincter m.)

FIGURE 5.19 Muscles of the Female Perineum. (From *Netter's atlas of human anatomy*, ed 8, Plate 397; S-224.)

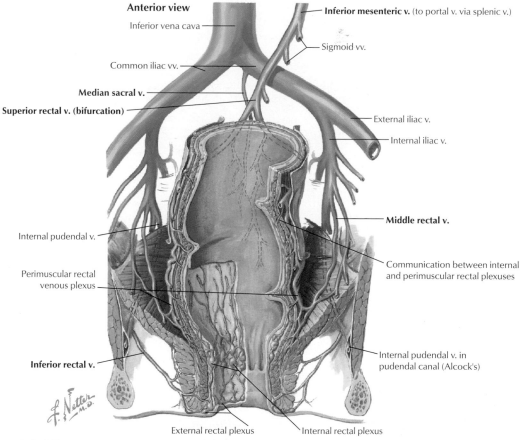

Anterior view

Inferior vena cava

Common iliac vv.

Median sacral v.

Superior rectal v. (bifurcation)

Internal pudendal v.

Perimuscular rectal
venous plexus

Inferior rectal v.

Inferior mesenteric v. (to portal v. via splenic v.)

Sigmoid vv.

External iliac v.

Internal iliac v.

Middle rectal v.

Communication between internal
and perimuscular rectal plexuses

Internal pudendal v. in
pudendal canal (Alcock's)

External rectal plexus

Internal rectal plexus

FIGURE 5.20 Veins of the Rectum and Anal Canal. (From *Netter's atlas of human anatomy*, ed 8, Plate 401; S-445.)

and 5.23). Medial to the labium majus, smaller skin folds comprise the hairless **labium minus**, whose boundaries define the vestibule (Table 5.10). Directly posterior to the vestibule is the **perineal body** (central tendon of the perineum), which is an

important fibromuscular support region lying just beneath the skin midway between the two ischial tuberosities and an important attachment point for the superficial and deep transverse perineal muscles (Figs. 5.19 and 5.22). The **deep pouch** is largely

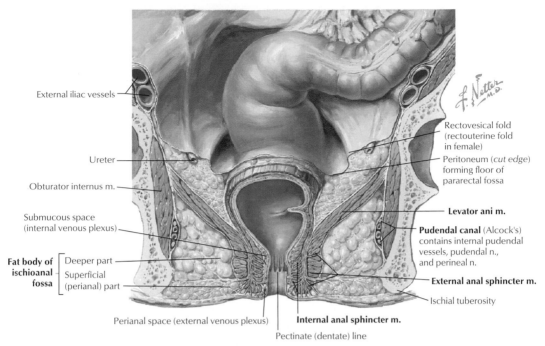

External iliac vessels

Ureter

Obturator internus m.

Submucous space
(internal venous plexus)

Fat body of
ischioanal
fossa
Deeper part
Superficial
(perianal) part

Rectovesical fold
(rectouterine fold
in female)

Peritoneum (*cut edge*)
forming floor of
pararectal fossa

Levator ani m.

Pudendal canal (Alcock's)
contains internal pudendal
vessels, pudendal n.,
and perineal n.

External anal sphincter m.

Ischial tuberosity

Perianal space (external venous plexus)   **Internal anal sphincter m.**

Pectinate (dentate) line

FIGURE 5.21   Anal Canal and Ischioanal Fossae. (From *Netter's atlas of human anatomy,* ed 8, Plate 394; S-225)

TABLE 5.9 Rectal Portosystemic Anastomoses

VEIN	COURSE AND STRUCTURES DRAINED
Superior rectal	Tributary of inferior mesenteric vein (portal system)
Middle rectal	Drains into internal iliac, vesical, or uterine (female) veins, draining pelvic diaphragm, rectum, and proximal anal canal
Inferior rectal	Drains into internal pudendal vein from external anal sphincter
Median sacral	Drains into the common iliac vein from the sacrum, coccyx, and rectum

occupied by the *urethrovaginalis–skeletal muscle sphincter* complex surrounding the urethra and vaginal apertures. Superior to the deep pouch lies the levator ani muscle, with an intervening anterior extension of the ischioanal fossae (fat) separating the deep pouch and muscle.

The **deep perineal pouch** contains the following (Fig. 5.23):

- **Urethra:** extends from the urinary bladder, runs through the deep pouch, and opens into the vestibule.
- **Vagina:** distal portion passes through the deep pouch and opens into the vestibule.
- **External urethral sphincter:** the voluntary skeletal muscle sphincter of the urethra.

- **Compressor urethrae:** two thin skeletal muscle bands that extend from the ischiopubic rami and fuse in the midline around the anterior aspect of the female urethra.
- **Sphincter urethrovaginalis muscle:** extends from the perineal body around the lateral sides of the vagina and fuses in the midline around the anterior aspect of the urethra.
- **Deep transversus perineal muscles:** extend from the ischial tuberosities and rami to the perineal body; stabilize the perineal body.

These structures, along with their respective neurovascular bundles, lie between the **perineal membrane** (thick fascial sheath) and the fascia covering the inferior aspect of the levator ani muscle. The neurovascular components include the following (Fig. 5.24):

- **Pudendal nerve:** passes out of the pelvis via the greater sciatic foramen and then passes around the sacrospinous ligament and into the lesser sciatic foramen, where it enters the **pudendal (Alcock's) canal;** provides the somatic innervation (S2-S4) to the skin and skeletal muscles of the perineum and gives rise to the inferior rectal (anal), perineal, labial, and dorsal clitoral nerve branches (Figs. 5.24 and 5.28)
- **Internal pudendal artery:** arises from the internal iliac artery and, along with the pudendal nerve, passes out of the *greater sciatic foramen;* it then passes around the sacrospinous ligament

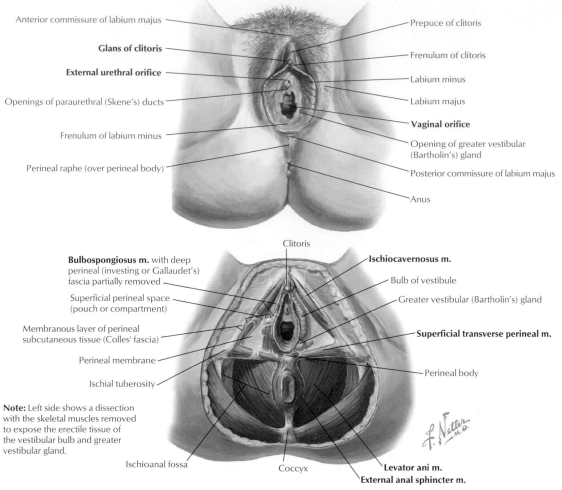

FIGURE 5.22 Female Perineum and Superficial Perineal Pouch. (From *Netter's atlas of human anatomy,* ed 8, Plates 377 and 379; S-491 and S-493.)

TABLE 5.10 Features of the Female External Genitalia

STRUCTURE	CHARACTERISTICS
Mons pubis	Anterior fatty eminence overlying pubic symphysis
Anterior labial commissure	Site where two labium majus meet anteriorly
Labium majus	Folds of pigmented skin, mainly fat and sebaceous glands; in the adult, covered with pubic hair externally but smooth and pink on internal aspect
Clitoris	Erectile tissue, distinguished by midline glans covered with prepuce (foreskin), body, and two crura (corpora cavernosa) that extend along ischiopubic rami, and covered by ischiocavernosus muscles
Labium minus	Fat-free hairless pink skin folds that contain some erectile tissue; course anteriorly to form frenulum and prepuce of clitoris; posteriorly, unite to form frenulum of labium minus (fourchette)
Vestibule	Space surrounded by labium minus that contains openings of urethra, vagina, and vestibular glands
Greater vestibular glands	Paired mucous glands lying posterior to bulbs of vestibule that produce secretions during arousal
Bulbs of vestibule	Paired erectile tissues lying deep and lateral to labium minus that flank vaginal and urethral openings and extend anteriorly to form small connection to glans of clitoris; covered by bulbospongiosus skeletal muscle
Posterior labial commissure	Site where two labium majus meet posteriorly; overlies perineal body

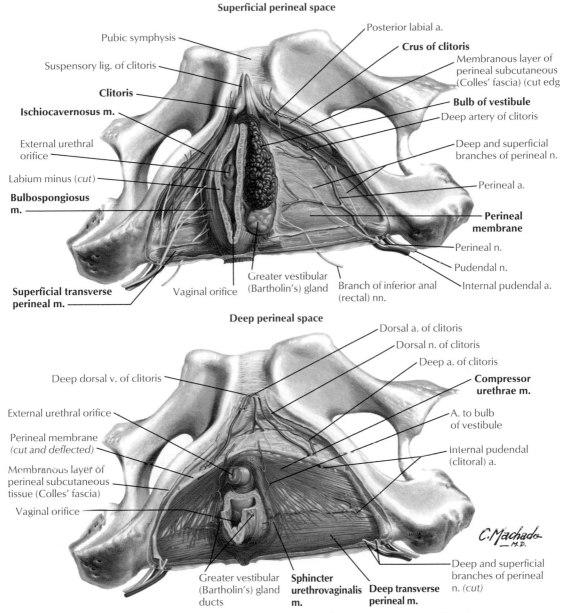

Superficial perineal space

Pubic symphysis

Suspensory lig. of clitoris

Clitoris

Ischiocavernosus m.

External urethral orifice

Labium minus (*cut*)

Bulbospongiosus m.

Superficial transverse perineal m.

Vaginal orifice

Greater vestibular (Bartholin's) gland

Posterior labial a.

Crus of clitoris

Membranous layer of perineal subcutaneous (Colles' fascia) (cut edg

Bulb of vestibule

Deep artery of clitoris

Deep and superficial branches of perineal n.

Perineal a.

Perineal membrane

Perineal n.

Pudendal n.

Internal pudendal a.

Branch of inferior anal (rectal) nn.

Deep perineal space

Deep dorsal v. of clitoris

External urethral orifice

Perineal membrane (cut and deflected)

Membranous layer of perineal subcutaneous tissue (Colles' fascia)

Vaginal orifice

Greater vestibular (Bartholin's) gland ducts

Sphincter urethrovaginalis m.

Deep transverse perineal m.

Dorsal a. of clitoris

Dorsal n. of clitoris

Deep a. of clitoris

Compressor urethrae m.

A. to bulb of vestibule

Internal pudendal (clitoral) a.

C.Machado —M.D.

Deep and superficial branches of perineal n. (*cut*)

FIGURE 5.23 Female Perineal Spaces. (From *Netter's atlas of human anatomy*, ed 8, Plates 375 and 380; S-486 and S-494.)

and into the *lesser sciatic foramen*, where it, too, enters the **pudendal (Alcock's) canal.** It provides arterial branches that distribute to the perineum and include the inferior rectal, perineal, and labial branches, the artery of the bulb, and the dorsal clitoral arterial branches (Figs. 5.23 and 5.24).

9. MALE PERINEUM

The boundaries of the perineum and the anal triangle in both genders are discussed in the previous section; this section focuses on the male urogenital triangle. The urogenital triangle is divided into a **superficial pouch** containing the external genitalia and associated skeletal muscles and a **deep pouch** largely occupied by the external urethral sphincter surrounding the membranous urethra.

The male external genitalia are shown in Fig. 5.25 and summarized in Table 5.11.

The bulb and crura form the root of the penis, whereas the **corpus spongiosum** and the two **corpora cavernosa** compose the shaft of the penis. They are bound tightly together by the **investing**

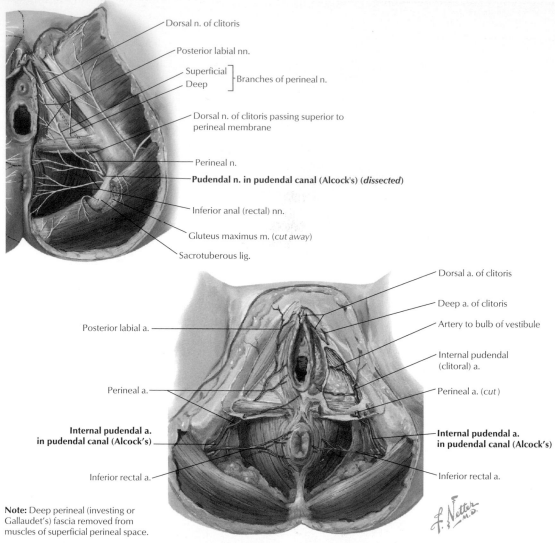

Dorsal n. of clitoris

Posterior labial nn.

Superficial ⎫
              ⎬ Branches of perineal n.
Deep   ⎭

Dorsal n. of clitoris passing superior to perineal membrane

Perineal n.

Pudendal n. in pudendal canal (Alcock's) (*dissected*)

Inferior anal (rectal) nn.

Gluteus maximus m. (*cut away*)

Sacrotuberous lig.

Dorsal a. of clitoris

Deep a. of clitoris

Artery to bulb of vestibule

Internal pudendal (clitoral) a.

Posterior labial a.

Perineal a.

Perineal a. (*cut*)

Internal pudendal a. in pudendal canal (Alcock's)

Internal pudendal a. in pudendal canal (Alcock's)

Inferior rectal a.

Inferior rectal a.

Note: Deep perineal (investing or Gallaudet's) fascia removed from muscles of superficial perineal space.

FIGURE 5.24 Neurovascular Supply to the Female Perineum. (From *Netter's atlas of human anatomy,* ed 8, Plates 406 and 415; S-511 and S-516.)

TABLE 5.11 Features of the Male External Genitalia	
STRUCTURE	**CHARACTERISTICS**
Bulb of penis	Erectile tissue anchored to perineal membrane; proximal part of corpus spongiosum; covered by bulbospongiosus skeletal muscle
Crura of penis	Paired erectile tissues attached to pubic arch that form proximal part of corpora cavernosa of penis; covered by ischiocavernosus skeletal muscles
Superficial transverse perineal muscle	Thin skeletal muscle extending from ischial tuberosity to perineal body; stabilizes perineal body

deep (Buck's) fascia of the penis and a **superficial (dartos) fascia** of the penis.

The superficial fascia (subcutaneous tissue) of the perineum includes a fatty and a membranous layer (Colles' fascia) similar to the anterior abdominal wall (Fig. 5.26). The fatty layer contributes to the labium majus and mons pubis in women but is minimal in men. In the male the membranous layer of the superficial fascia (called *Scarpa's fascia* on the abdominal wall but *Colles' fascia* in the perineum) is continuous with the **dartos** (smooth muscle) **fascia** of the penis and scrotum and envelops the superficial perineal pouch, thus providing a potential conduit for fluids or infections from the superficial pouch to the lower abdominal wall. The **deep perineal (Gallaudet's) fascia** invests

Clinical Focus 5.19

Hemorrhoids

Hemorrhoids (piles) are symptomatic varicose dilations of submucosal veins that protrude into the anal canal and can extend through the anal opening (external hemorrhoid). Hemorrhoids can bleed; the blood may pool and clot, yielding a "thrombosed" hemorrhoid.

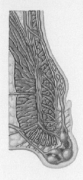
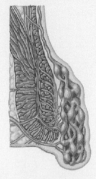

Origin below dentate line (external plexus)

Origin above dentate line (internal plexus)

Origin above and below dentate line (internal and external plexus)

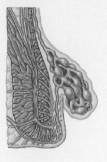
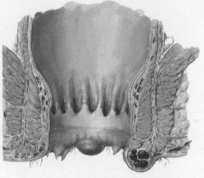

Thrombosed external hemorrhoid

External hemorrhoids and skin tabs

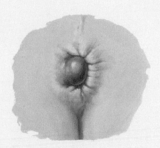
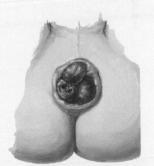

Internal hemorrhoids

Prolapsed "rosette" of internal hemorrhoids

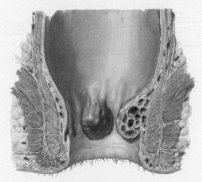

Characteristic	Description
Types	Internal: dilations of veins of internal rectal plexus. External: dilations of veins of external rectal plexus. Mixed: combination of internal and external
Prevalence	50–80% of all Americans; more common after pregnancy
Signs and symptoms	Perianal swelling, itching, pain, rectal bleeding, constipation, hematochezia, inflammation
Risk factors	Pregnancy, obesity, chronic cough, constipation, heavy lifting, sedentary work or lifestyle, hepatic disease, colon malignancy, portal hypertension, anal intercourse

Clinical Focus 5.20

Episiotomy

Occasionally, if there is danger of significant tearing of the perineal body during childbirth, the physician may perform an incision called an episiotomy to enlarge the vaginal opening to accommodate the head of the fetus. Despite the fact that nearly every primiparous birth results in at least a minor injury to the vagina, perineum, or vulva, routine episiotomy is performed much less frequently than it was several decades ago. When performed, episiotomies usually are either directly in the midline through the perineal body or posterolateral, to avoid the perineal body.

Posterolateral Approach
(one of two approaches normally used, posterolateral [shown here] or median)

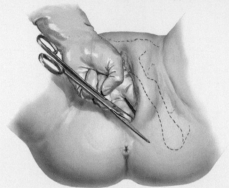

A. Scissors are directed from the midline to the tuberosity

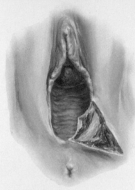

B. Incision in the bulbospongiosus muscle

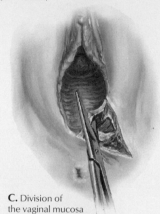

C. Division of the vaginal mucosa

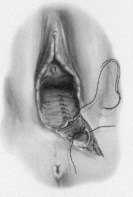

D. Continuous suture of vaginal mucosa

E. Inverted crown suture in perineal body

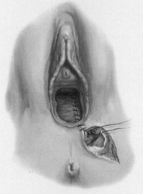

F. Running suture under hymen and continued in skin after approximation of perineal body

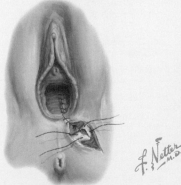

G. Closure of bulbospongiosus and fascia

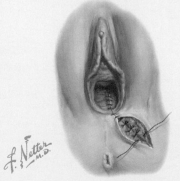

H. Closure of superficial tissues of perineum

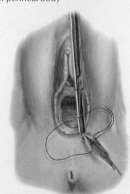

I. Subcuticular stitch in superficial fascia approximating the skin

Clinical Focus 5.21

Sexually Transmitted Diseases

Human papillomavirus (HPV) and *Chlamydia trachomatis* infections are the two most common STDs in the United States. HPV infections (>90% benign) are characterized in both genders by warty lesions caused most often by serotypes 6 and 11. The virus is typically spread by skin-to-skin contact; the incubation period is 3 weeks to 8 months. HPV is highly associated with **cervical cancer** in women. Chlamydial infection is the most common bacterial STD, with antibodies present in up to 40% of all sexually active women (which suggests prior infection). Infected structures include the urethra, cervix, greater vestibular glands, and uterine tubes in females and the urethra, epididymis, and prostate in males.

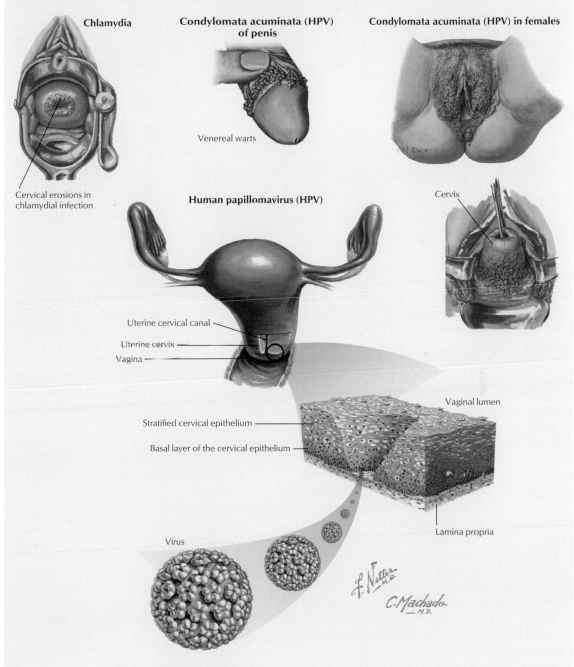

Chlamydia

Condylomata acuminata (HPV) of penis

Venereal warts

Condylomata acuminata (HPV) in females

Cervical erosions in chlamydial infection

Cervix

Human papillomavirus (HPV)

Uterine cervical canal

Uterine cervix

Vagina

Vaginal lumen

Stratified cervical epithelium

Basal layer of the cervical epithelium

Lamina propria

Virus

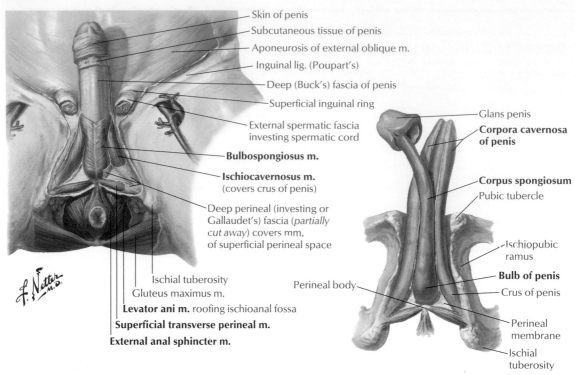

FIGURE 5.25 Male Perineum, Superficial Pouch, and Penis. (From *Netter's atlas of human anatomy,* ed 8, Plates 382 and 383; S-501 and S-502.)

the ischiocavernosus, bulbospongiosus, and superficial transverse perineal muscles in both genders and is continuous with the **deep (Buck's) fascia of the penis** and the deep investing fascia of the external abdominal oblique muscle and rectus sheath (Figs. 5.25 and 5.26). Depending on the clinical scenario, these fascial planes can inhibit or inadvertently facilitate the spread of fluids (e.g., pus, urine, or blood) throughout the perineum or into the lower abdominal wall (see Clinical Focus 5.23).

Features of the penis are summarized in Tables 5.11 and 5.12 and illustrated in Fig. 5.27. It is important to realize that the cavernous bodies in the male and female are *homologous structures,* although they vary in size.

Erection of the penis (and clitoris in the female) and ejaculation involve the following sequence of events:

1. Friction and sexual stimulation evoke the excitation of **parasympathetic fibers** (pelvic splanchnics from S2-S4), which leads to relaxation of the cavernous vessels and engorgement of the erectile tissue with blood (penis and clitoris).
2. **Sympathetic fibers** then initiate contraction of the smooth muscle of the epididymal ducts, ductus deferens, seminal vesicles, and prostate, in that order, to move sperm toward the prostatic urethra.

3. Sperm and the seminal and prostatic secretions (released by parasympathetic stimulation) enter the prostatic urethra and combine with secretions of the bulbourethral and penile urethral glands (the sperm and the collective secretions form the semen). (The seminal vesicles provide about 70% of the **seminal fluid** volume and produce a viscous alkaline fluid that nourishes and protects the sperm from the acidic environment of the vaginal tract.) **Prostatic secretions** also are slightly alkaline and include prostate-specific antigen, prostatic acid phosphatase, fibrinolysin (helps to liquefy the semen), and citric acid. In females, sexual arousal results in lubricating secretions from the greater vestibular glands.
4. Under sympathetic stimulation (L1-L2), the internal urethral sphincter contracts to prevent retrograde ejaculation into the urinary bladder. Through rhythmic contractions of the bulbospongiosus muscle and somatic stimulation from the pudendal nerve, the semen moves along the spongy urethra with help from parasympathetic stimulation of urethral smooth muscle and is ejaculated (orgasm).

The **deep (perineal) pouch** in males includes the following (Fig. 5.28):

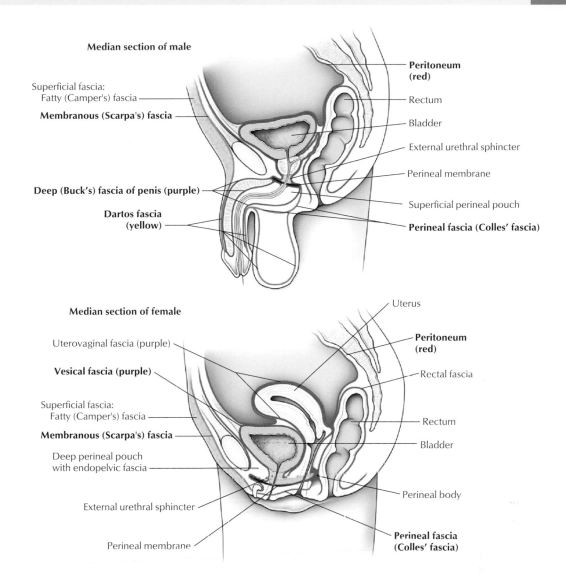

Median section of male

Superficial fascia:
Fatty (Camper's) fascia
Membranous (Scarpa's) fascia

Peritoneum (red)

Rectum

Bladder

External urethral sphincter

Perineal membrane

Deep (Buck's) fascia of penis (purple)

Superficial perineal pouch

Dartos fascia (yellow)

Perineal fascia (Colles' fascia)

Median section of female

Uterus

Uterovaginal fascia (purple)

Vesical fascia (purple)

Peritoneum (red)

Rectal fascia

Superficial fascia:
Fatty (Camper's) fascia

Membranous (Scarpa's) fascia

Rectum

Deep perineal pouch with endopelvic fascia

Bladder

External urethral sphincter

Perineal body

Perineal membrane

Perineal fascia (Colles' fascia)

FIGURE 5.26 Fasciae of the Male and Female Pelvis and Perineum.

- **Membranous urethra:** a continuation of the prostatic urethra.
- **Deep transverse perineal muscles:** extend from the ischial tuberosities and rami to the perineal body; stabilize the perineal body.
- **Bulbourethral (Cowper's) glands:** their ducts pass from the deep pouch to enter the proximal part of the spongy urethra; provide a mucus-like secretion that lubricates the spongy urethra.
- **External urethral sphincter:** skeletal muscle that encircles the membranous urethra is under voluntary control (via the pudendal nerve), and extends superiorly over the anterior aspect of the prostate gland but does not appear to possess sphincter-like action on the gland.

These structures, along with their respective neurovascular bundles, lie between the **perineal membrane** (thick fascial sheath) and the fascia covering the inferior aspect of the levator ani muscle. The neurovascular components include the following (Fig. 5.28):

- **Pudendal nerve:** passes out of the greater sciatic foramen with the internal pudendal vessels, around the sacrospinous ligament, and into the lesser sciatic foramen to enter the **pudendal (Alcock's) canal;** provides the somatic innervation (S2-S4) of the skin and skeletal muscles of the perineum and its branches; includes the inferior rectal (anal), perineal, scrotal, and dorsal nerves of the penis.

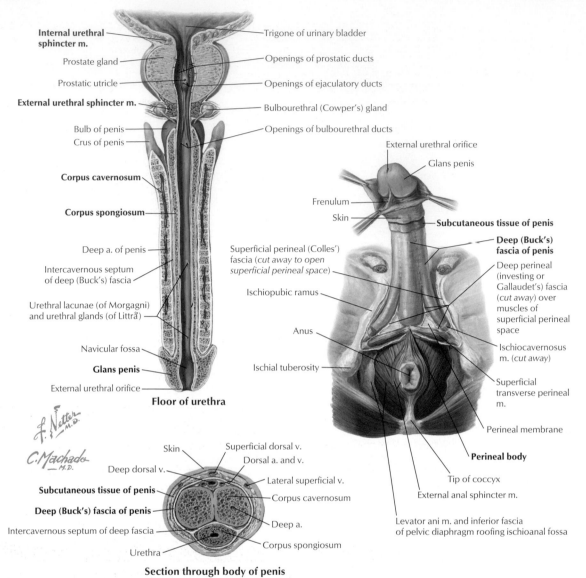

FIGURE 5.27 Penis and Urethra. (From *Netter's atlas of human anatomy,* ed 8, Plates 382, 383, 386; S-501, S-502, S-503)

TABLE 5.12 Features of the Penis			
STRUCTURE	**CHARACTERISTICS**	**STRUCTURE**	**CHARACTERISTICS**
Root of penis	Composed of bulb (proximal part of corpus spongiosum) and two crura (proximal part of corpora cavernosa)	Prepuce (foreskin)	Thin, double layer of skin that extends over most of glans penis; male circumcision removes foreskin to expose glans
Body of penis	Covered by skin, dartos fascia, and deep (Buck's) fascia of penis, which envelops the corpora cavernosa and corpus spongiosum, which contains spongy urethra	Suspensory ligament	Deep fascia that extends from dorsum of penis to pubic symphysis
		Fundiform ligament	Subcutaneous tissue that extends from dartos fascia superiorly to midline linea alba (see Fig. 5.9)
Glans penis	Expanded distal end of corpus spongiosum where spongy urethra expands (navicular fossa) and opens externally (external urethral meatus)		

Urethral Trauma in the Male

Although rare, direct trauma to the corpora cavernosa can occur. Rupture of the thick tunica albuginea usually involves the deep fascia of the penis (Buck's fascia), and blood can extravasate quickly, causing penile swelling. Urethral rupture is more common and involves one of three mechanisms:

- External trauma or a penetrating injury
- Internal injury (caused by a catheter, instrument, or foreign body)
- Spontaneous rupture (caused by increased intraurethral pressure or periurethral inflammation)

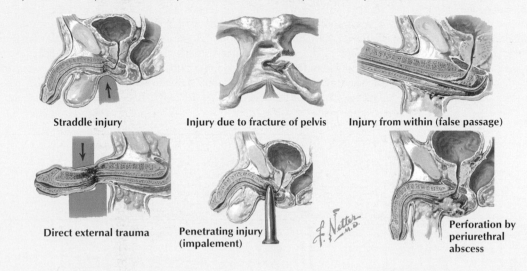

Straddle injury   Injury due to fracture of pelvis   Injury from within (false passage)

Direct external trauma   Penetrating injury (impalement)   Perforation by periurethral abscess

Urine Extravasation in the Male

Rupture of the male urethra can lead to urine extravasation into various pelvic or perineal spaces that are largely limited by the perineal, pelvic, and lower abdominal wall fascial planes.

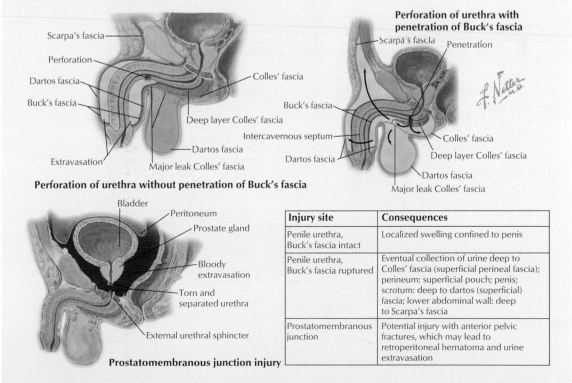

Perforation of urethra with penetration of Buck's fascia

Scarpa's fascia — Penetration

Buck's fascia
Intercavernous septum
Dartos fascia
Colles' fascia
Deep layer Colles' fascia
Dartos fascia
Major leak Colles' fascia

Scarpa's fascia
Perforation
Dartos fascia
Buck's fascia
Colles' fascia
Deep layer Colles' fascia
Extravasation
Dartos fascia
Major leak Colles' fascia

Perforation of urethra without penetration of Buck's fascia

Bladder
Peritoneum
Prostate gland
Bloody extravasation
Torn and separated urethra
External urethral sphincter

Prostatomembranous junction injury

Injury site	Consequences
Penile urethra, Buck's fascia intact	Localized swelling confined to penis
Penile urethra, Buck's fascia ruptured	Eventual collection of urine deep to Colles' fascia (superficial perineal fascia); perineum: superficial pouch; penis; scrotum: deep to dartos (superficial) fascia; lower abdominal wall: deep to Scarpa's fascia
Prostatomembranous junction	Potential injury with anterior pelvic fractures, which may lead to retroperitoneal hematoma and urine extravasation

Clinical Focus 5.24

Erectile Dysfunction

Erectile dysfunction (ED) is an inability to achieve and maintain penile erection sufficient for sexual intercourse. Its occurrence increases with age, and some of the probable causes are illustrated. Normal erectile function occurs when a sexual stimulus causes the release of *nitric oxide* from nerve endings and endothelial cells of the corpora cavernosa, thus relaxing the smooth muscle tone of the vessels and increasing blood flow into the erectile tissues. As the erectile tissue becomes engorged with blood, it compresses the veins in the tunica albuginea so that the blood remains in the cavernous bodies. The available drugs to treat ED aid in relaxing the smooth muscle of the blood vessels of the erectile tissues. Erectile dysfunction can also occur from damage to the nerves innervating the perineum (e.g., a complication of prostatic surgery). Afferent impulses conveying stimulation/arousal sensations are conveyed by the pudendal nerve (S2-S4, somatic fibers), whereas the autonomic efferent innervation of the cavernous vasculature is via the pelvic splanchnics (S2-S4, parasympathetic fibers).

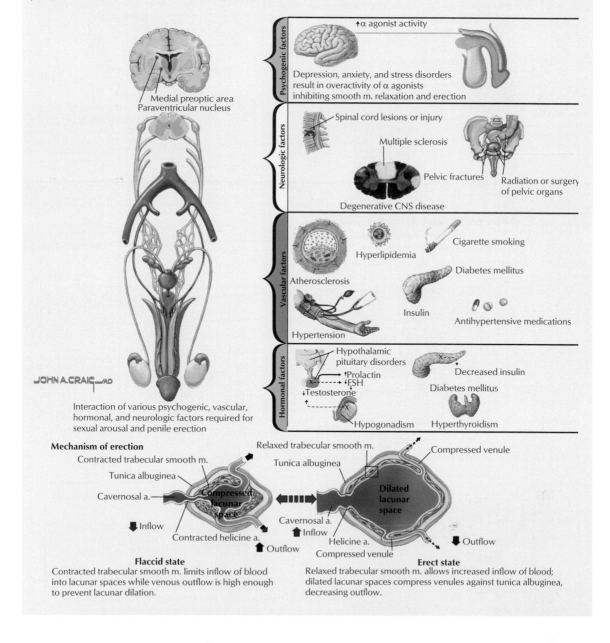

Interaction of various psychogenic, vascular, hormonal, and neurologic factors required for sexual arousal and penile erection

Mechanism of erection

Flaccid state
Contracted trabecular smooth m. limits inflow of blood into lacunar spaces while venous outflow is high enough to prevent lacunar dilation.

Erect state
Relaxed trabecular smooth m. allows increased inflow of blood; dilated lacunar spaces compress venules against tunica albuginea, decreasing outflow.

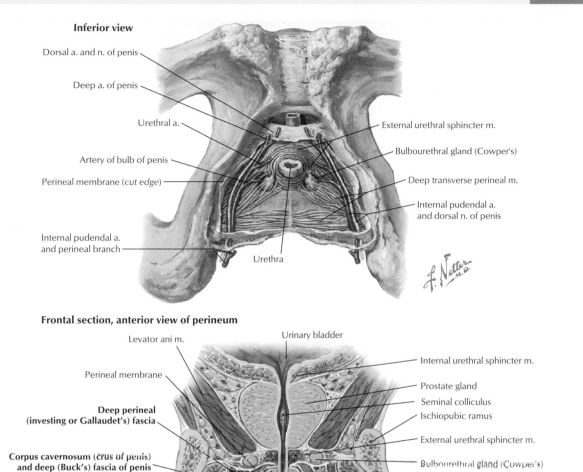

Inferior view

Dorsal a. and n. of penis

Deep a. of penis

Urethral a.

Artery of bulb of penis

Perineal membrane (*cut edge*)

Internal pudendal a.
and perineal branch

External urethral sphincter m.

Bulbourethral gland (Cowper's)

Deep transverse perineal m.

Internal pudendal a.
and dorsal n. of penis

Urethra

Frontal section, anterior view of perineum

Levator ani m.

Perineal membrane

**Deep perineal
(investing or Gallaudet's) fascia**

Corpus cavernosum (crus of penis)
and deep (Buck's) fascia of penis

Ischiocavernosus m.

**Membranous layer of perineal
subcutaneous tissue (Colles' fascia)
(closes superficial perineal space)**

Urinary bladder

Internal urethral sphincter m.

Prostate gland

Seminal colliculus

Ischiopubic ramus

External urethral sphincter m.

Bulbourethral gland (Cowper's)

**Bulb of penis (corpus spongiosum)
and deep (Buck's) fascia of penis**

Bulbospongiosus m.

FIGURE 5.28 Deeper Structures of the Male Perineum. (From *Netter's atlas of human anatomy*, ed 8, Plate 384; S-504.)

- **Internal pudendal artery:** arises from the internal iliac artery; passes out of the greater sciatic foramen with the pudendal nerve, around the sacrospinous ligament, and into the lesser sciatic foramen to enter the pudendal (Alcock's) canal. The internal pudendal artery distributes to the perineum as the *inferior rectal, perineal, scrotal, and dorsal arteries of the penis* as well as the artery of the bulb.

10. EMBRYOLOGY

Development of the Reproductive Organs

The reproductive systems of the female and male develop from a consolidation of intermediate mesoderm on the dorsal wall of the embryo that is called the **urogenital ridge** (Fig. 1.36). The genotype of the embryo is determined at fertilization (XX for females and XY for males), but sexual differentiation of each gender does not begin until after the sixth week of development.

The epithelium of the coelomic cavity and the underlying mesoderm form a gonadal ridge, which will become the definitive gonad. A dual duct system (mesonephric and paramesonephric ducts) associated with the urogenital ridge develops, with one of the duct systems becoming a major component of the reproductive system in each gender.

In genetic females, the mesonephric ducts degenerate and the **paramesonephric ducts** develop into the uterine tubes, uterus, and upper portion of the vagina (Fig. 5.29 and Table 5.13). The ovaries descend into the pelvis with the aid of a fibrous band of tissue called the *gubernaculum* (this descent probably results from the combined effects of the differential growth of the lower abdominopelvic region and the action of the *gubernaculum*). This ligament will persist as the **ovarian ligament** (which attaches the ovary to the lateral wall of the uterus) and will reflect off of the uterus to form the **round ligament of the uterus** (Fig. 5.7), which passes through the

deep inguinal ring and terminates in the labium majus (the female homologue of the male scrotum) (Table 5.14).

In genetic males, the **mesonephric ducts** persist and become the efferent ductules, duct of the epididymis, ductus deferens, seminal vesicles, and ejaculatory ducts (Table 5.13). Like the ovaries, the testes descend inferiorly, aided by the gubernaculum and differential growth, but enter the deep inguinal ring, and ultimately pass through the inguinal canal to descend into the scrotum. The testis is anchored to the bottom of the scrotum by the short remnant

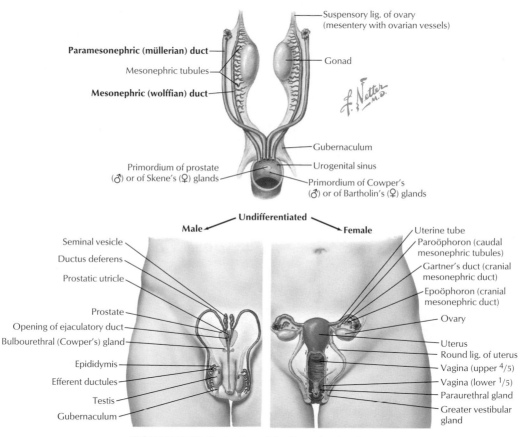

FIGURE 5.29 Derivation of the Reproductive Organs.

TABLE 5.13 Derivatives of the Urogenital System

MALE	FEMALE	MALE	FEMALE
From Urogenital Sinus		**From Mesonephric Duct and Tubules**	
Urinary bladder	Urinary bladder	Efferent ductules	Degenerates
Urethra (except navicular fossa)	Urethra	Duct of epididymis	(Ureter, renal pelvis, calyces, and collecting tubules in both genders)
Prostatic utricle	Lower vagina	Ductus deferens	
Prostate	Urethral and paraurethral glands	Seminal vesicles	
		Ejaculatory duct	
Bulbourethral glands	Greater vestibular glands	**From Paramesonephric Duct**	
		Degenerates	Uterine tubes, uterus, upper vagina

TABLE 5.14 Homologues of the External Genitalia

MALE	FEMALE
From Genital Tubercle/Phallus	
Penis	Clitoris
Glans penis	Glans clitoris
Corpora cavernosum penis	Corpora cavernosa clitoris
Corpus spongiosum penis	Vestibular bulbs
From Urogenital Folds	
Ventral raphe of penis	Labium minus
Most of the penile urethra	
Perineal raphe	Perineal raphe
Perianal tissue (and external sphincter)	Perianal tissue (and external anal sphincter)
From Labioscrotal Folds	
Scrotum	Labium majus
From Gubernaculum	
Gubernaculum testis	Ovarian ligament
	Round ligament of uterus

of the gubernaculum, called the gubernaculum testis (see Fig. 4.8). Undescended testis is the most common genital anomaly in males, occurring in about 3-4% of boys at birth in the United States. However, about 50% of undescended testes at birth subsequently descend during the first year of life.

Development of the External Genitalia

The female and male external genitalia develop from the **genital tubercle** (the phallic structures), paired **urogenital folds**, and **labioscrotal folds** (Fig. 5.30 and Table 5.14). Initially these tissues are undifferentiated, but after about the twelfth week recognizable external genital features associated with each sex begin to form. In Fig. 5.30, note the *homologous* color-coded features of the external genitalia.

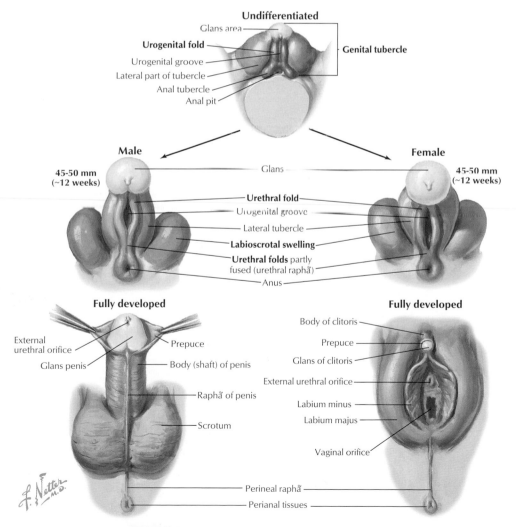

FIGURE 5.30 Development of the External Genitalia.

Clinical Focus 5.25

Hypospadias and Epispadias

Hypospadias and epispadias are congenital anomalies of the penis. *Hypospadias* is much more common (1 in 300 male births, but this figure varies widely from country to country) and is characterized by failure of fusion of the urogenital folds, which normally seal the penile (spongy) urethra within the penis. The defect occurs on the ventral aspect of the penis (corpus spongiosum). Hypospadias may be associated with inguinal hernias and undescended testes. *Epispadias* is rare (1 in 120,000 male births) and is characterized by a urethral orifice on the dorsal aspect of the penis. It is thought to occur from a defective migration of the genital tubercle primordia to the cloacal membrane early in development (fifth week).

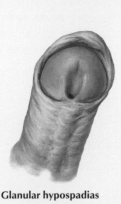

Glanular hypospadias

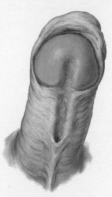

Penile hypospadias

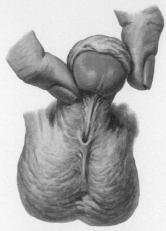

Penoscrotal hypospadias
(with chordee)

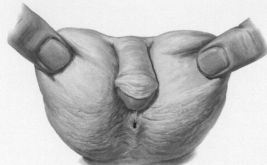

Scrotal hypospadias
(bifid scrotum, chordee)

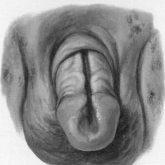

Complete epispadias

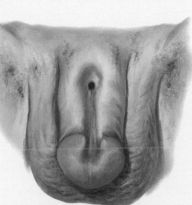

Penile epispadias

Uterine Anomalies

Incomplete fusion of the distal **paramesonephric (müllerian) ducts** can lead to septation of the uterus or partial or complete duplication of the uterus (bicornuate uterus). The prevalence is up to 3% for *septate* uterine anomalies but only about 0.1% for *bicornuate* anomalies. If only one paramesonephric duct persists and develops, a *unicornuate* uterus results. These conditions seem to be transmitted by a polygenic or multifactorial pattern and carry a higher risk for recurrent spontaneous abortions (15-25%), premature labor, uterine pain, breech or transverse deliveries, and dysmenorrhea.

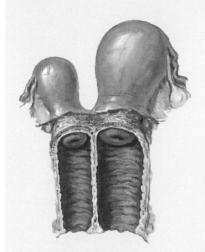

Complete septum
(with double uterus and double vagina)

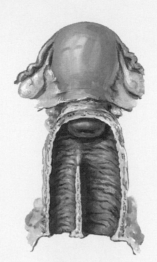

Partial septum

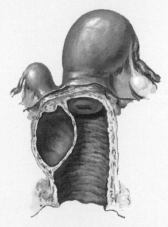

Rudimentary second vagina
(without external opening, forming cyst)

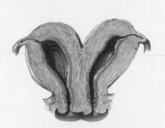

**Bicornuate uterus with
complete septum**
(double cervix)

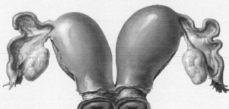

Double uterus

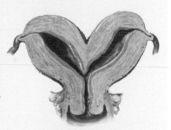

Bicornuate uterus

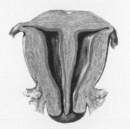

Septate uterus

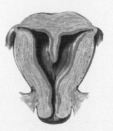

Partial septum

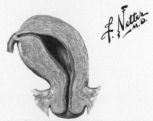

Unicornuate uterus

Clinical Focus 5.27

Male Circumcision (Newborn)

Male circumcision is the removal of the foreskin of the penis. Generally, this is not a medically indicated procedure but is done at the request of the parents or because of a religious preference.

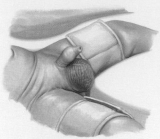

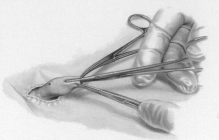

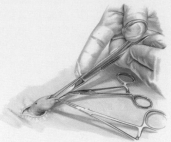

1. All circumcision techniques begin with the undiapered newborn restrained on an infant (papoose) board.

2. A hemostat is used to grasp the edge of the foreskin dorsal to the 3 and 9 o'clock positions (dorsal as 12 o'clock).

3. The crushed tissue is incised using scissors.

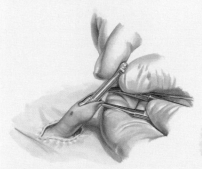

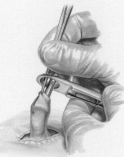

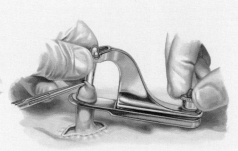

4. The bell of the Gomco clamp is placed under the foreskin, over the glans.

5. Placement of the bell through the baseplate may be facilitated by reaching through the opening with a hemostat.

6. The stem of the bell is placed into the top of the clamp and the thumb screw gently tightened.

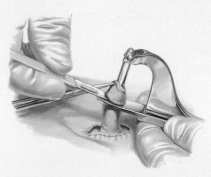

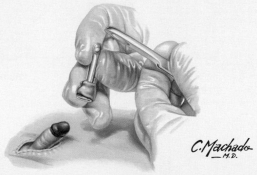

7. A scalpel is used to excise all of the tissue above the baseplate of the clamp.

8. The Gomco clamp is loosened and the bell freed to conclude the case.

Clinical Focus

Available Online

5.28 Ovarian Tumors

Additional figures available online (see inside front cover for details).

Challenge Yourself Questions

1. Cancer of the uterine cervix reaches an advanced stage and disseminates anteriorly. Which of the following structures is *most likely* to be involved in the spread of the tumor?

   A. Broad ligament
   B. Greater vestibular glands
   C. Perineal body
   D. Urinary bladder
   E. Uterine artery

2. A 14-year-old girl in an automobile crash has pelvic trauma. Ultrasound examination reveals that she has a bicornuate uterus with a complete septum and double cervix. Which of the following developmental events *best* accounts for this condition?

   A. Absence of a mesonephric duct on one side
   B. Division of the urogenital sinus
   C. Duplication of the gubernaculum
   D. Incomplete folding of the urogenital folds
   E. Malfusion of the distal paramesonephric ducts

3. A 41-year-old woman presents in the clinic with a uterine prolapse (cervix at introitus) in which the cervix is visible at the vaginal opening. She has delivered seven healthy children. Which of the following structures is the most important support structure of the uterus?

   A. Broad ligament
   B. Deep transverse perineal muscles
   C. Pubocervical ligaments
   D. Rectovaginal fascial condensations
   E. Transverse cervical ligaments

4. A 44-year-old woman is diagnosed with metastatic ovarian cancer. Which of the following lymph nodes will be the first to harbor disseminated ovarian cancer cells?

   A. Aortic (lumbar) nodes
   B. Deep inguinal nodes
   C. External iliac nodes
   D. Internal iliac nodes
   E. Superficial inguinal nodes

5. A 69-year-old man with a history of atherosclerotic disease and heavy smoking tells his physician that he is "impotent." Significant narrowing of which of the following arteries is most likely the cause of this patient's erectile dysfunction?

   A. External iliac
   B. Inferior epigastric
   C. Internal pudendal
   D. Lateral sacral
   E. Vas deferens

6. A 73-year-old woman is admitted to the hospital with significant abdominal ascites. When she sits upright on the side of her bed, the intraperitoneal fluid accumulates in her pelvis. Which of the following sites represents the lowest extent of the female abdominopelvic cavity where this fluid will collect?

   A. Left paracolic gutter
   B. Pararectal fossa
   C. Presacral space
   D. Rectouterine pouch
   E. Vesicouterine pouch

Multiple-choice and short-answer review questions available online; see inside front cover for details.

7. A male driver has sustained severe trauma to the pelvic region in a motor vehicle crash, resulting in a tearing of the prostatomembranous urethral junction (a tear just superior to the external urethral sphincter). Blood and urine from this injury would collect in which of the following spaces?

   A. Anterior lower abdominal wall deep to Scarpa's (membranous layer of superficial) fascia
   B. Beneath the deep (Buck's) fascia of the penis
   C. Beneath the superficial perineal (Colles') fascia
   D. Deep to the dartos fascia of the scrotum and penis
   E. Subperitoneal (retroperitoneal) space

8. After an automobile crash the teenage male driver presents to the emergency department with pelvic fractures and paralysis of his urinary bladder. Which of the following nerves was (were) most likely injured and caused this patient's condition?

   A. Ilioinguinal
   B. Lumbar splanchnics
   C. Pelvic splanchnics
   D. Pudendal
   E. Superior hypogastric

9. Biopsy of the inguinal lymph nodes reveals metastatic cancer. Which of the following pelvic structures is drained by these nodes?

   A. Distal rectum
   B. Ovaries
   C. Proximal anal canal
   D. Urinary bladder
   E. Uterine body

10. During surgery deep within the pelvis, the surgeon clamps the transverse cervical (cardinal) ligaments and the uterine arteries to provide hemostasis for a female patient. Which of the following structures lies close to these structures and must be preserved?

    A. Internal iliac artery
    B. Obturator nerve
    C. Pudendal nerve
    D. Superior gluteal nerve
    E. Ureter

11. Sexual arousal and orgasm employ a coordinated regulatory effort mediated by somatic and autonomic nerves, as well as by endocrine and central nervous system input. During male ejaculation, which of the following nerves contract the internal urethral sphincter and prevent the semen from entering the urinary bladder?

    A. Least splanchnic
    B. Lumbosacral trunk
    C. Pelvic splanchnics
    D. Pudendal
    E. Sacral splanchnics

12. The dissemination of cancer cells from the left testis would enter the testicular veins and then first enter which of the following veins?

    A. Inferior mesenteric
    B. Inferior vena cava
    C. Left inferior epigastric
    D. Left internal iliac
    E. Left internal pudendal
    F. Left renal

13. A forensic pathologist is asked to characterize the bony pelvis of an unidentified and largely decomposed human body. The pathologist identifies the bone as coming from a female. Which of the following pelvic features is unique to the female pelvis?

    A. The greater sciatic notch is narrow.
    B. The ischial tuberosities are inverted.
    C. The obturator foramen is round.
    D. The pelvic inlet is heart shaped.
    E. The pubic arch is wider.

For each of the descriptions below (14-20), select the muscle from the list (A-M) that is most closely associated.

(A) Bulbospongiosus
(B) Cremaster
(C) Compressor urethrae
(D) Coccygeus
(E) Detrusor
(F) External anal sphincter
(G) External urethral sphincter
(H) Gluteus maximus
(I) Internal urethral sphincter
(J) Ischiocavernosus
(K) Levator ani
(L) Obturator internus
(M) Piriformis

____ 14. This muscle is actually a derivative of one of the abdominal wall muscles.

_____ 15. Trauma injuring the pelvic splanchnic nerves would compromise this muscle's ability to contract.

_____ 16. The integrity of this muscle is critical for support of the pelvic viscera.

_____ 17. Contraction of this muscle expels the last few drops of urine from the male urethra.

_____ 18. An abscess in the ischioanal fossa is limited in its spread superiorly by this muscle.

_____ 19. Anterior rami of S2-S4 exit the anterior sacral foramina and then pass directly over (superficial to) this muscle.

_____ 20. Trauma to the L1-L2 sympathetic outflow would result in the inability to contract this muscle.

21. During pelvic surgery, the surgeon notices that the inferior gluteal artery and internal pudendal artery are leaving the pelvis just inferior to the piriformis muscle as they are headed for the gluteal region. Next they will pass through which of the following openings?
    A. Greater sciatic foramen
    B. Deep inguinal ring
    C. Femoral canal
    D. Pudendal canal
    E. Superficial inguinal ring

22. Surgeons operating in the perineal region must be cognizant of this structure, because it is the anchor point for many of the perineal structures. What is this structure?
    A. Perineal body
    B. Sacrotuberous ligament
    C. Superficial transverse perineal muscle
    D. Uterosacral ligament
    E. Vestibule

23. During a pelvic examination, the gynecologist feels a pulse adjacent to the vaginal fornix. Which of the following arteries is the physician feeling?
    A. External iliac artery
    B. Internal pudendal artery
    C. Ovarian artery
    D. Uterine artery
    E. Vaginal artery

24. A 33-year-old woman is being examined following an automobile accident. Abdominopelvic ultrasound reveals a collection of fluid in her peritoneal cavity. In which of the following spaces is this fluid most likely to be found?
    A. Lesser sac (omental bursa)
    B. Rectouterine pouch
    C. Rectovesical pouch
    D. Right paracolic gutter
    E. Vesicouterine pouch

25. An ultrasound examination of a 16-year-old girl shows that she has a double uterus. Failure of which of the following developmental events is responsible for this condition?
    A. Division of the urogenital sinus
    B. Failure of fusion of the labioscrotal folds
    C. Failure of fusion of the inferior paramesonephric duct
    D. Failure of fusion of the mesonephric duct
    E. Malformation of the genital tubercle

26. A 20-year-old male college student with testicular pain and swelling is seen in the university health clinic. CT examination reveals the collection of serous fluid within the cavity of the tunica vaginalis. Which of the following conditions is most likely the cause of the swelling and inflammation?
    A. Cystocele
    B. Epispadias
    C. Hydrocele
    D. Hypospadias
    E. Varicocele

27. A 48-year-old woman is diagnosed with cancer in the vestibule of her vagina. Which of the following lymph node collections is most likely to be involved first in the spread of this tumor?
    A. Aortic nodes
    B. External iliac nodes
    C. Internal iliac nodes
    D. Lumbar nodes
    E. Superficial inguinal nodes

28. During a difficult delivery, the physician decides to perform a posterolateral episiotomy to enlarge the vaginal opening. Which of the following structures will be completely or partially incised during this procedure?

    A. Bulbospongiosus muscle
    B. Crus (corpus cavernosa)
    C. Deep transverse perineal muscle
    D. Levator ani muscle
    E. Perineal body

29. During surgery to remove an ovary and its associated lymphatics, the surgeon must be particularly mindful of the close anatomical approximation of which of the following nerves?

    A. Femoral nerve
    B. Genitofemoral nerve
    C. Ilioinguinal nerve
    D. Lumbosacral trunk nerve
    E. Obturator nerve

30. Rupture of the male urethra can lead to the extravasation of urine into various pelvic or perineal spaces. If the injury perforates the penile urethra and Buck's fascia (deep fascia of the penis), into which of the following spaces might the collection of urine be found?

    A. Beneath the dartos fascia and the investing deep (Buck's) fascia of the penis
    B. Between the fatty (Camper's) superficial fascia and membranous (Scarpa's) fascia of the lower abdominal wall
    C. Deep to the membranous (Scarpa's) fascia of the lower abdominal wall
    D. External to the dartos fascia of the scrotum
    E. In the retroperitoneum of the lower pelvis

For each of the questions below (31-37), select one vessel from the list (A-L) that best fits the structure described. Each vessel in the list may be used once, more than once, or not at all.

(A) External iliac vein
(B) Inferior gluteal artery
(C) Internal pudendal artery
(D) Middle rectal vein
(E) Ovarian artery
(F) Pampiniform plexus of veins
(G) Prostatic venous plexus
(H) Superior gluteal artery
(I) Testicular artery
(J) Umbilical artery
(K) Uterine artery
(L) Vaginal veins

_____ 31. This vessel forms an important portosystemic anastomosis.

_____ 32. This vessel passes through both the greater and lesser sciatic foramina.

_____ 33. This vessel and its branches can become engorged and form hemorrhoids.

_____ 34. A portion of this vessel becomes a ligament postnatally.

_____ 35. This vessel can be found in the inguinal canal.

_____ 36. This vessel passes immediately over the ureter deep in the pelvis.

_____ 37. This vessel usually passes between the lumbosacral trunk and the first sacral nerve.

For each of the structures listed below (38-40), select the label (A-F) that identifies it on the axial MR scan of the female pelvis.

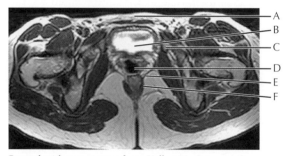

Reused with permission from Kelley LL, Petersen C: *Sectional anatomy for imaging professionals*, 2nd ed., St Louis, 2007, Elsevier.

_____ 38. Rectum

_____ 39. Urinary bladder

_____ 40. Vagina

Answers to Challenge Yourself Questions

1. **D.** The urinary bladder is directly anterior to the uterine cervix, lying just deep to the vesico-uterine pouch.

2. **E.** Incomplete fusion of the distal paramesoneph-ric (müllerian) ducts can lead to septation of the uterus, resulting in a partial or complete duplication of the uterus.

3. **E.** The transverse cervical (cardinal or Macken-rodt's) ligaments are fibrous condensations of the subperitoneal pelvic fascia and are the most important of the supporting structures for the uterus.

4. **A.** The ovaries descend into the pelvis from their original embryonic origin from the abdominal urogenital ridge. They drag their vessels (ovarian artery from the aorta and ovarian veins draining into the IVC on the right and into the left renal vein and then the IVC on the left) with them. Thus, the lymphatic drainage courses back to the aortic (lumbar) nodes (the same is true for the male testes).

5. **C.** The internal pudendal arteries give rise to the arteries of the bulb of the penis and the corpora cavernosa, which supply the erectile tissues. Narrowing of these vessels by atherosclerosis can be just one of several problems that may lead to erectile dysfunction (ED).

6. **D.** The space between the rectum and uterus, called the rectouterine pouch (of Douglas), is the lowest point in the female abdominopelvic cavity in the upright position. Fluids within the cavity will eventually percolate down and collect in this space.

7. **E.** This rupture occurs before the prostatic urethra is completely surrounded by the external urethral sphincter, so blood and urine would collect primarily in the subperitoneal space beneath the pelvic floor. Excessive fluids in this space will allow it to expand superiorly and stretch the peritoneal floor of the pelvis.

8. **C.** The pelvic splanchnic nerves arise from the S2-S4 spinal nerves and convey the preganglionic parasympathetic fibers that innervate the urinary bladder. Those fibers destined to innervate the bladder enter the inferior hypogastric plexus of nerves and then enter the vesical plexus on the bladder wall where they synapse on their postganglionic parasympathetic neurons.

9. **E.** While most of the listed structures do not drain to the inguinal nodes, some lymph can track along the broad ligament of the uterus and enter the inguinal nodes. First, one must eliminate the possibility of perineal cancer, cancer of the distal anal canal, and cancer of the lower limb before focusing on the uterus.

10. **E.** The ureters pass just inferior to the uterine vessels ("water flows under the bridge") and must be identified before anything in this region is clamped and/or incised.

11. **E.** The sacral splanchnic nerves convey preganglionic sympathetic fibers to the inferior hypogastric plexus, where they synapse and send postganglionic fibers to innervate the internal urethral sphincter at the neck of the male urinary bladder (females do not have an internal urethral sphincter).

12. **F.** The cancer cells from the left testis would course along the left testicular vein(s) to the left renal vein and then into the IVC. On the right side, the right testicular vein drains directly into the IVC.

13. **E.** The easiest way to identify the female pelvis is by the width of the pubic arch. Most of the adaptations that differentiate the female from the male pelvis pertain to its relationship to childbirth.

14. **B.** As the testis descends through the inguinal canal, it becomes covered by three layers of spermatic fascia. The middle spermatic fascia is the cremasteric fascia or muscle and is derived from the internal abdominal oblique muscle. The cremaster muscle is innervated by the genital branch of the genitofemoral nerve.

15. **E.** The pelvic splanchnic nerves (parasympathetics) would innervate a smooth muscle. The only smooth muscle in the list that is innervated by them, resulting in contraction, is the detrusor muscle of the bladder wall. Contraction of this muscle empties the urinary bladder and is under parasympathetic control.

16. **K.** The levator ani is one of two muscles comprising the pelvic diaphragm (the other one is the coccygeus), and is itself really the amalgam of three separate but closely associated muscles (the puborectalis, pubococcygeus, and iliococcygeus) that is commonly referred to as the levator ani. It is critical in supporting the pelvic viscera.

17. **A.** Contraction of the bulbospongiosus muscle following voiding helps evacuate the remaining urine in the penile urethra.

18. **K.** The levator ani muscle is the "roof" of the ischioanal fossa; it extends up the sides of the pelvic wall to contact the obturator internus muscle. This fossa is largely filled with fat; however, infections in this area can spread anteriorly, superior to the deep perineal pouch.

19. **M.** The anterior rami of S2-S4 lie on the surface of the piriformis muscle. They are joined by the anterior rami of L4-S1 from above to form the sciatic nerve (L4-S3), which then exits the pelvic cavity via the greater sciatic foramen and enters the gluteal region.

20. **I.** The internal urethral sphincter is one of two smooth muscles in the list (the other is the detrusor) and the only one innervated by the sympathetic nerves of the ANS. This muscle contracts during ejaculation, thus preventing the semen from entering the urinary bladder.

21. **A.** The piriformis muscle, the gluteal arteries and nerves (superior and inferior), the pudendal nerve, and the internal pudendal artery all pass through the greater sciatic foramen to reach the gluteal region. The internal pudendal artery and pudendal nerve then pass through the lesser sciatic foramen to enter the pudendal (Alcock's) canal as they move toward the perineum.

22. **A.** The perineal body, or central tendon of the perineum, is an important fibromuscular support region and an attachment point for the perineal muscles and the female urethro-vaginalis complex.

23. **D.** The uterine artery lies within the cardinal ligament at the inferior aspect of the broad ligament (mesometrium) and contacts the uterus near the cervix. Thus, its pulse may be felt near the lateral vaginal fornix. All the other arteries are much farther away in the lower pelvis.

24. **B.** The rectouterine pouch (of Douglas) is the lowest point in the female abdominopelvic cavity and is where the peritoneum reflects off of the anterior rectum and is continuous with the broad ligament of the uterus. When a person is in the upright position, fluid in the cavity will ultimately flow into this low point.

25. **C.** Incomplete fusion of the lower or distal portion of the paramesonephric (müllerian) duct can lead to partial or complete duplication of the uterus (bicornuate uterus). See Fig. 5.29 and Clinical Focus 5.26.

26. **C.** One of the most common causes of scrotal enlargement is hydrocele (excessive serous fluid within the tunica vaginalis). This usually occurs because of an inflammatory process, trauma, or the presence of a tumor. A small pouch of the processus vaginalis called the tunica vaginalis persists and partially envelops the testis. It is a piece of parietal peritoneum that envelops a portion of the testis as it passes through the deep inguinal ring.

27. **E.** Much of the lymphatic drainage of the pelvic viscera follows the venous drainage of the same structures. However, some lymph from the perineum and the vestibule of the vagina and lymph that courses along the round ligament of the uterus (which passes through the inguinal canal) also drains into the superficial inguinal nodes. Physicians must be aware of this possibility when these nodes are enlarged.

28. **A.** Although episiotomies are not routinely performed in the United States today, there are occasions when it is necessary to enlarge the vaginal opening, either with a midline episiotomy or a posterolateral approach. In the posterolateral approach, the incision usually will bisect the most posterior portion of the bulbospongiosus muscle; this is preferable to incising the perineal body.

29. **E.** The obturator nerve and usually the artery pass along the deep lateral aspect of the pelvic wall on their way to the obturator foramen. In this location, they are closer to the ovary and its vessels than any of the other nerves in the option list. Damage to the nerve will weaken the adductor muscles of the medial thigh, which the nerve innervates.

30. **C.** The fluid (blood and/or urine) may pass into the lower abdominal wall deep to the membranous (Scarpa's) fascia. Around the penis itself, the fluid would be between the dartos fascia and the investing deep (Buck's) fascia of the penis, not beneath both fascial layers. See Clinical Focus 5.23.

31. **D.** The middle (and inferior) rectal veins and their branches are part of the caval system and anastomose with the branches of the superior rectal vein, a tributary of the inferior mesenteric vein, which is part of the portal venous drainage.

32. **C.** The only vessel in the list that travels through both the greater and lesser sciatic foramina is the internal pudendal artery. It passes through the greater sciatic foramen, around the sacrospinous ligament, through the lesser sciatic foramen, and then into the pudendal (Alcock's) canal on its way to supply blood to the perineum.

33. **D.** Hemorrhoids are symptomatic varicose dilations of the submucosal veins that protrude into the anal canal (internal hemorrhoids) or extend through the anal opening (external hemorrhoids). These rectal veins are tributaries of the middle rectal veins from the internal iliac veins and from the inferior rectal veins draining into the internal pudendal veins.

34. **J.** The umbilical artery arises from the internal iliac artery and courses toward the abdominal wall, where it becomes a ligament. In the fetus, the two umbilical arteries returned blood to the placenta, but postnatally the arteries form the medial umbilical ligaments visible on the internal aspect of the lower abdominal wall.

35. **I.** The only vessel in the list that can be found in the inguinal canal is the testicular artery, a branch of the abdominal aorta. As each testis descends through the inguinal canal and enters the scrotum, it drags its artery with it. The artery of the ductus deferens and the cremasteric artery also pass through the canal; they are not on the list, however.

36. **K.** The ureter passes just under the uterine artery as it travels to the urinary bladder (like water passing under a bridge). Hence, the uterine artery has a close relationship to the ureter. Every surgeon working in the pelvis must be careful to avoid damaging the uterine artery.

37. **H.** The superior gluteal artery usually can be identified as it passes between the large lumbosacral trunk (L4-L5) and the first sacral spinal nerve on its way to the greater sciatic foramen. The inferior gluteal artery often passes between the S2-S3 branches as it courses toward the greater sciatic foramen and enters the gluteal region (see Fig. 6.7).

38. **F.**

39. **B.**

40. **D.**

Lower Limb

1. INTRODUCTION

As with the upper limb in Chapter 7, this chapter approaches our study of the lower limb by organizing its anatomical structures into functional compartments. Although the upper limb is organized into two functional compartments (extensor and flexor compartments), the thigh and leg each are organized into three functional compartments, with their respective muscles and neurovascular bundles. The lower limb subserves the following important functions and features:

- The limb supports the weight of the body and transfers that support to the axial skeleton across the hip and sacroiliac joints.
- The hip and knee joints lock into position when one is standing still in anatomical position, adding stability and balance to the transfer of weight and conserving the muscles' energy; this allows one to stand erect for prolonged periods.
- The limb functions in locomotion through the process of walking (our gait).
- The limb is anchored to the axial skeleton by the pelvic girdle, which allows for less mobility but significantly more stability than the pectoral girdle of the upper limb.

Be sure to review the movements of the lower limb as described in Chapter 1 (see Fig. 1.3). Note the terms *dorsiflexion* (extension) and *plantarflexion* (flexion), and *inversion* (supination) and *eversion* (pronation), which are unique to the movements of the ankle.

2. SURFACE ANATOMY

The components of the lower limb include the gluteal region (buttocks and lateral hip), thigh, leg,

and foot. The key surface landmarks include the following (Fig. 6.1):

- **Inguinal ligament:** the folded, inferior edge of the external abdominal oblique aponeurosis that separates the abdominal region from the thigh (Poupart's ligament).
- **Greater trochanter:** the point of the hip and attachment site for several gluteal muscles.
- **Quadriceps femoris:** the muscle mass of the anterior thigh, composed of four muscles—rectus femoris and three vastus muscles—that extend the leg at the knee.
- **Patella:** the kneecap; largest sesamoid bone in the body.
- **Popliteal fossa:** the region posterior to the knee.
- **Gastrocnemius muscles:** the muscle mass that forms most of the calf.
- **Calcaneal (Achilles) tendon:** the prominent tendon of several calf muscles.
- **Small saphenous vein:** subcutaneous vein that drains blood from the lateral dorsal venous arch and posterior leg (calf) into the popliteal vein posterior to the knee.
- **Great saphenous vein:** subcutaneous vein that drains blood from the medial dorsal venous arch, leg, and thigh into the femoral vein just inferior to the inguinal ligament.

Superficial veins drain blood toward the heart and communicate with *deep veins* that parallel the arteries of the lower limb (Fig. 6.2). When vigorous muscle contraction compresses the deep veins, venous blood is shunted into superficial veins and returned to the heart. All these veins have **valves** to aid in the venous return to the heart. The great and small saphenous veins are analogous to the cephalic and basilic subcutaneous veins of the upper limb, respectively.

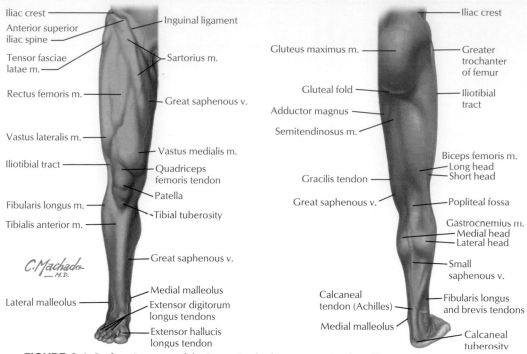

FIGURE 6.1 Surface Anatomy of the Lower Limb. (From *Netter's atlas of human anatomy*, ed 8, Plate 491; S-11.)

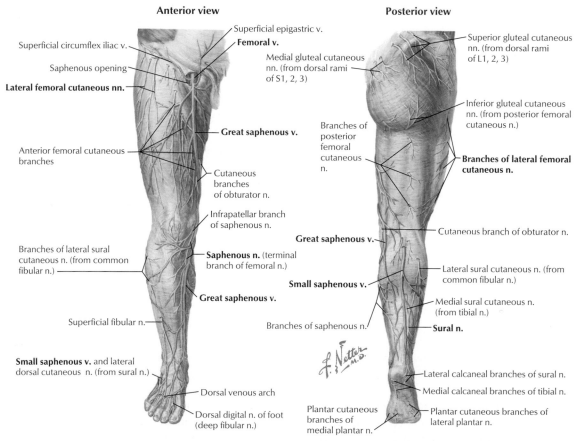

FIGURE 6.2 Superficial Veins and Nerves of the Lower Limb. (From *Netter's atlas of human anatomy*, ed 8, Plates 492 and 493; S-266 and S-267.)

Clinical Focus 6.1

Deep Venous Thrombosis

Although deep venous (or deep vein) thrombosis (DVT) may occur anywhere in the body, veins of the lower limb are most often involved. Three cardinal events account for the pathogenesis and risk of DVT: stasis, venous wall injury, and hypercoagulability. (See also Clinical Focus 3-8, Pulmonary Embolism.)

Clinical risk factors for DVT include the following:

- Postsurgical immobility
- Vessel trauma
- Infection
- Paralysis
- Malignancy
- Pregnancy

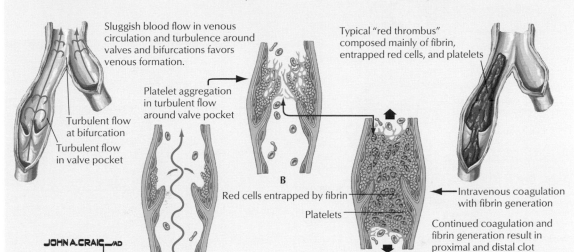

Sluggish blood flow in venous circulation and turbulence around valves and bifurcations favors venous formation.

Platelet aggregation in turbulent flow around valve pocket

Turbulent flow at bifurcation

Turbulent flow in valve pocket

JOHN A. CRAIG—AD

A

B

Red cells entrapped by fibrin

Platelets

Typical "red thrombus" composed mainly of fibrin, entrapped red cells, and platelets

Intravenous coagulation with fibrin generation

Continued coagulation and fibrin generation result in proximal and distal clot propagation.

C

Corresponding cutaneous nerves are terminal sensory branches of major lower limb nerves that arise from **lumbar (L1-L4)** and **sacral (L4-S4)** plexuses (Fig. 6.2). Note that the gluteal region has superior, middle, and inferior gluteal cutaneous nerves, and the thigh has posterior, lateral, anterior, and medial cutaneous nerves. The leg has lateral sural, superficial fibular, saphenous, and sural cutaneous nerves (named from the lateral leg to the posterior leg). The **sural nerve** (branch of the tibial nerve) on the posterior leg parallels the small saphenous vein, and the **saphenous nerve** (terminal portion of the femoral nerve) parallels the great saphenous vein from the level of the knee to the medial ankle.

3. HIP

Bones and Joints of the Pelvic Girdle and Hip

The pelvic girdle is the attachment point of the lower limb to the body's trunk and axial skeleton. The *pectoral girdle* is its counterpart for the attachment of the upper limb. The **sacroiliac ligaments**

(posterior, anterior, and interosseous) are among the strongest ligaments in the body and support its entire weight, almost pulling the sacrum into the pelvis. Note that the pelvis (sacrum and coxal bones) in anatomical position is tilted forward such that the pubic symphysis and the anterior superior iliac spines lie in the same vertical plane, placing great stress on the sacroiliac joints and ligaments (see Figs. 5.3 and 6.3). In fact, the body's center of gravity when standing upright lies just anterior to the S2 vertebra of the fused sacrum. These ligaments and joints of the pelvis are illustrated and described in Chapter 5 (Fig. 5.3 and Table 5.1).

The bones of the pelvis include the following (Fig. 6.3 and Table 6.1):

- **Right and left pelvic bones (coxal or hip bones):** the fusion of three separate bones called the *ilium, ischium,* and *pubis,* which join each other in the acetabulum (cup-shaped feature for articulation of the head of the femur).
- **Sacrum:** the fusion of the *five sacral vertebrae;* the two pelvic bones articulate with the sacrum posteriorly.

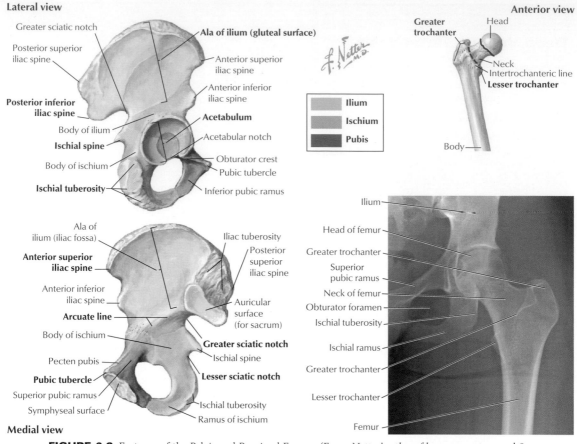

FIGURE 6.3 Features of the Pelvis and Proximal Femur. (From *Netter's atlas of human anatomy*, ed 8, Plate 495; S-153.)

TABLE 6.1 Features of the Pelvis and Proximal Femur

FEATURE	CHARACTERISTICS
Coxal (Hip) Bone	Fusion of three bones on each side to form the pelvis, which articulates with the sacrum to form the pelvic girdle
Ilium	Body fused to ischium and pubis, all meeting in the acetabulum (socket for articulation with femoral head) Ala (wing): weak spot of ilium
Ischium	Body fused with other two bones; ramus fused with pubis
Pubis	Body fused with other two bones; ramus fused with ischium
Femur (Proximal)	
Long bone	Longest bone in the body and very strong
Head	Point of articulation with acetabulum of coxal bone
Neck	Common fracture site
Greater trochanter	Point of the hip; attachment site for several gluteal muscles
Lesser trochanter	Attachment site of iliopsoas tendon (strong hip flexor)

- **Coccyx:** the terminal end of the vertebral column, and a remnant of our embryonic tail.

Additionally, the proximal **femur** (thigh bone) articulates with the pelvis at the acetabulum (see Fig. 6.3 and Table 6.1).

The hip joint is a classic **ball-and-socket synovial joint** that affords great stability, provided by both its bony anatomy and its strong ligaments (Fig. 6.4 and Table 6.2), but it also is a fairly mobile joint. It can flex, extend, adduct, abduct, and medially and laterally rotate, and it has limited circumduction, although not as much as the shoulder joint. As with most large joints, there is a rich vascular anastomosis around the hip joint, contributing a blood supply not only to the hip but also to the associated muscles (Fig. 6.5 and Table 6.3).

The other features of the pelvic girdle and its stabilizing lumbosacral and sacroiliac joints are illustrated and summarized in Chapter 5.

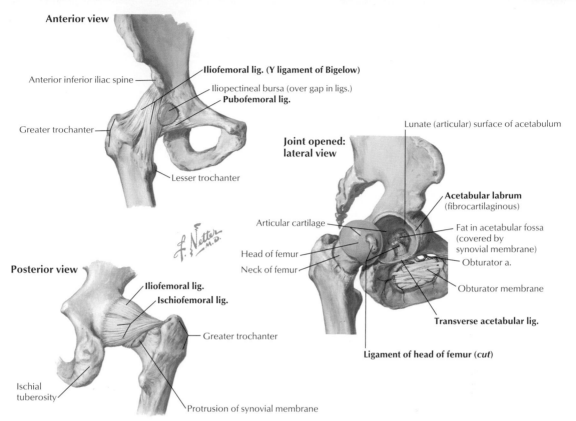

FIGURE 6.4 Hip Joint and Its Ligaments. (From *Netter's atlas of human anatomy,* ed 8, Plate 496; S-170.)

TABLE 6.2 Ligaments of the Hip Joint (Multiaxial Synovial Ball and Socket)

LIGAMENT	ATTACHMENT	COMMENT
Capsular	Acetabular margin to femoral neck	Encloses femoral head and part of neck; acts in flexion, extension, abduction, adduction, medial and lateral rotation, and circumduction
Iliofemoral	Iliac spine and acetabulum to intertrochanteric line	Forms inverted Y (of Bigelow); limits hyperextension and lateral rotation; the stronger ligament
Ischiofemoral	Acetabulum to femoral neck posteriorly	Limits extension and medial rotation; the weaker ligament
Pubofemoral	Pubic ramus to lower femoral neck	Limits extension and abduction
Labrum	Acetabulum	Fibrocartilage, deepens socket
Transverse acetabular	Acetabular notch inferiorly	Cups acetabulum to form a socket for femoral head
Ligament of head of femur	Acetabular notch and transverse ligament to femoral head	Artery to femoral head runs in ligament

TABLE 6.3 Arteries of the Hip Joint

ARTERY	COURSE AND STRUCTURES SUPPLIED	ARTERY	COURSE AND STRUCTURES SUPPLIED
Medial circumflex	Usually arises from deep artery of thigh; branches supply femoral head and neck; passes posterior to iliopsoas muscle tendon	Acetabular branch	Arises from obturator artery; runs in ligament of head of femur; supplies femoral head
Lateral circumflex	Usually arises from deep femoral artery of the thigh	Gluteal branches (superior and inferior)	Form anastomoses with medial and lateral femoral circumflex branches

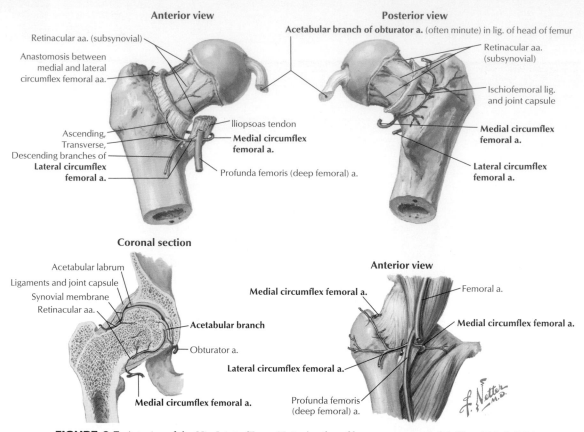

FIGURE 6.5 Arteries of the Hip Joint. (From *Netter's atlas of human anatomy*, ed 8, Plate 514; S-278.)

Clinical Focus 6.2

Developmental Dislocation of the Hip

In the United States, 10 in 1000 infants are born with developmental dislocation of the hip. With early diagnosis and treatment, about 96% of affected children have normal hip function. Girls are affected more often than boys. About 60% of affected children are firstborns, which may suggest that unstretched uterine and abdominal walls limit fetal movement. Thirty percent to 50% of the affected children are breech deliveries. *Ortolani's test* of hip abduction confirms the diagnosis.

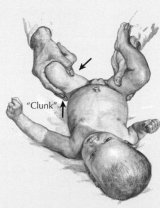

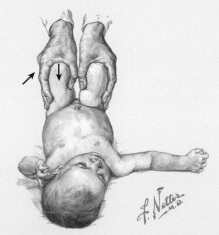

Ortolani's (reduction) test
With baby relaxed and content on firm surface, hips and knees flexed to 90 degrees. Hips examined one at a time. Examiner grasps baby's thigh with middle finger over greater trochanter and lifts thigh to bring femoral head from its dislocated posterior position to opposite the acetabulum. Simultaneously, thigh gently abducted, reducing femoral head into acetabulum. In positive finding, examiner senses reduction by palpable, nearly audible "clunk."

Barlow's (dislocation) test
Reverse of Ortolani's test. If femoral head is in acetabulum at time of examination, Barlow's test is performed to discover any hip instability. Baby's thigh grasped as shown and adducted with gentle downward pressure. Dislocation is palpable as femoral head slips out of acetabulum. Diagnosis confirmed with Ortolani's test.

Pelvic Fractures

Pelvic fractures are, by definition, limited to the **pelvic ring** (pelvis and sacrum), whereas *acetabular* fractures (caused by high-impact trauma such as falls and automobile crashes) are described and classified separately. *Stable* pelvic fractures involve only one side of the pelvic ring, whereas *unstable* fractures involve two portions of the pelvic ring and/or ligamentous disruption. Excessive bleeding, nerve injury, and soft tissue damage (muscle and viscera) may accompany pelvic fractures.

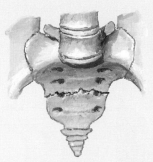
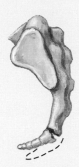

Transverse fracture of the sacrum that is minimally displaced

Fracture usually requires no treatment

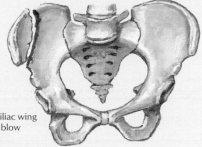
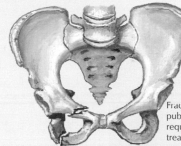

Fracture of iliac wing from direct blow

Fracture of ipsilateral pubic and ischial rami requires only symptomatic treatment

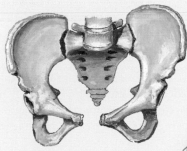
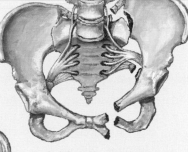

Open book fracture. Disruption of symphysis pubis with wide anterior separation of pelvic ring. Anterior sacroiliac ligaments are torn, with slight opening of sacroiliac joints. Intact posterior sacroiliac ligaments prevent vertical migration of the pelvis.

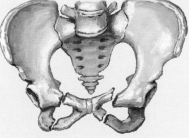

Straddle fracture. Double break in continuity of anterior pelvic ring causes instability but usually little displacement. Visceral (especially genitourinary) injury likely.

Vertical shear fracture. Upward and posterior dislocation of sacroiliac joint and fracture of both pubic rami on same side result in upward shift of hemipelvis. Note also fracture of transverse process of vertebra L5, avulsion of ischial spine, and stretching of sacral nerves.

Clinical Focus 6.4

Intracapsular Femoral Neck Fracture

Femoral neck fractures are common injuries. In young persons the fracture often results from trauma; in elderly people the cause is often related to osteoporosis and associated with a fall. The *Garden classification* identifies four fracture types:

- **I:** impaction of superior portion of femoral neck (incomplete fracture)
- **II:** nondisplaced fracture (complete fracture)
- **III:** partial displacement between femoral head and neck
- **IV:** complete displacement between femoral head and neck

The occurrence of complications related to nonunion and avascular necrosis of the femoral head increases from type I to IV.

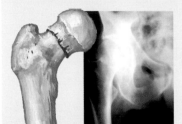

Type I. Impacted fracture

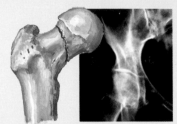

Type II. Nondisplaced fracture

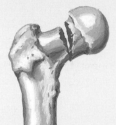

Type III. Partially displaced fracture

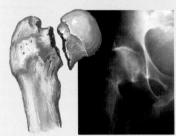

Type IV. Displaced fracture

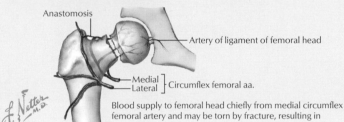

Anastomosis

Artery of ligament of femoral head

Medial ⎤
Lateral ⎦ Circumflex femoral aa.

Blood supply to femoral head chiefly from medial circumflex femoral artery and may be torn by fracture, resulting in osteonecrosis of femoral head. Artery of ligament usually insignificant.

Nerve Plexuses

Several nerve plexuses exist within the abdomino-pelvic cavity and send branches to somatic structures (skin and skeletal muscle) in the pelvis and lower limb. The **lumbar plexus** is composed of the anterior rami of spinal nerves L1-L4, which give rise to two large nerves, the femoral and obturator nerves, and several smaller branches (see Fig. 4.43, Table 4.13, and Fig. 6.6). The **femoral nerve** (L2-L4) innervates muscles of the anterior thigh, whereas the **obturator nerve** (L2-L4) innervates muscles of the medial thigh.

The **sacral plexus** is composed of the anterior rami of spinal nerves L4-S4. Its major branches are summarized in Fig. 6.7 and Table 6.4. The small **coccygeal plexus** has contributions from S4-Co1

and gives rise to small anococcygeal branches that innervate the coccygeus muscle and skin of the anal triangle (see Chapter 5). Often the lumbar and sacral plexuses are simply referred to as the **lumbosacral plexus**.

Access to the Lower Limb

Structures passing out of or into the lower limb from the abdominopelvic cavity may do so through one of the following *four passageways* (see Figs. 5.3 and 6.11):

- Anteriorly between the inguinal ligament and bony pelvis into the anterior thigh.
- Anteroinferiorly through the **obturator canal** into the medial thigh.
- Posterolaterally through the **greater sciatic foramen** into the gluteal region.

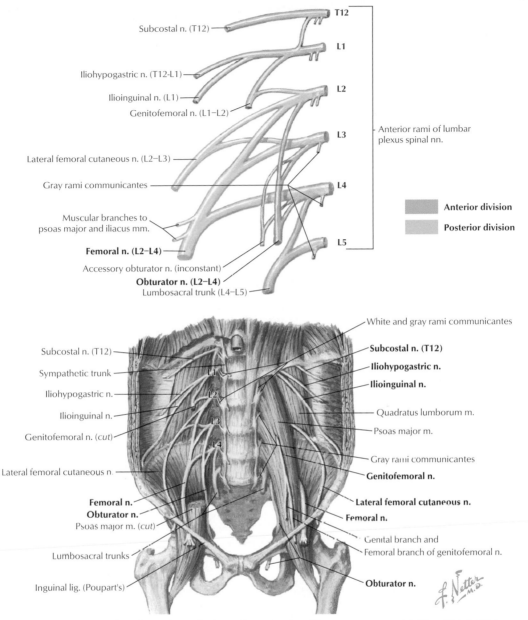

FIGURE 6.6 Lumbar Plexus (L1-L4). (From *Netter's atlas of human anatomy*, ed 8, Plate 507; S-113.)

TABLE 6.4 Major Branches of the Sacral Plexus (see Fig. 6.7)			
DIVISION AND NERVE	**INNERVATION**	**DIVISION AND NERVE**	**INNERVATION**
Anterior		**Posterior**	
Pudendal	Supplies motor and sensory innervation to perineum (S2-S4)	Superior gluteal	Innervates several gluteal muscles (L4-S1)
Tibial (part of sciatic nerve)	Innervates posterior thigh muscles, posterior leg muscles, and foot; part of sciatic nerve (largest nerve in body, L4-S3) with common fibular nerve	Inferior gluteal	Innervates gluteus maximus muscle (L5-S2)
		Common fibular (part of sciatic nerve)	Portion of sciatic nerve (with tibial nerve) that innervates lateral and anterior muscle compartments of leg (L4-S2)

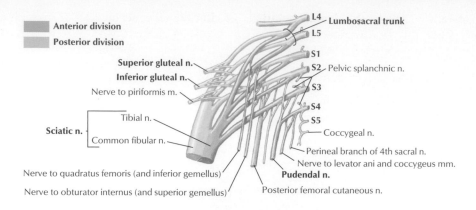

■ Anterior division
■ Posterior division

L4 — **Lumbosacral trunk**
L5
S1
S2 — Pelvic splanchnic n.
S3
S4
S5
Coccygeal n.

Superior gluteal n.
Inferior gluteal n.
Nerve to piriformis m.

Sciatic n. ⎨ Tibial n.
              ⎩ Common fibular n.

Perineal branch of 4th sacral n.
Nerve to levator ani and coccygeus mm.
Pudendal n.
Posterior femoral cutaneous n.

Nerve to quadratus femoris (and inferior gemellus)
Nerve to obturator internus (and superior gemellus)

Topography: medial and slightly anterior view of hemisected pelvis

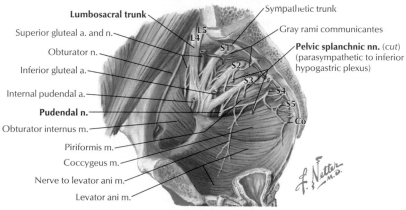

Lumbosacral trunk
Superior gluteal a. and n.
Obturator n.
Inferior gluteal a.
Internal pudendal a.
Pudendal n.
Obturator internus m.
Piriformis m.
Coccygeus m.
Nerve to levator ani m.
Levator ani m.

Sympathetic trunk
Gray rami communicantes
Pelvic splanchnic nn. (*cut*)
(parasympathetic to inferior hypogastric plexus)

L5
L4
S1
S2
S3
S4
S5
Co

FIGURE 6.7 Sacral and Coccygeal Plexuses. (From *Netter's atlas of human anatomy,* ed 8, Plate 508; S-114.)

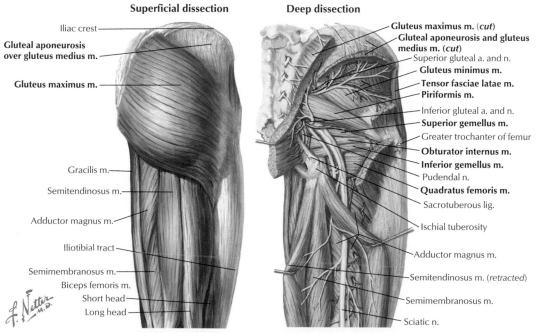

Superficial dissection

Iliac crest
Gluteal aponeurosis over gluteus medius m.
Gluteus maximus m.

Gracilis m.
Semitendinosus m.
Adductor magnus m.
Iliotibial tract
Semimembranosus m.
Biceps femoris m.
    Short head
    Long head

Deep dissection

Gluteus maximus m. (*cut*)
Gluteal aponeurosis and gluteus medius m. (*cut*)
Superior gluteal a. and n.
Gluteus minimus m.
Tensor fasciae latae m.
Piriformis m.
Inferior gluteal a. and n.
Superior gemellus m.
Greater trochanter of femur
Obturator internus m.
Inferior gemellus m.
Pudendal n.
Quadratus femoris m.
Sacrotuberous lig.
Ischial tuberosity
Adductor magnus m.
Semitendinosus m. (*retracted*)
Semimembranosus m.
Sciatic n.

FIGURE 6.8 Gluteal Muscles. (From *Netter's atlas of human anatomy,* ed 8, Plates 504 and 511; S-273 and S-274.)

- Posterolaterally through the **lesser sciatic foramen** from the gluteal region into the perineum (via the pudendal [Alcock's] canal).

4. GLUTEAL REGION

Muscles

The muscles of the gluteal (buttock) region are arranged into superficial and deep groups, as follows (Fig. 6.8 and Table 6.5):

- Superficial muscles include the three gluteal muscles and the tensor fasciae latae laterally.

- Deep muscles act on the hip, primarily as lateral rotators of the thigh at the hip, and assist in stabilizing the hip joint.

The **gluteus maximus muscle** is one of the strongest muscles in the body in absolute terms and is a powerful extensor of the thigh at the hip (Fig. 6.8). It is especially important in extending the hip when one rises from a squatting or sitting position and when one is climbing stairs. The gluteus maximus muscle also stabilizes and laterally (externally) rotates the hip joint. The **gluteus medius** and **gluteus minimus muscles** are primarily abductors and medial (internal) rotators of the thigh

TABLE 6.5 Gluteal Muscles

MUSCLE	PROXIMAL ATTACHMENT	DISTAL ATTACHMENT	INNERVATION	MAIN ACTIONS
Gluteus maximus	Ilium posterior to posterior gluteal line, dorsal surface of sacrum and coccyx, and sacrotuberous ligament	Most fibers end in iliotibial tract that inserts into lateral condyle of tibia; some fibers insert on gluteal tuberosity of femur	Inferior gluteal nerve (L5-S2)	Extends flexed thigh at the hip and assists in its lateral rotation; abducts and assists in raising trunk from flexed position
Gluteus medius	Lateral surface of ilium	Lateral surface of greater trochanter of femur	Superior gluteal nerve (L4-S1)	Abducts and medially rotates thigh at hip; steadies pelvis on limb when opposite limb is raised
Gluteus minimus	Lateral surface of ilium	Anterior surface of greater trochanter of femur	Superior gluteal nerve (L4-S1)	Abducts and medially rotates thigh at hip; steadies pelvis on limb when opposite limb is raised
Tensor fasciae latae	Anterior superior iliac spine and anterior iliac crest	Iliotibial tract that attaches to lateral condyle of tibia	Superior gluteal nerve (L4-S1)	Abducts, medially rotates, and flexes thigh at hip; helps to keep knee extended
Piriformis	Anterior surface of sacrum and sacrotuberous ligament	Superior border of greater trochanter of femur	Branches of anterior rami (L5-S2)	Laterally rotates extended thigh at hip and abducts flexed thigh at hip; steadies femoral head in acetabulum
Obturator internus	Pelvic surface of obturator membrane and surrounding bones	Medial surface of greater trochanter of femur	Nerve to obturator internus (L5-S2)	Laterally rotates extended thigh at hip and abducts flexed thigh at hip; steadies femoral head in acetabulum
Gemelli, superior and inferior	*Superior:* ischial spine *Inferior:* ischial tuberosity	Medial surface of greater trochanter of femur	*Superior gemellus:* same nerve supply as obturator internus *Inferior gemellus:* same nerve supply as quadratus femoris	Laterally rotate extended thigh at the hip and abducts flexed thigh at the hip; steady femoral head in acetabulum
Quadratus femoris	Lateral border of ischial tuberosity	Quadrate tubercle on intertrochanteric crest of femur	Nerve to quadratus femoris (L4-S1)	Laterally rotates thigh at hip

Variations in spinal nerve contributions to the innervation of muscles, their attachments, and their actions are common in human anatomy. Therefore, expect differences between texts and realize that anatomical variation is normal.

Clinical Focus 6.5

Pressure (Decubitus) Ulcers

Pressure ulcers **(bedsores)** are common complications in patients confined to beds or wheelchairs. They form when soft tissue is compressed between a bony eminence (e.g., greater trochanter) and the bed or wheelchair. Comatose, paraplegic, or debilitated patients cannot sense discomfort caused by pressure from prolonged contact with hard surfaces. Common ulcer sites are shown in the figure, with more than half associated with the pelvic girdle (sacrum, iliac crest, ischium, and greater trochanter of femur). The four stages of these ulcers are as follows:

- **Stage I:** Changes in skin temperature, consistency, or sensation; persistent redness
- **Stage II:** Partial-thickness skin loss, similar to an abrasion with a shallow crater or blister
- **Stage III:** Full-thickness skin loss with subcutaneous tissue damage and a deep crater
- **Stage IV:** Full-thickness skin loss with necrosis or damage to muscle, bone, or adjacent structures

Sites and incidence of pressure ulcers

Occiput 1%
Chin 0.5%
Scapula 0.5%
Elbow 3%
Spinous processes 1%
Iliac crest 4%
Sacrum 23%
Trochanter 15%
Ischium 24%
Knee 6%
Pretibial crest 2%
Malleolus 7%
Heel 8%

Prone position
Supine position
Sitting position
Lateral position
Leader line key

Early deep ulceration

Extensive epidermal reaction
Cicatrization of rolled ulcer edges
Eschar
Inflammation and bacterial invasion superficial to still-intact fascial plane

Late deep ulceration

Sinus tract
Breakdown of fascial plane
Chronic inflammation and fibrosis of deep tissue (bursa formation)
Septic arthritis
Thrombosis of deep blood vessels

JOHN A.CRAIG—AD

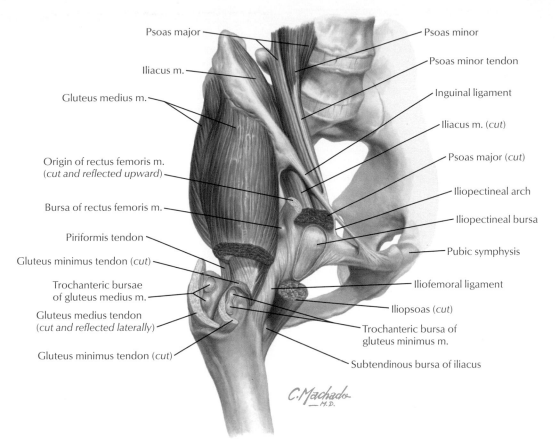

FIGURE 6.9 Hip Bursae: Posterior View. (From *Atlas of human anatomy,* ed 7, Plate 494.)

at the hip, steadying the pelvis over the lower limb when the opposite lower limb is raised off the ground.

The **tensor fasciae latae muscle** abducts, medially (internally) rotates, and stabilizes the extended knee. The deep fascia of the thigh *(fascia lata)* is especially thickened laterally and is known as the *iliotibial tract* (or band by most clinicians). Both the tensor fasciae latae muscle and most of the gluteus maximus muscles insert into this tract and help stabilize the hip, and knee extension, when one is standing. People may shift their weight from one lower limb to the other and stabilize the limb they are standing on by placing tension on this iliotibial tract.

Gluteal bursae are closed sacs that are lined with a synovial membrane and contain synovial fluid. They are located in the gluteal region and elsewhere throughout the body in regions that are subject to friction, especially where a muscle slides

across a bony prominence. Their presence reduces friction and allows the contracted muscle to slide over the bony prominence more freely. The major bursae in the gluteal region include the following (Fig. 6.9 and Clinical Focus 6.9):

- **Trochanteric bursae** of the gluteal muscles.
- **Sciatic bursae**.
- **Superior (ischial) bursa of the biceps femoris muscle (long head).**

Neurovascular Structures

The nerves innervating the gluteal muscles arise from the **sacral plexus** (see Figs. 6.7 and 6.8 and Tables 6.4 and 6.5) and gain access to the gluteal region largely by passing through the greater sciaticforamen. The blood supply to this region is via the **superior** and **inferior gluteal arteries,** which are branches of the internal iliac artery in the pelvis (see also Figs. 5.23, 5.24 and Table 5.6); these arteries also gain access to the gluteal region

Clinical Focus 6.6

Iliotibial Tract (Band) Syndrome

Iliotibial tract syndrome is common in runners and presents as lateral knee pain, often in the midrange of flexion, between 20 and 70 degrees of knee flexion. The iliotibial tract, often referred to as "iliotibial band" by clinicians, rubs across the lateral femoral condyle, and this pain also may be associated with more proximal pain from **greater trochanteric bursitis.**

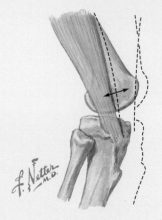

As knee flexes and extends, iliotibial tract glides back and forth over lateral femoral epicondyle, causing friction

TABLE 6.6 Features of the Femur	
STRUCTURE	**CHARACTERISTICS**
Long bone	Longest bone in the body; very strong
Head	Point of articulation with acetabulum of coxal bone
Neck	Common fracture site
Greater trochanter	Point of hip; attachment site for several gluteal muscles
Lesser trochanter	Attachment site of iliopsoas tendon (strong hip flexor)
Distal condyles	Medial and lateral (smaller) sites that articulate with tibial condyles
Patella	Sesamoid bone (largest) embedded in quadriceps femoris tendon

muscle and skin of the perineum (see Tables 5.8 and 6.4). The internal pudendal artery is the major blood supply to the perineum and external genitalia (Fig. 5.24).

5. THIGH

The thigh is the region of the lower limb between the hip and knee. As you learn the anatomical arrangement of the thigh and leg, organize your study around the functional muscular compartments. The thigh is divided into *three muscular compartments* by intermuscular septae: an anterior (extensor) compartment, a medial (adductor) compartment, and a posterior (flexor) compartment.

Bones

The **femur,** the longest bone in the body, is the bone of the thigh. It is slightly bowed anteriorly and runs slightly diagonally, lateral to medial, from the hip to the knee (Fig. 6.10 and Table 6.6). Proximally the femur articulates with the pelvis, and distally it articulates with the **tibia** and the **patella** (kneecap), which is the largest sesamoid bone in the body. The proximal femur is supplied with blood by the medial and lateral femoral circumflex branches of the deep femoral artery (see Figs. 6.5 and 6.14), by an acetabular branch of the obturator artery, and by anastomotic branches of the inferior gluteal artery (Table 6.3). The shaft and distal femur are supplied by femoral nutrient arteries and by anastomotic branches of the popliteal artery, the distal continuation of the femoral artery posterior to the knee (Fig. 6.14).

via the greater sciatic foramen. These superior and inferior gluteal neurovascular elements pass in the plane between the gluteus medius muscle (superior gluteal neurovascular bundle) and the gluteus minimus muscles, and run deep to the gluteus maximus muscle (inferior gluteal neurovascular structures). Also passing through the gluteal region is the largest nerve in the body, the **sciatic nerve** (L4-S3), which exits the greater sciatic foramen, passes through or more often inferior to the piriformis muscle, and enters the posterior thigh, passing deep to the long head of the biceps femoris muscle (see Fig. 6.8).

The **internal pudendal artery** and **pudendal nerve** (a somatic nerve, S2-S4) pass out of the greater sciatic foramen, wrap around the sacrospinous ligament, and reenter the lesser sciatic foramen to gain access to the **pudendal (Alcock's) canal** (see Figs. 5.22, 5.23, and 6.8). The pudendal nerve innervates the skeletal

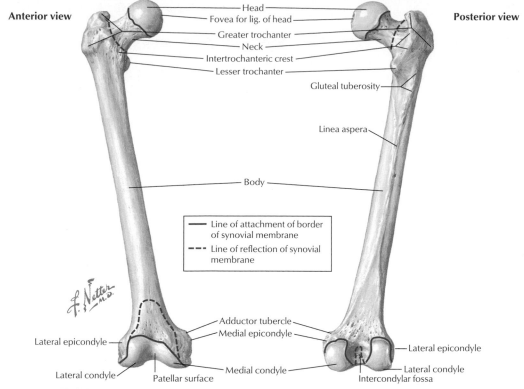

Anterior view

Head
Fovea for lig. of head
Greater trochanter
Neck
Intertrochanteric crest
Lesser trochanter

Posterior view

Gluteal tuberosity

Linea aspera

Body

— Line of attachment of border of synovial membrane
--- Line of reflection of synovial membrane

Adductor tubercle
Medial epicondyle
Lateral epicondyle
Lateral condyle
Medial condyle
Patellar surface

Lateral epicondyle
Lateral condyle
Intercondylar fossa

FIGURE 6.10 Femur. (From *Netter's atlas of human anatomy,* ed 8, Plate 500; S-172.)

Clinical Focus 6.7

Fractures of the Shaft and Distal Femur

Femoral shaft fractures occur in all age groups but are especially common in young and elderly persons. Spiral fractures usually occur from torsional forces rather than direct forces. Fractures of the distal femur are divided into two groups depending on whether the joint surface is involved. If reduction and fixation of intraarticular fractures are not satisfactory, osteoarthritis is a common posttraumatic complication.

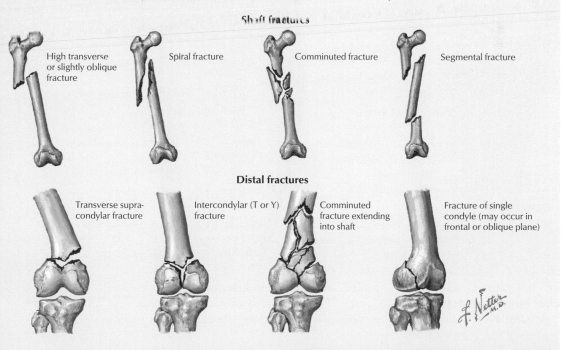

Shaft fractures

High transverse or slightly oblique fracture

Spiral fracture

Comminuted fracture

Segmental fracture

Distal fractures

Transverse supracondylar fracture

Intercondylar (T or Y) fracture

Comminuted fracture extending into shaft

Fracture of single condyle (may occur in frontal or oblique plane)

Anterior Compartment Thigh Muscles, Vessels, and Nerves

Muscles of the anterior compartment exhibit the following characteristics (Figs. 6.11 and 6.12 and Table 6.7):

- Include the **quadriceps muscles,** which attach to the patella by the quadriceps femoris tendon and to the tibia by the patellar ligament (clinicians often refer to this ligament as the "patellar tendon").
- Are primarily extensors of the leg at the knee.
- Two can secondarily flex the thigh at the hip (sartorius and rectus femoris muscles).
- Are innervated by the **femoral nerve.**
- Are supplied by the **femoral artery** and its **deep femoral artery.**

Additionally, the psoas major and iliacus muscles (which form the *iliopsoas muscle*) pass from the posterior abdominal wall to the anterior thigh by passing deep to the inguinal ligament to insert on the lesser trochanter of the femur. These muscles act jointly as powerful flexors of the thigh at the hip joint (Table 6.7; see also Fig. 4.32).

Medial Compartment Thigh Muscles, Vessels, and Nerves

Muscles of the medial compartment exhibit the following characteristics (see Figs. 6.11 and 6.12 and Table 6.8):

- Are primarily adductors of the thigh at the hip.
- Most of the muscles can secondarily flex and/or rotate the thigh.
- Are largely innervated by the **obturator nerve.**
- Are supplied by the **obturator artery** and **deep femoral artery** of the thigh.

The *pectineus muscle*, while residing in the medial compartment, is largely innervated by the femoral nerve, although it also may receive a branch from the obturator nerve. The *adductor magnus muscle*,

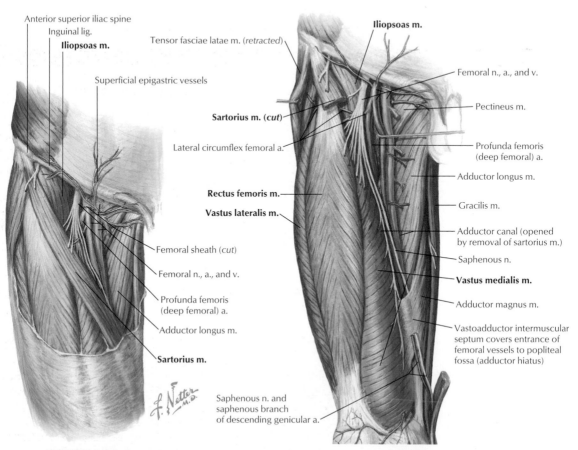

FIGURE 6.11 Anterior Compartment Thigh Muscles and Nerves. (From *Netter's atlas of human anatomy*, ed 8, Plate 490; S-270.)

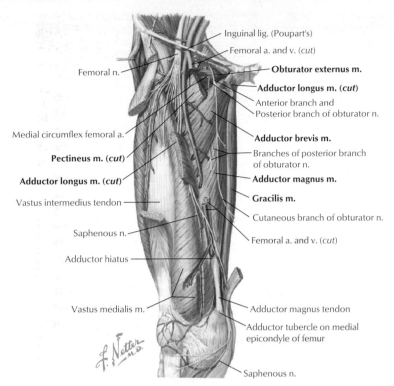

FIGURE 6.12 Medial Compartment Thigh Muscles and Nerves. (From *Netter's atlas of human anatomy,* ed 8, Plate 510; S-271.)

TABLE 6.7 Anterior Compartment Thigh Muscles

MUSCLE	PROXIMAL ATTACHMENT	DISTAL ATTACHMENT	INNERVATION	MAIN ACTIONS
Psoas major (iliopsoas)	Sides of T12-L5 vertebrae and discs between them; transverse processes of all lumbar vertebrae	Lesser trochanter of femur	Anterior rami of lumbar nerves (L1-L3)	Acts jointly with iliacus in flexing thigh at hip joint and in stabilizing hip joint
Iliacus (iliopsoas)	Iliac crest, iliac fossa, ala of sacrum, and anterior sacroiliac ligaments	Tendon of psoas major, lesser trochanter, and femur	Femoral nerve (L2-L4)	Acts jointly with psoas major in flexing thigh at hip joint and in stabilizing hip joint
Sartorius	Anterior superior iliac spine and superior part of notch inferior to it	Superior part of medial surface of tibia	Femoral nerve (L2-L3)	Flexes, abducts, and laterally rotates thigh at hip joint; flexes knee joint
Quadriceps Femoris				
Rectus femoris	Anterior inferior iliac spine and ilium superior to acetabulum	Base of patella and by patellar ligament to tibial tuberosity	Femoral nerve (L2-L4)	Extends leg at knee joint; also steadies hip joint and helps iliopsoas to flex thigh at hip
Vastus lateralis	Greater trochanter and lateral lip of linea aspera and gluteal tuberosity	Base of patella and by patellar ligament to tibial tuberosity	Femoral nerve (L2-L4)	Extends leg at knee joint
Vastus medialis	Intertrochanteric line, greater trochanter, and medial lip of linea aspera of femur	Base of patella and by patellar ligament to tibial tuberosity	Femoral nerve (L2-L4)	Extends leg at knee joint
Vastus intermedius	Anterior and lateral surfaces of femoral shaft	Base of patella and by patellar ligament to tibial tuberosity	Femoral nerve (L2-L4)	Extends leg at knee joint

Variations in spinal nerve contributions to the innervation of muscles, their attachments, and their actions are common in human anatomy. Therefore, expect differences between texts and realize that anatomical variation is normal.

TABLE 6.8 Medial Compartment Thigh Muscles

MUSCLE	PROXIMAL ATTACHMENT	DISTAL ATTACHMENT	INNERVATION	MAIN ACTIONS
Pectineus	Superior ramus of pubis	Pectineal line of femur, just inferior to lesser trochanter	Femoral nerve; may receive a branch from obturator nerve	Adducts and flexes thigh at hip
Adductor longus	Body of pubis inferior to pubic crest	Middle third of linea aspera of femur	Obturator nerve (L2-L4)	Adducts thigh at hip
Adductor brevis	Body and inferior ramus of pubis	Pectineal line and proximal part of linea aspera of femur	Obturator nerve (L2-L4)	Adducts thigh at hip and, to some extent, flexes it
Adductor magnus	Inferior ramus of pubis, ramus of ischium, and ischial tuberosity	*Adductor part:* gluteal tuberosity, linea aspera, medial supracondylar line *Hamstring part:* adductor tubercle of femur	*Adductor part:* obturator nerve *Hamstring part:* tibial part of sciatic nerve	Adducts thigh at hip *Adductor part:* also flexes thigh at hip *Hamstring part:* extends thigh
Gracilis	Body and inferior ramus of pubis	Superior part of medial surface of tibia	Obturator nerve (L2-L3)	Adducts thigh at hip; flexes leg at knee and helps to rotate it medially
Obturator externus	Margins of obturator foramen and obturator membrane	Trochanteric fossa of femur	Obturator nerve (L3-L4)	Rotates thigh laterally at hip; steadies femoral head in acetabulum

Variations in spinal nerve contributions to the innervation of muscles, their attachments, and their actions are common in human anatomy. Therefore, expect differences between texts and realize that anatomical variation is normal.

Clinical Focus 6.8

Thigh Muscle Injuries

Muscle injuries are common and may include **pulled muscles** (muscle "strain," actually a partial tearing of a muscle-tendon unit) from overstretching, or actual **muscle tears,** which can cause significant focal bleeding. **Groin injuries** usually involve muscles of the medial compartment, especially the adductor longus muscle. Because the hamstring muscles cross two joints and are actively used in walking and running, they can become pulled or torn if not adequately stretched and loosened before vigorous use. Likewise, a "charley horse" is muscle pain or stiffness often felt in the quadriceps muscles of the anterior compartment or in the hamstrings. Additionally, quadriceps muscle tears and tendon disruptions can occur, especially in athletes (see images).

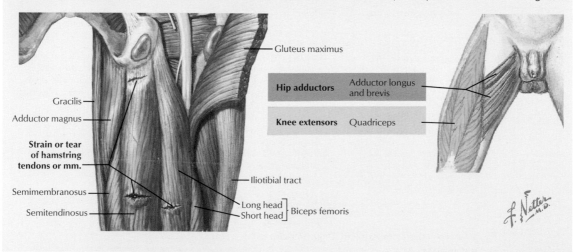

being an exceptionally large and powerful muscle, also receives some innervation via the *tibial portion of the sciatic nerve*, which runs in the posterior compartment of the thigh (Table 6.8).

Posterior Compartment Thigh Muscles, Vessels, and Nerves

Muscles of the posterior compartment exhibit the following characteristics (Figs. 6.13 and 6.8, Table 6.9):

- Are largely flexors of the leg at the knee and extensors of the thigh at the hip (except the short head of the biceps femoris muscle).
- Are collectively referred to as the *hamstrings;* can also rotate the knee and are attached proximally to the ischial tuberosity (except the short head of the biceps femoris muscle, which is *not* a hamstring muscle).
- Are innervated by the **tibial division of the sciatic nerve** (except the short head of the biceps femoris muscle, which is innervated by the common fibular division of the *sciatic nerve*).

- Are supplied by the **femoral artery** and the **deep femoral artery.**

Femoral Triangle

The **femoral triangle** is located on the anterosuperior aspect of the thigh and is bound by the following structures (see Fig. 6.11):

- **Inguinal ligament:** forms the base of the triangle.
- **Sartorius muscle:** forms the lateral boundary of the triangle.
- **Adductor longus muscle:** forms the medial boundary of the triangle.

Inferiorly, a fascial sleeve extends from the apex of the femoral triangle and is continuous with the **adductor (Hunter's) canal;** the femoral vessels course through this canal and become the *popliteal vessels* posterior to the knee. The **femoral triangle** contains the femoral nerve and vessels as they pass beneath the inguinal ligament and gain access to the anterior thigh (see Fig. 6.11). Within this triangle is a fascial sleeve called the **femoral sheath,**

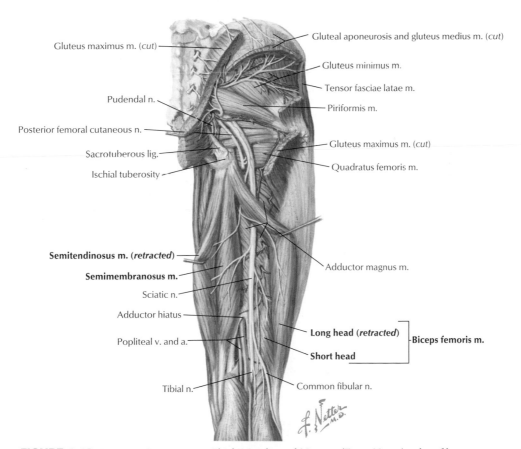

Gluteus maximus m. (*cut*)

Pudendal n.

Posterior femoral cutaneous n.

Sacrotuberous lig.

Ischial tuberosity

Gluteal aponeurosis and gluteus medius m. (*cut*)

Gluteus minimus m.

Tensor fasciae latae m.

Piriformis m.

Gluteus maximus m. (*cut*)

Quadratus femoris m.

Semitendinosus m. (*retracted*)

Semimembranosus m.

Sciatic n.

Adductor hiatus

Popliteal v. and a.

Tibial n.

Adductor magnus m.

Long head (*retracted*)

Short head

Biceps femoris m.

Common fibular n.

FIGURE 6.13 Posterior Compartment Thigh Muscles and Nerves. (From *Netter's atlas of human anatomy*, ed 8, Plate 511; S-274.)

TABLE 6.9 Posterior Compartment Thigh Muscles

MUSCLE	PROXIMAL ATTACHMENT	DISTAL ATTACHMENT	INNERVATION	MAIN ACTIONS
Semitendinosus	Ischial tuberosity	Medial surface of superior part of tibia	Tibial division of sciatic nerve (L5-S2)	Extends thigh at hip; flexes leg at knee and rotates it medially; with flexed hip and knee, extends trunk
Semimembranosus	Ischial tuberosity	Posterior part of medial condyle of tibia	Tibial division of sciatic nerve (L5-S2)	Extends thigh at hip; flexes leg at knee and rotates it medially; with flexed hip and knee, extends trunk
Biceps femoris	*Long head:* ischial tuberosity *Short head:* linea aspera and lateral supracondylar line of femur	Lateral side of head of fibula; tendon at this site split by fibular collateral ligament of knee	*Long head:* tibial division of sciatic nerve (L5-S2) *Short head:* common fibular division of sciatic nerve (L5-S2)	Flexes leg at knee and rotates it laterally; extends thigh at hip (e.g., when starting to walk)

Variations in spinal nerve contributions to the innervation of muscles, their attachments, and their actions are common in human anatomy. Therefore, expect differences between texts and realize that anatomical variation is normal.

Clinical Focus 6.9

Diagnosis of Hip, Buttock, and Back Pain

Athletically active individuals may report hip pain when the injury may actually be related to the lumbar spine (herniated disc), buttocks (bursitis or hamstring injury), or pelvic region (intrapelvic disorder). Careful follow-up should examine all potential causes of the pain to determine whether it is *referred pain* and thus originates from another source.

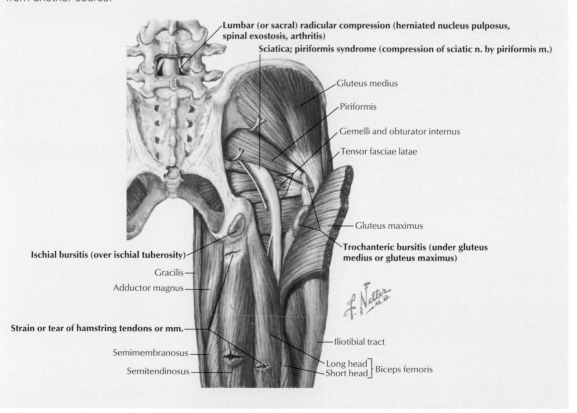

a continuation of transversalis fascia and iliac fascia of the abdomen. The femoral sheath contains the femoral artery and vein and medially the lymphatics. Laterally the femoral nerve lies within the femoral triangle but *outside* this femoral sheath. The most medial portion of the femoral sheath is called the **femoral canal** and contains the lymphatics that drain through the **femoral ring** and into the external iliac lymph nodes. The femoral canal and ring are a weak point and the site for **femoral hernias.** The femoral ring is narrow, and consequently, femoral hernias may be difficult to reduce and may be prone to strangulation.

Femoral Artery

The femoral artery supplies the tissues of the thigh and then descends into the adductor canal to gain access to the popliteal fossa (Fig. 6.14 and Table 6.10). The superomedial aspect of the thigh also is supplied by the *obturator artery.* These vessels form anastomoses around the hip (see Fig. 6.5) and, in the case of the femoral-popliteal artery, around the knee as well (see Fig. 6.14).

TABLE 6.10 Key Arteries of the Thigh

ARTERY	COURSE AND STRUCTURES SUPPLIED
Obturator	Arises from internal iliac artery (pelvis); has anterior and posterior branches; passes through obturator foramen
Femoral	Continuation of external iliac artery with numerous branches to perineum, hip, thigh, and knee
Deep femoral artery	Arises from femoral artery; supplies hip and thigh

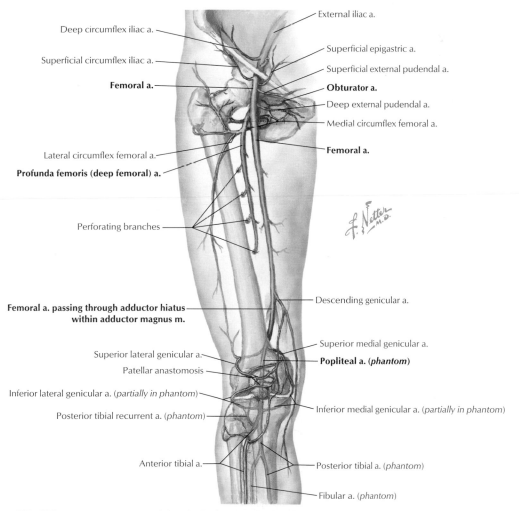

Deep circumflex iliac a.

Superficial circumflex iliac a.

Femoral a.

Lateral circumflex femoral a.

Profunda femoris (deep femoral) a.

Perforating branches

Femoral a. passing through adductor hiatus within adductor magnus m.

Superior lateral genicular a.

Patellar anastomosis

Inferior lateral genicular a. (*partially in phantom*)

Posterior tibial recurrent a. (*phantom*)

Anterior tibial a.

External iliac a.

Superficial epigastric a.

Superficial external pudendal a.

Obturator a.

Deep external pudendal a.

Medial circumflex femoral a.

Femoral a.

Descending genicular a.

Superior medial genicular a.

Popliteal a. (*phantom*)

Inferior medial genicular a. (*partially in phantom*)

Posterior tibial a. (*phantom*)

Fibular a. (*phantom*)

FIGURE 6.14 Key Arteries of the Thigh. (From *Netter's atlas of human anatomy,* ed 8, Plate 522; S-333.)

Clinical Focus 6.10

Revascularization of the Lower Limb

Peripheral vascular disease and claudication can usually be managed medically by reducing the associated risk factors. However, patients who are refractory to medical management have the following invasive options:

- Percutaneous angioplasty: balloon dilation (with or without an endovascular stent) for recanalization of a stenosed artery (percutaneous revascularization)
- Surgical bypass: bypassing a diseased segment of the artery with a graft (operative mortality rate of 1% to 3%)

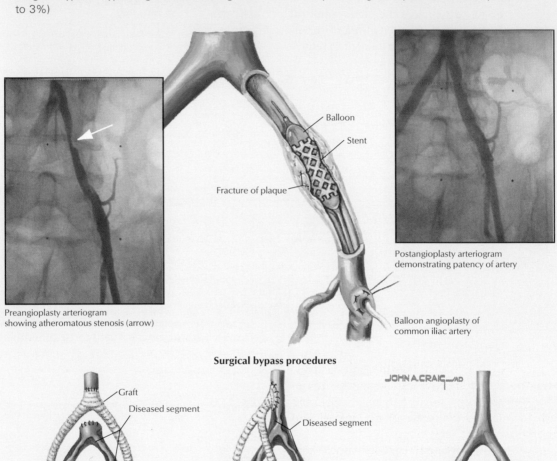

Balloon

Stent

Fracture of plaque

Preangioplasty arteriogram
showing atheromatous stenosis (arrow)

Postangioplasty arteriogram
demonstrating patency of artery

Balloon angioplasty of
common iliac artery

Surgical bypass procedures

JOHN A.CRAIG—MD

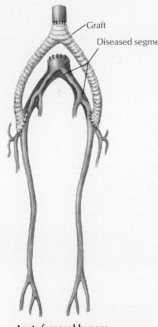

Graft

Diseased segment

Aortofemoral bypass

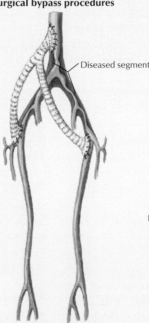

Diseased segment

Aortofemoral bypass

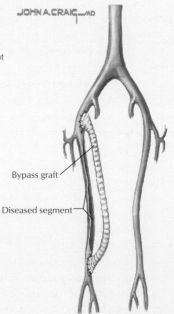

Bypass graft

Diseased segment

Femoral-popliteal bypass

Clinical Focus 6.11

Femoral Pulse and Vascular Access

The femoral pulse is felt at about the midpoint of the inguinal ligament. The femoral artery at this point lies directly over or just medial to the femoral head, just lateral to the femoral vein and about a finger's breadth medial to the femoral nerve (see Figs. 6.11 and 6.14). The femoral artery and vein may be used to gain access to major vessels of the limbs, abdominopelvic cavity, and thorax (e.g., catheter threaded through femoral artery and into aorta for coronary artery angiography and angioplasty). Similarly, access to the larger veins of the inferior vena cava and the right side of the heart and pulmonary veins may be obtained through the femoral vein.

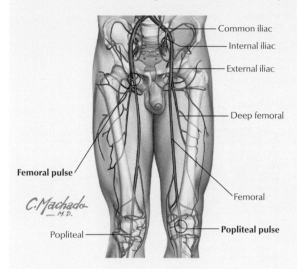

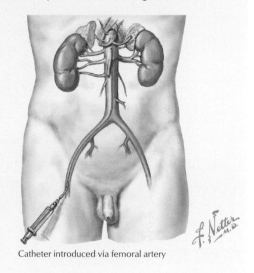

Catheter introduced via femoral artery

Thigh in Cross Section

Cross sections of the thigh show the three compartments and their respective muscles and neurovascular elements (Fig. 6.15). Lateral, medial, and posterior *intermuscular septae* divide the thigh into the following three sections:

- **Anterior compartment:** contains muscles that primarily extend the leg at the knee and are innervated by the *femoral nerve.*
- **Medial compartment:** contains muscles that primarily adduct the thigh at the hip and are innervated largely by the *obturator nerve.*
- **Posterior compartment:** contains muscles that primarily extend the thigh at the hip and flex the leg at the knee and are innervated by the *sciatic nerve* (tibial portion).

Refer to the muscle tables to note several exceptions to these general divisions. However, *learning the primary action and general innervation of the muscles by functional compartments will help you organize your study.* Also, note that the large **sciatic nerve** usually begins to separate into its two component nerves—the **tibial nerve** and the

common fibular nerve—in the thigh, although this separation may occur proximally in the gluteal region in some cases.

6. LEG

Bones

The bones of the leg (defined as the portion of the lower limb extending from the knee to the ankle) are the medially placed **tibia** and lateral **fibula** (Fig. 6.16 and Table 6.11). The tibia is *weight-bearing* in the leg, and the two bones are joined by a fibrous interosseous membrane. The tibia is subcutaneous from the knee to the ankle (our shin) and vulnerable to injury along its length. The fibula functions primarily for *muscle attachments,* forms part of the ankle joint, and acts as a pulley for the fibularis longus and fibularis brevis muscle tendons (everting the foot at the ankle).

Knee Joint

The knee is the most sophisticated joint in the body and the largest of the synovial joints. It participates in flexion, extension, and some gliding

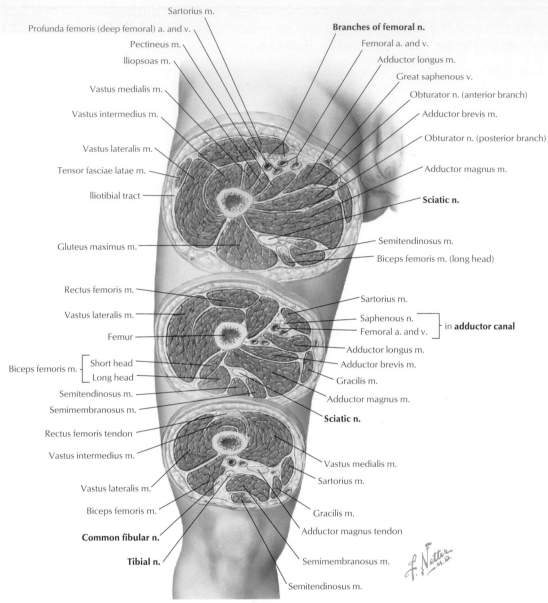

FIGURE 6.15 Serial Cross Sections of the Thigh. (From *Netter's atlas of human anatomy*, ed 8, Plate 476; S-153.)

TABLE 6.11 Features of the Tibia and Fibula

FEATURE	CHARACTERISTICS	FEATURE	CHARACTERISTICS
Tibia		Medial malleolus	Prominence on medial aspect of ankle
Long bone	Large, weight-bearing bone		
Proximal facets	Large plateau for articulation with femoral condyles	**Fibula**	
		Long bone	Slender bone, primarily for muscle attachment
Tibial tuberosity	Insertion site for patellar ligament		
Inferior articular surface	Surface for cupping talus at ankle joint	Neck	Possible damage to common fibular nerve if fracture occurs here

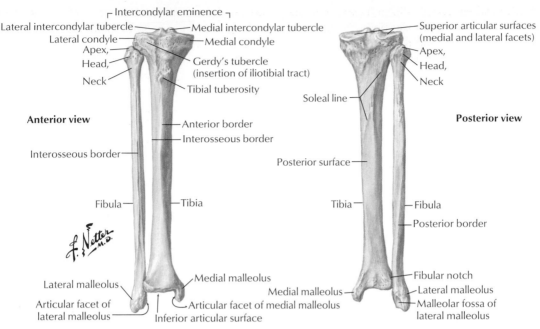

Intercondylar eminence
Lateral intercondylar tubercle
Lateral condyle
Apex,
Head,
Neck

Medial intercondylar tubercle
Medial condyle
Gerdy's tubercle
(insertion of iliotibial tract)
Tibial tuberosity

Superior articular surfaces
(medial and lateral facets)
Apex,
Head,
Neck

Anterior view

Anterior border
Interosseous border

Soleal line

Posterior view

Interosseous border

Posterior surface

Fibula   Tibia

Tibia   Fibula

Posterior border

Lateral malleolus

Articular facet of
lateral malleolus

Medial malleolus

Medial malleolus

Articular facet of medial malleolus
Inferior articular surface

Fibular notch
Lateral malleolus
Malleolar fossa of
lateral malleolus

FIGURE 6.16 Tibia and Fibula of the Right Leg. (From *Netter's atlas of human anatomy,* ed 8, Plate 524; S-174.)

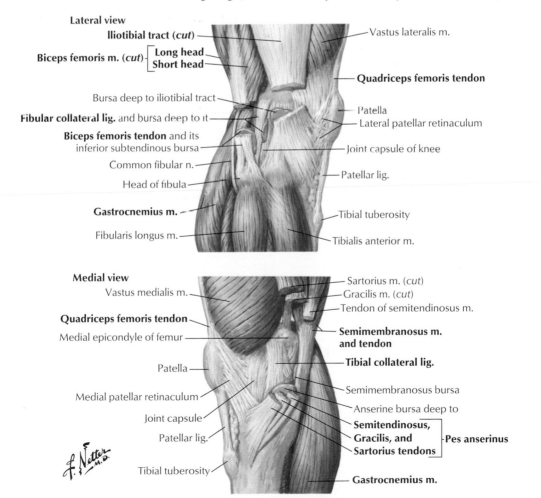

Lateral view
Iliotibial tract (*cut*)
Biceps femoris m. (*cut*) [**Long head** / **Short head**]

Vastus lateralis m.

Quadriceps femoris tendon

Bursa deep to iliotibial tract
Fibular collateral lig. and bursa deep to it
Biceps femoris tendon and its
inferior subtendinous bursa
Common fibular n.
Head of fibula

Patella
Lateral patellar retinaculum

Joint capsule of knee

Patellar lig.

Gastrocnemius m.
Fibularis longus m.

Tibial tuberosity
Tibialis anterior m.

Medial view
Vastus medialis m.

Sartorius m. (*cut*)
Gracilis m. (*cut*)
Tendon of semitendinosus m.

Quadriceps femoris tendon
Medial epicondyle of femur

**Semimembranosus m.
and tendon**

Tibial collateral lig.

Patella
Medial patellar retinaculum
Joint capsule
Patellar lig.

Semimembranosus bursa
Anserine bursa deep to
**Semitendinosus,
Gracilis, and
Sartorius tendons**] **Pes anserinus**

Tibial tuberosity

Gastrocnemius m.

FIGURE 6.17 Muscle Tendon Support of the Knee. (From *Netter's atlas of human anatomy,* ed 8, Plate 516; S-279.)

and rotation when flexed. With full extension, the *femur rotates medially* on the tibia, the supporting ligaments tighten, and the knee is *locked* into position. The knee consists of the articulation between the femur and the tibia (biaxial condylar synovial joint), and between the patella and the femur.

Features of the knee joint are shown in Figs. 6.17 (muscle tendon support), 6.18 and 6.20 (ligaments), 6.19 (radiographs), and 6.20 (bursae) and are summarized in Tables 6.12 to 6.14. Because of the number of muscle-tendon units running across the knee joint, several bursae protect the underlying structures from friction (Figs. 6.17, 6.18 and 6.20). The first four of the bursae listed in Table 6.14 also communicate with the synovial cavity of the knee joint. The vascular supply to the knee primarily arises from genicular branches of the **popliteal artery,** the inferior continuation of the femoral artery (Fig. 6.14).

The innervation to the knee joint is via articular branches from the *femoral, obturator, tibial, and common fibular nerves.*

The **proximal (superior) tibiofibular joint** is a plane synovial joint between the fibular head and the lateral condyle of the tibia (Fig. 6.21). The joint is stabilized by a wider and stronger anterior ligament and a narrow weaker posterior ligament; this joint allows for some minimal gliding movement.

Popliteal Fossa

The popliteal fossa is a "diamond-shaped" region behind the knee and contains the popliteal vessels

Text continued on p. 324.

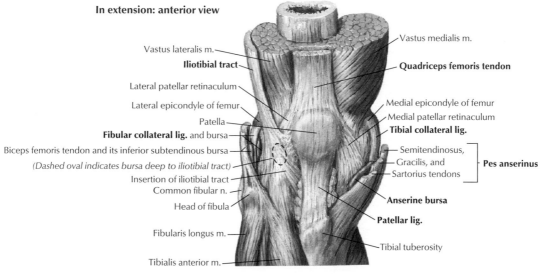

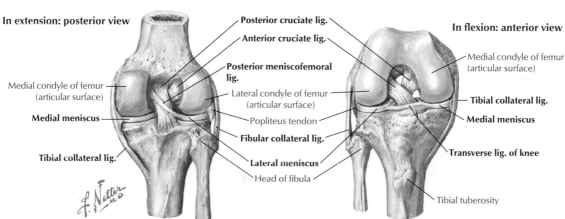

FIGURE 6.18 Ligaments of the Right Knee. (From *Netter's atlas of human anatomy,* ed 8, Plates 517 and 519; S-280 and S-173.)

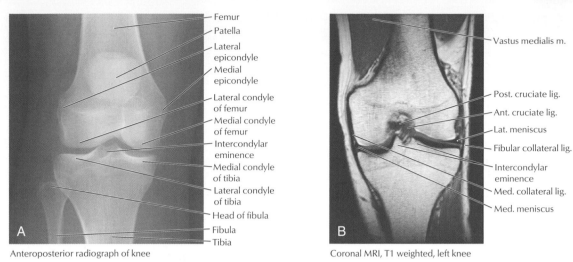

Anteroposterior radiograph of knee   Coronal MRI, T1 weighted, left knee

FIGURE 6.19 Radiograph and MR Image of Knee. (**B** from Bo W et al: *Basic atlas of sectional anatomy*, ed 4, Philadelphia, 2007, Saunders.)

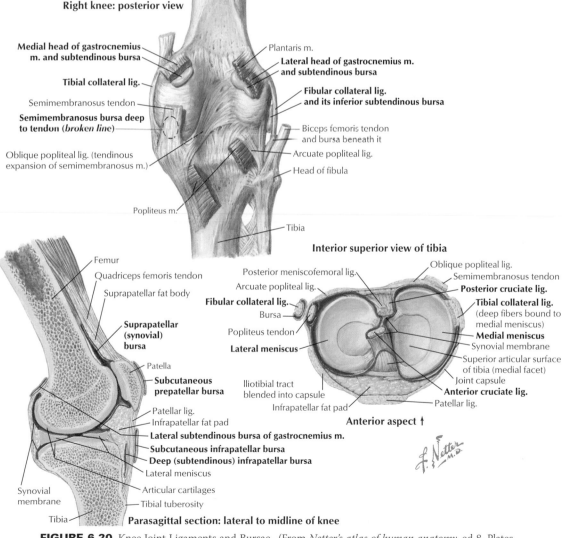

FIGURE 6.20 Knee Joint Ligaments and Bursae. (From *Netter's atlas of human anatomy*, ed 8, Plates 518 and 521; S-281 and S-282.)

TABLE 6.12 Muscle Tendon Support of the Knee

MUSCLE AND TENDON	COMMENT
Lateral Aspect	
Biceps femoris	Posterolateral support, attaching to fibular head
Gastrocnemius (lateral)	Support somewhat more posteriorly
Iliotibial tract	Lateral support and stabilization
Popliteus	Located posterolaterally beneath the fibular collateral ligament
Medial Aspect	
Semimembranosus	Posteromedial support
Gastrocnemius (medial)	Support somewhat more posteriorly
Pes anserinus	Semitendinosus, gracilis, and sartorius tendons (looks like a goose's foot), attaching to medial tibial condyle

TABLE 6.14 Features of the Knee Joint Bursae

BURSA	LOCATION
Suprapatellar	Between quadriceps tendon and femur
Popliteus	Between popliteus tendon and lateral tibial condyle
Anserine	Between pes anserinus and tibia and tibial collateral ligament
Subtendinous	Deep to heads of the gastrocnemius muscles
Semimembranosus	Deep to the tendon of the semimembranosus muscle
Prepatellar	Between skin and patella
Subcutaneous infrapatellar	Between skin and tibia
Deep infrapatellar	Between patellar ligament and tibia

TABLE 6.13 Ligaments of the Knee

LIGAMENT	ATTACHMENT	COMMENT
Knee (Biaxial Condylar Synovial) Joint		
Capsule	Surrounds femoral and tibial condyles and patella	Is fibrous, weak (offers little support); flexion, extension, some gliding and medial rotation
Extracapsular Ligaments		
Tibial collateral	Medial femoral epicondyle to medial tibial condyle	Limits extension and abduction of leg; attached to medial meniscus
Fibular collateral	Lateral femoral epicondyle to fibular head	Limits extension and adduction of leg; overlies popliteus tendon
Patellar	Patella to tibial tuberosity	Acts in extension of quadriceps tendon
Arcuate popliteal	Fibular head to capsule	Passes over popliteus muscle
Oblique popliteal	Semimembranosus tendon to posterior knee	Limits hyperextension and lateral rotation
Intracapsular Ligaments		
Medial meniscus	Interarticular area of tibia, lies over medial facet, attached to tibial collateral	Is semicircular (C-shaped); acts as cushion; often torn
Lateral meniscus	Interarticular area of tibia, lies over lateral facet	Is more circular and smaller than medial meniscus; acts as cushion
Anterior cruciate	Anterior intercondylar tibia to lateral femoral condyle	Prevents posterior slipping of femur on tibia; torn in hyperextension
Posterior cruciate	Posterior intercondylar tibia to medial femoral condyle	Prevents anterior slipping of femur on tibia; shorter and stronger than anterior cruciate
Transverse	Anterior aspect of menisci	Binds and stabilizes menisci
Posterior meniscofemoral (of Wrisberg)	Posterior lateral meniscus to medial femoral condyle	Is strong
Patellofemoral (Biaxial Synovial Saddle) Joint		
Quadriceps tendon	Muscles to superior patella	Is part of extension mechanism
Patellar	Patella to tibial tuberosity	Acts in extension of quadriceps tendon; patella stabilized by medial and lateral ligament (retinaculum) attachment to tibia and femur

Anterior view with ligament attachments

Superior view

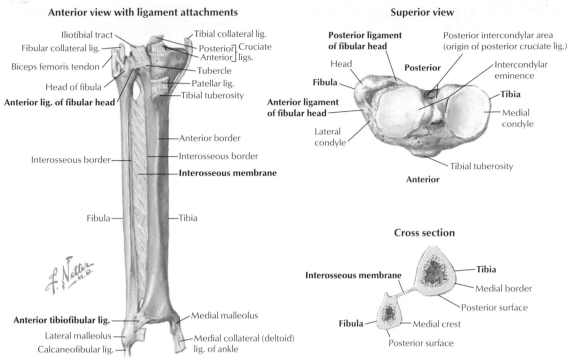

FIGURE 6.21 Tibiofibular Joint and Ligaments. (From *Netter's atlas of human anatomy*, ed 8, Plate 525; S-175.)

Clinical Focus 6.12

Multiple Myeloma

Multiple myeloma, a **tumor of plasma cells**, is the most malignant type of primary bone tumor. This painful tumor is sensitive to radiation therapy, and newer chemotherapeutic agents and bone marrow transplantation offer hope for improved survival. Fever, weight loss, fatigue, anemia, thrombocytopenia, and renal failure are associated with this cancer, which usually occurs in middle age.

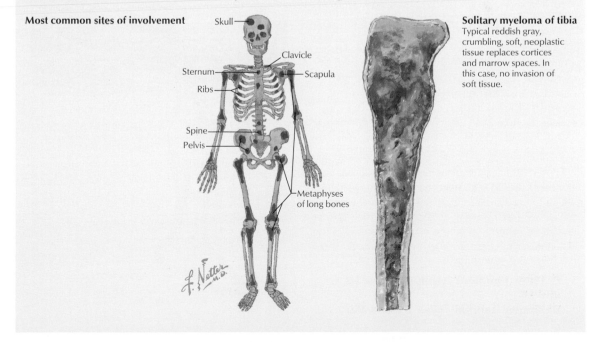

Most common sites of involvement

Solitary myeloma of tibia
Typical reddish gray, crumbling, soft, neoplastic tissue replaces cortices and marrow spaces. In this case, no invasion of soft tissue.

Tibial Fractures

Six types of tibial plateau fractures are recognized, most of which involve the lateral tibial condyle (plateau). Most result from direct trauma and, because they involve the articular surface, must be stabilized. Fractures of the tibial shaft are the *most common fractures* of a long bone. Because the tibia is largely subcutaneous along its medial border, many of these fractures are open injuries. Often, both tibia and fibula are fractured.

Tibial plateau fracture

 I. Split fracture of lateral tibial plateau

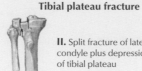 **II.** Split fracture of lateral condyle plus depression of tibial plateau

 III. Depression of lateral tibial plateau without split fracture

 IV. Comminuted split fracture of medial tibial plateau and tibial spine

 V. Bicondylar fracture involving both tibial plateaus with widening

 VI. Fracture of lateral tibial plateau with separation of metaphyseal-diaphyseal junction

Fracture of shaft of tibia

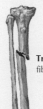 **Transverse fracture;** fibula intact

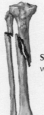 **Spiral fracture** with shortening

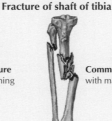 **Comminuted fracture** with marked shortening

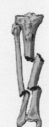 **Segmental fracture** with marked shortening

Deep Tendon Reflexes

A brisk tap to a partially stretched muscle tendon near its point of insertion elicits a myotactic (muscle stretch) deep tendon reflex (DTR) that is dependent on the following:

- Intact afferent (sensory) nerve fibers
- Normal functional synapses in the spinal cord at the appropriate level
- Intact efferent (motor) nerve fibers
- Normal functional neuromuscular junctions on the tapped muscle
- Normal muscle fiber functioning (contraction)

The DTR usually involves only several spinal cord segments (and their afferent and efferent nerve fibers). If a pathologic process is involved at the level tested, the reflex may be weak or absent, requiring further testing to determine where along the pathway the lesion occurred. For the lower limb, you should know the following segmental levels for the DTR:

- **Patellar ligament (tendon) reflex L3 and L4**
- **Calcaneal tendon reflex S1 and S2**

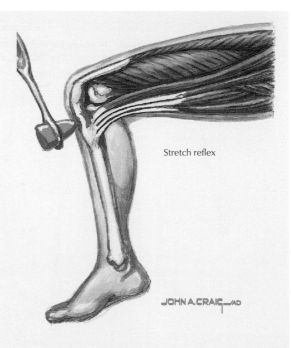

Stretch reflex

Patellar Injuries

Subluxation of the patella, usually laterally, is a fairly common occurrence, especially in adolescent girls and young women. It often presents with tenderness along the medial patellar aspect and atrophy of the quadriceps tendon, especially the oblique portion medially derived from the vastus medialis. **Patellar ligament rupture** usually occurs just inferior to the patella as a result of direct trauma in younger people. **Quadriceps tendon rupture** occurs mostly in older individuals, from either minor trauma or age-related degenerative changes, including the following:

- Arthritis
- Arteriosclerosis
- Chronic renal failure
- Corticosteroid therapy
- Diabetes
- Hyperparathyroidism
- Gout

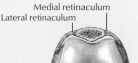

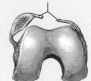

Skyline view. Normally, patella rides in groove between medial and lateral femoral condyles.

In subluxation, patella deviates laterally because of weakness of vastus medialis muscle and tightness of lateral retinaculum.

In dislocation, patella is displaced completely out of intercondylar groove.

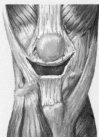

Patellar ligament rupture
Rupture of patellar ligament at inferior margin of patella

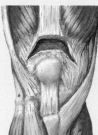

Quadriceps tendon rupture
Rupture of quadriceps femoris tendon at superior margin of patella

Rupture of the Anterior Cruciate Ligament

Rupture of the anterior cruciate ligament (ACL) is a common athletic injury usually related to sharp turns, when the knee is twisted while the foot is firmly on the ground. The patient may hear a popping sound and feel a tearing sensation associated with acute pain. Joint stability can be assessed by using the Lachman and **anterior drawer tests**. With an ACL injury, the tibia moves anteriorly (the ACL normally limits knee hyperextension) in the anterior drawer test and back and forth in the Lachman test.

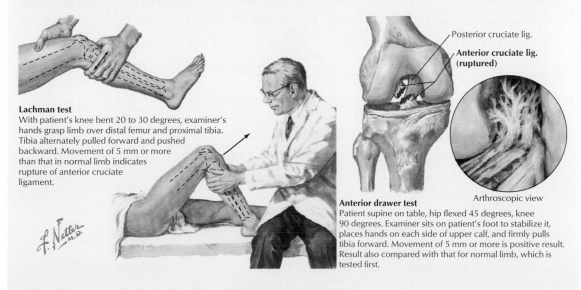

Lachman test
With patient's knee bent 20 to 30 degrees, examiner's hands grasp limb over distal femur and proximal tibia. Tibia alternately pulled forward and pushed backward. Movement of 5 mm or more than that in normal limb indicates rupture of anterior cruciate ligament.

Posterior cruciate lig.

Anterior cruciate lig. (ruptured)

Arthroscopic view

Anterior drawer test
Patient supine on table, hip flexed 45 degrees, knee 90 degrees. Examiner sits on patient's foot to stabilize it, places hands on each side of upper calf, and firmly pulls tibia forward. Movement of 5 mm or more is positive result. Result also compared with that for normal limb, which is tested first.

Sprains of the Knee Ligaments

Ligament injuries (sprains) of the knee are common in athletes and can be characterized as:

- First degree: stretched ligament with little or no tearing
- Second degree: partial tearing of the ligament with joint laxity
- Third degree: complete rupture of the ligament, resulting in an unstable joint

Damage to the tibial collateral ligament may also involve a tear of the medial meniscus, as the meniscus is attached to the ligament. The **"unhappy triad"**—tears of these structures and the ACL—is usually the result of a direct blow to the lateral aspect of the knee with the foot on the ground.

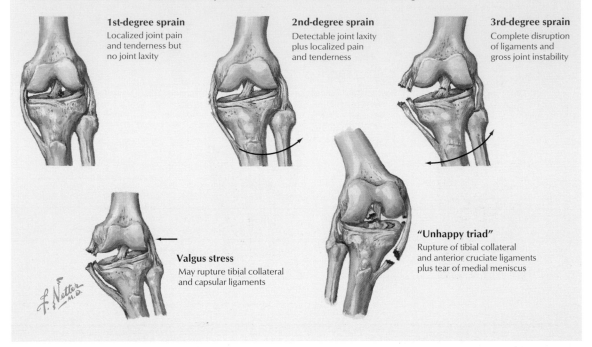

1st-degree sprain
Localized joint pain and tenderness but no joint laxity

2nd-degree sprain
Detectable joint laxity plus localized pain and tenderness

3rd-degree sprain
Complete disruption of ligaments and gross joint instability

Valgus stress
May rupture tibial collateral and capsular ligaments

"Unhappy triad"
Rupture of tibial collateral and anterior cruciate ligaments plus tear of medial meniscus

Tears of the Meniscus

The fibrocartilaginous menisci are often torn when the knee undergoes a twisting injury. Patients complain of pain at the joint line, and the involved knee "gives way" when flexed or extended. Rupture of the tibial collateral ligament often involves a tear of the medial meniscus because the ligament and meniscus are attached.

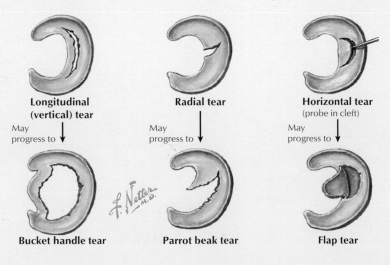

Longitudinal (vertical) tear
May progress to ↓

Radial tear
May progress to ↓

Horizontal tear
(probe in cleft)
May progress to ↓

Bucket handle tear

Parrot beak tear

Flap tear

Osgood-Schlatter Lesion

Osgood-Schlatter lesion (OSL) is a *partial avulsion of the tibial tuberosity*. During normal fetal development, the tuberosity develops as a distinct anterior segment of the epiphysis of the proximal tibia. After birth, this segment develops its own growth plate composed mostly of fibrocartilage instead of hyaline cartilage, the fibrocartilage perhaps serving as a means to handle the tensile stress placed on the tuberosity by the patellar ligament. The tuberosity normally ossifies and joins with the tibial epiphysis, but in OSL, repetitive stress on the tuberosity may cause it to separate (avulse) from the tibia. The avulsed fragment continues to grow, with the intervening space filled with new bone or fibrous connective tissue, so that the tibial tuberosity is enlarged. At times, a painful prominence occurs. OSL is usually more common in children who engage in vigorous physical activity than in less active children.

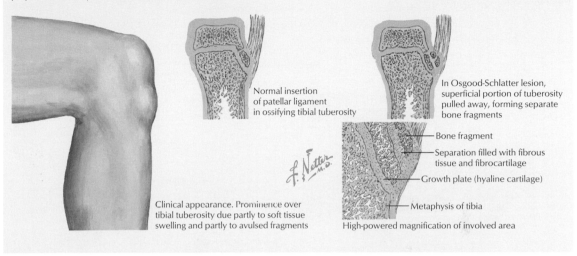

Normal insertion of patellar ligament in ossifying tibial tuberosity

In Osgood-Schlatter lesion, superficial portion of tuberosity pulled away, forming separate bone fragments

Bone fragment

Separation filled with fibrous tissue and fibrocartilage

Growth plate (hyaline cartilage)

Metaphysis of tibia

Clinical appearance. Prominence over tibial tuberosity due partly to soft tissue swelling and partly to avulsed fragments

High-powered magnification of involved area

Osteoarthritis of the Knee

As with arthritis of the hip, osteoarthritis of the knee is a painful condition associated with activity, although other causes may also precipitate painful episodes, including changes in the weather. Stiffness after inactivity and decreased range of motion are common. With time, subluxation of the knee may occur with a varus **(bowleg) deformity.**

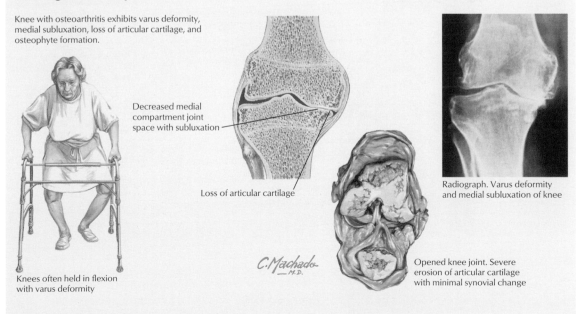

Knee with osteoarthritis exhibits varus deformity, medial subluxation, loss of articular cartilage, and osteophyte formation.

Decreased medial compartment joint space with subluxation

Loss of articular cartilage

Radiograph. Varus deformity and medial subluxation of knee

Knees often held in flexion with varus deformity

Opened knee joint. Severe erosion of articular cartilage with minimal synovial change

Clinical Focus 6.21

Septic Bursitis and Arthritis

Humans have more than 150 bursae in their subcutaneous tissues. With increased irritation, these bursae, which are lined with synovium and contain synovial fluid, produce more fluid until significant swelling and bacterial infection occur. The result is septic bursitis, characterized by the following:

- Heat over the affected area
- Swelling
- Local tenderness
- Limited range of motion

  Septic arthritis occurs when infection gains entry to the joint space. If initial therapy fails, surgical debridement and lengthy antibiotic treatment may be needed.

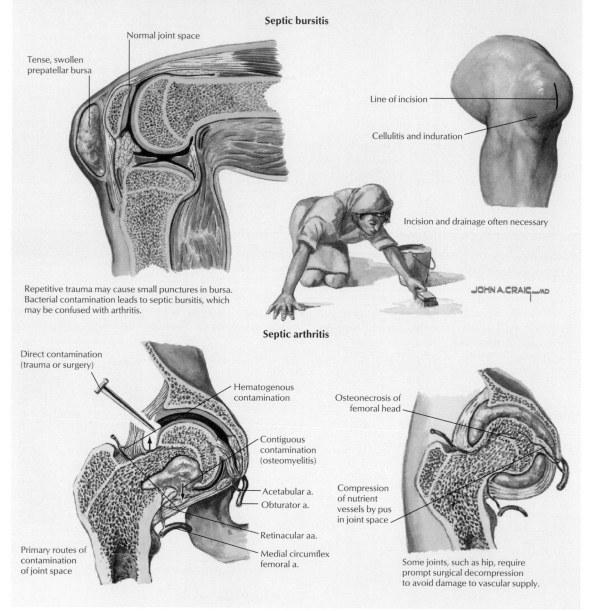

Septic bursitis

Normal joint space

Tense, swollen
prepatellar bursa

Line of incision

Cellulitis and induration

Incision and drainage often necessary

Repetitive trauma may cause small punctures in bursa.
Bacterial contamination leads to septic bursitis, which
may be confused with arthritis.

JOHN A. CRAIG—AD

Septic arthritis

Direct contamination
(trauma or surgery)

Hematogenous
contamination

Osteonecrosis of
femoral head

Contiguous
contamination
(osteomyelitis)

Acetabular a.
Obturator a.

Compression
of nutrient
vessels by pus
in joint space

Retinacular aa.

Medial circumflex
femoral a.

Primary routes of
contamination
of joint space

Some joints, such as hip, require
prompt surgical decompression
to avoid damage to vascular supply.

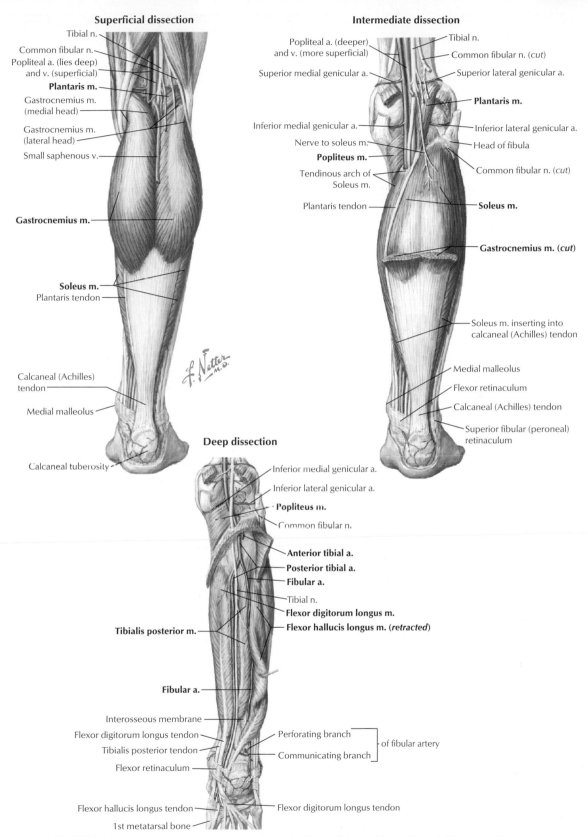

Superficial dissection

Tibial n.
Common fibular n.
Popliteal a. (lies deep) and v. (superficial)
Plantaris m.
Gastrocnemius m. (medial head)
Gastrocnemius m. (lateral head)
Small saphenous v.

Gastrocnemius m.

Soleus m.
Plantaris tendon

Calcaneal (Achilles) tendon

Medial malleolus

Calcaneal tuberosity

Intermediate dissection

Popliteal a. (deeper) and v. (more superficial)
Superior medial genicular a.

Inferior medial genicular a.
Nerve to soleus m.
Popliteus m.
Tendinous arch of Soleus m.
Plantaris tendon

Tibial n.
Common fibular n. (cut)
Superior lateral genicular a.
Plantaris m.
Inferior lateral genicular a.
Head of fibula
Common fibular n. (cut)
Soleus m.
Gastrocnemius m. (cut)

Soleus m. inserting into calcaneal (Achilles) tendon
Medial malleolus
Flexor retinaculum
Calcaneal (Achilles) tendon
Superior fibular (peroneal) retinaculum

Deep dissection

Inferior medial genicular a.
Inferior lateral genicular a.
Popliteus m.
Common fibular n.
Anterior tibial a.
Posterior tibial a.
Fibular a.
Tibial n.
Flexor digitorum longus m.
Flexor hallucis longus m. (retracted)

Tibialis posterior m.

Fibular a.

Interosseous membrane
Flexor digitorum longus tendon
Tibialis posterior tendon
Flexor retinaculum

Perforating branch
Communicating branch
} of fibular artery

Flexor hallucis longus tendon
1st metatarsal bone
Flexor digitorum longus tendon

FIGURE 6.22 Posterior Compartment Leg Muscles (Superficial and Deep Group), Vessels, and Nerves. (From *Netter's atlas of human anatomy*, ed 8, Plates 527 to 529; S-284 to S-286.)

and the tibial and common fibular nerves (Fig. 6.22). This fossa marks the transition region between the thigh and the leg, where the neurovascular components of the thigh pass to the flexor side of the knee joint. *(At most joints, the neurovascular bundles pass on the flexor side of the joint.)* The superior margins of this diamond-shaped fossa are formed medially by the distal portions of the semitendinosus and semimembranosus muscles,

and laterally by the distal end of the long head of the biceps femoris muscle. The lower margins of the diamond are formed medially by the medial head of the gastrocnemius muscle and laterally by the plantaris and lateral head of the gastrocnemius muscles (see Figs. 6.13 and 6.22). The small saphenous vein courses subcutaneously upward toward the knee in the midline of the calf and drains into the popliteal vein (see Fig. 6.2).

Clinical Focus 6.22
Shin Splints

Shin splints cause pain along the inner or medial distal two-thirds of the tibial shaft. The syndrome is common in athletes. The primary cause is repetitive pulling of the tibialis posterior tendon as one pushes off the foot during running (see Clinical Focus 6.25 for description of anterior or lateral shin splints). Stress on the muscle occurs at its attachment to the tibia and interosseous membrane. Chronic conditions can produce periostitis and bone remodeling or can lead to stress fractures. Pain usually begins as soreness after running that worsens and then occurs while walking or climbing stairs.

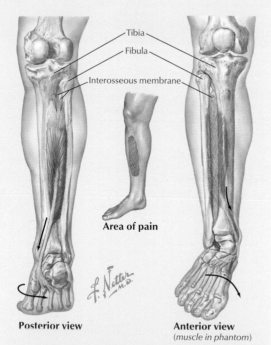

Tibia
Fibula
Interosseous membrane

Area of pain

Posterior view

Anterior view
(muscle in phantom)

Tibialis posterior muscle originates at posterior surface of tibia, interosseous membrane, and fibula and inserts on undersurface of navicular bone, cuboid, all three cuneiform bones, and 2nd, 3rd, and 4th metatarsal bones. Upper arrows indicate direction of excessive traction of tendon on tibial periosteum and interosseous membrane caused by hypereversion (lower arrows).

Clinical Focus 6.23
Osteosarcoma of the Tibia

Osteosarcoma is the most common malignant bone tumor of mesenchymal origin. It is more common in males and usually occurs before 30 years of age, often in the distal femur or proximal tibia. Other sites include the proximal humerus, proximal femur, and pelvis. Most tumors appear in the metaphysis of long bones at areas of greatest growth. The tumors often invade cortical bone in this region because of its rich vascular supply and then infiltrate surrounding soft tissue. These tumors are aggressive and require immediate attention.

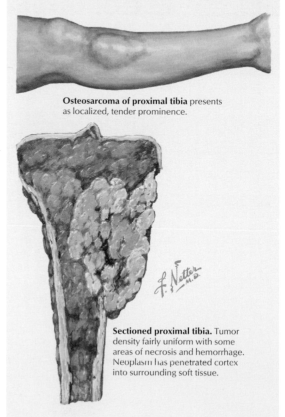

Osteosarcoma of proximal tibia presents as localized, tender prominence.

Sectioned proximal tibia. Tumor density fairly uniform with some areas of necrosis and hemorrhage. Neoplasm has penetrated cortex into surrounding soft tissue.

Posterior Compartment Leg Muscles, Vessels, and Nerves

The posterior compartment leg muscles are arranged into a *superficial group* (gastrocnemius, plantaris, soleus) and a *deep group* (remaining posterior compartment muscles). These muscles exhibit the following general features (Fig. 6.22 and Table 6.15):

- Are primarily flexors of the foot at the ankle (plantarflexion) and flexors of the toes.
- Several of these muscles can flex the leg at the knee or invert the foot.
- Are innervated by the **tibial nerve.**
- Are supplied by the **posterior tibial artery** (the popliteal artery divides into the anterior and posterior tibial arteries) with some supply from the **fibular artery** (a branch of the posterior tibial artery).

Anterior Compartment Leg Muscles, Vessels, and Nerves

The muscles of the anterior compartment exhibit the following features (Fig. 6.23 and Table 6.16):

- Are primarily extensors of the foot at the ankle (dorsiflexion) and extensors of the toes.
- Several of these muscles can invert the foot, and one muscle (fibularis tertius) can weakly evert the foot.
- Are innervated by the **deep fibular nerve** (the common fibular nerve divides into the superficial and deep branches).
- Are supplied by the **anterior tibial artery.**

Lateral Compartment Leg Muscles, Vessels, and Nerves

The two muscles of the lateral compartment exhibit the following features (Figs. 6.22 and 6.24; Table 6.17):

- Are primarily able to evert the foot, and can weakly plantarflex the foot at the ankle.
- Are innervated by the **superficial fibular nerve.**
- Are supplied by the **fibular artery,** a branch of the posterior tibial artery (see Fig. 6.22).

Leg in Cross Section

The interosseous membrane and intermuscular septae divide the leg into three compartments. The

TABLE 6.15 Posterior Compartment Leg Muscles and Nerves

MUSCLE	PROXIMAL ATTACHMENT	DISTAL ATTACHMENT	INNERVATION	MAIN ACTIONS
Gastrocnemius	*Lateral head:* lateral aspect of lateral condyle of femur *Medial head:* popliteal surface of femur, superior to medial condyle	Posterior surface of calcaneus via calcaneal tendon	Tibial nerve (S1-S2)	Plantarflexes foot at ankle; flexes leg at knee joint
Soleus	Posterior aspect of head of fibula, superior fourth of posterior surface of fibula, soleal line and medial border of tibia	Posterior surface of calcaneus via calcaneal tendon	Tibial nerve (S1-S2)	Plantarflexes foot at ankle; steadies leg over foot
Plantaris	Inferior end of lateral supracondylar line of femur and oblique popliteal ligament	Posterior surface of calcaneus via calcaneal tendon	Tibial nerve (L5-S1)	Weakly assists gastrocnemius in plantarflexing foot at ankle and flexing knee
Popliteus	Lateral condyle of femur and lateral meniscus	Posterior surface of tibia, superior to soleal line	Tibial nerve (L4-S1)	Weakly flexes leg at knee and unlocks it (rotates femur on fixed tibia)
Flexor hallucis longus	Inferior two-thirds of posterior surface of fibula and inferior interosseous membrane	Base of distal phalanx of great toe (big toe)	Tibial nerve (L5-S2)	Flexes great toe at all joints and plantarflexes foot at ankle
Flexor digitorum longus	Medial part of posterior surface of tibia inferior to soleal line	Plantar bases of distal phalanges of lateral four digits	Tibial nerve (L5-S2)	Flexes lateral four digits and plantarflexes foot at ankle; supports longitudinal arches of foot
Tibialis posterior	Interosseous membrane, posterior surface of tibia inferior to soleal line, and posterior surface of fibula	Tuberosity of navicular, cuneiform, and cuboid and bases of metatarsals 2, 3, and 4	Tibial nerve (L4-L5)	Plantarflexes foot at ankle and inverts foot

Variations in spinal nerve contributions to the innervation of muscles, their attachments, and their actions are common in human anatomy. Therefore, expect differences between texts and realize that anatomical variation is normal.

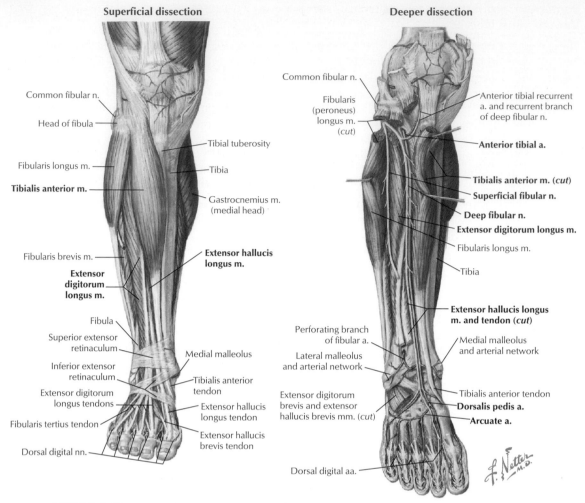

Superficial dissection

Common fibular n.

Head of fibula

Fibularis longus m.

Tibialis anterior m.

Fibularis brevis m.

Extensor digitorum longus m.

Fibula

Superior extensor retinaculum

Inferior extensor retinaculum

Extensor digitorum longus tendons

Fibularis tertius tendon

Dorsal digital nn.

Tibial tuberosity

Tibia

Gastrocnemius m. (medial head)

Extensor hallucis longus m.

Medial malleolus

Tibialis anterior tendon

Extensor hallucis longus tendon

Extensor hallucis brevis tendon

Deeper dissection

Common fibular n.

Fibularis (peroneus) longus m. (*cut*)

Perforating branch of fibular a.

Lateral malleolus and arterial network

Extensor digitorum brevis and extensor hallucis brevis mm. (*cut*)

Dorsal digital aa.

Anterior tibial recurrent a. and recurrent branch of deep fibular n.

Anterior tibial a.

Tibialis anterior m. (*cut*)

Superficial fibular n.

Deep fibular n.

Extensor digitorum longus m.

Fibularis longus m.

Tibia

Extensor hallucis longus m. and tendon (*cut*)

Medial malleolus and arterial network

Tibialis anterior tendon

Dorsalis pedis a.

Arcuate a.

FIGURE 6.23 Anterior Compartment Leg Muscles, Vessels, and Nerves. (From *Netter's atlas of human anatomy,* ed 8, Plates 531 and 532; S-288 and S-289.)

TABLE 6.16 Anterior Compartment Leg Muscles and Nerves

MUSCLE	PROXIMAL ATTACHMENT	DISTAL ATTACHMENT	INNERVATION	MAIN ACTIONS
Tibialis anterior	Lateral condyle and superior half of lateral tibia and interosseous membrane	Medial plantara surfaces of medial cuneiform and base of 1st metatarsal	Deep fibular nerve (L4-L5)	Dorsiflexes foot at ankle and inverts foot
Extensor hallucis longus	Middle part of anterior surface of fibula and interosseous membrane	Dorsal aspect of base of distal phalanx of great toe	Deep fibular nerve (L5-S1)	Extends great toe and dorsiflexes foot at ankle
Extensor digitorum longus	Lateral condyle of tibia and superior three-fourths of anterior surface of interosseous membrane and fibula	Middle and distal phalanges of lateral four digits	Deep fibular nerve (L5-S1)	Extends lateral four digits and dorsiflexes foot at ankle
Fibularis tertius	Inferior third of anterior surface of fibula and interosseous membrane	Dorsum of base of 5th metatarsal	Deep fibular nerve (L5-S1)	Dorsiflexes foot at ankle and aids in eversion of foot

Variations in spinal nerve contributions to the innervation of muscles, their attachments, and their actions are common in human anatomy. Therefore, expect differences between texts and realize that anatomical variation is normal.

TABLE 6.17 Lateral Compartment Leg Muscles and Nerves

MUSCLE	PROXIMAL ATTACHMENT	DISTAL ATTACHMENT	INNERVATION	MAIN ACTIONS
Fibularis longus	Head and superior two-thirds of lateral surface of fibula	Plantar base of 1st metatarsal and medial cuneiform	Superficial fibular nerve (L5-S2)	Everts foot and weakly plantarflexes foot at ankle
Fibularis brevis	Inferior two-thirds of lateral surface of fibula	Dorsal surface of tuberosity on lateral side of 5th metatarsal	Superficial fibular nerve (L5-S2)	Everts foot and weakly plantarflexes foot at ankle

Variations in spinal nerve contributions to the innervation of muscles, their attachments, and their actions are common in human anatomy. Therefore, expect differences between texts and realize that anatomical variation is normal.

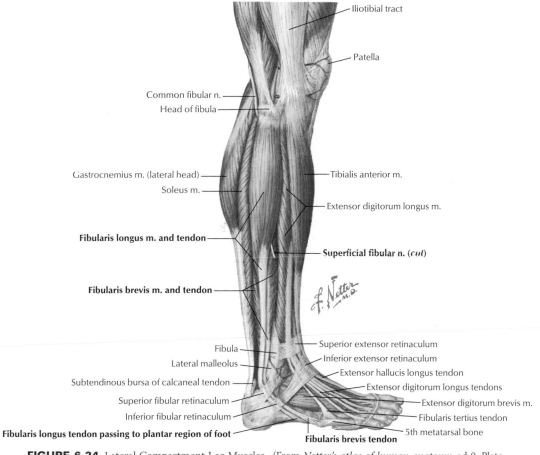

FIGURE 6.24 Lateral Compartment Leg Muscles. (From *Netter's atlas of human anatomy,* ed 8, Plate 530; S-287.)

posterior compartment is further subdivided into the superficial and deep compartments. Moreover, the leg is ensheathed in a *tight deep fascia,* and some of the underlying muscle fibers actually attach to this fascial sleeve. These muscle compartments may be summarized as follows (Fig. 6.25):

- **Posterior compartment:** muscles that plantarflex and invert the foot at the ankle and flex the toes, are innervated by the **tibial nerve,** and are supplied largely by the **posterior tibial artery**.

- **Anterior compartment:** muscles that dorsiflex (extend) and invert/evert the foot at the ankle and extend the toes, are innervated by the **deep fibular nerve,** and are supplied by the anterior **tibial artery**.

- **Lateral compartment:** muscles that evert the foot at the ankle and weakly plantarflex the foot, are innervated by the **superficial fibular nerve,** and are supplied by the **fibular artery**.

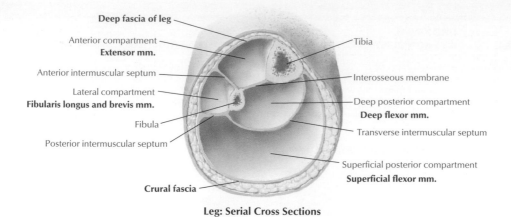

Leg: Serial Cross Sections

Deep fascia of leg
Anterior compartment
Extensor mm.
Anterior intermuscular septum
Lateral compartment
Fibularis longus and brevis mm.
Fibula
Posterior intermuscular septum
Crural fascia

Tibia
Interosseous membrane
Deep posterior compartment
Deep flexor mm.
Transverse intermuscular septum
Superficial posterior compartment
Superficial flexor mm.

Tibialis anterior m.
Tibialis posterior m.
Anterior tibial a.

Common fibular n.
Flexor hallucis longus m.
Fibularis longus m.
Fibularis brevis m.
Fibula

Tibialis anterior m.
Extensor hallucis longus m.
Extensor digitorum longus m.
Superficial fibular n.
Deep fibular n.
Anterior tibial a.
Interosseus membrane
Fibularis longus m.
Fibularis brevis m.

Tibialis anterior m. and t.
Extensor digitorum longus and fibularis tertius mm.
Deep fibular n.
Fibularis longus m.
Anterior tibial a.
Fibularis brevis m.

Tibia
Posterior tibial a. and v.
Saphenous n.
Great saphenous v.
Popliteus m.
Tibial n.
Soleus m.
Gastrocnemius m. (lateral and medial heads)
Medial sural cutaneous n.

Tibialis posterior m.
Fibular a.
Flexor digitorum longus m.
Tibial n.
Posterior tibial a.
Flexor hallucis longus m.
Soleus m.
Gastrocnemius m. (lateral and medial heads)

Flexor digitorum longus m.
Tibialis posterior m.
Fibular a.
Posterior tibial a.
Tibial n.
Flexor hallucis longus m.
Calcaneal t.
Soleus m.
Sural communicating branch of lateral sural cutaneous n.

FIGURE 6.25 Cross Section of the Right Leg. (From *Netter's atlas of human anatomy,* ed 8, Plate 534; S-555.)

Genu Varum and Valgum

The knee of a standing patient should look symmetric and level. The tibia normally has a slight valgus angulation compared with the femur. *Valgus* is used to describe the bone distal to the examined joint; a *valgus angulation* refers to a slight lateral angle. Excessive valgus angulation is called *genu valgum*, or **knock-knee**, and an excessive varus angulation is called *genu varum,* or **bowleg**. These deformities occur in growing children and are often related to rickets, skeletal dysplasia, or trauma. Most resolve without treatment.

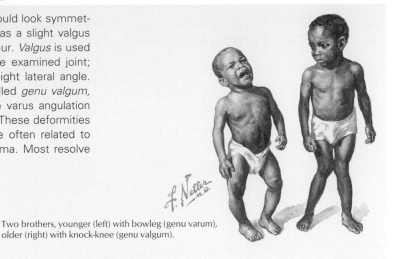

Two brothers, younger (left) with bowleg (genu varum), older (right) with knock-knee (genu valgum).

Exertional Compartment Syndromes

Anterior (tibial) compartment syndrome (or *anterior or lateral shin splints*) occurs from excessive contraction of anterior compartment muscles; pain over these muscles radiates down the ankle and dorsum of the foot overlying the extensor tendons. *Lateral compartment syndrome* occurs in people with excessively mobile ankle joints in which hypereversion irritates the lateral compartment muscles. These conditions are usually chronic, and expansion of the compartment may lead to nerve and vessel compression. In the acute syndrome (rapid, unrelenting expansion), the compartment may have to be opened surgically (fasciotomy) to relieve pressure. **The five Ps of acute anterior compartment syndrome are:**

- Pain
- Pallor
- Paresis (footdrop, caused by compression of deep fibular nerve)
- Paresthesia
- Pulselessness (variable)

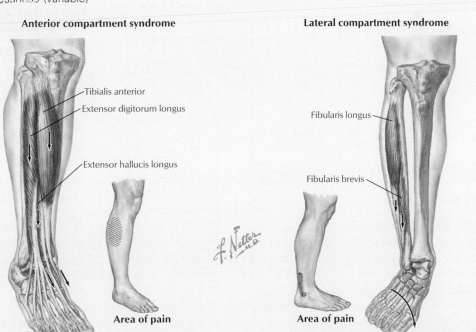

Anterior compartment syndrome

Tibialis anterior
Extensor digitorum longus

Extensor hallucis longus

Area of pain

Lateral compartment syndrome

Fibularis longus

Fibularis brevis

Area of pain

Clinical Focus 6.26

Achilles Tendinitis and Bursitis

Tendinitis of the calcaneal (Achilles) tendon is a painful inflammation that often occurs in runners who run on hills or uneven surfaces. Repetitive stress on the tendon occurs as the heel strikes the ground and when plantarflexion lifts the foot and toes. Tendon rupture is a serious injury, and the avascular tendon heals slowly. Retrocalcaneal bursitis, an inflammation of the subtendinous bursa between the overlying tendon and the calcaneus, presents as a tender area just anterior to the tendon attachment.

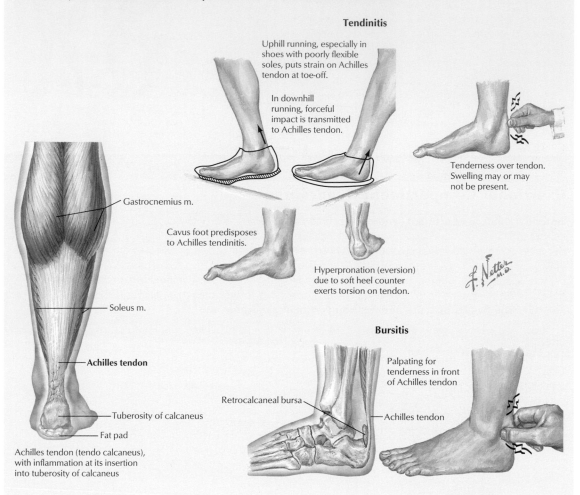

Tendinitis

Uphill running, especially in shoes with poorly flexible soles, puts strain on Achilles tendon at toe-off.

In downhill running, forceful impact is transmitted to Achilles tendon.

Tenderness over tendon. Swelling may or may not be present.

Gastrocnemius m.

Cavus foot predisposes to Achilles tendinitis.

Hyperpronation (eversion) due to soft heel counter exerts torsion on tendon.

Soleus m.

Achilles tendon

Tuberosity of calcaneus

Fat pad

Achilles tendon (tendo calcaneus), with inflammation at its insertion into tuberosity of calcaneus

Bursitis

Palpating for tenderness in front of Achilles tendon

Retrocalcaneal bursa

Achilles tendon

7. ANKLE AND FOOT

Bones and Joints

The ankle connects the foot to the leg and is composed of seven **tarsal bones** arranged in a proximal group *(talus and calcaneus)*, intermediate group *(navicular)*, and distal group *(cuboid and three cuneiform bones)*. The foot includes five **metatarsals** and the five digits and their **phalanges** (Figs. 6.26 and 6.27 and Table 6.18).

The **ankle (talocrural) joint** is a uniaxial synovial hinge joint between the talus and the tibia (inferior surface and medial malleolus) and fibula (lateral malleolus). The combination forms a mortise that is then covered by the capsule of the joint and reinforced medially and laterally by ligaments. The ankle joint functions primarily in **plantarflexion** and **dorsiflexion.** Intertarsal, tarsometatarsal, intermetatarsal, metatarsophalangeal, and interphalangeal joints complete the ankle and foot joint complex

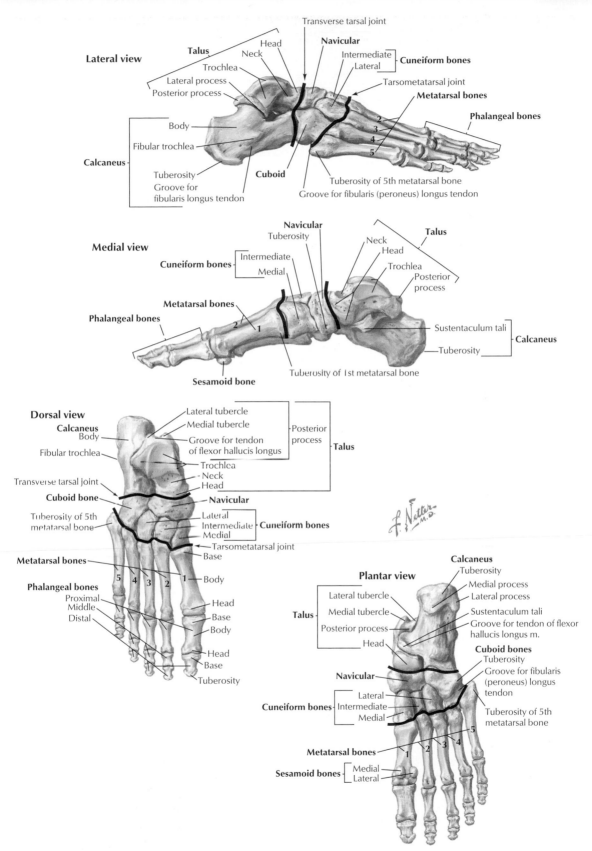

FIGURE 6.26 Bones of the Ankle and Foot. (From *Netter's atlas of human anatomy,* ed 8, Plate 536; S-177.)

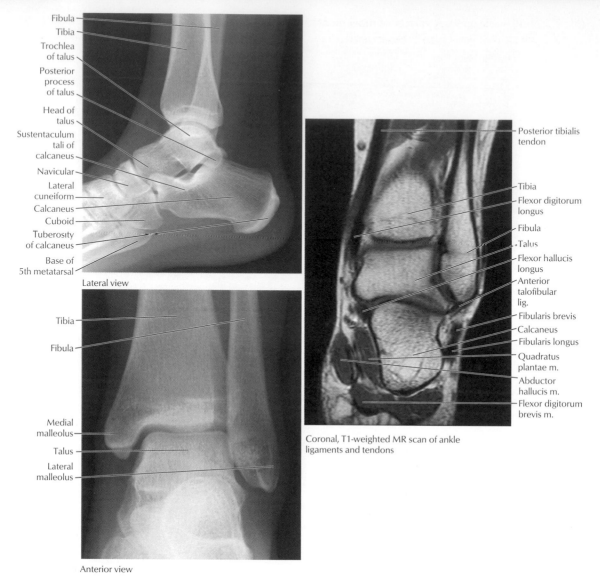

FIGURE 6.27 Radiographs of the Ankle. (Left images from *Netter's atlas of human anatomy*, ed 8, Plate 556; S-179; right image from Kelley LL, Petersen C: *Sectional anatomy for imaging professionals*, Philadelphia, 2007, Mosby.)

TABLE 6.18 Features of the Bones of the Ankle and Foot

STRUCTURE	CHARACTERISTICS	STRUCTURE	CHARACTERISTICS
Talus (ankle bone)*	Transfers weight from tibia to foot; no muscle attachment	Groove	For fibularis longus tendon
Trochlea	Articulates with tibia and fibula	*Cuneiforms**	Three wedge-shaped bones
Head	Articulates with navicular bone	**Metatarsals**	
Calcaneus (heel bone)*	Articulates with talus superiorly and cuboid anteriorly	Numbered 1 to 5, from great toe to little toe	Possess base, shaft, and head Fibularis brevis tendon inserts on 5th metatarsal
Sustentaculum tali	Medial shelf that supports talar head	Two sesamoid bones	Associated with flexor hallucis brevis tendons
*Navicular**	Boat shaped, between talar head and three cuneiforms	**Phalanges**	
Tuberosity	If large, can cause medial pain in tight-fitting shoe	Three for each digit except great toe	Possess base, shaft, and head Termed *proximal, middle,* and *distal*
*Cuboid**	Most lateral tarsal bone		Stubbed 5th toe common injury

*Tarsal bones.

(Fig. 6.28 and Table 6.19). A variety of movements are possible at these joints, and the ankle and foot can provide a stable but flexible platform for standing, walking, and running. Because of the shape of the talus (the anterior portion of its superior articular aspect is wider), the *ankle is more stable when dorsiflexed than when plantarflexed.*

The bones of the foot do not lie in a flat plane but are arranged to form the following arches (see Fig. 6.26):

- **Longitudinal arch:** extends from the posterior calcaneus to the metatarsal heads; is higher medially (medial longitudinal arch) than laterally (lateral longitudinal arch).
- **Transverse arch:** extends from lateral to medial across the cuboid, cuneiforms, and base of the metatarsals; is higher medially than laterally.

These arches are supported by muscles and ligaments. Supporting muscles include the tibialis anterior, tibialis posterior, and fibularis longus.

TABLE 6.19 Features of the Joints and Ligaments of the Ankle and Foot

LIGAMENT	ATTACHMENT	COMMENT
Distal Tibiofibular (Fibrous [Syndesmosis]) Joint		
Anterior tibiofibular	Anterior distal tibia and fibula	Runs obliquely
Posterior tibiofibular	Posterior distal tibia and fibula	Is weaker than anterior ligament
Inferior transverse	Medial malleolus to fibula	Is deep continuation of posterior ligament
Talocrural (Uniaxial Synovial Hinge [Ginglymus]) Joint		
Capsule	Tibia and fibula to talus	Functions in plantarflexion and dorsiflexion
Medial (deltoid)	Medial malleolus to talus, calcaneus, and navicular	Limits eversion of foot; maintains medial longitudinal arch; has four parts
Lateral (collateral)	Lateral malleolus to talus and calcaneus	Is weak and often sprained; resists inversion of foot; has three parts
Intertarsal Joints (Next Three Joints)		
Talocalcaneal (Subtalar Plane Synovial) Joints		
Capsule	Margins of articulation	Functions in inversion and eversion
Talocalcaneal	Talus to calcaneus	Has medial, lateral, and posterior parts
Interosseous talocalcaneal	Talus to calcaneus	Is strong; binds bones together
Talocalcaneonavicular (Partial Ball-and-Socket Synovial) Joint		
Capsule	Encloses part of joint	Functions in gliding and rotational movements
Plantar calcaneonavicular	Sustentaculum tali to navicular	Is strong plantar support for head of talus (called *spring ligament*)
Dorsal talonavicular	Talus to navicular	Is dorsal support to talus
Calcaneocuboid (Plane Synovial) Joint		
Capsule	Encloses joint	Functions in inversion and eversion
Calcaneocuboid	Calcaneus to cuboid	Are dorsal, plantar (short plantar, strong), and long plantar ligaments
Tarsometatarsal (Plane Synovial) Joints		
Capsule	Encloses joint	Functions in gliding or sliding movements
Tarsometatarsal	Tarsals to metatarsals	Are dorsal, plantar, interosseous ligaments
Intermetatarsal (Plane Synovial) Joints		
Capsule	Base of metatarsals	Provides little movement, supports transverse arch
Intermetatarsal	Adjacent metatarsals	Are dorsal, plantar, interosseous ligaments
Deep transverse	Adjacent metatarsals	Connect adjacent heads
Metatarsophalangeal (Multiaxial Condyloid Synovial) Joints		
Capsule	Encloses joint	Functions in flexion, extension, some abduction and adduction, and circumduction
Collateral	Metatarsal heads to base of proximal phalanges	Are strong ligaments
Plantar (plates)	Plantar side of capsule	Are part of weight-bearing surface
Interphalangeal (Uniaxial Hinge Synovial) Joints		
Capsule	Encloses each joint	Functions in flexion and extension
Collateral	Head of one to base of other	Support the capsule
Plantar (plates)	Plantar side of capsule	Support the capsule

Cuboideonavicular, cuneonavicular, intercuneiform, and cuneocuboid joints: dorsal, plantar, and interosseous ligaments are present, but little movement occurs at these joints.

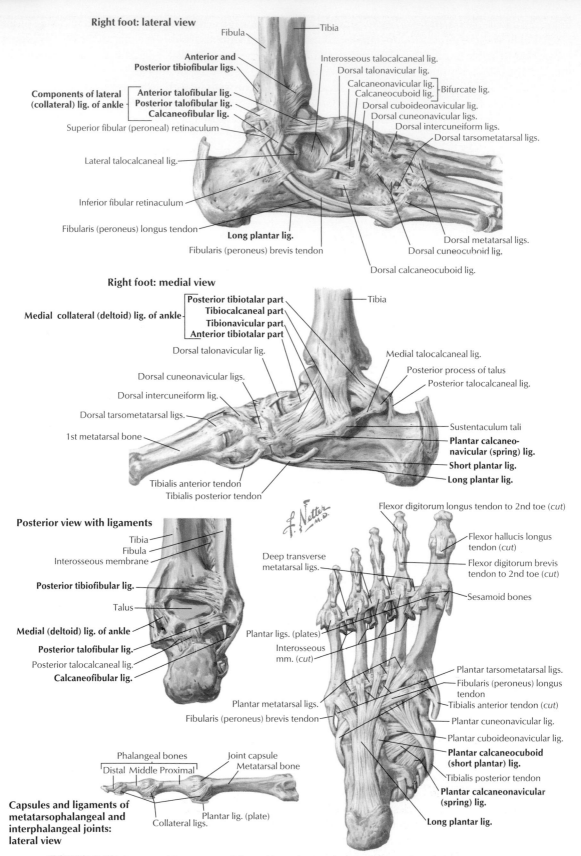

Right foot: lateral view

Fibula

Tibia

Anterior and Posterior tibiofibular ligs.

Interosseous talocalcaneal lig.

Dorsal talonavicular lig.

Components of lateral (collateral) lig. of ankle
- **Anterior talofibular lig.**
- **Posterior talofibular lig.**
- **Calcaneofibular lig.**

Calcaneonavicular lig.
Calcaneocuboid lig. ⎫ Bifurcate lig.

Dorsal cuboideonavicular lig.

Dorsal cuneonavicular ligs.

Superior fibular (peroneal) retinaculum

Dorsal intercuneiform ligs.

Dorsal tarsometatarsal ligs.

Lateral talocalcaneal lig.

Inferior fibular retinaculum

Fibularis (peroneus) longus tendon

Long plantar lig.

Fibularis (peroneus) brevis tendon

Dorsal metatarsal ligs.

Dorsal cuneocuboid lig.

Dorsal calcaneocuboid lig.

Right foot: medial view

Medial collateral (deltoid) lig. of ankle
- **Posterior tibiotalar part**
- **Tibiocalcaneal part**
- **Tibionavicular part**
- **Anterior tibiotalar part**

Tibia

Dorsal talonavicular lig.

Medial talocalcaneal lig.

Posterior process of talus

Posterior talocalcaneal lig.

Dorsal cuneonavicular ligs.

Dorsal intercuneiform lig.

Dorsal tarsometatarsal ligs.

1st metatarsal bone

Sustentaculum tali

Plantar calcaneo-navicular (spring) lig.

Short plantar lig.

Long plantar lig.

Tibialis anterior tendon

Tibialis posterior tendon

Posterior view with ligaments

Tibia
Fibula
Interosseous membrane

Deep transverse metatarsal ligs.

Flexor digitorum longus tendon to 2nd toe (*cut*)

Flexor hallucis longus tendon (*cut*)

Flexor digitorum brevis tendon to 2nd toe (*cut*)

Posterior tibiofibular lig.

Talus

Medial (deltoid) lig. of ankle

Posterior talofibular lig.

Posterior talocalcaneal lig.

Calcaneofibular lig.

Sesamoid bones

Plantar ligs. (plates)

Interosseous mm. (*cut*)

Plantar tarsometatarsal ligs.

Fibularis (peroneus) longus tendon

Tibialis anterior tendon (*cut*)

Plantar cuneonavicular lig.

Plantar cuboideonavicular lig.

Plantar calcaneocuboid (short plantar) lig.

Tibialis posterior tendon

Plantar calcaneonavicular (spring) lig.

Long plantar lig.

Plantar metatarsal ligs.

Fibularis (peroneus) brevis tendon

Phalangeal bones
Distal Middle Proximal

Joint capsule
Metatarsal bone

Capsules and ligaments of metatarsophalangeal and interphalangeal joints: lateral view

Collateral ligs.

Plantar lig. (plate)

FIGURE 6.28 Joints and Ligaments of the Ankle and Foot. (From *Netter's atlas of human anatomy,* ed 8, Plates 538 and 539; S-180 and S-181.)

Clinical Focus 6.27

Footdrop

An inability to dorsiflex the foot at the ankle resulting in a foot that cannot be raised is characterized as footdrop. A patient with footdrop must raise the knee during the swing phase of gait to avoid dragging the affected foot on the ground or to avoid tripping. This distinctive gait pattern is called **"steppage" gait,** and at the end of the swing phase, the foot slaps down to the ground. Typically, footdrop results from injury to the *common fibular nerve* or *deep fibular nerve*. The common fibular nerve is vulnerable to injury because it lies superficially beneath the skin where the nerve passes around the fibular neck (coffee table or car bumper height). This nerve also may be affected by a herniated disc that compresses the L5 nerve root (L4-L5 herniated disc; see Clinical Focus 2.6.

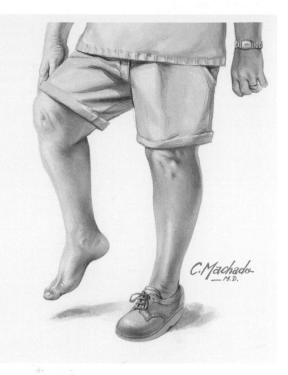

Ligaments include the plantar calcaneonavicular (spring) ligament, plantar calcaneocuboid (short plantar) ligament, and long plantar ligament. The plantar aponeurosis also provides some support (Fig. 6.28 and Table 6.19).

Synovial sheaths provide protection and lubrication for muscle tendons passing from the leg to the foot. Various fibrous bands, called *retinacula*, tether the tendons at the ankle (Fig. 6.29):

- **Flexor retinaculum:** extends from the medial malleolus to the calcaneus (tethers the plantarflexor tendons).
- **Extensor retinaculum:** superior and inferior bands (tethers the dorsiflexor tendons).
- **Fibular retinacula:** superior and inferior bands (tethers the fibularis tendons of the lateral compartment).

Muscles, Vessels, and Nerves of the Dorsum of the Foot

The dorsum (top) of the foot consists of two intrinsic muscles, the extensor digitorum brevis muscles and the extensor hallucis brevis muscles, innervated by the deep fibular nerve as it passes from the leg into the foot (Fig. 6.23). These muscles function to extend the toes and are supplied by the anterior tibial artery from the leg via its **dorsalis pedis branch** (Figs. 6.23

and 6.30). A **dorsal venous arch** drains most of the blood from the foot (similar to the dorsal aspect of the hand), ultimately carrying the blood to the medially located great saphenous vein or laterally and posteriorly to the small saphenous vein (see Fig. 6.2).

Muscles, Vessels, and Nerves of the Sole of the Foot

The sole of the foot is protected by a thick layer of the deep fascia called the **plantar aponeurosis,** which extends from the calcaneal tuberosity to individual bands of fascia that attach to the toes anteriorly (Fig. 6.31).

Beneath the plantar aponeurosis, the intrinsic muscles of the foot are arranged into four layers, shown in sequence in Figs. 6.31, 6.32, and 6.33 and Tables 6.20, 6.21, and 6.22. These muscles functionally assist the long muscle tendons that pass from the leg into the foot. The **lumbrical muscles** and the **interosseus muscles** have the same actions as their counterparts in the hand. The lumbricals flex the metatarsophalangeal joints and extend the interphalangeal joints via the extensor hood. The plantar interossei adduct (**PAD**) the digits (2-4) and help flex the metatarsophalangeal joints, while the **dorsal** interossei abduct (**DAB**) the digits and help flex the metatarsophalangeal joints. In the foot, the reference toe for adduction and

Clinical Focus 6.28

Ankle Sprains

Most ankle sprains involve an inversion injury when the foot is plantarflexed, placing stress on the components of the lateral collateral ligament (see Fig. 6.28). Often the severity of the injury occurs from anterior to posterior, involving first the **anterior talofibular ligament,** then the **calcaneofibular ligament,** and finally, if especially severe, the **posterior talofibular ligament.** The anterior drawer test, in which the tibia is held steady while the heel is pulled anteriorly with the foot in about 10 to 20 degrees of plantarflexion, will confirm the injury to the anterior talofibular ligament if the translation of the foot anteriorly is excessive compared with that of the uninjured contralateral ankle.

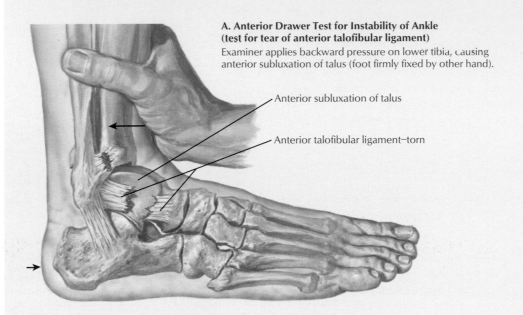

**A. Anterior Drawer Test for Instability of Ankle
(test for tear of anterior talofibular ligament)**
Examiner applies backward pressure on lower tibia, causing anterior subluxation of talus (foot firmly fixed by other hand).

Anterior subluxation of talus

Anterior talofibular ligament–torn

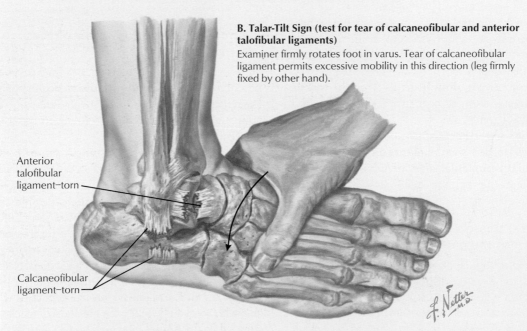

B. Talar-Tilt Sign (test for tear of calcaneofibular and anterior talofibular ligaments)
Examiner firmly rotates foot in varus. Tear of calcaneofibular ligament permits excessive mobility in this direction (leg firmly fixed by other hand).

Anterior talofibular ligament–torn

Calcaneofibular ligament–torn

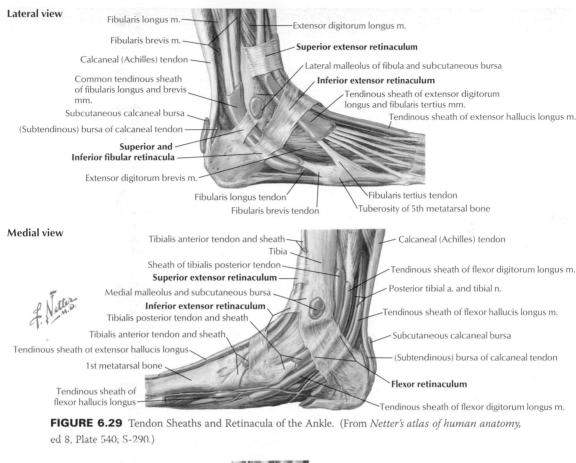

FIGURE 6.29 Tendon Sheaths and Retinacula of the Ankle. (From *Netter's atlas of human anatomy*, ed 8, Plate 540; S-290.)

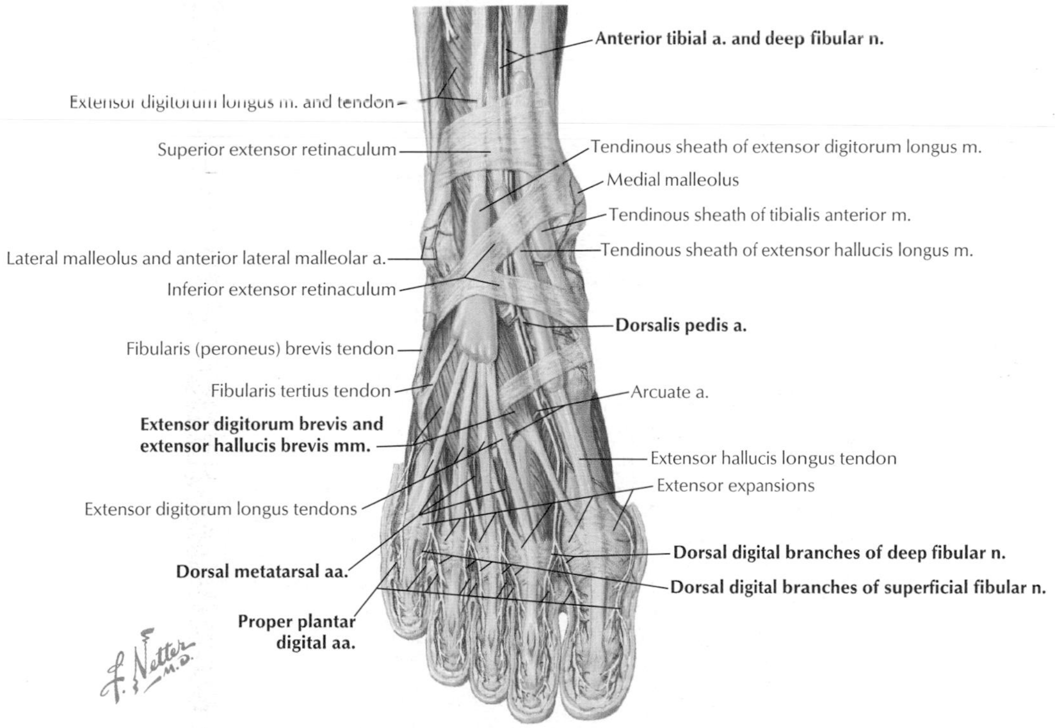

FIGURE 6.30 Muscles, Nerves, and Arteries of the Dorsum of the Foot. (From *Netter's atlas of human anatomy*, ed 8, Plate 541; S-291.)

Clinical Focus 6.29

Rotational Fractures

Most ankle injuries are caused by twisting, so that the talus rotates in the frontal plane and impinges on either the lateral or medial malleolus. This causes it to fracture and places tension on supporting ligaments of the opposite side. The following three types are recognized:

- **Type A:** Medial rotation of the talus
- **Type B:** Lateral rotation of the talus
- **Type C:** Injury extends proximally, with torn tibiofibular ligament and interosseous membrane (a variant is the Maisonneuve fracture)

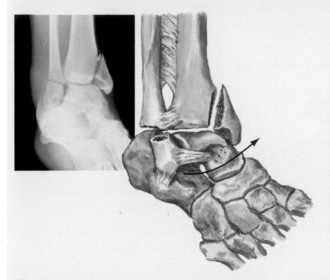

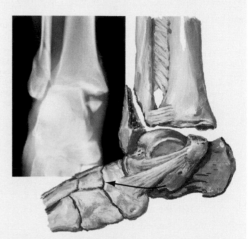

Type A. Avulsion fracture of lateral malleolus and shear fracture of medial malleolus caused by medial rotation of talus. **Tibiofibular ligaments intact.**

Type B. Shear fracture of lateral malleolus and small avulsion fracture of medial malleolus caused by lateral rotation of talus. **Tibiofibular ligaments intact or only partially torn.**

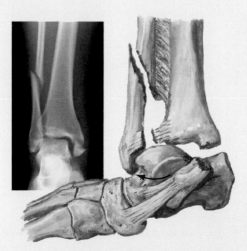

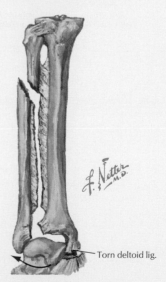

Torn deltoid lig.

Type C. Disruption of tibiofibular ligaments with diastasis of syndesmosis caused by external rotation of talus. Force transmitted to fibula results in oblique fracture at higher level. In this case, avulsion of medial malleolus has also occurred.

Maisonneuve fracture. Complete disruption of tibiofibular syndesmosis with diastasis caused by external rotation of talus and transmission of force to proximal fibula, resulting in high fracture of fibula. **Interosseous membranes torn longitudinally.**

Fractures of the Calcaneus

Calcaneal fractures (the most common tarsal fracture) are extraarticular or intraarticular. Extraarticular fractures include the following:

- **Anterior process fracture:** stress on the bifurcate ligament (calcaneocuboid and calcaneonavicular ligaments) caused by landing on an adducted plantarflexed foot
- **Avulsion fracture of the calcaneal tuberosity:** sudden forceful contraction of the gastrocnemius and soleus muscles
- **Fracture of the sustentaculum tali:** jumping and landing on an inverted foot
- **Fracture of the body:** jumping and landing on a heel

Most calcaneal fractures are intraarticular (forceful landing on a heel); the talus is "driven" down into the calcaneus, which cannot withstand the force because it is cancellous bone.

Extraarticular fracture of calcaneus

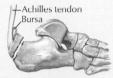
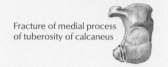
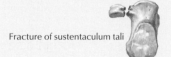
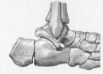

Avulsion fracture of anterior process of calcaneus caused by tension on bifurcate ligament (calcaneocuboid and calcaneonavicular)

Comminuted fracture of anterior process of calcaneus due to compression by cuboid in forceful abduction of forefoot

Achilles tendon
Bursa

Avulsion fracture of tuberosity of calcaneus due to sudden, violent contraction of Achilles tendon

Fracture of medial process of tuberosity of calcaneus

Fracture of sustentaculum tali

Fracture of body of calcaneus with no involvement of subtalar articulation

Intraarticular fracture of calcaneus

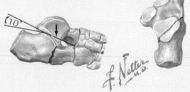

Primary fracture line
Talus driven down into calcaneus, usually by fall and landing on heel

Primary fracture line runs across posterior facet, forming anteromedial and posterolateral fragments.

abduction is the *second toe,* which in most people is the *longest toe.* All these intrinsic muscles of the sole are innervated by the **medial or lateral plantar nerves** (from the tibial nerve) (Tables 6.20, 6.21, and 6.22) and are supplied with blood from the **medial** and **lateral plantar arteries** (derived from the posterior tibial artery). **Arterial pulses** may be palpated between the medial malleolus and the heel (from the **posterior tibial artery**) and on the dorsum of the foot just lateral to the extensor hallucis longus tendon (from the **dorsalis pedis artery**).

8. LOWER LIMB MUSCLE SUMMARY AND GAIT

Table 6.23 summarizes the actions of major muscles on the joints. *The list is not exhaustive and highlights only major muscles responsible for each movement;* the separate muscle tables provide more detail. Realize that most joints move because of the action of multiple muscles working on that joint, and that this list only focuses on the more important of these muscles for each joint.

Text continued on p. 348.

Superficial dissection

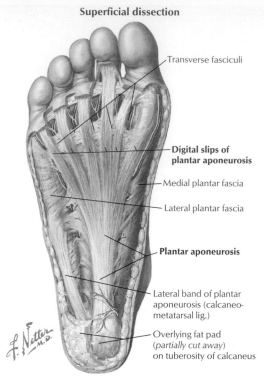

Transverse fasciculi

**Digital slips of
plantar aponeurosis**

Medial plantar fascia

Lateral plantar fascia

Plantar aponeurosis

Lateral band of plantar
aponeurosis (calcaneo-
metatarsal lig.)

Overlying fat pad
(*partially cut away*)
on tuberosity of calcaneus

FIGURE 6.31 Plantar Aponeurosis. (From *Netter's atlas
of human anatomy,* ed 8, Plate 543; S-293.)

First layer

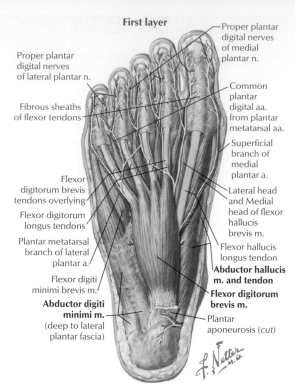

Proper plantar
digital nerves
of lateral plantar n.

Fibrous sheaths
of flexor tendons

Flexor
digitorum brevis
tendons overlying

Flexor digitorum
longus tendons

Plantar metatarsal
branch of lateral
plantar a.

Flexor digiti
minimi brevis m.

**Abductor digiti
minimi m.**
(deep to lateral
plantar fascia)

Proper plantar
digital nerves
of medial
plantar n.

Common
plantar
digital aa.
from plantar
metatarsal aa.

Superficial
branch of
medial
plantar a.

Lateral head
and Medial
head of flexor
hallucis
brevis m.

Flexor hallucis
longus tendon

**Abductor hallucis
m. and tendon**

**Flexor digitorum
brevis m.**

Plantar
aponeurosis (*cut*)

FIGURE 6.32 Muscles, Nerves, and Arteries of the
Sole: First Layer. (From *Netter's atlas of human anatomy,*
ed 8, Plate 544; S-294.)

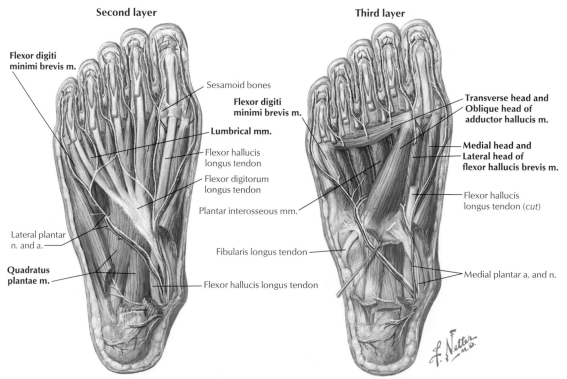

Second layer

Flexor digiti
minimi brevis m.

Sesamoid bones

**Flexor digiti
minimi brevis m.**

Lumbrical mm.

Flexor hallucis
longus tendon

Flexor digitorum
longus tendon

Plantar interosseous mm.

Lateral plantar
n. and a.

**Quadratus
plantae m.**

Flexor hallucis longus tendon

Third layer

**Transverse head and
Oblique head of
adductor hallucis m.**

**Medial head and
Lateral head of
flexor hallucis brevis m.**

Flexor hallucis
longus tendon (*cut*)

Fibularis longus tendon

Medial plantar a. and n.

FIGURE 6.33 Muscles, Nerves, and Arteries of the Sole: Second and Third Layers. (From *Netter's
atlas of human anatomy,* ed 8, Plates 545 and 546; S-295 and S-296.)

TABLE 6.20 Muscles of the Sole: First Layer*

MUSCLE	PROXIMAL ATTACHMENT	DISTAL ATTACHMENT	INNERVATION	MAIN ACTIONS
Abductor hallucis	Medial tubercle of tuberosity of calcaneus, flexor retinaculum, and plantar aponeurosis	Medial side of base of proximal phalanx of 1st digit	Medial plantar nerve (S1-S2)	Abducts and flexes great toe
Flexor digitorum brevis	Medial tubercle of tuberosity of calcaneus, plantar aponeurosis, and intermuscular septa	Both sides of middle phalanges of lateral four digits	Medial plantar nerve (S1-S2)	Flexes lateral four digits
Abductor digiti minimi	Medial and lateral tubercles of tuberosity of calcaneus, plantar aponeurosis, and intermuscular septa	Lateral side of base of proximal phalanx of 5th digit	Lateral plantar nerve (S1-S3)	Abducts and flexes little toe

TABLE 6.21 Muscles of the Sole: Second and Third Layers*

MUSCLE	PROXIMAL ATTACHMENT	DISTAL ATTACHMENT	INNERVATION	MAIN ACTIONS
Quadratus plantae	Medial surface and lateral margin of plantar surface of calcaneus	Posterolateral margin of tendon of flexor digitorum longus	Lateral plantar nerve (S1-S3)	Assist flexor digitorum longus in flexing lateral four digits
Lumbricals	Tendons of flexor digitorum longus	Medial aspect of dorsal expansion over lateral four digits	*Medial one:* medial plantar nerve *Lateral three:* lateral plantar nerve	Flex metatarso-phalangeal joints and extend interphalangeal joints of lateral four digits
Flexor hallucis brevis	Plantar surfaces of cuboid and lateral cuneiform	Both sides of base of proximal phalanx of 1st digit	Medial plantar nerve (S1-S2)	Flexes proximal phalanx of great toe
Adductor hallucis	*Oblique head:* bases of metatarsals 2-4 *Transverse head:* plantar ligaments of metatarsophalangeal joints of digits 3-5	Tendons of both heads attach to lateral side of base of proximal phalanx of 1st digit	Deep branch of lateral plantar nerve (S2-S3)	Adducts great toe; assists in maintaining transverse arch of foot
Flexor digiti minimi brevis	Base of 5th metatarsal	Lateral base of proximal phalanx of 5th digit	Superficial branch of lateral plantar nerve (S2-S3)	Flexes proximal phalanx of little toe, thereby assisting with its flexion

TABLE 6.22 Muscles of the Sole: Fourth Layer*

MUSCLE	PROXIMAL ATTACHMENT	DISTAL ATTACHMENT	INNERVATION	MAIN ACTIONS
Plantar interossei (three muscles)	Bases and medial sides of metatarsals 3-5	Medial sides of bases of proximal phalanges of digits 3-5	Lateral plantar nerve (S2-S3)	Adduct digits 3-5, flex metatarsophalangeal joints, and extend phalanges
Dorsal interossei (four muscles)	Adjacent sides of metatarsals 1-5	*First:* medial side of proximal phalanx of second digit *Second to fourth:* lateral sides of digits 2-4	Lateral plantar nerve (S2-S3)	Abduct digits 2-4, flex metatarsophalangeal joints, and extend phalanges

*Variations in spinal nerve contributions to the innervation of muscles, their attachments, and their actions are common in human anatomy. Therefore, expect differences between texts and realize that anatomical variation is normal.

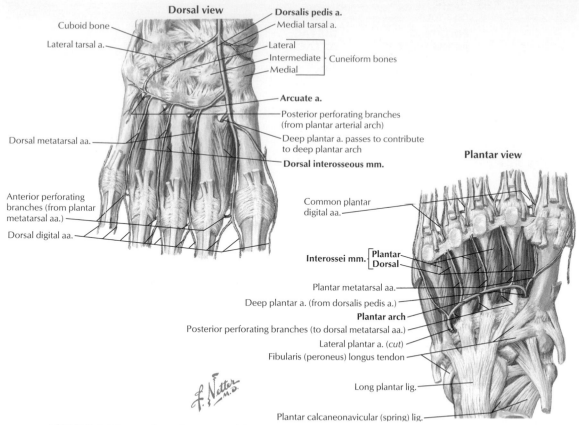

Dorsal view

Cuboid bone
Lateral tarsal a.

Dorsalis pedis a.
Medial tarsal a.

Lateral
Intermediate } Cuneiform bones
Medial

Arcuate a.

Posterior perforating branches
(from plantar arterial arch)

Deep plantar a. passes to contribute
to deep plantar arch

Dorsal interosseous mm.

Dorsal metatarsal aa.

Anterior perforating
branches (from plantar
metatarsal aa.)

Dorsal digital aa.

Plantar view

Common plantar
digital aa.

Interossei mm. [**Plantar** / **Dorsal**]

Plantar metatarsal aa.

Deep plantar a. (from dorsalis pedis a.)

Plantar arch

Posterior perforating branches (to dorsal metatarsal aa.)

Lateral plantar a. (*cut*)

Fibularis (peroneus) longus tendon

Long plantar lig.

Plantar calcaneonavicular (spring) lig.

FIGURE 6.34 Muscles and Arteries of the Sole: Fourth Layer. (From *Netter's atlas of human anatomy,* ed 8, Plate 547; S-297.)

Clinical Focus 6.31

Congenital Clubfoot

Congenital clubfoot *(congenital equinovarus)* is a structural defect in which the entire foot is plantarflexed (equinus) and the hindfoot and forefoot are inverted (varus). This deformity has a strong genetic link; males are more frequently affected, but females often have a more severe deformity. The bones not only are misaligned with each other but also may have an abnormal shape and size. Thus, after correction, the true clubfoot is smaller than normal. Management may be conservative or may require splinting, casting, or even surgery.

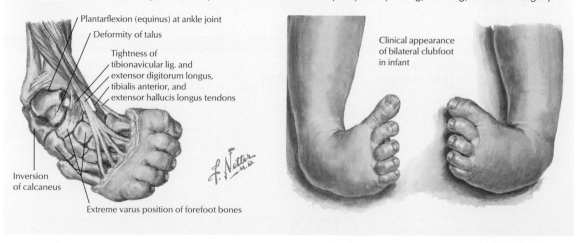

Plantarflexion (equinus) at ankle joint
Deformity of talus
Tightness of tibionavicular lig. and extensor digitorum longus, tibialis anterior, and extensor hallucis longus tendons
Inversion of calcaneus
Extreme varus position of forefoot bones
Clinical appearance of bilateral clubfoot in infant

Plantar Fasciitis

Plantar fasciitis *(heel spur syndrome)* is the most common cause of heel pain, especially in joggers, and results from inflammation of plantar aponeurosis (fascia) at its point of attachment to the calcaneus. Generally, it is more common in females and obese persons. A bony spur may develop with plantar fasciitis, but the inflammation causes most of the pain, mediated by the medial calcaneal branch of the tibial nerve. Most patients can be managed nonsurgically, but relief from the pain may take 6 to 12 months. Exercises and orthotic devices are usually recommended in the initial course of treatment.

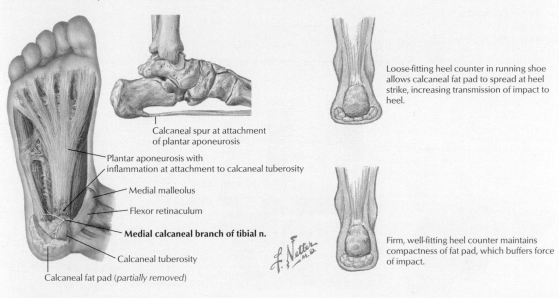

Loose-fitting heel counter in running shoe allows calcaneal fat pad to spread at heel strike, increasing transmission of impact to heel.

Calcaneal spur at attachment of plantar aponeurosis

Plantar aponeurosis with inflammation at attachment to calcaneal tuberosity

Medial malleolus

Flexor retinaculum

Medial calcaneal branch of tibial n.

Calcaneal tuberosity

Calcaneal fat pad *(partially removed)*

Firm, well-fitting heel counter maintains compactness of fat pad, which buffers force of impact.

Deformities of the Toes

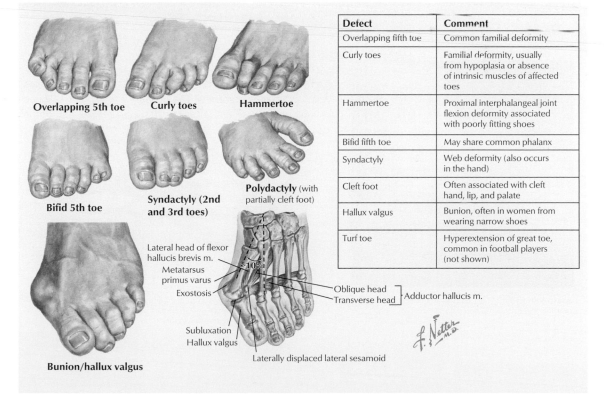

Overlapping 5th toe

Curly toes

Hammertoe

Bifid 5th toe

Syndactyly (2nd and 3rd toes)

Polydactyly (with partially cleft foot)

Bunion/hallux valgus

Lateral head of flexor hallucis brevis m.
Metatarsus primus varus
Exostosis
±10°
Oblique head
Transverse head — Adductor hallucis m.
Subluxation
Hallux valgus
Laterally displaced lateral sesamoid

Defect	Comment
Overlapping fifth toe	Common familial deformity
Curly toes	Familial deformity, usually from hypoplasia or absence of intrinsic muscles of affected toes
Hammertoe	Proximal interphalangeal joint flexion deformity associated with poorly fitting shoes
Bifid fifth toe	May share common phalanx
Syndactyly	Web deformity (also occurs in the hand)
Cleft foot	Often associated with cleft hand, lip, and palate
Hallux valgus	Bunion, often in women from wearing narrow shoes
Turf toe	Hyperextension of great toe, common in football players (not shown)

Clinical Focus 6.34

Fractures of the Talar Neck

The talar neck is the most common site for fractures of this tarsal. Injury usually results from direct trauma or landing on the foot after a fall from a great height. The foot is hyperdorsiflexed so that the neck impinges on the distal tibia. The three types of fractures are as follows:

- **Type I:** Nondisplaced fractures
- **Type II:** Neck fracture with subluxation or dislocation of the subtalar joint
- **Type III:** Neck fracture with dislocation of the subtalar and tibiotalar joints

These fractures can lead to **avascular necrosis of the talus body** because most of the blood supply to the talus passes through the talar neck.

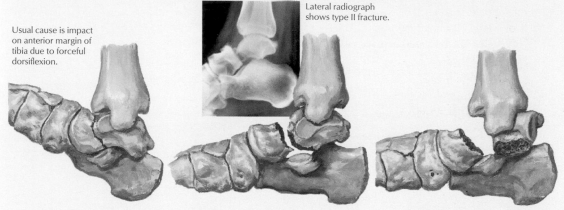

Usual cause is impact on anterior margin of tibia due to forceful dorsiflexion.

Lateral radiograph shows type II fracture.

Type I. No displacement

Type II. Fracture of talar neck with subluxation or dislocation of subtalar joint

Type III. Fracture of talar neck with dislocation of subtalar and tibiotalar joints

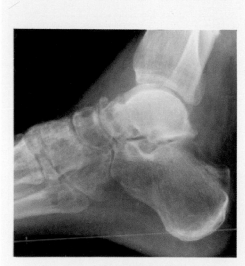

Avascular necrosis of talar body evidenced by increased density (sclerosis) compared with other tarsal bones

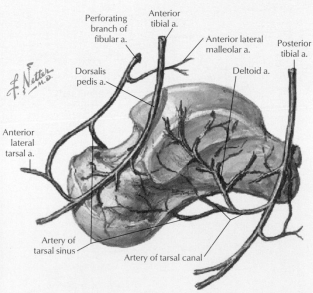

Because of profuse intraosseous anastomoses, avascular necrosis commonly occurs only when surrounding soft tissue is damaged, as in type II and III fractures of talar neck.

Common Foot Infections

Ingrown toenail

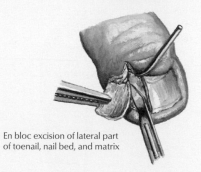

Broken lines show lines of incision for excision of lateral one-fourth of toenail, nail bed, and matrix.

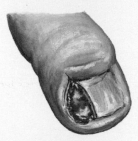

Area of excision

En bloc excision includes nail matrix.

En bloc excision of lateral part of toenail, nail bed, and matrix

After excision, wound allowed to granulate

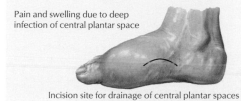

Pain and swelling due to deep infection of central plantar space

Incision site for drainage of central plantar spaces

Puncture wound or perforating ulcer may penetrate deep central plantar spaces, leading to abscess.

Distal and lateral subungual onychomycosis (DLSO)

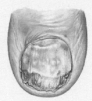

DLSO due to *Trichophyton rubrum*

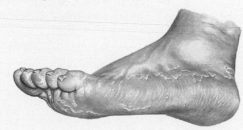

DLSO may be found with tinea pedis.

Additional clinical features of DLSO

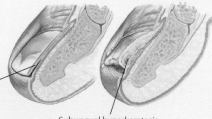

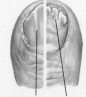

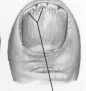

Onycholysis (detachment of the nail from its bed)

Subungual hyperkeratosis

Yellow longitudinal spikes   Crumbling   Splitting

Condition	Comment
Ingrown toenail	Usually great toe, medial or lateral aspect; can lead to an inflamed area that becomes secondarily infected
Onychomycosis	Fungal nail infection, which makes a toenail thick and brittle
Puncture wound	Common injury; can lead to deep infection; requires check of tetanus status

Clinical Focus 6.36

Diabetic Foot Lesions

Diabetes mellitus (DM), a common complex metabolic disorder characterized by hyperglycemia, affects over 18 million people in the United States. The skin is one of many organ systems affected, especially the skin of the leg and foot. **Microvascular disease** may result in a decreased cutaneous blood flow. **Peripheral sensory neuropathy** may render the skin susceptible to injury and may blunt healing. Hyperglycemia predisposes the extremity to bacterial and fungal infection. Associated complications in the lower limb include Charcot joint (progressive destructive arthropathy caused by neuropathy), ulceration, infection, gangrene, and amputation. DM accounts for most nontraumatic foot and lower leg amputations, which total more than 80,000 per year.

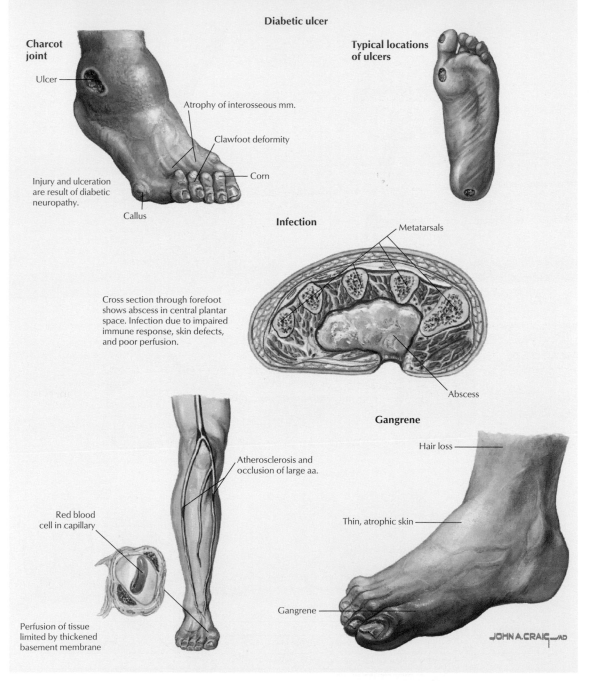

Diabetic ulcer

Charcot joint

Ulcer

Atrophy of interosseous mm.

Clawfoot deformity

Corn

Injury and ulceration are result of diabetic neuropathy.

Callus

Typical locations of ulcers

Infection

Metatarsals

Cross section through forefoot shows abscess in central plantar space. Infection due to impaired immune response, skin defects, and poor perfusion.

Abscess

Gangrene

Hair loss

Atherosclerosis and occlusion of large aa.

Red blood cell in capillary

Thin, atrophic skin

Gangrene

Perfusion of tissue limited by thickened basement membrane

JOHN A.CRAIG_AD

Arterial Occlusive Disease

Atherosclerosis can affect not only the coronary and cerebral vasculature but also the arteries that supply the kidneys, intestines, and lower limbs. The resulting arterial stenosis (narrowing) or occlusion in the leg leads to *peripheral vascular disease* (PVD), a disorder largely associated with increasing age. PVD produces symptoms of claudication, which should be a warning sign of atherosclerosis elsewhere that may produce myocardial infarction and stroke (see also Clinical Focus 6.10).

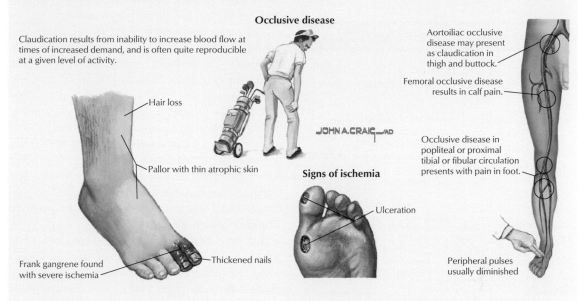

Occlusive disease

Claudication results from inability to increase blood flow at times of increased demand, and is often quite reproducible at a given level of activity.

Aortoiliac occlusive disease may present as claudication in thigh and buttock.

Femoral occlusive disease results in calf pain.

Occlusive disease in popliteal or proximal tibial or fibular circulation presents with pain in foot.

Hair loss

Pallor with thin atrophic skin

Signs of ischemia

Ulceration

JOHN A.CRAIG—AD

Frank gangrene found with severe ischemia

Thickened nails

Peripheral pulses usually diminished

Gout

Uric acid (ionized urate in plasma) is a by-product of purine metabolism and is largely eliminated from the body by renal secretion and excretion. An abnormally elevated serum urate concentration may lead to gout. Gout is caused by precipitation of sodium urate crystals within the joint's *synovial or tenosynovial spaces*, which produces inflammation. About 85% to 90% of clinical gout cases are caused by underexcretion of urate by the kidneys. The disorder may be caused by genetic or renal disease or diseases that affect renal function. Chronic gout presents with deforming arthritis that affects the hands, wrists, feet (especially the great toe), knees, and shoulders.

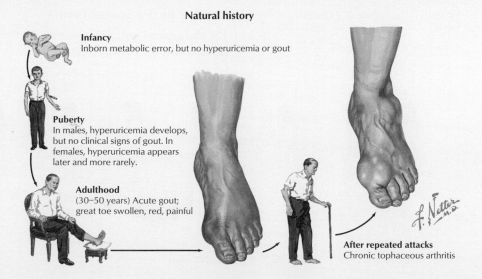

Natural history

Infancy
Inborn metabolic error, but no hyperuricemia or gout

Puberty
In males, hyperuricemia develops, but no clinical signs of gout. In females, hyperuricemia appears later and more rarely.

Adulthood
(30–50 years) Acute gout; great toe swollen, red, painful

After repeated attacks
Chronic tophaceous arthritis

f. Netter M.D.

Gait

The gait (walking) cycle involves both a **swing phase** and a **stance phase** (when the foot is weight-bearing). Additionally, walking produces pelvic tilt and rotation, hip and knee flexion and extension,

---

TABLE 6.23 Summary of Actions of Major Lower Limb Muscles

HIP

Flex: iliopsoas, rectus femoris, sartorius

Rotate medially: gluteus medius and gluteus minimus

Extend: hamstrings, gluteus maximus

Rotate laterally: gluteus maximus, obturator internus, gemelli, piriformis

Abduct: gluteus medius, gluteus minimus, tensor fasciae latae

Adduct: adductor muscles of medial thigh

KNEE

Flex: hamstrings, gracilis, sartorius, gastrocnemius

Rotate medially: semitendinosus, semimembranosus

Extend: quadriceps femoris

Rotate laterally: biceps femoris

ANKLE

Plantarflex: gastrocnemius, soleus, tibialis posterior, flexor digitorum longus, flexor hallucis longus

Dorsiflex: tibialis anterior, extensor digitorum longus, extensor hallucis longus, fibularis tertius

INTERTARSAL

Evert: fibularis longus, brevis, and tertius

Invert: tibialis anterior and posterior

METATARSOPHALANGEAL

Flex: interossei and lumbricals

Abduct: dorsal interossei

Extend: extensor digitorum longus and brevis

Adduct: plantar interossei

INTERPHALANGEAL

Flex: flexor digitorum longus and brevis

Extend: extensor digitorum longus and brevis, lumbricals

---

and a smoothly coordinated interaction among the pelvis, hip, knee, ankle, and foot.

The **swing phase** occurs from pre-swing toe-off (TO) position (Fig. 6.35, No. 5), in which the push-off of the toes occurs by the powerful plantarflexion of the ankle and the forward swing of the hips. The "ball" of the big toe, with its two sesamoid bones, provides the last push needed to accelerate into the swing phase. The foot then accelerates through the initial swing to the midswing (MSW) and terminal swing phase. (Follow the girl's right lower limb in Nos. 6 and 7 of Fig. 6.35.) When the right foot is off the ground, drooping of the pelvis (pelvic dip or tilt) to the unsupported side (right side) is prevented by the action of left hip abductors, primarily the gluteus medius and minimus muscles. *Paralysis of these muscles* (e.g., from polio or pelvic fractures that damage the superior gluteal nerves) can lead to a "gluteal or pelvic dip" and a **positive Trendelenburg sign**.

The limb then decelerates to the heel strike (HS) phase (Fig. 6.35, No. 8 and then back to No. 1) when the foot meets the ground. The heel strike phase is the only point in the gait cycle where the knee is fully extended. The **stance phase** occurs from the HS position, to the flat foot (FF) position, to the midstance (MST) phase, and then the heel-off (HO) phase (forward thrust to TO position and, correspondingly, the HS position for the opposite foot; follow the girl's right lower limb in Nos. 1 to 4 in Fig. 6.35). Table 6.24 summarizes the major muscles involved in the gait cycle.

9. LOWER LIMB ARTERY AND VEIN SUMMARY

Arteries of the Lower Limb

The **abdominal aorta (1)** gives rise to the **left** and **right common iliac arteries (2).** These arteries

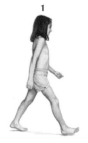 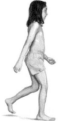 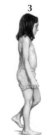 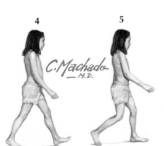 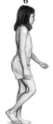 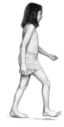 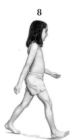

1 Heel strike   2 Foot flat   3 Midstance   4 Opposite heel strike   5 Pre-swing   6 Initial swing   7 Terminal swing   8 Heel strike

FIGURE 6.35 Phases of Gait.

TABLE 6.24 Major Muscles Involved in the Gait Cycle	
GAIT CYCLE	**MUSCLE ACTIONS**
Toe-off (TO) to midswing (MSW)	Hip flexors accelerate the thigh, knee is passively flexed, and foot is dorsiflexed to clear the ground (**swing phase**).
MSW to heel strike (HS)	Knee is extended rapidly, foot is dorsiflexed, and knee is in full extension as heel strikes the ground (**swing phase**).
HS to flat foot (FF)	Hip is flexed, knee is extended, and ankle is in neutral position, but the knee then flexes and the foot then plantarflexes flat on the ground, and limb extensors stabilize the weight-bearing joints (**stance phase**).
FF to midstance (MST)	Body moves forward on planted foot; plantarflexion and hip flexion are eliminated, extensors support limb while other limb is in the swing phase, and hip abductors control pelvic tilt (**stance phase**).
MST to heel-off (HO)	Body continues forward; hip and knee extend, ground force shifts from heel to metatarsal heads, and plantarflexors contract to lift heel off the ground; hip abductors remain active until opposite leg is planted on the ground (**stance phase**).
HO to TO	Push-off as opposite heel strikes the ground, plantarflexors exert thrust, and knee flexes; foot goes into dorsiflexed position at beginning of HO to plantarflexed position as toes push off at TO, and hip abductors relax while hip flexors prepare for the swing phase (**stance phase**).

ankle, and it continues onto the dorsum of the foot as the **dorsal artery of the foot (dorsalis pedis artery) (8)** (Fig. 6.36).

Anastomoses occur around the hip joint, largely supplied by the deep artery of thigh (medial and lateral circumflex femoral arteries) with contributions from several other arteries (e.g., a branch from the obturator artery). The knee and ankle joints also have a rich vascular supply from the genicular arteries (knee) and malleolar and tarsal arteries (ankle). Many of these arteries have small muscular branches (not listed) to supply the muscles of the limb and nutrient arteries to the adjacent bones (not named). **Arteriovenous (AV) anastomoses** are direct connections between small arteries and veins, and usually are involved in *cutaneous thermoregulation.*

Major pulse points of the lower limb include:

- **Femoral pulse:** palpated just inferior to the inguinal ligament.
- **Popliteal pulse:** felt deep behind the knee (very difficult to feel).
- **Posterior tibial pulse:** palpated on the medial aspect of the ankle as it passes through the tarsal tunnel posterior to the medial malleolus.
- **Dorsalis pedis pulse** *(farthest pulse from the heart)*: palpated just lateral to the flexor hallucis longus tendon when pressed against the intermediate cuneiform bone.

In the outline of arteries, major vessels often dissected in anatomy courses include the first-order arteries (in **bold** and numbered) and their second-order major branches. Only more detailed courses in anatomy will dissect the third-order or fourth-order arteries.

Veins of the Lower Limb

Note that the venous drainage of the lower limb begins largely on the dorsum of the foot, with venous blood returning proximally in both a **superficial (1)** and **deep (2)** venous pattern (Fig. 6.37). The **small saphenous vein (3)** drains most of the foot. This same vein and the **deep veins (2)** drain the leg, both largely terminating in the **popliteal vein (4)**. *Variable connections between these veins are common,* so the flow patterns should never be considered absolute; the pattern outlined details the major flow pattern from distal to proximal.

Genicular veins, draining into the popliteal vein, drain the arterial anastomosis around the knee joint. The **great saphenous vein (5)** courses up the medial aspect of the leg and also has connections

divide into internal and external iliac arteries (Fig. 6.36). The internal iliac artery generally supplies the pelvis, perineum, and gluteal regions, while the **external iliac artery (3)** passes deep to the inguinal ligament and into the thigh to become the **femoral artery (4).** The femoral artery gives off a **deep femoral artery (5)** and then continues inferiorly by passing through the adductor hiatus to become the **popliteal artery (6)** posterior to the knee. The popliteal artery divides in the leg to give rise to the **anterior tibial artery (7)** and **posterior tibial artery (9).** The posterior tibial artery gives rise to the small **fibular artery (10)** and passes into the sole of the foot, where it divides into the **medial plantar artery (11)** and **lateral plantar artery (12).** The anterior tibial artery supplies the anterior compartment of the leg, as well as the

1. **Abdominal Aorta***
2. **Right Common Iliac Artery/Left Common Iliac Artery**
3. **Right External Iliac Artery**
4. **Femoral Artery**
   Superficial epigastric artery
   Superficial circumflex iliac artery
   Superficial external pudendal artery
   Deep external pudendal artery
   Descending genicular artery (knee)
5. **Deep Femoral Artery**
   Medial circumflex femoral artery
   Lateral circumflex femoral artery
   Perforating aa. (muscles/bone)
6. **Popliteal Artery**
   Superior lateral and medial geniculate aa.
   Inferior lateral and medial geniculate aa.
   Genicular and patellar anastomoses
7. **Anterior Tibial Artery**
   Ant. and post. tibial recurrent aa.
   Ant. lateral and medial malleolar aa.
   Lateral malleolar network
8. **Dorsal Artery of Foot (Dorsalis Pedis Artery)**
   Lateral and medial tarsal aa.
   Dorsal metatarsal aa.
   Dorsal digital aa.
   Deep plantar artery
9. **Posterior Tibial Artery**
   Medial malleolar aa.
   Calcaneal aa.
   Tibial nutrient artery
10. **Fibular Artery**
    Perforating branches
    Communicating branch
    Lateral malleolar artery
    Calcaneal branches
    Fibular nutrient artery
11. **Medial Plantar Artery**
    Superficial and deep branches
12. **Lateral Plantar Artery**
    Deep plantar artery
       Metatarsal and perforating aa.
          Common plantar digital aa.
             Proper plantar digital arteries
*Direction of blood flow from proximal to distal.

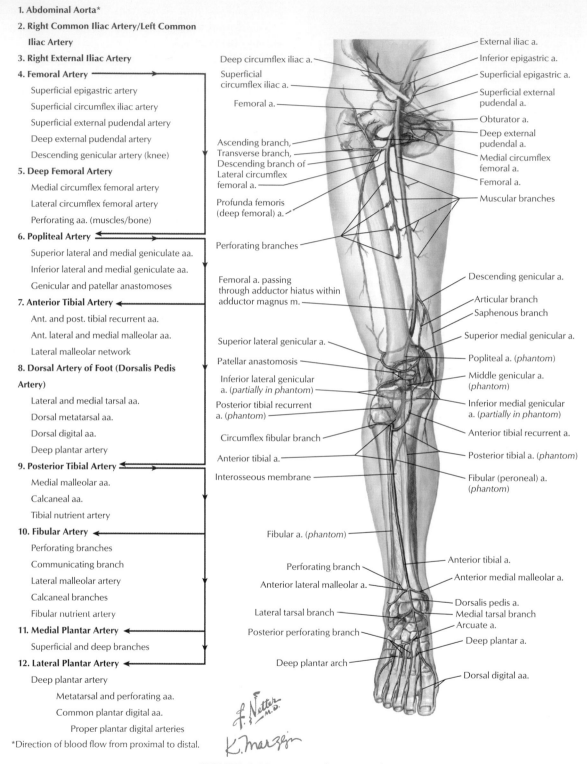

Deep circumflex iliac a.
Superficial circumflex iliac a.
Femoral a.
Ascending branch,
Transverse branch,
Descending branch of
Lateral circumflex femoral a.
Profunda femoris (deep femoral) a.
Perforating branches
Femoral a. passing through adductor hiatus within adductor magnus m.
Superior lateral genicular a.
Patellar anastomosis
Inferior lateral genicular a. (partially in phantom)
Posterior tibial recurrent a. (phantom)
Circumflex fibular branch
Anterior tibial a.
Interosseous membrane
Fibular a. (phantom)
Perforating branch
Anterior lateral malleolar a.
Lateral tarsal branch
Posterior perforating branch
Deep plantar arch

External iliac a.
Inferior epigastric a.
Superficial epigastric a.
Superficial external pudendal a.
Obturator a.
Deep external pudendal a.
Medial circumflex femoral a.
Femoral a.
Muscular branches
Descending genicular a.
Articular branch
Saphenous branch
Superior medial genicular a.
Popliteal a. (phantom)
Middle genicular a. (phantom)
Inferior medial genicular a. (partially in phantom)
Anterior tibial recurrent a.
Posterior tibial a. (phantom)
Fibular (peroneal) a. (phantom)
Anterior tibial a.
Anterior medial malleolar a.
Dorsalis pedis a.
Medial tarsal branch
Arcuate a.
Deep plantar a.
Dorsal digital aa.

FIGURE 6.36 Arteries of Lower Limb.

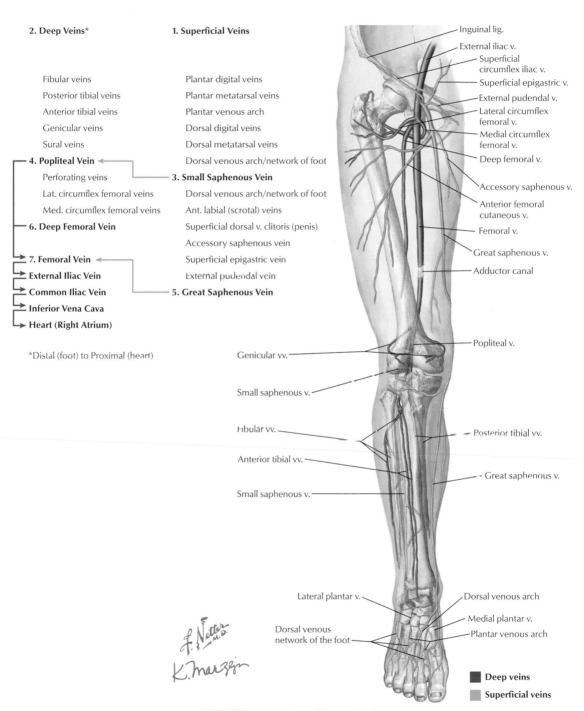

2. Deep Veins*

Fibular veins
Posterior tibial veins
Anterior tibial veins
Genicular veins
Sural veins
4. Popliteal Vein ←
    Perforating veins
    Lat. circumflex femoral veins
    Med. circumflex femoral veins
6. Deep Femoral Vein

7. Femoral Vein ←
External Iliac Vein
Common Iliac Vein
Inferior Vena Cava
Heart (Right Atrium)

*Distal (foot) to Proximal (heart)

1. Superficial Veins

Plantar digital veins
Plantar metatarsal veins
Plantar venous arch
Dorsal digital veins
Dorsal metatarsal veins
Dorsal venous arch/network of foot
3. Small Saphenous Vein
Dorsal venous arch/network of foot
Ant. labial (scrotal) veins
Superficial dorsal v. clitoris (penis)
Accessory saphenous vein
Superficial epigastric vein
External pudendal vein
5. Great Saphenous Vein

Inguinal lig.
External iliac v.
Superficial circumflex iliac v.
Superficial epigastric v.
External pudendal v.
Lateral circumflex femoral v.
Medial circumflex femoral v.
Deep femoral v.
Accessory saphenous v.
Anterior femoral cutaneous v.
Femoral v.
Great saphenous v.
Adductor canal

Popliteal v.
Genicular vv.
Small saphenous v.
Fibular vv.
Anterior tibial vv.
Small saphenous v.
Posterior tibial vv.
Great saphenous v.

Lateral plantar v.
Dorsal venous network of the foot
Dorsal venous arch
Medial plantar v.
Plantar venous arch

■ Deep veins
■ Superficial veins

FIGURE 6.37 Veins of Lower Limb.

with the deep veins of the leg. It continues to run superiorly into the medioanterior thigh to drain into the **femoral vein (7).** The **great saphenous vein (5)** receives tributaries from the superficial perineal structures (labia and clitoris/scrotum and penis) and lower anterior abdominal wall adjacent to the inguinal region. The **deep femoral vein (6)** drains the deep thigh structures (muscles and bone) and is a major tributary draining into the **femoral vein (7).** The femoral vein then drains into the **external iliac vein**, which combined with the **internal iliac vein**, forms the **common iliac vein**. This then drains into the **inferior vena cava**, which drains into the **right atrium of the heart** (Fig. 6.37).

In the human body, the venous system is the compliance system, and, at rest, about 65% of the blood resides in the low-pressure venous system. Veins generally are larger than their corresponding arteries and they have thinner walls. Additionally, they are variable, and multiple veins often accompany

a single artery (the body has many more veins than arteries).

10. LOWER LIMB NERVE SUMMARY

Femoral Nerve

The femoral nerve (L2-L4) innervates the muscles in the anterior compartment of the thigh, which are largely extensors of the leg at the knee (Fig. 6.38). The **patellar tendon reflex** (L3-L4) (knee extension) tests the integrity of this nerve. Injury to this nerve can lead to an *inability to fully extend the knee* unless one pushes on the anterior thigh with one's hand. Major cutaneous branches include the separate lateral cutaneous nerve of the thigh and, from the femoral nerve directly, the following:

- Anterior cutaneous branches to the anterior thigh.
- Saphenous nerve (terminal branch of the femoral nerve) to the medial knee, leg, and ankle.

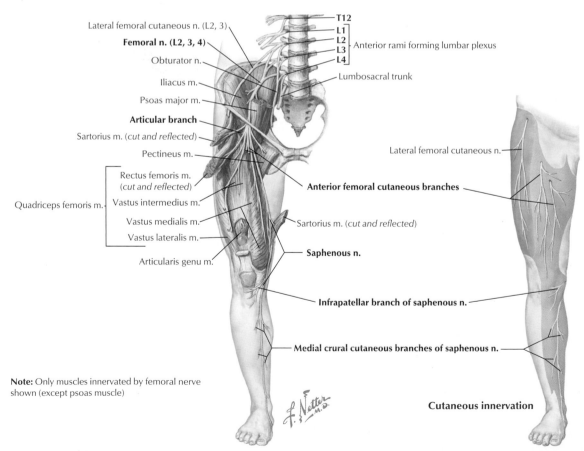

FIGURE 6.38 Course of Femoral Nerve. (From *Netter's atlas of human anatomy,* ed 8, Plate 550; S-115.)

Obturator Nerve

The obturator nerve (L2-L4) innervates the muscles of the medial compartment of the thigh, which are largely adductors of the thigh at the hip (Fig. 6.39). The nerve divides into anterior and posterior branches on both sides of the obturator externus and adductor brevis muscles (the anterior and posterior branches, in effect, "scissors" these two muscles). A small field of cutaneous innervation exists on the medial thigh. Injury to this nerve usually occurs inside the pelvis or close to its origin from the lumbar spine (e.g., from a herniated disc or spinal stenosis). Injury to the nerve can lead to a *weakened ability to adduct the thigh.*

Sciatic Nerve

The sciatic nerve (L4-S3) is the *largest nerve in the body* and is composed of the **tibial** and **common fibular (peroneal) nerves** (Fig. 6.40). The sciatic nerve innervates muscles of the posterior compartment of the thigh (tibial component), which are largely extensors of the thigh at the hip and flexors of the leg at the knee. It also innervates all muscles below the knee, via its tibial and common fibular components.

Tibial Nerve

The tibial nerve (L4-S3), the larger of the two components of the **sciatic nerve,** innervates muscles of the posterior compartment of the leg and all muscles of the plantar foot (Fig. 6.41). These muscles are largely plantarflexors, and some have an inversion function. A lesion to this nerve may result in the loss of plantarflexion and weakened inversion of the foot, and thus a *shuffling gait.* The **calcaneal (Achilles) tendon reflex** (S1-S2) (plantarflexion) tests this nerve.

Fibular Nerve

The common fibular nerve (L4-S2) innervates muscles of the lateral compartment of the leg (everts the foot) via its superficial branch, and muscles of the anterior compartment of the leg and dorsum of the foot via its deep branch, the deep fibular nerve

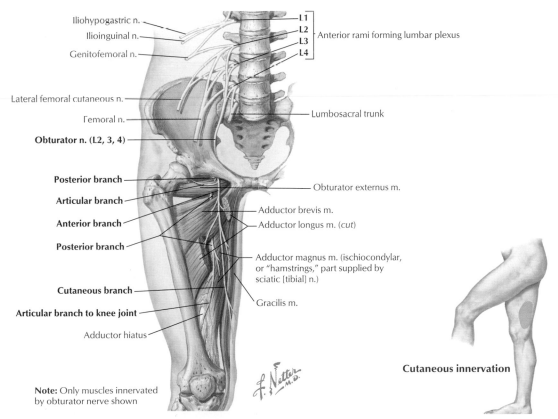

Iliohypogastric n.
Ilioinguinal n.
Genitofemoral n.
L1
L2
L3
L4
Anterior rami forming lumbar plexus

Lateral femoral cutaneous n.
Femoral n.
Obturator n. (L2, 3, 4)
Lumbosacral trunk

Posterior branch
Articular branch
Anterior branch
Posterior branch
Obturator externus m.
Adductor brevis m.
Adductor longus m. (*cut*)
Adductor magnus m. (ischiocondylar, or "hamstrings," part supplied by sciatic [tibial] n.)

Cutaneous branch
Articular branch to knee joint
Adductor hiatus
Gracilis m.

Cutaneous innervation

Note: Only muscles innervated by obturator nerve shown

FIGURE 6.39 Course of Obturator Nerve. (From *Netter's atlas of human anatomy,* ed 8, Plate 551; S-116.)

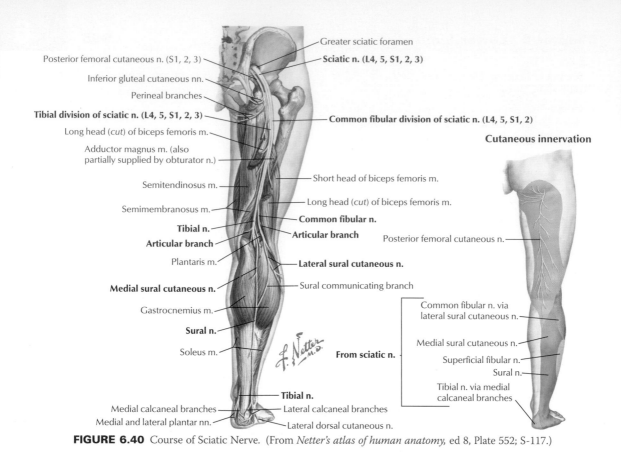

FIGURE 6.40 Course of Sciatic Nerve. (From *Netter's atlas of human anatomy*, ed 8, Plate 552; S-117.)

FIGURE 6.40 labels

Greater sciatic foramen
Posterior femoral cutaneous n. (S1, 2, 3)
Sciatic n. (L4, 5, S1, 2, 3)
Inferior gluteal cutaneous nn.
Perineal branches
Tibial division of sciatic n. (L4, 5, S1, 2, 3)
Common fibular division of sciatic n. (L4, 5, S1, 2)
Long head (*cut*) of biceps femoris m.
Adductor magnus m. (also partially supplied by obturator n.)
Short head of biceps femoris m.
Semitendinosus m.
Long head (*cut*) of biceps femoris m.
Semimembranosus m.
Common fibular n.
Tibial n.
Articular branch
Articular branch
Plantaris m.
Lateral sural cutaneous n.
Medial sural cutaneous n.
Sural communicating branch
Gastrocnemius m.
Sural n.
Soleus m.
From sciatic n.
Tibial n.
Medial calcaneal branches
Lateral calcaneal branches
Medial and lateral plantar nn.
Lateral dorsal cutaneous n.

Cutaneous innervation
Posterior femoral cutaneous n.
Common fibular n. via lateral sural cutaneous n.
Medial sural cutaneous n.
Superficial fibular n.
Sural n.
Tibial n. via medial calcaneal branches

FIGURE 6.41 labels

Tibial n. (L4, 5, S1, 2, 3)
Common fibular n.
Articular branch
Medial sural cutaneous n. (*cut*)
Lateral sural cutaneous n. (*cut*)
Articular branches
Plantaris m.
Gastrocnemius m. (*cut*)
Muscular branch of tibial n.
Popliteus m.
Crural interosseous n.
Soleus m. (*cut and partly retracted*)
Flexor digitorum longus m.
Tibialis posterior m.
Flexor hallucis longus m.
Tibial n.
Sural n. (*cut*)
Medial calcaneal branch
Lateral calcaneal branch
Lateral dorsal cutaneous n.

From tibial n.
Medial calcaneal branches (S1, 2)
Medial plantar n. (L4, 5)
Lateral plantar n. (S1, 2)
Saphenous n. (L3, 4)
Sural n. (S1, 2) via lateral calcaneal and lateral dorsal cutaneous branches

Cutaneous innervation of plantar region

Tibial n.
Lateral plantar n.
Medial plantar n.
Nerve to abductor digiti minimi m.
Flexor digitorum brevis m. (*cut*) and n.
Quadratus plantae m. and n.
Abductor digiti minimi m.
Abductor hallucis m. and n.
Deep branch to 2nd, 3rd, and 4th lumbrical mm. and interossei mm.
Adductor hallucis m.
Flexor hallucis brevis m. and n.
Superficial branch to 4th interosseous m. and Flexor digiti minimi brevis m.
1st lumbrical m. and n.
Common plantar digital nn.
Proper plantar digital nn.

Note: Articular branches not shown

FIGURE 6.41 Course of Tibial Nerve. (From *Netter's atlas of human anatomy*, ed 8, Plate 553; S-118.)

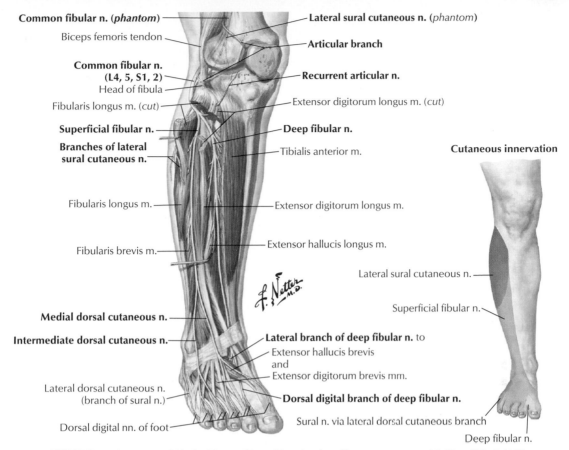

Common fibular n. (*phantom*)

Biceps femoris tendon

Common fibular n.
(L4, 5, S1, 2)
Head of fibula

Fibularis longus m. (*cut*)

Superficial fibular n.

**Branches of lateral
sural cutaneous n.**

Fibularis longus m.

Fibularis brevis m.

Medial dorsal cutaneous n.

Intermediate dorsal cutaneous n.

Lateral dorsal cutaneous n.
(branch of sural n.)

Dorsal digital nn. of foot

Lateral sural cutaneous n. (*phantom*)

Articular branch

Recurrent articular n.

Extensor digitorum longus m. (*cut*)

Deep fibular n.

Tibialis anterior m.

Extensor digitorum longus m.

Extensor hallucis longus m.

Lateral branch of deep fibular n. to
Extensor hallucis brevis
and
Extensor digitorum brevis mm.

Dorsal digital branch of deep fibular n.

Sural n. via lateral dorsal cutaneous branch

Cutaneous innervation

Lateral sural cutaneous n.

Superficial fibular n.

Deep fibular n.

FIGURE 6.42 Course of Fibular Nerve. (From *Netter's atlas of human anatomy,* ed 8, Plate 554; S-119.)

(Fig. 6.42). These muscles are largely dorsiflexors. *Footdrop* and *steppage gait* (high stepping) may occur if this nerve or its deep branch is injured (see Clinical Focus 6.27). The common fibular nerve is most vulnerable as it passes around the fibular neck, where it can be injured by direct trauma or a tight-fitting plaster cast.

Dermatomes

The spiral dermatome pattern of the lower limb is the result of its embryonic medial rotation (Fig. 6.43). Because of the stability of the hip joint, the spiral dermatome pattern is similar to the stripes seen on a barbershop pole. Considerable overlap and some variability in the dermatome pattern are to be expected. However, the following key dermatome regions are generally constant:

- Inguinal region: L1.
- Anterior knee: L4.
- Second toe: L5.
- Posterior leg and thigh: S1-S2.

Zones of autonomous sensory testing (virtually pure dermatome areas) and spinal cord levels

involved in primary movements of the joints are illustrated in Fig. 6.43.

11. EMBRYOLOGY

While the upper limb rotates 90 degrees laterally, the lower limb rotates about **90 degrees medially** so that the knee and elbow are oriented about 180 degrees from each other (Fig. 6.44; see also Figs. 7.43 and 7.44). The thumb lies laterally in anatomical position, but the great toe lies medially. Knee, ankle, and toe flexor muscles are on the posterior aspect of the lower limb. Knee, ankle, and toe extensor muscles are on the anterior aspect. The hip is unaffected, so hip flexors are anterior and extensors are posterior. This limb rotation pattern produces a spiral (barbershop pole) arrangement of the dermatomes as one moves distally along the limb (Fig. 6.44). All the muscles of the lower limb are from **hypaxial** (hypomeres) embryonic ventral mesoderm (see Fig. 2.22) and are innervated by anterior rami and their respective lumbosacral nerves (gluteal, obturator, femoral, and sciatic).

Schematic demarcation of dermatomes (according to Keegan and Garrett) shown as distinct segments. There is considerable overlap between any two adjacent dermatomes. Autonomous sensory zones mark areas of virtually pure dermatome demarcation for sensory testing clinically.

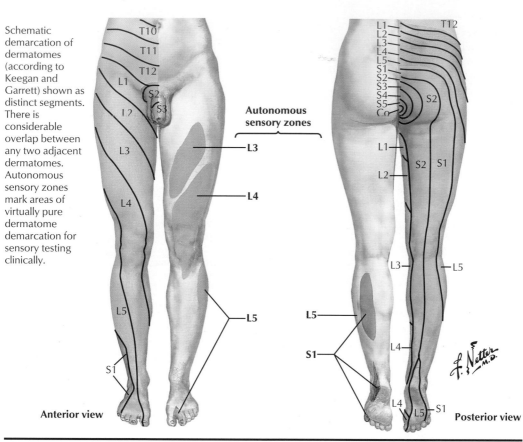

Autonomous sensory zones

Anterior view

Posterior view

Segmental innervation of lower limb movements

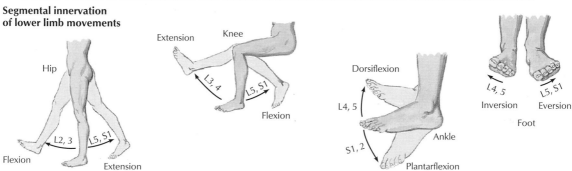

FIGURE 6.43 Dermatomes of the Lower Limb.

Changes in position of limbs before birth

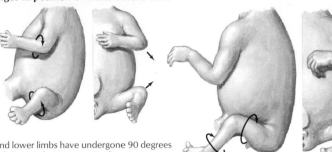

At 7 weeks. Upper and lower limbs have undergone 90 degrees of torsion about their long axes but in opposite directions, so elbows point caudally and knees cranially.

At 8 weeks. Torsion of lower limbs results in twisted or "barber pole" arrangement of their cutaneous innervation.

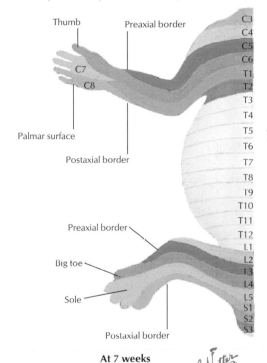

Dermatome pattern

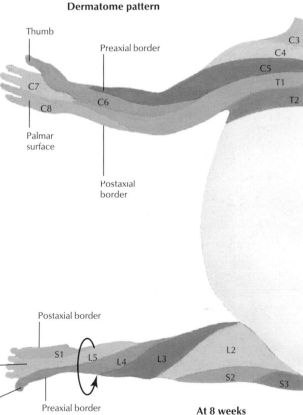

At 7 weeks

At 8 weeks

FIGURE 6.44 Lower Limb Rotation.

Available Online

6.39 Healing of Fractures

Additional figures available online (see inside front cover for details).

Challenge Yourself Questions

1. An elderly patient who has been minimally ambulatory is transported to the clinic with a swollen lower limb and evidence of a deep vein thrombosis. Your examination reveals a sizable clot in her small saphenous vein, and you are concerned that a thromboembolus might originate from this clot and pass to her heart and lungs. After it exits the small saphenous vein, the thromboembolus would next pass into which of the following veins on its journey to the heart?

   A. Deep femoral
   B. External iliac
   C. Femoral
   D. Great saphenous
   E. Popliteal

2. An obese 48-year-old woman presents with a painful lump in her proximal thigh, just medial to the femoral vessels. Examination reveals the herniation of some abdominal viscera, which passes under the inguinal ligament. Through which of the following openings has this hernia passed to enter her thigh?

   A. Deep inguinal ring
   B. Femoral ring
   C. Fossa ovalis
   D. Obturator canal
   E. Superficial inguinal ring

3. The hip is a stable ball-and-socket synovial joint with several strong supporting ligaments. Hip flexion exhibits a significant range of motion, but hip extension is more limited. Which of the following hip ligaments is the strongest ligament and the one that limits hip extension?

   A. Iliofemoral
   B. Ischiofemoral
   C. Ligament of head of femur
   D. Pubofemoral
   E. Transverse acetabular

4. A football player receives a blow to the lateral aspect of his weight-bearing right leg and immediately feels his knee give way. Under extreme pain, he is carried from the field and immediately examined by the team physician, who is able to move the player's right tibia forward excessively compared with the uninjured leg. Which of the following ligaments is injured?

   A. Anterior cruciate
   B. Fibular collateral
   C. Posterior cruciate
   D. Tibial collateral
   E. Transverse

5. During a routine physical exam, the physician taps a patient's patellar ligament with a reflex hammer and elicits a knee-jerk reflex. Which of the following nerves mediates this patellar reflex?

   A. Common fibular
   B. Femoral
   C. Obturator
   D. Saphenous
   E. Tibial

6. A long-distance runner is examined by her physician after complaining of pain along the anteromedial aspect of her left leg, extending from just below the knee to just above the ankle. She has been running on a hard surface and notices that the pain is especially acute as she pushes off from the ground with the affected limb. Which of the following muscles of the leg is most likely affected by this stress injury?

   A. Extensor digitorum longus
   B. Fibularis longus
   C. Gastrocnemius
   D. Popliteus
   E. Tibialis posterior

Multiple-choice and short-answer review questions available online; see inside front cover for details.

7. A stab injury to the buttocks results in the patient's inability to rise from a seated position without the use of his arms, as well as weakness in climbing stairs. A nerve injury is suspected. Which of the following muscles was most likely affected by this stab injury?

   A. Gluteus maximus
   B. Gluteus medius
   C. Obturator internus
   D. Piriformis
   E. Semitendinosus

8. An inversion ankle injury results in the tearing of two of the three major ligaments that stabilize this joint. Which of the following pairs of ligaments are most likely injured?

   A. Anterior talofibular and calcaneofibular
   B. Calcaneofibular and deltoid
   C. Deltoid and long plantar
   D. Long plantar and posterior talofibular
   E. Posterior talofibular and anterior talofibular

9. An 11-year-old boy jumps from a tree house 15 feet above the ground and lands on his feet before rolling forward, immediately feeling extreme pain in his right ankle. Radiographic examination reveals that he has broken the most frequently fractured tarsal bone in the body. Which of the following tarsal bones is most likely fractured?

   A. Calcaneus
   B. Cuboid
   C. Medial cuneiform
   D. Navicular
   E. Talus

10. A laceration across the back of the lower leg results in numbness over the site of the laceration that extends inferiorly over the heel and the lateral back of the sole. Which of the following nerves was mostly likely injured?

   A. Lateral plantar
   B. Medial plantar
   C. Saphenous
   D. Superficial fibular
   E. Sural

11. A 54-year-old man presents with an inability to fully dorsiflex his foot at the ankle, although he can invert and evert his foot. Which of the following nerves may be affected?

   A. Common fibular
   B. Deep fibular
   C. Medial plantar
   D. Superficial fibular
   E. Tibial

12. A man is seen in the clinic waiting room who enters with a "shuffling" gait and a weakened ability to plantarflex his foot. Which of the following nerve-muscle combinations is most likely involved?

   A. Deep fibular nerve and tibialis anterior muscle
   B. Deep fibular nerve and tibialis posterior muscle
   C. Superficial fibular nerve and fibularis longus muscle
   D. Tibial nerve and tibialis anterior muscle
   E. Tibial nerve and tibialis posterior muscle

13. A first-year medical student is asked to demonstrate the location of the dorsalis pedis pulse. Which of the following landmarks would be a reliable guide for finding this artery?

   A. Lateral to the extensor hallucis longus tendon
   B. Medial to the extensor digitorum longus tendons
   C. Over the intermediate cuneiform bone
   D. Over the second metatarsal bone
   E. Web space between toes 1 and 2

14. A 38-year-old woman complains of pain in her feet when walking. Examination reveals the presence of bunions on the medial aspect of both her great (first) toes, from wearing shoes with a very narrow toe. Which of the following clinical terms is used to describe this condition?

   A. Cleft foot
   B. Genu vara
   C. Hallux valgus
   D. Hammertoes
   E. Syndactyly

15. Irritation of the knee in a cleaning lady who scrubs floors on her knees results in septic bursitis and "housemaid's knee." Which of the following bursae is most likely involved?

   A. Anserine
   B. Deep infrapatellar
   C. Prepatellar
   D. Subcutaneous infrapatellar
   E. Suprapatellar

For each condition described below (16-20), select the muscle from the list (A-N) that is most likely responsible or affected.

(A) Adductor longus	**(H)** Piriformis
(B) Biceps femoris (short head)	**(I)** Quadratus femoris
	(J) Rectus femoris
(C) Gluteus maximus	**(K)** Sartorius
(D) Gluteus medius	**(L)** Semimembranosus
(E) Gracilis	**(M)** Semitendinosus
(F) Obturator externus	**(N)** Tensor fasciae latae
(G) Obturator internus	

_____ 16. Pain over the lateral knee leads to a common muscle-tendon injury in runners called ITB (iliotibial tract or band) syndrome.

_____ 17. A dipping of the pelvis during the stance phase of walking may occur if there is an injury to the nerves innervating this important abductor of the femur at the hip.

_____ 18. Weakened flexion of the thigh and abduction at the hip, and flexion of the leg at the knee would suggest an injury to this muscle or to the nerves innervating this muscle.

_____ 19. An orthopedic surgeon examining the integrity of the medial aspect of the knee palpates the tendons of the pes anserinus (goose's foot), including the tendons of the sartorius, semitendinosus, and this muscle.

_____ 20. An athlete "pulls" her hamstring muscles while sprinting. Although this muscle is a muscle of the posterior compartment of the thigh and does flex the leg at the knee, it is not a true hamstring.

21. A 15-year-old adolescent boy suffers a skateboard accident while "showing off" to friends. Examination reveals a sagging left pelvis or dip when he places his weight on his right leg while walking. Which of the following nerve-muscle combinations is most likely responsible for this presentation?

   A. Left inferior gluteal nerve and gluteus maximus muscle
   B. Left inferior gluteal nerve and gluteus medius and minimus muscles
   C. Left superior gluteal nerve and gluteus medius and minimus muscles
   D. Right inferior gluteal nerve and gluteus maximus muscle
   E. Right inferior gluteal nerve and gluteus medius and minimus muscles
   F. Right superior gluteal nerve and gluteus medius and minimus muscles

22. A 14-year-old high school track athlete has pain in his foot, which becomes more and more intense throughout the track season. Examination by an orthopedic surgeon reveals that the cause of his pain is flat feet. Which of the following ligaments is most likely weakened, accounting for this condition?

   A. Anterior talofibular ligament
   B. Medial deltoid ligament
   C. Long plantar ligament
   D. Plantar calcaneocuboid (short plantar) ligament
   E. Plantar calcaneonavicular (spring) ligament

23. Following an accident at home when she walked into a coffee table, a 59-year-old woman presents with footdrop and a weakened ability to dorsiflex and evert her foot at the ankle. Which of the following nerves has she most likely injured?

   A. Common fibular nerve
   B. Deep fibular nerve
   C. Femoral nerve
   D. Superficial fibular nerve
   E. Tibial nerve

24. During a routine examination, you notice that your patient has a weakened calcaneal (Achilles) tendon reflex. Which of the following spinal cord levels is associated with this tendon reflex?

    A. L2-L3
    B. L3-L4
    C. L4-L5
    D. L5-S1
    E. S1-S2

25. A number of important arterial branches supply the hip joint. Each of the following arteries can supply the hip joint, but one of these arteries supplies a small branch that travels in the ligament of the femur and supplies the femoral head. Which of these arteries gives rise to this acetabular branch?

    A. Deep femoral artery
    B. Femoral artery
    C. Inferior gluteal artery
    D. Obturator artery
    E. Superior gluteal artery

26. The tibial nerve and its plantar branches innervate the numerous sweat glands on the sole of the foot. Which of the following nerve fibers innervate these glands?

    A. Pelvic splanchnics
    B. Preganglionic parasympathetics from S2-S4
    C. Preganglionic sympathetics
    D. Postganglionic sympathetics
    E. Somatic efferents from L5

27. Fractures of the talar neck are the most common fractures associated with this tarsal bone. A neck fracture with dislocation may be especially problematic because of which of the following complications?

    A. Avascular necrosis of the talar body
    B. Deep venous thrombosis
    C. Disruption of the tibialis posterior insertion
    D. Rupture of the calcaneal tendon
    E. Rupture of the spring ligament

28. During the normal gait cycle, what is the position of the foot as it pushes off the ground prior to beginning the swing phase?

    A. Dorsiflexed
    B. Everted
    C. Inverted
    D. Plantarflexed

29. A 48-year-old construction worker suffers a knee injury while on the job. When he is examined, it is evident that he has great difficulty unlocking his knee when it is in full extension. Which of the following muscles is most likely involved in this instance?

    A. Adductor magnus muscle
    B. Gastrocnemius muscle
    C. Popliteus muscle
    D. Short head of biceps femoris muscle
    E. Vastus lateralis muscle

For each condition described in questions 30 to 36, select the nerve from the list (A-K) that is most likely responsible for the condition or affected by it.

(A) Common fibular nerve
(B) Deep fibular nerve
(C) Femoral nerve
(D) Inferior gluteal nerve
(E) Lateral plantar nerve
(F) Medial plantar nerve
(G) Obturator nerve
(H) Sciatic nerve
(I) Superficial fibular nerve
(J) Superior gluteal nerve
(K) Tibial nerve

_____ 30. Trauma to the medial pelvic wall results in weakness of adduction of the thigh at the hip.

_____ 31. A patient presents with obvious tenderness on the dorsum of the foot.

_____ 32. Sharp trauma to the popliteal fossa results in presentation of a patient with the foot dorsiflexed and everted. Which nerve has been damaged?

_____ 33. Following a sharp, penetrating injury to the sole of the foot, a patient notices that she is having difficulty flexing her big toe.

_____ 34. Trauma to the leg following an automobile accident results in the loss of sensation on the dorsal skin between the first and second toes.

_____ 35. A patient has difficulty rising from a sitting or squatting position and climbing stairs, but has little difficulty walking on level ground.

_____36. A 27-year-old man has a compound fracture of his lower tibia and is unable to spread (abduct) his lateral four toes.

For each site or point described in questions 37 and 38, select the label (A-F) from the radiographic image of the hip that best matches that description.

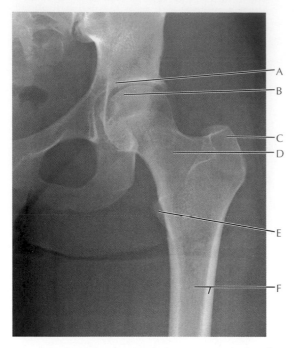

_____ 37. The most common site of a hip fracture in an elderly person.

_____ 38. The insertion point for the most powerful hip flexor muscle.

For each of the bones described in questions 39 and 40, select the label (A-I) from the radiograph of the ankle that best matches that description.

Lateral view

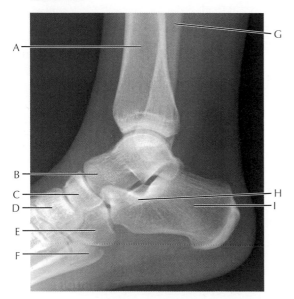

_____ 39. This bone transfers weight from the leg to the foot and has no muscle attachments associated with it.

_____ 40. This bone is the most lateral tarsal bone in the ankle.

Answers to Challenge Yourself Questions

1. **E.** The small saphenous vein drains superiorly along the posterior aspect of the leg and then dives deeply to drain into the popliteal vein deep within the knee.

2. **B.** This woman has a femoral hernia, which gains access to the anterior thigh via the femoral ring. The femoral ring is the abdominal opening in the femoral canal.

3. **A.** The iliofemoral ligament forms an inverted "Y" (of Bigelow) configuration. It is the strongest of the hip ligaments and limits hyperextension.

4. **A.** Excessive movement of the tibia forward on a fixed femur suggests rupture of the anterior cruciate ligament, which limits hyperextension. The posterior cruciate ligament is shorter and the stronger of the two cruciate ligaments.

5. **B.** Extension of the knee occurs with the contraction of the quadriceps femoris group of muscles, which are innervated by the femoral nerve (L2-L4). The patellar reflex tests the L3-L4 component of the femoral nerve.

6. **E.** The leg muscles are encased in a strong and tight crural fascia, and overuse of these muscles can lead to swelling and pain or damage to the muscles in this tight compartment. The muscle most often affected by pushing off the ground is the tibialis posterior muscle during the action of plantarflexion at the ankle.

7. **A.** The inferior gluteal nerves were probably injured and they innervate the most powerful extensor of the hip, the gluteus maximus. We use this muscle especially when climbing stairs or rising from a sitting position. One can exercise on a "stair master" and build up this muscle of the buttock ("buns of steel").

8. **A.** These two ligaments are the most susceptible to inversion injuries of the ankle. In a very severe injury, the posterior talofibular ligament also may be injured.

9. **A.** The calcaneus is a rather soft (cancellous) bone compared with the denser talus. A fall from a great height that includes landing on the feet will result in the talus being driven down into the calcaneus, causing an intraarticular fracture.

10. **E.** The sural nerve is a cutaneous nerve (contains only somatic afferent fibers and postganglionic sympathetic fibers) and lies subcutaneously along the posterior aspect of the leg and close to the small saphenous vein. It innervates the skin of the calf, heel, and posterior sole.

11. **B.** Since the man can evert and invert but cannot fully dorsiflex at the ankle, he most likely has injured his deep fibular nerve. If he had lost eversion alone, he would have injured the superficial fibular nerve and if dorsiflexion and eversion were weakened, then one would suspect an injury of the common fibular nerve.

12. **E.** The tibial nerve innervates the muscles that plantarflex the foot at the ankle. The major muscle that accomplishes this action is the tibialis posterior muscle.

13. **A.** The dorsalis pedis pulse can be reliably and most easily found just lateral to the extensor hallucis longus tendon (points the big toe up), where this artery can be palpated by pressing it against the underlying navicular or intermediate cuneiform bone.

14. **C.** Hallux valgus is the clinical term for a bunion. Bunions result from a medial angling of the distal first metatarsal (varus) coupled with a subluxation and proximal lateral displacement (valgus) of the first phalanx (big toe).

15. **C.** The prepatellar bursa lies right over the lower aspect of the patella and the patellar ligament when the knee is flexed. Thus, it is in the perfect position to bear the brunt of the pressure on the bended knee.

16. **N.** The iliotibial tract (IT; often called "band" by clinicians) is the lower extension and insertion of the tensor fasciae latae muscle on the lateral condyle of the tibia. The IT tract rubs on the lateral epicondyle of the femur.

17. **D.** The gluteus medius muscle is a powerful abductor of the femur at the hip and maintains a relatively stable pelvis when the opposite foot is off the ground. The "gluteal dip" or lurch is seen when the patient stands on the injured limb and the pelvis dips on the other side when that limb is off the ground (a positive Trendelenburg sign). The gluteus medius (and minimus) cannot abduct the hip on the affected side (stance side) to prevent the dip. Usually, this denotes an injury to the superior gluteal nerves innervating the medius and minimus.

18. **K.** The sartorius ("tailor's") muscle flexes and abducts the hip and flexes the knee (think about the action of sitting in a chair with one thigh crossed over the other, as a "tailor" might do while stitching). Thus, it acts on both joints and is innervated by branches of the femoral nerve.

19. **E.** The gracilis is the third muscle of the pes anserinus (three toes of a goose's foot). These muscle tendons help to stabilize the medial aspect of the knee.

20. **B.** The biceps femoris (short head) is a muscle of the posterior compartment of the thigh but only flexes the leg at the knee and does not cross the hip joint and extend the thigh at the hip, like the other three "hamstring" muscles. Therefore, it is not a true hamstring muscle and not as commonly injured.

21. **F.** This is a positive Trendelenburg sign and indicates paralysis (usually from polio, hip surgery, or a pelvic fracture) of the hip adductors (gluteus medius and minimus muscles) innervated by the superior gluteal nerves on the side of the limb that is weight-bearing, in this case, the right lower limb. The opposite hip "dips," and the patient may actually lurch to the weakened side to maintain a level pelvis when walking. Thus, when one is standing on the right leg and the left pelvis dips or drops, a positive right Trendelenburg sign is present (i.e., the contralateral side dips because the ipsilateral hip adductors [in this case, those on the right side] cannot stabilize the pelvis to prevent the dip [see the Gait section in this chapter]).

22. **E.** The arch is stabilized by several ligaments and muscle tendons, but the most important support for the medial arch is the plantar calcaneonavicular (spring) ligament.

23. **A.** Footdrop and weakened eversion of the foot are associated with weakness of the anterior and lateral compartment muscles of the leg, all innervated by the common fibular nerve. This nerve is the most commonly injured nerve of the lower limb.

24. **E.** Tapping the calcaneal tendon elicits the reflex contraction of the gastrocnemius and soleus muscles, and is associated with the S1-S2 nerve roots. Level L3-L4 is associated with the patellar ligament reflex.

25. **D.** The acetabular branch runs in the ligament of the femur, supplies the head of the femur, and is a branch of the obturator artery (see Table 6.3). However, the medial and lateral circumflex branches of the deep femoral artery supply most of the blood to the hip.

26. **D.** Sweat glands on the sole of the foot are innervated by the postganglionic sympathetic fibers found in the medial and lateral plantar somatic nerves. Somatic nerves contain somatic efferents, afferents, and postganglionic sympathetic fibers, which innervate the glands of the skin, hair follicles, and smooth muscle of the blood vessels. These sympathetics originate as preganglionic fibers from the lateral cell column of the L1-L2 spinal cord.

27. **A.** The blood supply to the talus usually occurs through the talar neck. Fracture of the neck accompanied by subluxation or dislocation can lead to avascular necrosis of the remainder of the tarsal (see Clinical Focus 6.34).

28. **D.** In the normal gait cycle, as one pushes off the ground with the toes (at toe-off), the foot undergoes powerful plantarflexion of the ankle and the hips swing forward. The foot is dorsiflexed during the swing phase to clear the ground.

29. **C.** In order for the knee to be unlocked prior to flexion, the femur must be rotated laterally and flexion initiated by the popliteus muscle (it pops the knee).

30. **G.** The obturator nerve passes through the pelvic cavity near its medial wall and then moves out of the obturator foramen; it supplies the adductor muscles of the thigh's medial compartment. The pathway of the nerve in the pelvic cavity may place the nerve in jeopardy if pelvic trauma is significant.

31. **I.** Sensation on the dorsum of the foot is largely conveyed by the medial and intermediate dorsal cutaneous nerves of the superficial fibular nerve. A small area of skin between the first and second toes is supplied by the medial branch of the deep fibular nerve.

32. **K.** The tibial nerve passes through the popliteal fossa behind the knee. It innervates muscles of the leg that are largely plantarflexors of the ankle and toes and muscles that are invertors at the ankle. Loss of these functions due to tibial nerve damage places the relaxed foot in eversion and dorsiflexion at the ankle, mediated by the common fibular nerve.

33. **F.** The medial plantar nerve in the sole innervates the short intrinsic flexors of the big toe. The tibial nerve resides in the leg but divides into the medial and lateral plantar nerves at the ankle, so the best answer is the medial plantar nerve. Some weakened flexion may still be present, however, because the flexor hallucis longus muscle of the leg continues to be innervated, as the injury occurred distal to this point on the side of the foot.

34. **B.** The deep fibular nerve, via its medial branch, innervates the dorsal skin between the first and second toes.

35. **D.** The gluteus maximus muscle is the "power extensor" of the hip, and it is innervated by the large inferior gluteal nerve. This is especially evident when one is rising from a squatting or sitting position, or climbing stairs.

36. **E.** The tibial nerve divides into its medial and lateral plantar nerves at the ankle. It is the lateral plantar nerve that innervates the muscles that abduct the lateral four toes (the dorsal interossei muscles abduct toes 2 to 4, and the abductor digiti minimi muscle abducts the 5th toe).

37. **D.** The femoral neck is the most common site for hip fractures, especially in an elderly person, whose bones may be weakened by osteoporosis. The strong pull of muscles on a weakened bone may cause femoral neck fractures.

38. **E.** The most powerful flexor of the thigh at the hip is the iliopsoas muscle, which inserts on the lesser trochanter of the femur.

39. **B.** The talus transfers the weight from the tibia to the foot. It is much denser than the lighter calcaneus and has no muscle tendons attaching to it.

40. **E.** The large cuboid tarsal bone is the most lateral of the tarsals and is easily visible because of the transverse arch of the foot, which extends from the cuboid, across the cuneiforms, and the base of the metatarsals.

Upper Limb

1. INTRODUCTION

The upper limb is part of the **appendicular skeleton** and includes the shoulder, arm, forearm, and hand. It is continuous with the lower neck and is suspended from the trunk at the shoulder. It is anatomically and clinically convenient and beneficial to divide the limb into its functional muscle compartments and to review the nerve(s) and vessels supplying these compartments. Thus, for each component of the upper limb, this chapter focuses on organizing the clinical anatomy into functional compartments and understanding how that anatomy is ideally suited for a wide range of motion, thereby allowing us to manipulate our surrounding environment.

To prepare for your study, review the movements of the upper limb at the shoulder, elbow, wrist, and fingers in Chapter 1 (Fig. 1.3).

2. SURFACE ANATOMY

Much of the underlying anatomy of the upper limb can be appreciated by a careful inspection of the surface features (Fig. 7.1). The following surface features are of special note:

- **Acromion:** attachment site of the trapezius and deltoid muscles; easily palpable.
- **Clavicle:** long bone that lies subcutaneously throughout its length.
- **Olecranon:** elbow and proximal portion of the ulna.
- **Deltoid muscle:** muscle that caps the shoulder.
- **Flexor tendons:** wrist and finger flexor tendons are visible at the distal anterior forearm.
- **Extensor tendons:** wrist and finger extensor tendons are visible on the dorsum of the hand.

- **Thenar eminence:** cone of muscles at the base of the thumb.
- **Hypothenar eminence:** cone of muscles at the base of the little finger.
- **Dorsal venous network:** veins seen on the dorsum of the hand.
- **Cephalic vein:** subcutaneous vein that drains the lateral forearm and arm into the axillary vein.
- **Basilic vein:** subcutaneous vein that drains the medial forearm and distal arm into the axillary vein.
- **Median cubital vein:** subcutaneous vein that lies in the cubital fossa (anterior aspect of the elbow); often used for venipuncture.

As seen elsewhere in the body, a set of **superficial and deep veins** drain the upper limb. Superficial veins drain blood toward the heart and communicate with deep veins that parallel the major arteries of the upper limb (Fig. 7.2). When vigorous muscle contraction increases the blood flow to the limb and compresses the deep veins, venous blood is shunted into the superficial veins and then returned to the heart. (The veins become more prominent as the limb is being exercised, e.g., when lifting weights.) The superficial and deep veins have **valves** to assist in venous return. Cutaneous nerves also lie in the superficial fascia and are the terminal sensory branches of the major nerves arising from the brachial plexus (anterior rami of C5-T1 spinal levels) (Fig. 7.2).

3. SHOULDER

Bones and Joints of Pectoral Girdle and Shoulder

The pectoral girdle is composed of the following structures:

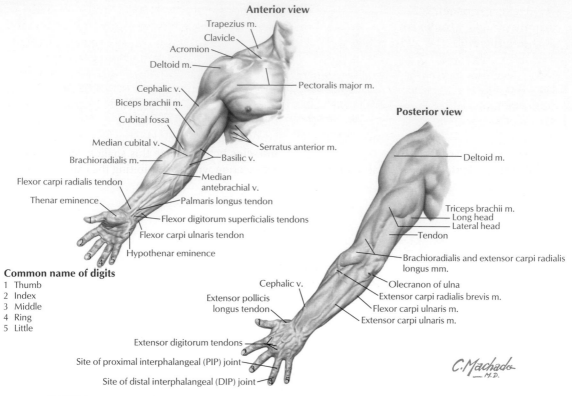

Anterior view

Trapezius m.
Clavicle
Acromion
Deltoid m.
Cephalic v.
Biceps brachii m.
Cubital fossa
Median cubital v.
Brachioradialis m.
Flexor carpi radialis tendon
Thenar eminence
Palmaris longus tendon
Flexor digitorum superficialis tendons
Flexor carpi ulnaris tendon
Hypothenar eminence
Pectoralis major m.
Serratus anterior m.
Basilic v.
Median antebrachial v.

Posterior view

Deltoid m.
Triceps brachii m.
Long head
Lateral head
Tendon
Brachioradialis and extensor carpi radialis longus mm.
Olecranon of ulna
Extensor carpi radialis brevis m.
Flexor carpi ulnaris m.
Extensor carpi ulnaris m.

Common name of digits
1 Thumb
2 Index
3 Middle
4 Ring
5 Little

Cephalic v.
Extensor pollicis longus tendon
Extensor digitorum tendons
Site of proximal interphalangeal (PIP) joint
Site of distal interphalangeal (DIP) joint

C. Machado
M.D.

FIGURE 7.1 Key Surface Landmarks of Upper Limb. (From *Netter's atlas of human anatomy*, ed 8, Plate 422; S-10.)

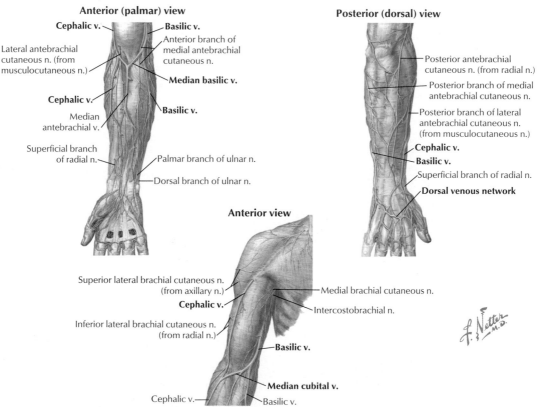

Anterior (palmar) view

Cephalic v.
Basilic v.
Anterior branch of medial antebrachial cutaneous n.
Lateral antebrachial cutaneous n. (from musculocutaneous n.)
Median basilic v.
Cephalic v.
Basilic v.
Median antebrachial v.
Superficial branch of radial n.
Palmar branch of ulnar n.
Dorsal branch of ulnar n.

Posterior (dorsal) view

Posterior antebrachial cutaneous n. (from radial n.)
Posterior branch of medial antebrachial cutaneous n.
Posterior branch of lateral antebrachial cutaneous n. (from musculocutaneous n.)
Cephalic v.
Basilic v.
Superficial branch of radial n.
Dorsal venous network

Anterior view

Superior lateral brachial cutaneous n. (from axillary n.)
Cephalic v.
Inferior lateral brachial cutaneous n. (from radial n.)
Medial brachial cutaneous n.
Intercostobrachial n.
Basilic v.
Median cubital v.
Cephalic v.
Basilic v.

f. Netter
M.D.

FIGURE 7.2 Superficial Veins and Nerves of Upper Limb. (From *Netter's atlas of human anatomy*, ed 8, Plates 424 and 425; S-228 and S-229.)

- **Clavicle** (collar bone).
- **Scapula** (shoulder blade).

The **humerus**, or arm bone, articulates with the scapula and forms the shoulder joint (the glenohumeral ball-and-socket synovial joint). These bones are shown in Fig. 7.3 and listed in Table 7.1. The joints contributing to the pectoral girdle and shoulder are described in Table 7.2 (acromioclavicular and glenohumeral joints) and Table 3.2 (sternoclavicular joint).

The **sternoclavicular** and **acromioclavicular joints** of the pectoral girdle allow for a significant amount of movement of the limb and combined with the shallow ball-and-socket **glenohumeral joint** permit extension, flexion, abduction, adduction, medial (internal) rotation, lateral (external) rotation, protraction, retraction, and circumduction movements (see Fig. 1.3 for examples of these movements). This flexibility and range of movement greatly enhance our ability to interact with our environment. The tendons of the four **rotator cuff muscles** help stabilize this shallow glenohumeral articulation without inhibiting the extensive range of motion that we enjoy at the shoulder (Fig. 7.4).

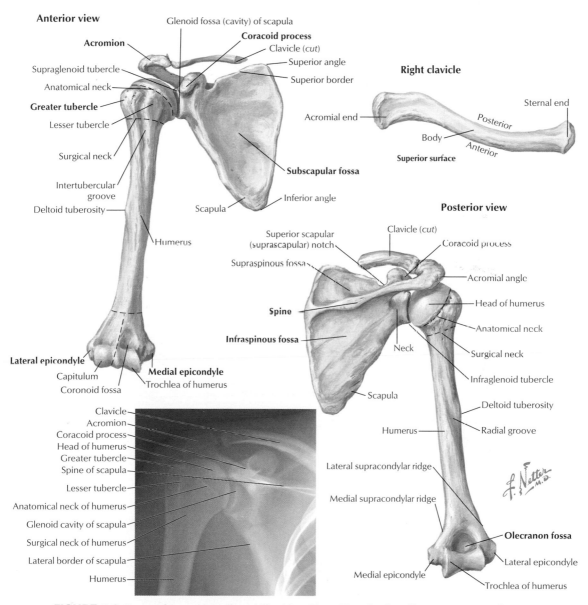

FIGURE 7.3 Bones of Pectoral Girdle and Shoulder. (From *Netter's atlas of human anatomy*, ed 8, Plates 427 to 430; S-155, S-156, S-158, S-264.)

368

Chapter 7   Upper Limb

TABLE 7.1 Features of the Clavicle, Scapula, and Humerus

CLAVICLE	SCAPULA	HUMERUS
Cylindrical bone with slight S-shaped curve; has no medullary cavity Middle third: narrowest portion First bone to ossify but last to fuse; formed by intramembranous ossification Most frequently fractured long bone; acts as a strut to keep limb away from trunk	Flat triangular bone Shallow glenoid cavity Attachment locations for 16 muscles Fractures relatively uncommon	Long bone Proximal head: articulates with glenoid cavity of scapula Distal medial and lateral condyles: articulate at elbow with ulna and radius Surgical neck is common fracture site, endangering axillary nerve Midshaft fracture: radial nerve vulnerable

Clinical Focus 7.1

Glenohumeral Dislocations

Almost 95% of shoulder (glenohumeral joint) dislocations occur in an anterior or anteroinferior direction. They are most common in adolescents and young adults, often as athletic injuries. Abduction, extension, and lateral (external) rotation of the arm at the shoulder (e.g., the throwing motion) place stress on the capsule and anterior elements of the rotator cuff (subscapularis tendon). The types of anterior dislocations include the following:

- Subcoracoid (most common; anterior)
- Subglenoid (anteroinferior)
- Subclavicular (rare) (anterosuperior)

The **axillary** (most often; usually a traction type of injury) and **musculocutaneous nerves** may be injured during such dislocations.

Anterior dislocation of glenohumeral joint

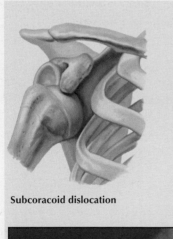

Subcoracoid dislocation

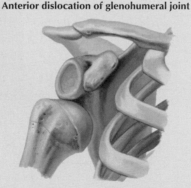

Subglenoid dislocation

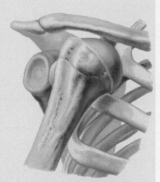

Subclavicular dislocation

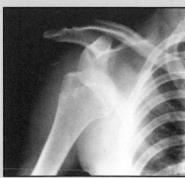

Subcoracoid dislocation. Anteroposterior radiograph

Acromion prominent

Humeral head prominent

Testing sensation in areas of (1■) axillary and (2 ■) musculocutaneous nerves

Arm in slight abduction

Elbow flexed

Forearm internally rotated, supported by other hand

Clinical appearance

C. Machado M.D.

TABLE 7.2 Acromioclavicular and Glenohumeral Joints

LIGAMENT OR BURSA	ATTACHMENT	COMMENT
Acromioclavicular (Synovial Plane) Joint		
Capsule and articular disc	Surrounds joint	Allows gliding movement as arm is raised and scapula rotates
Acromioclavicular	Acromion to clavicle	Supports joint superiorly
Coracoclavicular (conoid and trapezoid ligaments)	Coracoid process to clavicle	Reinforces the joint by stabilizing the clavicle
Glenohumeral (Multiaxial Synovial Ball-and-Socket) Joint		
Fibrous capsule	Surrounds joint	Permits flexion, extension, abduction, adduction, protraction, retraction, circumduction; most commonly dislocated joint
Coracohumeral	Coracoid process to greater tubercle of humerus	Strong ligament
Glenohumeral	Supraglenoid tubercle to lesser tubercle of humerus	Composed of superior, middle, and inferior thickenings
Transverse humeral	Spans greater and lesser tubercles of humerus	Holds long head of biceps tendon in intertubercular groove
Glenoid labrum	Margin of glenoid cavity of scapula	Is fibrocartilaginous ligament that deepens glenoid cavity
Bursae		
Subacromial		Between coracoacromial arch and suprascapular muscle
Subdeltoid		Between deltoid muscle and capsule
Subscapular		Between subscapularis tendon and scapular neck

Clinical Focus 7.2

Fracture of the Proximal Humerus

Fractures of the proximal humerus often occur from a fall on an outstretched hand or from direct trauma to the area. They are especially common in elderly persons, in whom osteoporosis is a factor. The most common site is the **surgical neck of the humerus,** because the bone begins to taper down at this point and is structurally weaker (see Fig. 7.3).

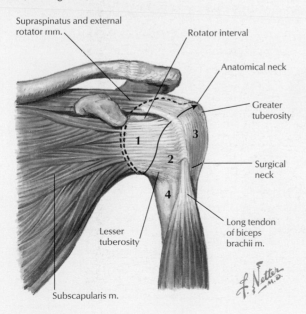

Supraspinatus and external rotator mm.

Rotator interval

Anatomical neck

Greater tuberosity

Surgical neck

Long tendon of biceps brachii m.

Lesser tuberosity

Subscapularis m.

Neer four-part classification of fractures of proximal humerus. 1. Articular fragment (humeral head). 2. Lesser tuberosity. 3. Greater tuberosity. 4. Shaft. If no fragments displaced, fracture considered stable (most common) and treated with minimal external immobilization and early range-of-motion exercise. Displacement of 1 cm or angulation of 45 degrees of one or more fragments necessitates open reduction and internal fixation or prosthetic replacement.

Clinical Focus 7.3

Clavicular Fractures

Fracture of the clavicle is quite common, especially in children. Clavicular fracture usually results from a fall on an outstretched hand or from direct trauma to the shoulder. Fractures of the medial third of the clavicle are rare (about 5%), but *fractures of the middle third* are common (about 80%). Fractures of the lateral third can involve coracoclavicular ligament tears.

Fractures of lateral third of clavicle

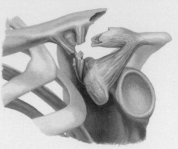

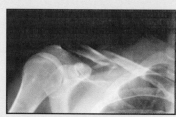

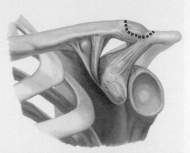

Type I. Fracture with no disruption of ligaments and therefore no displacement.

Type II. Fracture with tear of coracoclavicular ligament and upward displacement of medial fragment.

Type III. Fracture through acromioclavicular joint; no displacement

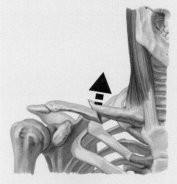

Fractures of middle third of clavicle (most common). Medial fragment displaced upward by pull of sterno-cleidomastoid muscle; lateral fragment displaced downward by weight of shoulder. Fractures occur most often in children.

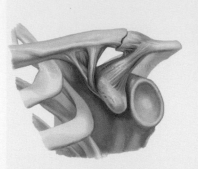

Anteroposterior radiograph.
Fracture of middle third of clavicle

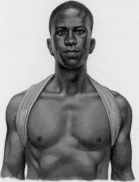

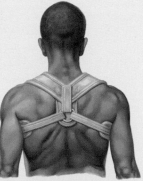

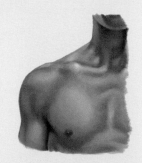

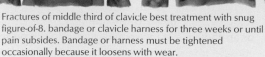

Fractures of middle third of clavicle best treatment with snug figure-of-8. bandage or clavicle harness for three weeks or until pain subsides. Bandage or harness must be tightened occasionally because it loosens with wear.

Healed fracture of clavicle. Even with proper treatment, small lump may remain.

Joint opened: lateral view

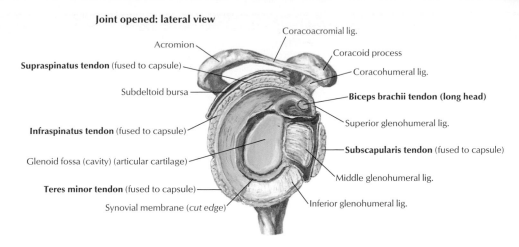

Coracoacromial lig.

Acromion

Coracoid process

Supraspinatus tendon (fused to capsule)

Coracohumeral lig.

Subdeltoid bursa

Biceps brachii tendon (long head)

Superior glenohumeral lig.

Infraspinatus tendon (fused to capsule)

Subscapularis tendon (fused to capsule)

Glenoid fossa (cavity) (articular cartilage)

Middle glenohumeral lig.

Teres minor tendon (fused to capsule)

Inferior glenohumeral lig.

Synovial membrane (*cut edge*)

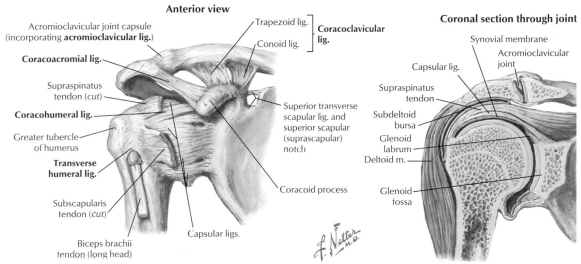

Anterior view

Coronal section through joint

Acromioclavicular joint capsule (incorporating **acromioclavicular lig.**)

Trapezoid lig.
Conoid lig.
Coracoclavicular lig.

Synovial membrane

Acromioclavicular joint

Coracoacromial lig.

Capsular lig.

Supraspinatus tendon (*cut*)

Supraspinatus tendon

Superior transverse scapular lig. and superior scapular (suprascapular) notch

Subdeltoid bursa

Coracohumeral lig.

Greater tubercle of humerus

Glenoid labrum

Deltoid m.

Transverse humeral lig.

Coracoid process

Glenoid fossa

Subscapularis tendon (*cut*)

Capsular ligs.

Biceps brachii tendon (long head)

FIGURE 7.4 Shoulder Joint Tendons and Ligaments. (From *Netter's atlas of human anatomy*, ed 8, Plate 431; S-157.)

The glenohumeral joint is both the *most mobile* of the body's joints and *one of the most frequently dislocated joints* in the body (see Clinical Focus 7.1).

Muscles

Muscles of the shoulder include the superficial back muscles, the deltoid and teres major muscles, the four rotator cuff muscles, and the superficial muscles of the pectoral region (anterior chest wall) (Fig. 7.5 and Table 7.3). It is important to note that 16 different muscles attach to the scapula (back, limb, and neck muscles) and account for the range of movement of the scapula as the upper limb is abducted (the scapula rotates), adducted, flexed, extended, and rotated.

Note that abduction at the shoulder is initiated by the **supraspinatus muscle** up to about 15 degrees of abduction and then abduction to 90 degrees is achieved largely by the action of the **deltoid muscle.** For full elevation to 180 degrees, the scapula must laterally rotate upward (the inferior angle swings laterally) by the action of the superior portion of the trapezius muscle, levator scapulae muscle, and serratus anterior muscle. In reality, abduction at the shoulder is a smooth movement, and even as one initiates abduction, the scapula begins to rotate laterally as well. During adduction at the shoulder, the scapula is brought back into its resting position primarily by the actions of the medial and lower fibers of the trapezius muscle, the pectoralis minor muscle, and the rhomboid muscles.

Because of its broad encapsulation of the shoulder, the **deltoid muscle** functions primarily as an abductor of the shoulder, although its posterior muscle fibers also assist in *extension* and *lateral rotation.* Its medial fibers assist in flexion and medial rotation at the shoulder. Many of these muscles

TABLE 7.3 Shoulder Muscles

MUSCLE	PROXIMAL ATTACHMENT	DISTAL ATTACHMENT	INNERVATION	MAIN ACTIONS
Trapezius	Medial third of superior nuchal line; external occipital protuberance, ligamentum nuchae, and spinous processes of C7-T12	Lateral third of clavicle, acromion, and spine of scapula	Accessory nerve (cranial nerve XI)	Elevates, retracts, and rotates scapula; superior fibers elevate, middle fibers retract, and inferior fibers depress scapula
Latissimus dorsi	Spinous processes of T7-L5, thoracolumbar fascia, iliac crest, and inferior three ribs	Intertubercular sulcus of humerus	Thoracodorsal nerve (C6-C8)	Extends, adducts, and medially rotates humerus at shoulder
Levator scapulae	Transverse processes of C1-C4 vertebrae	Superior part of medial border of scapula	Dorsal scapular and cervical (C3 and C4) nerves	Elevates scapula and tilts its glenoid cavity inferiorly by rotating scapula
Rhomboid minor and major	*Minor:* ligamentum nuchae, spinous processes of C7 and T1 *Major:* spinous processes, T2-T5	Medial border of scapula from level of spine to inferior angle	Dorsal scapular nerve (C4-C5)	Retracts scapula and rotates it to depress glenoid cavity; fixes scapula to thoracic wall
Deltoid	Lateral third of clavicle, acromion, and spine of scapula	Deltoid tuberosity of humerus	Axillary nerve (C5-C6)	*Anterior part:* flexes and medially rotates arm at shoulder *Middle part:* abducts arm at shoulder *Posterior part:* extends and laterally rotates arm at shoulder
Supraspinatus (rotator cuff muscle)	Supraspinous fossa of scapula and deep fascia	Greater tubercle of humerus	Suprascapular nerve (C5-C6)	Initiates abduction, helps deltoid abduct arm at shoulder and acts with rotator cuff muscles
Infraspinatus (rotator cuff muscle)	Infraspinous fossa of scapula and deep fascia	Greater tubercle of humerus	Suprascapular nerve (C5-C6)	Laterally rotates arm at shoulder; helps to hold head in glenoid cavity
Teres minor (rotator cuff muscle)	Lateral border of scapula	Greater tubercle of humerus	Axillary nerve (C5-C6)	Laterally rotates arm at shoulder; helps to hold head in glenoid cavity
Teres major	Dorsal surface of inferior angle of scapula	Medial lip of intertubercular sulcus of humerus	Lower subscapular nerve (C5-C6)	Adducts arm and medially rotates arm
Subscapularis (rotator cuff muscle)	Subscapular fossa of scapula	Lesser tubercle of humerus	Upper and lower subscapular nerves (C5-C6)	Medially rotates arm at shoulder and adducts it; helps to hold humeral head in glenoid cavity
Pectoralis major	Medial half of clavicle; sternum; superior six costal cartilages; aponeurosis of external abdominal oblique	Lateral lip of intertubercular sulcus of humerus	Lateral (C5-C7) and medial pectoral (C8-T1) nerves	Flexes, adducts, and medially rotates arm at shoulder
Pectoralis minor	3rd to 5th ribs and deep fascia	Coracoid process of scapula	Medial pectoral nerve (C8-T1)	Depresses and protracts scapula
Serratus anterior	Upper eight ribs	Medial border of scapula	Long thoracic nerve (C5-C7)	Rotates and protracts scapula; pulls it anteriorly toward thoracic wall
Subclavius	Junction of 1st rib and costal cartilage	Inferior surface of clavicle	Nerve to subclavius (C5-C6)	Depresses and anchors clavicle

Variations in spinal nerve contributions to the innervation of muscles, their attachments, and their actions are common in human anatomy. Therefore, expect differences between texts and realize that anatomical variation is normal.

Posterior view

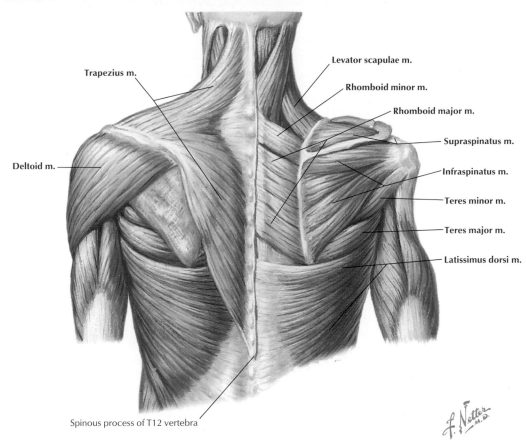

Trapezius m.

Deltoid m.

Levator scapulae m.

Rhomboid minor m.

Rhomboid major m.

Supraspinatus m.

Infraspinatus m.

Teres minor m.

Teres major m.

Latissimus dorsi m.

Spinous process of T12 vertebra

Anterior view

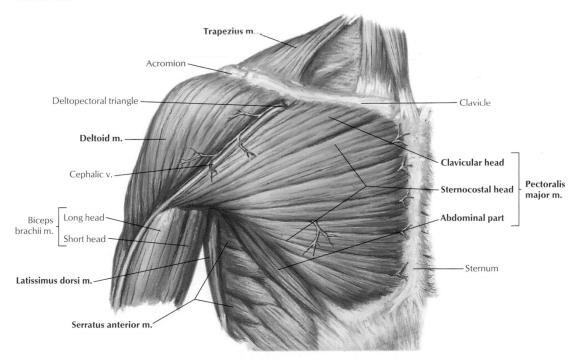

Trapezius m.

Acromion

Deltopectoral triangle

Deltoid m.

Cephalic v.

Biceps brachii m. { Long head / Short head

Latissimus dorsi m.

Serratus anterior m.

Clavicle

Clavicular head

Sternocostal head

Abdominal part

Pectoralis major m.

Sternum

FIGURE 7.5 Muscles Acting on the Shoulder. (From *Netter's atlas of human anatomy,* ed 8, Plate 413; S-230.)

Clinical Focus 7.4

Rotator Cuff Injury

The tendons of insertion of the rotator cuff muscles form a musculotendinous cuff about the shoulder joint on its anterior, superior, and posterior aspects. The muscles of the rotator cuff group are as follows:

- Subscapularis
- Infraspinatus
- Supraspinatus
- Teres minor

Repeated abduction and flexion (e.g., a throwing motion) cause wear and tear on the tendons as they rub on the acromion and coracoacromial ligament, which may lead to cuff tears or rupture. The tendon of the supraspinatus is most vulnerable to injury.

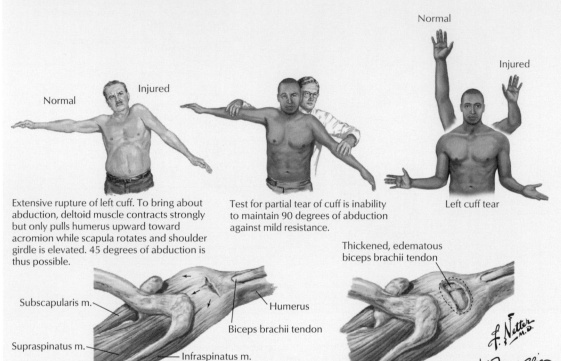

Extensive rupture of left cuff. To bring about abduction, deltoid muscle contracts strongly but only pulls humerus upward toward acromion while scapula rotates and shoulder girdle is elevated. 45 degrees of abduction is thus possible.

Test for partial tear of cuff is inability to maintain 90 degrees of abduction against mild resistance.

Left cuff tear

Acute rupture (superior view). Often associated with splitting tear parallel to tendon fibers. Further retraction results in crescentic defect as shown at right.

Retracted tear, commonly found in surgery. Broken line indicates extent of débridement of degenerated tendon for repair.

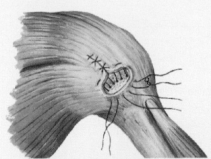

Repair. If freshened edges of tear cannot be brought together, notch is created in humerus just beneath articular surface to allow attachment of tendon through drill holes in bone, using strong sutures.

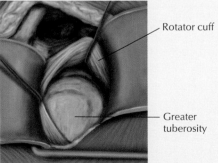

Open surgery for rotator cuff tendon tear. The open rotator cuff repair view demonstrates a large tear of the supraspinatus and infraspinatus tendons.

Clinical Focus 7.5

Shoulder Tendinitis and Bursitis

Movement at the shoulder joint (or almost any joint) can lead to inflammation of the tendons surrounding that joint and secondary inflammation of the bursa that cushions the joint from the overlying muscle or tendon. A painful joint can result, possibly even with calcification within the degenerated tendon. The **supraspinatus muscle tendon** is especially vulnerable because it can become pinched by the greater tubercle of the humerus, the acromion, and the coracoacromial ligament.

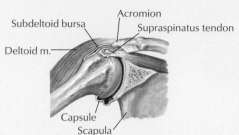
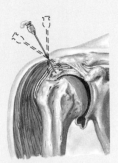

Subdeltoid bursa
Acromion
Supraspinatus tendon
Deltoid m.
Capsule
Scapula

Abduction of arm causes repeated impingement of greater tubercle of humerus on acromion, leading to degeneration and inflammation of supraspinatus tendon, secondary inflammation of bursa, and pain on abduction of arm. Calcific deposit in degenerated tendon produces elevation that further aggravates inflammation and pain.

Needle rupture of deposit in acute tendinitis promptly relieves acute symptoms. After administration of local anesthetic, needle introduced at point of greatest tenderness. Toothpaste-like deposit may ooze from needle. Irrigation of bursa with saline solution using two needles often done to remove more calcific material. Corticosteroid may be injected for additional relief.

have several actions affecting movements at the shoulder (see Table 7.3); the primary actions of the muscles on shoulder movements are summarized at the end of this chapter (see Table 7.19).

4. AXILLA

The axilla (armpit) is a four-sided pyramid-shaped region that contains important neurovascular structures that pass through the shoulder region. These neurovascular elements are enclosed in a fascial sleeve called the **axillary sheath**, which is a direct continuation of the prevertebral fascia of the neck. The axilla is a passageway from the neck to the arm and has the following six boundaries (Fig. 7.6):

- **Base (floor):** axillary fascia and skin of armpit.
- **Apex (inlet):** passageway for structures entering or leaving the shoulder and arm; bounded by the first rib, clavicle, and superior part of the scapula.
- **Anterior wall:** pectoralis major and minor muscles and clavipectoral fascia.
- **Posterior wall:** subscapularis, teres major, latissimus dorsi, and long head of the triceps muscle.

- **Medial wall:** upper rib cage and intercostal and serratus anterior muscles.
- **Lateral wall:** humerus (intertubercular sulcus).

  Important structures in the axilla include the following:
- **Axillary artery:** divided into three parts for descriptive purposes.
- **Axillary vein(s):** usually multiple veins paralleling the axillary artery.
- **Axillary lymph nodes:** five major collections of nodes embedded in a considerable amount of fat.
- **Brachial plexus of nerves:** anterior rami of C5-T1.
- **Biceps and coracobrachialis muscle:** proximal portions of these muscles.
- **Axillary tail (of Spence):** an extension of the female breast's upper outer quadrant (see Chapter 3).

  Axillary fasciae include the following:
- **Pectoral fascia:** invests the pectoralis major muscle; attaches to the sternum and clavicle.
- **Clavipectoral fascia:** invests the subclavius and pectoralis minor muscles.
- **Axillary fascia:** forms the base (floor) of the axilla.

Anterior view

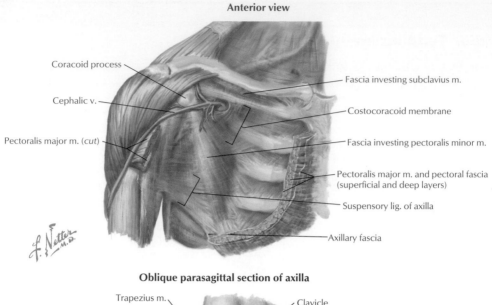

Coracoid process

Cephalic v.

Pectoralis major m. (*cut*)

Fascia investing subclavius m.

Costocoracoid membrane

Fascia investing pectoralis minor m.

Pectoralis major m. and pectoral fascia (superficial and deep layers)

Suspensory lig. of axilla

Axillary fascia

Oblique parasagittal section of axilla

Trapezius m.

Brachial plexus — Lateral cord / Posterior cord / Medial cord

Supraspinatus m.

Scapula

Infraspinatus m.

Subscapularis m.

Teres minor m.

Teres major m.

Latissimus dorsi m.

Axillary lymph nodes

Clavicle

Subclavius m. and fascia

Costocoracoid lig.

Costocoracoid membrane

Axillary a. and v.

Pectoralis major m. and fascia

Pectoralis minor m. and fascia

Suspensory lig. of axilla

Axillary fascia (fenestrated)

FIGURE 7.6 Boundaries and Features of the Axilla. (From *Netter's atlas of human anatomy,* ed 8, Plate 435; S-231.)

- **Axillary sheath:** invests the axillary neurovascular structures; derivative of the prevertebral fascia of the neck.

Axillary Vessels

The **axillary artery** is the distal continuation of the subclavian artery and begins at the first rib and is *divided into three descriptive parts* by the anterior presence of the pectoralis minor muscle (Fig. 7.7 and Table 7.4). It continues in the arm as the brachial artery distally at the level of the inferior border of the teres major muscle.

As with most joints, the shoulder joint has a rich vascular **anastomosis.** This anastomosis not only supplies the 16 muscles attaching to the scapula and other shoulder muscles but also provides collateral circulation to the upper limb should

the proximal part of the axillary artery become occluded or avulsed (proximal to the subscapular branch). This **scapular anastomosis** includes the following important component arteries (Figs. 7.7 and 7.8):

- **Dorsal scapular (transverse cervical) artery,** a branch of the subclavian artery (arises from the thyrocervical trunk).
- **Suprascapular artery** from the subclavian (thyrocervical trunk) artery.
- **Subscapular artery** and its circumflex scapular and thoracodorsal branches.
- **Posterior and anterior humeral circumflex arteries** passing around the surgical neck of the humerus.
- **Acromial branch of the thoracoacromial artery** from the second part of the axillary artery.

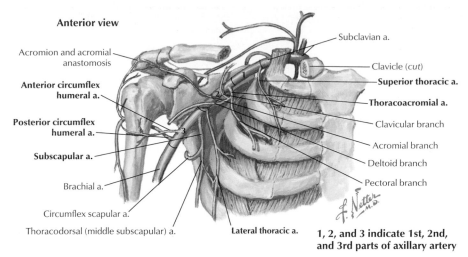

Anterior view

Acromion and acromial anastomosis

Anterior circumflex humeral a.

Posterior circumflex humeral a.

Subscapular a.

Brachial a.

Circumflex scapular a.

Thoracodorsal (middle subscapular) a.

Subclavian a.

Clavicle (*cut*)

Superior thoracic a.

Thoracoacromial a.

Clavicular branch

Acromial branch

Deltoid branch

Pectoral branch

Lateral thoracic a.

1, 2, and 3 indicate 1st, 2nd, and 3rd parts of axillary artery

FIGURE 7.7 Branches of Axillary Artery. (From *Netter's atlas of human anatomy*, ed 8, Plate 437; S-234.)

TABLE 7.4 Branches of Axillary Artery in Its Three Parts

PART	BRANCH	COURSE AND STRUCTURES SUPPLIED	PART	BRANCH	COURSE AND STRUCTURES SUPPLIED
1	Superior thoracic	Supplies first two intercostal spaces	3	Subscapular	Divides into thoracodorsal and circumflex scapular branches
2	Thoracoacromial	Has clavicular, pectoral, deltoid, and acromial branches		Anterior circumflex humeral	Passes around surgical neck of humerus
	Lateral thoracic	Runs with long thoracic nerve and supplies muscles that it traverses		Posterior circumflex humeral	Runs with axillary nerve through quadrangular space to anastomose with anterior circumflex branch

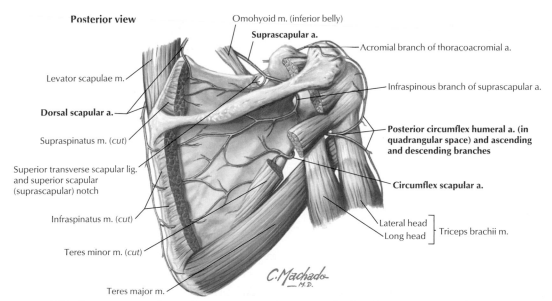

Posterior view

Levator scapulae m.

Dorsal scapular a.

Supraspinatus m. (*cut*)

Superior transverse scapular lig. and superior scapular (suprascapular) notch

Infraspinatus m. (*cut*)

Teres minor m. (*cut*)

Teres major m.

Omohyoid m. (inferior belly)

Suprascapular a.

Acromial branch of thoracoacromial a.

Infraspinous branch of suprascapular a.

Posterior circumflex humeral a. (in quadrangular space) and ascending and descending branches

Circumflex scapular a.

Lateral head
Long head } Triceps brachii m.

FIGURE 7.8 Arteries of Scapular Anastomosis. (From *Netter's atlas of human anatomy*, ed 8, Plate 437; S-234.)

Clinical Focus 7.6

Brachial Plexopathy

Damage (trauma, inflammation, tumor, radiation damage, bleeding) to the brachial plexus may present as pain, loss of sensation, and motor weakness. Clinical findings depend on the site of the lesion:

- **Upper plexus lesions:** usually affect the distribution of C5-C6 nerve roots, with the deltoid and biceps muscles affected, and sensory changes that extend below the elbow to the hand.
- **Lower plexus lesions:** usually affect the distribution of C8-T1 nerve roots, with radial and ulnar innervated muscles affected; hand weakness and sensory changes involve most of the medial hand, with weakness of finger abduction and finger extension.

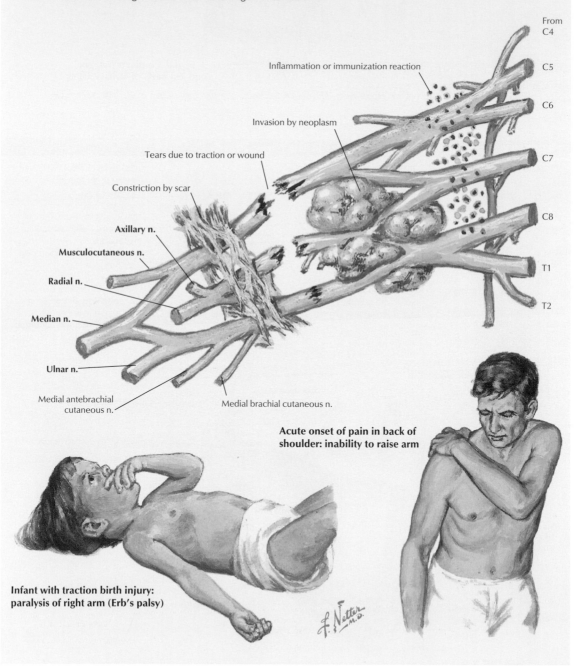

From C4

Inflammation or immunization reaction

C5

C6

Invasion by neoplasm

Tears due to traction or wound

C7

Constriction by scar

Axillary n.

Musculocutaneous n.

C8

Radial n.

T1

Median n.

T2

Ulnar n.

Medial antebrachial cutaneous n.

Medial brachial cutaneous n.

Acute onset of pain in back of shoulder: inability to raise arm

Infant with traction birth injury: paralysis of right arm (Erb's palsy)

The **axillary vein** begins at the inferior border of the *teres major muscle* and is the proximal continuation of the basilic vein (and/or the brachial venae comitantes, which include several small brachial veins that parallel the brachial artery in the arm). When the axillary vein meets the first rib, it becomes the **subclavian vein,** which then drains into the **brachiocephalic vein** on each side; these two veins then form the **superior vena cava**, which enters the right atrium of the heart (see Fig. 3.15).

Brachial Plexus

The *axillary artery, axillary vein* (which lies somewhat medial and inferior to the artery), and *cords of the brachial plexus* are all bound in the **axillary sheath** (see Fig. 7.6), a continuation of the prevertebral fascia of the neck. In Fig. 7.9 the sheath and some parts of the axillary vein have been removed and several muscles reflected for better visualization of the plexus as it invests the axillary artery. Key nerves and branches of the axillary artery also are shown supplying muscles.

Nerves that innervate most of the shoulder muscles and all the muscles of the upper limb arise from the **brachial plexus.** The plexus arises from anterior rami of spinal nerves C5-T1 (Fig. 7.10). The plexus is descriptively divided into **five roots** (anterior rami), **three trunks, six divisions** (three anterior, three posterior), **three cords** (named for their relationship to the axillary artery), and **five large terminal branches**. Important motor branches of the brachial plexus are described in Table 7.5. The designated anterior root (rami) axons contributing to each nerve are generally accurate, although *minor variations are normal*, as reflected in different textbooks.

The **sensory innervation** of the upper limb also comes from the brachial plexus, with a small contribution from T2 (the T2 dermatome via the intercostobrachial nerve from T1 and T2) on the skin of the anterior and posterior aspects of the proximal arm (see Figs. 2.17 and 7.44).

Specific nerve lesions related to the brachial plexus (or distal to the plexus) are fairly common and can occur during obstetric procedures, direct

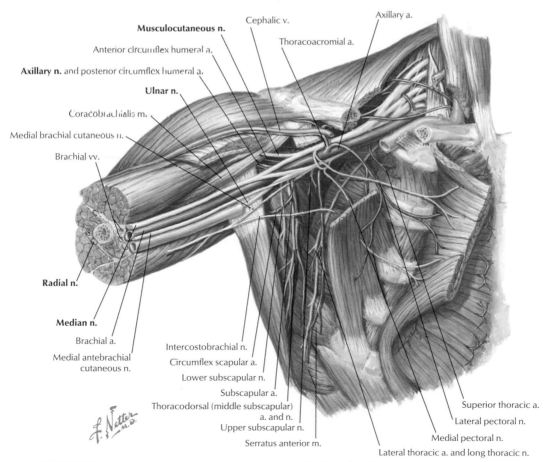

FIGURE 7.9 Brachial Plexus (Terminal Branches Highlighted) and Axillary Artery. (From *Netter's atlas of human anatomy,* ed 8, Plate 438; S-237.)

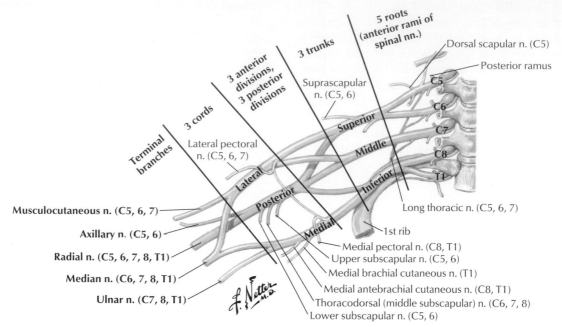

FIGURE 7.10 Schematic of Brachial Plexus. (From *Netter's atlas of human anatomy*, ed 8, Plate 439; S-106.)

TABLE 7.5 Major Motor Branches of Brachial Plexus

ARISE FROM	NERVE	MUSCLES INNERVATED
Roots	Dorsal scapular	Levator scapulae and rhomboids
	Long thoracic	Serratus anterior
Superior trunk	Suprascapular	Supraspinatus and infraspinatus
	Subclavius	Subclavius
Lateral cord	Lateral pectoral	Pectoralis major
	Musculocutaneous	Anterior compartment muscles of arm
Medial cord	Medial pectoral	Pectoralis minor and major
	Ulnar	Some forearm and most hand muscles
Medial and lateral cords	Median	Most forearm and some hand muscles
Posterior cord	Upper subscapular	Subscapularis
	Thoracodorsal	Latissimus dorsi
	Lower subscapular	Subscapularis and teres major
	Axillary	Deltoid and teres minor
	Radial	Posterior compartment muscles of arm and forearm

trauma from a cervical rib (extra rib), compression by a neoplasm, radiation injury, bone fractures, joint dislocations, or autoimmune plexopathies. Examples of several nerve lesions are featured in Section 10 (Upper Limb Nerve Summary) and in the Clinical Focus boxes later in this chapter.

Despite the complexity of the brachial plexus, its *sensory (dermatome) distribution* throughout the upper limb is segmental, beginning proximally and laterally over the deltoid muscle and radiating down the lateral arm and forearm to the lateral aspect of the hand. The segmental distribution then courses to the medial side of the hand, back up the medial aspect of the forearm and arm. This distribution is as follows (see also Figs. 2.17 and 7.44):

- **C4:** from the cervical plexus (anterior rami of C1-C4) over the shoulder.
- **C5:** lateral arm over the deltoid and triceps muscles.
- **C6:** lateral forearm over the brachioradialis muscle, thenar eminence, and thumb.
- **C7:** skin of the hand, primarily second through third or fourth digits.
- **C8:** medial two digits (fourth and fifth digits), hypothenar eminence, and medial forearm.
- **T1:** medial arm (some dermatome charts also include anterior forearm).
- **T2:** from the intercostobrachial nerve to the skin of the axilla (not part of the brachial plexus).

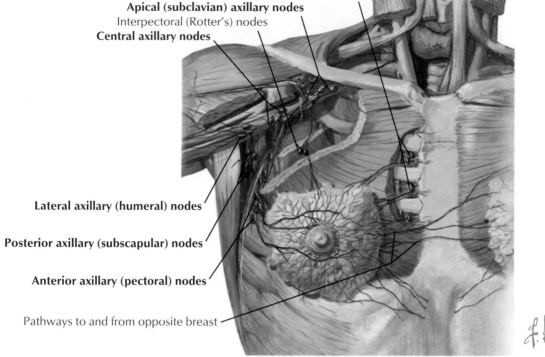

Parasternal nodes
Apical (subclavian) axillary nodes
Interpectoral (Rotter's) nodes
Central axillary nodes

Lateral axillary (humeral) nodes

Posterior axillary (subscapular) nodes

Anterior axillary (pectoral) nodes

Pathways to and from opposite breast

FIGURE 7.11 Axillary Lymph Nodes and Lymph Drainage of the Breast. (From *Netter's atlas of human anatomy*, ed 8, Plate 207; S-348.)

Axillary Lymph Nodes

The axillary lymph nodes lie in the fatty connective tissue of the axilla and are the major collection nodes for all lymph draining from the upper limb and portions of the thoracic wall, especially the breast. About 75% of lymphatic drainage from the breast passes through the axillary nodes. The 20 to 30 nodes are divided into the following five groups (Fig. 7.11):

- **Central nodes:** receive lymph from several of the other groups.
- **Lateral (brachial, humeral) nodes:** receive most of the upper limb drainage.
- **Posterior (subscapular) nodes:** drain the upper back, neck, and shoulder.
- **Anterior (pectoral) nodes:** drain the breast and anterior trunk.
- **Apical (subclavian) nodes:** connect with infraclavicular nodes.

Lymph from the breast also can drain superiorly into infraclavicular nodes, into pectoral nodes, medially into parasternal nodes, and inferiorly into abdominal trunk nodes (see Clinical Focus 3.4).

5. ARM

As you study the anatomical arrangement of the arm and forearm, organize your study around the *functional muscular compartments*. We have already discussed the **humerus**, which is the long bone of the arm (see Fig. 7.3 and Table 7.1).

The arm is divided into an **anterior (flexor) compartment** and a **posterior (extensor) compartment** by an *intermuscular septum*, which is attached medially and laterally to the deep (investing) fascia surrounding the muscles.

Anterior Compartment Arm Muscles, Vessels, and Nerves

Muscles of the anterior compartment exhibit the following features (Fig. 7.12 and Table 7.6):

- Are primarily flexors of the forearm at the elbow.
- Are secondarily flexors of the arm at the shoulder (biceps and coracobrachialis muscles).
- Can supinate the flexed forearm (biceps muscle only).
- Are innervated by the **musculocutaneous nerve.**

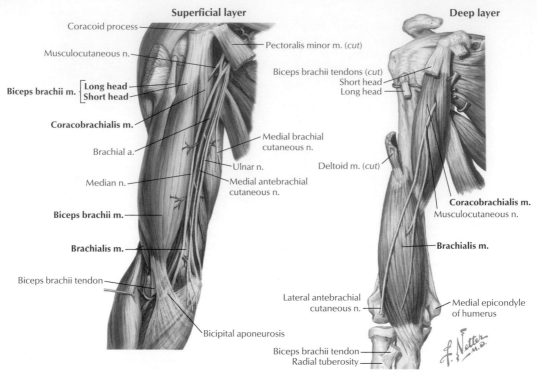

FIGURE 7.12 Anterior Compartment Arm Muscles and Nerves. (From *Netter's atlas of human anatomy,* ed 8, Plates 440 and 442; S-238 and S-239)

TABLE 7.6 Anterior Compartment Arm Muscles

MUSCLE	PROXIMAL ATTACHMENT	DISTAL ATTACHMENT	INNERVATION	MAIN ACTIONS
Biceps brachii	*Short head:* apex of coracoid process of scapula *Long head:* supraglenoid tubercle of scapula	Tuberosity of radius and fascia of forearm via bicipital aponeurosis	Musculocutaneous nerve (C5-C6)	Supinates flexed forearm; flexes forearm at elbow
Brachialis	Distal half of anterior humerus	Coronoid process and tuberosity of ulna	Musculocutaneous nerve (C5-C6), and contribution from radial nerve (C7)	Flexes forearm at elbow in all positions
Coracobrachialis	Tip of coracoid process of scapula	Middle third of medial surface of humerus	Musculocutaneous nerve (C5-C7)	Helps to flex and adduct arm at shoulder

Variations in spinal nerve contributions to the innervation of muscles, their attachments, and their actions are common in human anatomy. Therefore, expect differences between texts and realize that anatomical variation is normal.

● Are supplied by the brachial artery and its muscular branches.

Posterior Compartment Arm Muscles, Vessels, and Nerves

Muscles of the posterior compartment exhibit the following features (Fig. 7.13 and Table 7.7):
● Are primarily extensors of the forearm at the elbow.
● Are supplied with blood from the profunda brachii (deep brachial) artery and its muscular branches.
● Are innervated by the **radial nerve.**

The artery of the arm is the **brachial artery** and its branches. The brachial artery extends from the inferior border of the teres major muscle to just below the anterior elbow, where it divides into the **ulnar** and **radial arteries** (Fig. 7.14 and Table 7.8). A *rich anastomosis* exists around the elbow joint between branches of the brachial artery and branches of the radial and ulnar arteries. One can feel a **brachial pulse** by pressing the artery medially at the midarm against the underlying humerus.

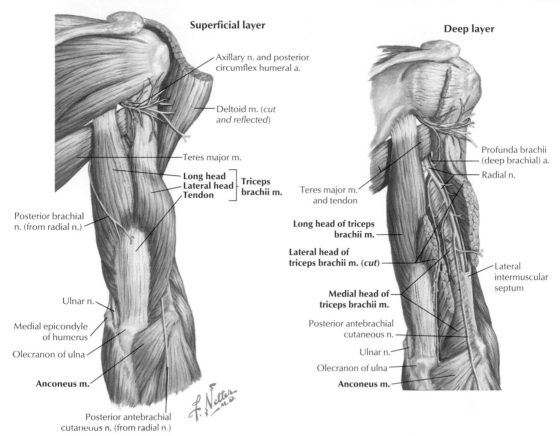

FIGURE 7.13 Posterior Compartment Arm Muscles and Nerves. (From *Netter's atlas of human anatomy*, ed 8, Plate 441; S-240.)

TABLE 7.7 Posterior Compartment Arm Muscles

MUSCLE	PROXIMAL ATTACHMENT	DISTAL ATTACHMENT	INNERVATION	MAIN ACTIONS
Triceps brachii	*Long head:* infraglenoid tubercle of scapula *Lateral head:* posterior surface of humerus *Medial head:* posterior surface of humerus, inferior to radial groove	Posterior surface of olecranon of ulna and fascia of forearm	Radial nerve (C6-C8)	Extends forearm at elbow; is chief extensor of elbow; steadies head of abducted humerus (long head)
Anconeus	Posterior surface of lateral epicondyle of humerus	Lateral surface of olecranon and superior part of posterior surface of ulna	Radial nerve (C6-C8)	Assists triceps in extending elbow; abducts ulna during pronation

Variations in spinal nerve contributions to the innervation of muscles, their attachments, and their actions are common in human anatomy. Therefore, expect differences between texts and realize that anatomical variation is normal.

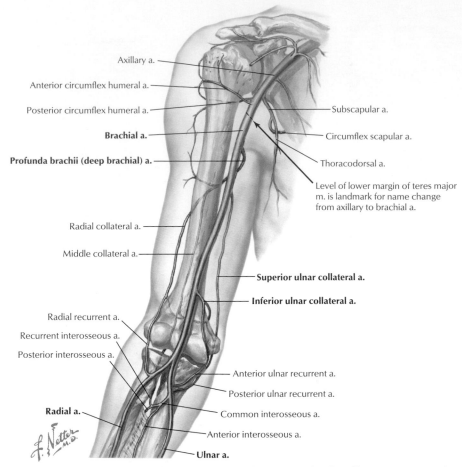

FIGURE 7.14 Brachial Artery and Its Anastomoses. (From *Netter's atlas of human anatomy,* ed 8, Plate 443; S-331.)

TABLE 7.8 Branches of Brachial Artery

ARTERY	COURSE	ARTERY	COURSE
Brachial	Begins at inferior border of teres major and ends at its bifurcation in cubital fossa	Inferior ulnar collateral	Passes anterior to medial epicondyle of humerus
		Radial	Is smaller lateral terminal branch of brachial artery
Profunda brachii (deep brachial) artery	Runs with radial nerve around humeral shaft	Ulnar	Is larger medial terminal branch of brachial artery
Superior ulnar collateral	Runs with ulnar nerve		

As shown in Figs. 7.2 and 7.35, the superficial **cephalic** and **basilic veins** course in the subcutaneous tissues of the arm and drain proximally into the axillary vein. The **deep brachial veins** usually consist of either paired veins or *venae comitantes* (multiple small veins) that surround the brachial artery. These veins also drain into the **axillary vein** (see Fig. 7.35).

Arm in Cross Section

Cross sections of the arm show the anterior and posterior compartments and their respective flexor and extensor muscles (Fig. 7.15). Note the nerve of each compartment and the medially situated neurovascular bundle containing the brachial artery, median nerve, and ulnar nerve. The *median and ulnar nerves* do not innervate arm muscles but

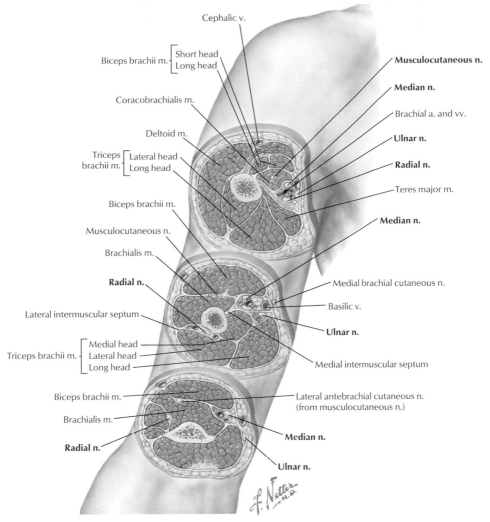

Cephalic v.

Biceps brachii m. — Short head / Long head

Musculocutaneous n.

Median n.

Coracobrachialis m.

Brachial a. and vv.

Deltoid m.

Ulnar n.

Triceps brachii m. — Lateral head / Long head

Radial n.

Biceps brachii m.

Teres major m.

Musculocutaneous n.

Median n.

Brachialis m.

Radial n.

Medial brachial cutaneous n.

Lateral intermuscular septum

Basilic v.

Triceps brachii m. — Medial head / Lateral head / Long head

Ulnar n.

Medial intermuscular septum

Biceps brachii m.

Lateral antebrachial cutaneous n. (from musculocutaneous n.)

Brachialis m.

Median n.

Radial n.

Ulnar n.

FIGURE 7.15 Serial Cross Sections of the Arm. (From *Netter's atlas of human anatomy,* ed 8, Plate 445; S-551)

simply pass through the arm to reach the forearm and hand.

6. FOREARM

Bones and Elbow Joint

The bones of the forearm (defined as the portion of the arm from the elbow to the wrist) are the laterally placed **radius** and medial **ulna** (Fig. 7.16 and Table 7.9). The radioulnar fibrous (syndesmosis) joint unites both bones by an **interosseous membrane,** which also divides the forearm functionally into an *anterior flexor-pronator compartment* and a *posterior extensor-supinator compartment.*

The elbow joint is composed of the **humeroulnar** and **humeroradial joints** for flexion and extension, and the **proximal radioulnar joint** for pronation and supination (Figs. 7.17 and 7.18 and Table 7.10).

Anterior Compartment Forearm Muscles, Vessels, and Nerves

The muscles of the anterior compartment of the forearm are arranged in two layers, with the muscles of the superficial layer largely arising from the **medial epicondyle** of the humerus, although several muscles also arise from the ulna and/or radius or interosseous membrane (Fig. 7.19 and Table 7.11). Specifically, it is the deeper group of anterior forearm muscles that typically arise from the ulna, the radius, and/or the interosseous membrane. The anterior forearm muscles exhibit the following general features:

Text continued on page 392

Deep Tendon Reflexes

A brisk tap to a partially stretched muscle tendon near its point of insertion elicits a deep tendon (muscle stretch) reflex (DTR) dependent on the following:

- Intact afferent (sensory) nerve fibers
- Normal functional synapses in the spinal cord at the appropriate level
- Intact efferent (motor) nerve fibers
- Normal functional neuromuscular junctions on the tapped muscle
- Normal muscle fiber functioning (contraction)

Characteristically, the DTR only involves several spinal cord segments (and their afferent and efferent nerve fibers). If pathology is involved at the level tested, the reflex may be weak or absent, requiring further testing to determine where along the pathway the lesion occurred. For the arm, you should know the following segmental levels for the DTR:

- **Biceps brachii** reflex C5 and C6
- **Triceps brachii** reflex C7 and C8

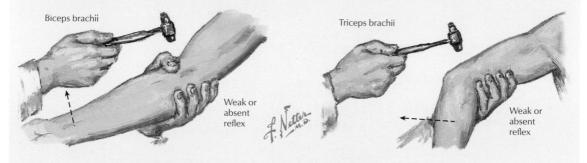

Fractures of the Humerus

Fractures of the humerus may occur *proximally* (e.g., surgical neck fractures, which are common in older persons from a fall on an outstretched hand). Humeral fractures also may occur along the *midshaft,* usually from direct trauma, or *distally* (uncommon in adults). Proximal fractures mainly occur at the following four sites:

- Humeral head (articular fragment)
- Lesser tuberosity
- Greater tuberosity
- Proximal shaft (surgical neck)

Midshaft fractures usually heal well but may involve entrapment of the **radial nerve** as it spirals around the shaft to reach the arm's posterior muscle compartment (triceps muscle).

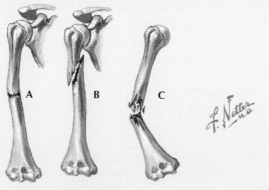

A. Transverse fracture of midshaft
B. Oblique (spiral) fracture
C. Comminuted fracture with marked angulation

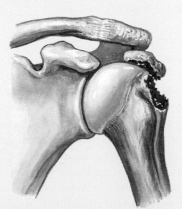

Displaced fracture of greater tuberosity

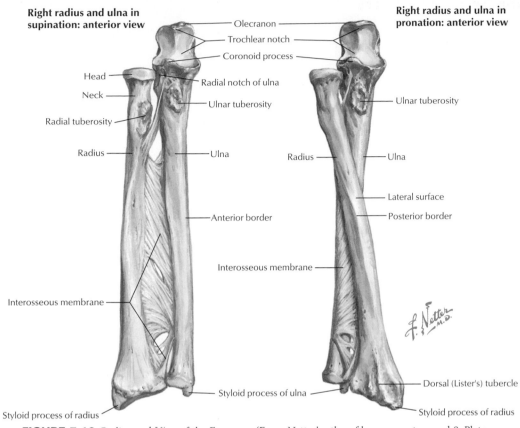

Right radius and ulna in supination: anterior view

- Olecranon
- Trochlear notch
- Coronoid process
- Head
- Neck
- Radial notch of ulna
- Ulnar tuberosity
- Radial tuberosity
- Radius
- Ulna
- Anterior border
- Interosseous membrane
- Styloid process of ulna
- Styloid process of radius

Right radius and ulna in pronation: anterior view

- Ulnar tuberosity
- Radius
- Ulna
- Lateral surface
- Posterior border
- Interosseous membrane
- Dorsal (Lister's) tubercle
- Styloid process of radius

f. Netter m.o.

FIGURE 7.16 Radius and Ulna of the Forearm. (From *Netter's atlas of human anatomy*, ed 8, Plate 449, S-162.)

TABLE 7.9 Features of Radius and Ulna

STRUCTURE	DESCRIPTION
Radius	
Long bone	Is shorter than ulna
Proximal head	Articulates with capitulum of humerus and radial notch of ulna
Distal radius and styloid process	Articulates with scaphoid, lunate, and triquetrum carpal bones
Ulna	
Long bone	Is longer than radius
Proximal olecranon	Is attachment point of triceps tendon
Proximal trochlear notch	Articulates with trochlea of humerus
Radial notch	Articulates with head of radius
Distal head	Articulates with disc at distal radioulnar joint

TABLE 7.10 Forearm Joints

LIGAMENT	ATTACHMENT	COMMENT
Humeroulnar (Uniaxial Synovial Hinge [Ginglymus]) Joint		
Capsule	Surrounds joint	Provides flexion and extension
Ulnar (medial) collateral	Medial epicondyle of humerus to coronoid process and olecranon of ulna	Is triangular ligament with anterior, posterior, and oblique bands
Humeroradial Joint		
Capsule	Surrounds joint	Capitulum of humerus to head of radius
Radial (lateral) collateral	Lateral epicondyle of humerus to radial notch of ulna and anular ligament	Is weaker than ulnar collateral ligament but provides posterolateral stability
Proximal Radioulnar (Uniaxial Synovial Pivot) Joint		
Anular ligament	Surrounds radial head and radial notch of ulna	Keeps radial head in radial notch; allows pronation and supination

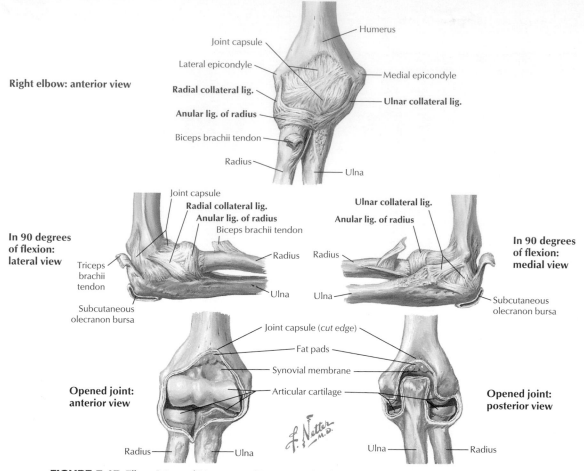

FIGURE 7.17 Elbow Joint and Ligaments. (From *Netter's atlas of human anatomy,* ed 8, Plate 428; S-161.)

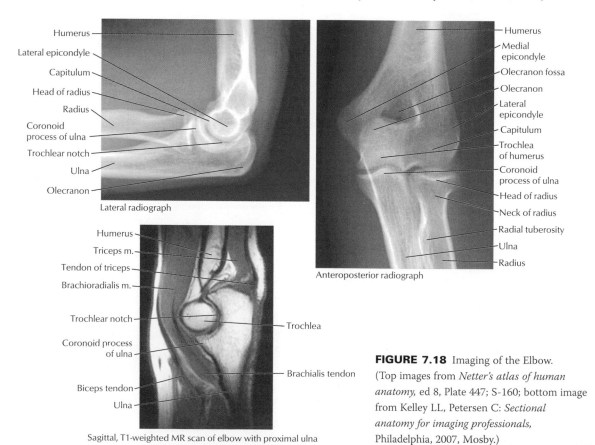

FIGURE 7.18 Imaging of the Elbow. (Top images from *Netter's atlas of human anatomy,* ed 8, Plate 447; S-160; bottom image from Kelley LL, Petersen C: *Sectional anatomy for imaging professionals,* Philadelphia, 2007, Mosby.)

Clinical Focus 7.9

Biceps Brachii Rupture

Rupture of the biceps brachii muscle may occur at the tendon (or rarely the muscle belly). It has a high rate of *spontaneous rupture* compared with most muscle tendons. Rupture is seen most often in patients older than 40, in association with rotator cuff injuries (as the tendon begins to undergo degenerative changes), and with repetitive lifting (e.g., weight lifters). Rupture of the long head of the biceps brachii tendon is most common and may occur in the following locations:

- Shoulder joint
- Intertubercular (bicipital) sulcus of the humerus
- Musculotendinous junction

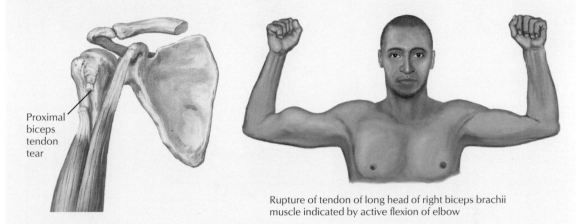

Proximal biceps tendon tear

Rupture of tendon of long head of right biceps brachii muscle indicated by active flexion of elbow

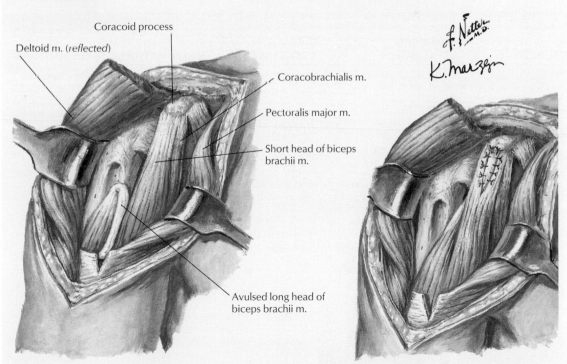

Coracoid process

Deltoid m. (*reflected*)

Coracobrachialis m.

Pectoralis major m.

Short head of biceps brachii m.

Avulsed long head of biceps brachii m.

Exposure shows tendon of long head of biceps brachii muscle avulsed.

For repair, long head tendon brought through slit in short head tendon and sutured to margins and to coracoid process.

Elbow Dislocation

Elbow dislocations occur third in frequency after shoulder and finger dislocations. Dislocation often results from a fall on an outstretched hand and includes the following types:

- Posterior (most common)
- Anterior (rare; may lacerate brachial artery)
- Lateral (uncommon)
- Medial (rare)

Dislocations may be accompanied by fractures of the humeral medial epicondyle, olecranon (ulna), radial head, or coronoid process of the ulna. Injury to the **ulnar nerve** (most common) or **median nerve** may accompany these dislocations.

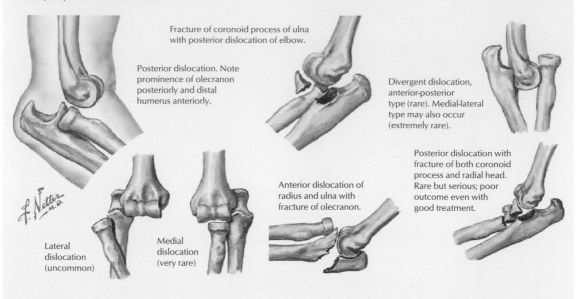

Fracture of coronoid process of ulna with posterior dislocation of elbow.

Posterior dislocation. Note prominence of olecranon posteriorly and distal humerus anteriorly.

Divergent dislocation, anterior-posterior type (rare). Medial-lateral type may also occur (extremely rare).

Posterior dislocation with fracture of both coronoid process and radial head. Rare but serious; poor outcome even with good treatment.

Anterior dislocation of radius and ulna with fracture of olecranon.

Lateral dislocation (uncommon)

Medial dislocation (very rare)

TABLE 7.11 Anterior Compartment Forearm Muscles

MUSCLE	PROXIMAL ATTACHMENT	DISTAL ATTACHMENT	INNERVATION	MAIN ACTIONS
Pronator teres	Medial epicondyle of humerus and coronoid process of ulna	Middle of lateral surface of radius	Median nerve (C6-C7)	Pronates forearm and flexes elbow
Flexor carpi radialis	Medial epicondyle of humerus	Base of 2nd metacarpal bone	Median nerve (C6-C7)	Flexes hand at wrist and abducts it
Palmaris longus	Medial epicondyle of humerus	Distal half of flexor retinaculum and palmar aponeurosis	Median nerve (C7-C8)	Flexes hand at wrist and tightens palmar aponeurosis
Flexor carpi ulnaris	*Humeral head:* medial epicondyle of humerus *Ulnar head:* olecranon and posterior border of ulna	Pisiform bone, hook of hamate bone, and 5th metacarpal bone	Ulnar nerve (C7-T1)	Flexes hand at wrist and adducts it
Flexor digitorum superficialis	*Humeroulnar head:* medial epicondyle of humerus, ulnar collateral ligament, and coronoid process of ulna *Radial head:* superior half of anterior radius	Bodies of middle phalanges of medial four digits	Median nerve (C8-T1)	Flexes middle phalanges of medial four digits; also weakly flexes proximal phalanges, forearm, and wrist
Flexor digitorum profundus	Proximal three-fourths of medial and anterior surfaces of ulna and interosseous membrane	Palmar bases of distal phalanges of medial four digits	*Medial part:* ulnar nerve *Lateral part:* median nerve	Flexes distal phalanges of medial four digits; assists with flexion of wrist
Flexor pollicis longus	Anterior surface of radius and adjacent interosseous membrane	Base of distal phalanx of thumb	Median nerve (anterior interosseous)	Flexes phalanges of 1st digit (thumb)
Pronator quadratus	Distal one-fourth of anterior surface of ulna	Distal one-fourth of anterior surface of radius	Median nerve (anterior interosseous) (C8-T1)	Pronates forearm and hand

Variations in spinal nerve contributions to the innervation of muscles, their attachments, and their actions are common in human anatomy. Therefore, expect differences between texts and realize that anatomical variation is normal.

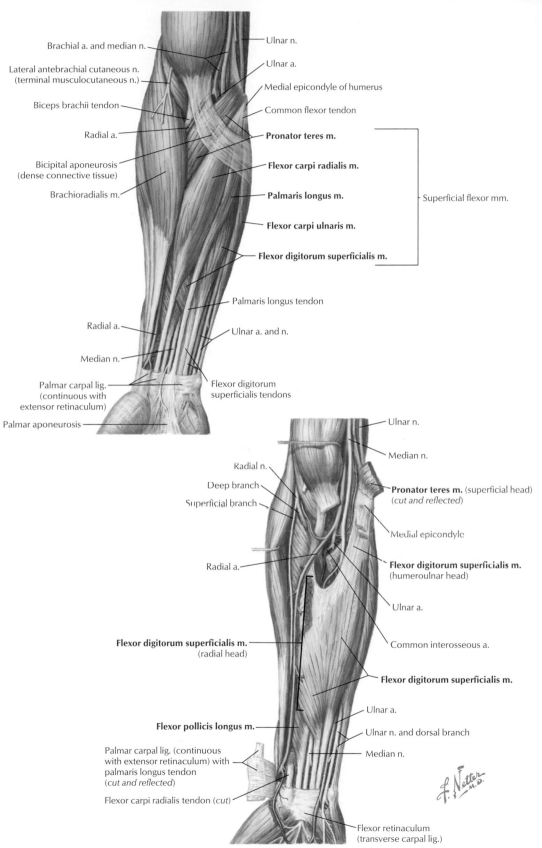

Brachial a. and median n.
Lateral antebrachial cutaneous n. (terminal musculocutaneous n.)
Biceps brachii tendon
Radial a.
Bicipital aponeurosis (dense connective tissue)
Brachioradialis m.

Ulnar n.
Ulnar a.
Medial epicondyle of humerus
Common flexor tendon
Pronator teres m.
Flexor carpi radialis m.
Palmaris longus m.
Flexor carpi ulnaris m.
Flexor digitorum superficialis m.
Superficial flexor mm.

Palmaris longus tendon
Radial a.
Median n.
Palmar carpal lig. (continuous with extensor retinaculum)
Palmar aponeurosis

Ulnar a. and n.
Flexor digitorum superficialis tendons

Radial n.
Deep branch
Superficial branch
Radial a.

Flexor digitorum superficialis m. (radial head)

Flexor pollicis longus m.
Palmar carpal lig. (continuous with extensor retinaculum) with palmaris longus tendon (cut and reflected)
Flexor carpi radialis tendon (cut)

Ulnar n.
Median n.
Pronator teres m. (superficial head) (cut and reflected)
Medial epicondyle
Flexor digitorum superficialis m. (humeroulnar head)
Ulnar a.
Common interosseous a.
Flexor digitorum superficialis m.
Ulnar a.
Ulnar n. and dorsal branch
Median n.

Flexor retinaculum (transverse carpal lig.)

FIGURE 7.19 Anterior Compartment Forearm Muscles and Nerves. (From *Netter's atlas of human anatomy,* ed 8, Plates 456 and 457; S-244 and S-247.)

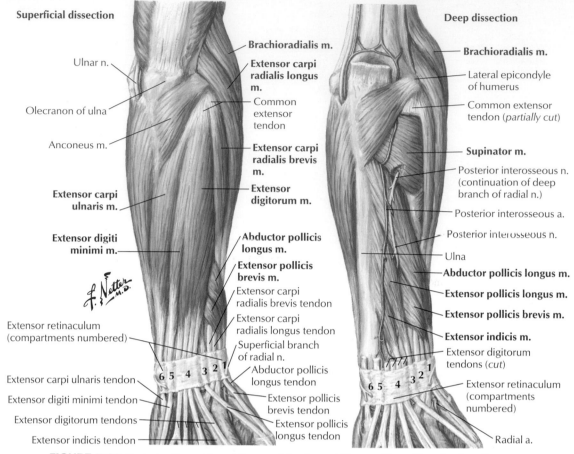

FIGURE 7.20 Posterior Compartment Forearm Muscles and Nerves. (From *Netter's atlas of human anatomy,* ed 8, Plates 454 and 455; S-241 and S-242.)

- Are primarily flexors of the hand at the wrist and/or finger flexors.
- Two are pronators of the hand.
- Secondarily, several of the muscles can abduct and adduct the hand at the wrist.
- Muscle bellies reside in the forearm, but tendons extend to the wrist or into the hand (except for the pronator muscles).
- Muscles are supplied by the **ulnar** and **radial arteries.**
- All except two of the muscles are innervated by the **median nerve** (the flexor carpi ulnaris muscle and medial half of the flexor digitorum profundus muscle are innervated by the **ulnar nerve**).

The **cubital fossa** is a depression anterior to the elbow and is demarcated by the brachioradialis muscle laterally and the pronator teres muscle medially (Fig. 7.19). The floor of the cubital fossa is formed by the brachialis muscle. The **median nerve** and brachial vessels traverse the cubital fossa

and are covered by the bicipital aponeurosis. The **brachial artery** divides into its **radial** and **ulnar branches** in the fossa, and the biceps brachii tendon inserts into the radial tuberosity.

Posterior Compartment Forearm Muscles, Vessels, and Nerves

The muscles of the posterior compartment of the forearm also are arranged in superficial and deep layers, with the superficial layer of muscles largely arising from the **lateral epicondyle** of the humerus (Fig. 7.20 and Table 7.12). The deeper muscles of the posterior forearm compartment arise from the radius, the ulna, and/or the interosseous membrane connecting these two forearm bones. The posterior forearm muscles exhibit the following general features:

- Are primarily extensors of the hand at the wrist and/or finger extensors; several can adduct or abduct the thumb.

TABLE 7.12 Posterior Compartment Forearm Muscles and Nerves

MUSCLE	PROXIMAL ATTACHMENT	DISTAL ATTACHMENT	INNERVATION	MAIN ACTIONS
Brachioradialis	Proximal two-thirds of lateral supracondylar ridge of humerus	Lateral surface of distal end of radius	Radial nerve (C5-C6)	Flexes midpronated forearm at elbow
Extensor carpi radialis longus	Lateral supracondylar ridge of humerus	Base of 2nd metacarpal bone	Radial nerve (C6-C7)	Extends and abducts hand at wrist
Extensor carpi radialis brevis	Lateral epicondyle of humerus	Base of 3rd metacarpal bone	Radial nerve (deep branch) (C7)	Extends and abducts hand at wrist
Extensor digitorum	Lateral epicondyle of humerus	Extensor expansions of medial four digits	Radial nerve (posterior interosseous) (C7-C8)	Extends medial four digits at MCP joints; extends hand at wrist joint
Extensor digiti minimi	Lateral epicondyle of humerus	Extensor expansion of 5th digit	Radial nerve (posterior interosseous)	Extends 5th digit at MCP and IP joints
Extensor carpi ulnaris	Lateral epicondyle of humerus and posterior border of ulna	Base of 5th metacarpal bone	Radial nerve (posterior interosseous)	Extends and adducts hand at wrist
Supinator	Lateral epicondyle of humerus; radial collateral and anular ligaments; supinator fossa; and crest of ulna	Lateral, posterior, and anterior surfaces of proximal third of radius	Radial nerve (deep branch) (C7-C8)	Supinates forearm (i.e., rotates radius to turn palm anteriorly)
Abductor pollicis longus	Posterior surfaces of ulna, radius, and interosseous membrane	Base of 1st metacarpal bone	Radial nerve (posterior interosseous)	Abducts thumb and extends it at CMC joint
Extensor pollicis brevis	Posterior surfaces of radius and interosseous membrane	Base of proximal phalanx of thumb	Radial nerve (posterior interosseous)	Extends proximal phalanx of thumb at CMC joint
Extensor pollicis longus	Posterior surfaces of middle third of ulna and interosseous membrane	Base of distal phalanx of thumb	Radial nerve (posterior interosseous) (C7-C8)	Extends distal phalanx of thumb at MCP and IP joints
Extensor indicis	Posterior surfaces of ulna and interosseous membrane	Extensor expansion of 2nd digit	Radial nerve (posterior interosseous) (C7-C8)	Extends 2nd digit and helps to extend hand at wrist

CMC, Carpometacarpal; IP, interphalangeal; MCP, metacarpophalangeal.
Variations in spinal nerve contributions to the innervation of muscles, their attachments, and their actions are common in human anatomy. Therefore, expect differences between texts and realize that anatomical variation is normal.

- One is a supinator.
- Secondarily, several of the muscles can abduct and adduct the hand at the wrist.
- Muscle bellies reside largely in the forearm, but tendons extend to the wrist or into the dorsum of the hand.
- Muscles are supplied by the **radial** and **ulnar arteries** (the posterior interosseous branch of the common interosseous artery from the ulnar artery).
- All of the muscles are innervated by the **radial nerve.**

Importantly, the *brachioradialis muscle* is unique because it lies between the anterior and posterior compartments; it actually flexes the forearm when it is midpronated.

The muscles of the forearm are supplied by the **radial** and **ulnar arteries** (see Figs. 7.14, 7.19, and 7.21; Table 7.13). Deeper muscles also receive blood from the **common interosseous** branch of the ulnar artery via the anterior and posterior interosseous arteries. **Deep veins** parallel the radial and ulnar arteries and have connections with the superficial veins in the subcutaneous tissue of the forearm (tributaries draining into the *basilic and cephalic veins*) (Figs. 7.2 and 7.35).

Forearm in Cross Section

Cross sections of the forearm demonstrate the **anterior** (flexor-pronator) and **posterior** (extensor-supinator) compartments and their respective neurovascular structures (Fig. 7.22). The **median nerve** innervates all the muscles except the flexor carpi ulnaris muscle and the ulnar half of the flexor digitorum profundus muscle (which is innervated by the **ulnar nerve**) in the anterior compartment.

Clinical Focus 7.11

Fracture of the Radial Head and Neck

Fractures to the *proximal radius* often involve either the head or the neck of the radius. These fractures can result from a fall on an outstretched hand (indirect trauma) or a direct blow to the elbow. Fracture of the radial head is more common in adults, whereas fracture of the neck is more common in children.

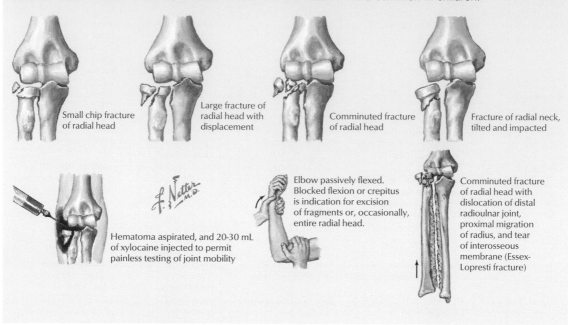

Small chip fracture of radial head

Large fracture of radial head with displacement

Comminuted fracture of radial head

Fracture of radial neck, tilted and impacted

Hematoma aspirated, and 20-30 mL of xylocaine injected to permit painless testing of joint mobility

Elbow passively flexed. Blocked flexion or crepitus is indication for excision of fragments or, occasionally, entire radial head.

Comminuted fracture of radial head with dislocation of distal radioulnar joint, proximal migration of radius, and tear of interosseous membrane (Essex-Lopresti fracture)

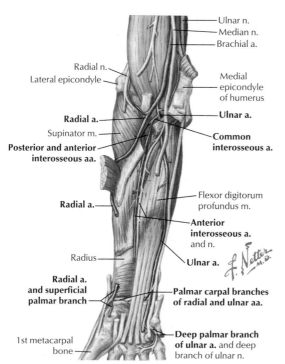

FIGURE 7.21 Forearm Arteries. (From *Netter's atlas of human anatomy*, ed 8, Plate 458; S-249.)

Ulnar n.
Median n.
Brachial a.

Radial n.
Lateral epicondyle

Medial epicondyle of humerus

Radial a.
Supinator m.
Posterior and anterior interosseous aa.

Ulnar a.
Common interosseous a.

Flexor digitorum profundus m.
Radial a.

Anterior interosseous a. and n.

Radius
Ulnar a.

Radial a. and superficial palmar branch

Palmar carpal branches of radial and ulnar aa.

1st metacarpal bone

Deep palmar branch of ulnar a. and deep branch of ulnar n.

TABLE 7.13 Major Branches of the Radial and Ulnar Arteries in Forearm

ARTERY	COURSE
Radial	Arises from brachial artery in cubital fossa
Radial recurrent branch	Anastomoses with radial collateral artery in arm
Palmar carpal branch	Anastomoses with carpal branch of ulnar artery
Ulnar	Arises from brachial artery in cubital fossa
Anterior ulnar recurrent	Anastomoses with inferior ulnar collateral in arm
Posterior ulnar recurrent	Anastomoses with superior ulnar collateral in arm
Common interosseous	Gives rise to anterior and posterior interosseous arteries
Palmar carpal branch	Anastomoses with carpal branch of radial artery

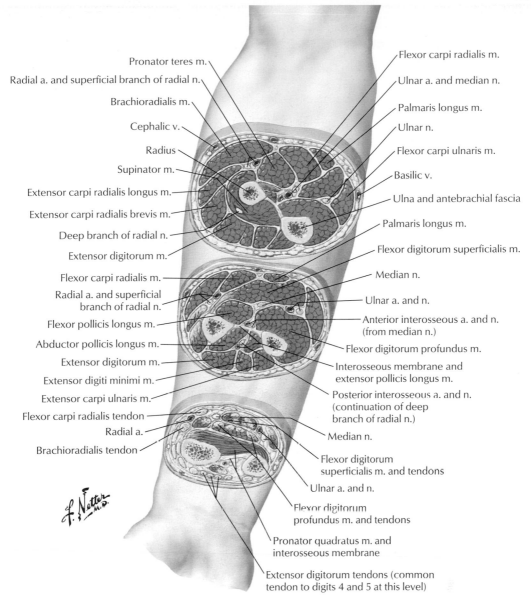

FIGURE 7.22 Serial Cross Sections of the Forearm. (From *Netter's atlas of human anatomy,* ed 8, Plate 461; S-552.)

The **radial nerve** innervates all the posterior compartment muscles.

The attachment of the superficial forearm muscles to the medial (flexors) and lateral (extensors) humeral epicondyles is noteworthy, especially when these muscles are overused in sports such as tennis and golf. Generally, pain from overuse of the forearm extensors is known as **"tennis elbow,"** with the pain felt over the lateral epicondyle and distally into the proximal forearm. Overuse of the forearm flexors may cause pain over the medial epicondyle that radiates into the proximal anterior forearm and is known as **"golfer's elbow."**

7. WRIST AND HAND

Bones and Joints

The wrist connects the hand to the forearm and is composed of eight **carpal bones** aligned in proximal and distal rows (four carpals in each row). The hand includes the metacarpus (the palm, with five **metacarpal bones**) and five digits with their **phalanges** (Fig. 7.23 and Table 7.14).

The wrist joint is a **radiocarpal synovial joint** between the radius and an articular disc covering the distal ulna, and the proximal articular surfaces

Clinical Focus 7.12

Biomechanics of Forearm Radial Fractures

The ulna is a *straight bone* with a stable articulation (elbow), but the radius is not uniform in size, proximal to distal. Natural *lateral bowing of the radius* is essential for optimal pronation and supination. However, when the radius is fractured, the muscles attaching to the bone deform this alignment. Careful reduction of the fracture should attempt to replicate the normal anatomy to maximize pronation and supination, as well as to maintain the integrity of the interosseous membrane.

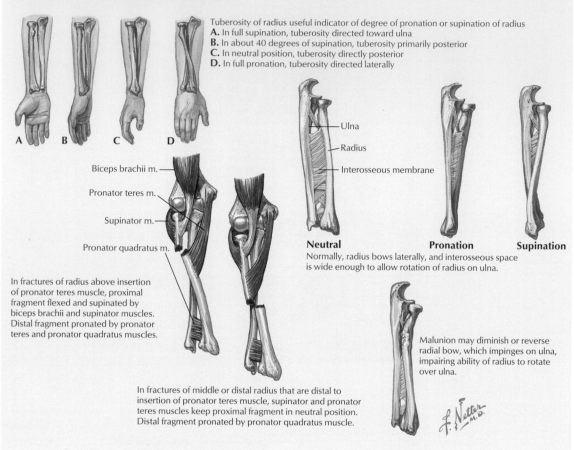

Tuberosity of radius useful indicator of degree of pronation or supination of radius
A. In full supination, tuberosity directed toward ulna
B. In about 40 degrees of supination, tuberosity primarily posterior
C. In neutral position, tuberosity directly posterior
D. In full pronation, tuberosity directed laterally

Biceps brachii m.

Pronator teres m.

Supinator m.

Pronator quadratus m.

In fractures of radius above insertion of pronator teres muscle, proximal fragment flexed and supinated by biceps brachii and supinator muscles. Distal fragment pronated by pronator teres and pronator quadratus muscles.

Ulna
Radius
Interosseous membrane

Neutral   **Pronation**   **Supination**
Normally, radius bows laterally, and interosseous space is wide enough to allow rotation of radius on ulna.

Malunion may diminish or reverse radial bow, which impinges on ulna, impairing ability of radius to rotate over ulna.

In fractures of middle or distal radius that are distal to insertion of pronator teres muscle, supinator and pronator teres muscles keep proximal fragment in neutral position. Distal fragment pronated by pronator quadratus muscle.

---

of the scaphoid, lunate, and triquetrum (radiocarpal and distal radioulnar joints); it permits a wide range of movements (Figs. 7.24 and 7.25). Although the **carpal joints** (intercarpal and midcarpal) are within the wrist, they provide for gliding movements and significant wrist extension and flexion.

Carpometacarpal (CMC, carpals to metacarpals), **metacarpophalangeal** (MCP), and **proximal interphalangeal** (PIP) and **distal interphalangeal** (DIP) **joints** complete the joints of the hand (Figs. 7.24, 7.26; Table 7.15). Note that the thumb (the biaxial saddle joint of the first digit) possesses only one interphalangeal joint. Finger and thumb movements are shown in Figure 7.27. Table 7.15 summarizes the

ligaments, attachments, and movements at each of these wrist and hand joints, along with a clinical comment.

Carpal Tunnel and the Extensor Compartments

The **carpal tunnel** is formed by the arching alignment of the carpal bones and the thick **flexor retinaculum** (transverse carpal ligament), which covers this fascioosseous tunnel on its anterior surface (Fig. 7.28). Structures passing through the carpal tunnel include the following:

- Four flexor digitorum superficialis tendons.
- Four flexor digitorum profundus tendons.

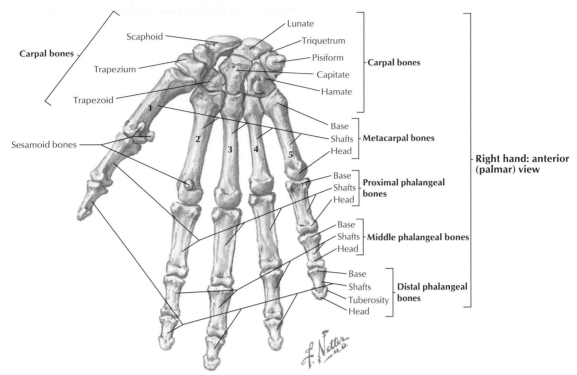

Carpal bones

Scaphoid

Trapezium

Trapezoid

Sesamoid bones

Lunate

Triquetrum

Pisiform

Capitate

Hamate

Carpal bones

1

2   3   4   5

Base
Shafts
Head

Base
Shafts
Head

Base
Shafts
Head

Base
Shafts
Tuberosity
Head

Metacarpal bones

Proximal phalangeal
bones

Middle phalangeal bones

Distal phalangeal
bones

Right hand: anterior
(palmar) view

FIGURE 7.23 Wrist and Hand Bones. (From *Netter's atlas of human anatomy,* ed 8, Plate 466; S-167.)

TABLE 7.14 Features of the Wrist and Hand Bones

FEATURE	CHARACTERISTICS
Proximal Row of Carpals	
Scaphoid (boat shaped)	Lies beneath anatomical snuffbox; is most commonly fractured carpal
Lunate (moon or crescent shaped)	Broader anteriorly than posteriorly
Triquetrum (triangular)	All three bones (scaphoid, lunate, triquetrum) articulate with distal radius
Pisiform (pea shaped)	Lies on the palmar aspect of the triquetrum
Distal Row of Carpals	
Trapezium (four sided)	Distal row articulates with proximal row of carpals and distally with metacarpals; trapezium articulates with metacarpal of thumb (saddle joint)
Trapezoid	
Capitate (round bone)	
Hamate (hooked bone)	Wedge-shaped bone
	Largest carpal bone
Metacarpals	
Numbered 1-5 (thumb to little finger)	Possess a base, shaft, and head
	Are triangular in cross section
	Fifth metacarpal most often fractured
Two sesamoid bones	Are associated with head of first metacarpal
Phalanges	
Three for each digit except thumb	Possess base, shaft, and head
	Termed *proximal, middle,* and *distal*
	Distal phalanx of middle finger often fractured

- One flexor pollicis longus tendon.
- Median nerve.

The tendon of the flexor carpi radialis lies outside the carpal tunnel but is encased within its own fascial sleeve in the lateral flexor retinaculum (Fig. 7.28). **Synovial sheaths** surround the muscle tendons within the carpal tunnel and permit sliding movements as the muscles contract and relax. The **palmar carpal ligament** (a thickening of the deep antebrachial fascia) and the **flexor retinaculum** (transverse carpal ligament) prevent "bow-stringing" of the tendons as they cross the anterior aspect of the wrist (Fig. 7.28).

The **extensor tendons** and their synovial sheaths enter the hand by passing on the medial, dorsal, and lateral aspects of the wrist beneath the **extensor retinaculum,** which segregates the tendons into six compartments (Fig. 7.29). These tendons are enclosed in dorsal carpal synovial sheaths (shown in blue in Fig. 7.29), which permit the tendons to slide smoothly beneath the extensor retinaculum.

Intrinsic Hand Muscles

The intrinsic hand muscles originate and insert in the hand and carry out *fine precision movements,* whereas the forearm muscles and their tendons that pass into the hand are more important for

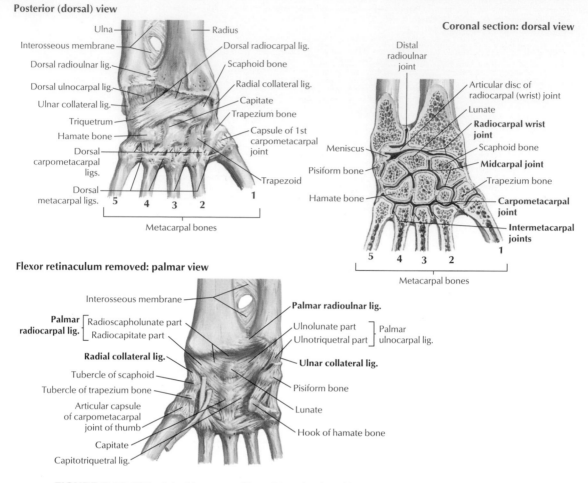

Posterior (dorsal) view

Ulna
Interosseous membrane
Dorsal radioulnar lig.
Dorsal ulnocarpal lig.
Ulnar collateral lig.
Triquetrum
Hamate bone
Dorsal carpometacarpal ligs.
Dorsal metacarpal ligs.
Metacarpal bones
5 4 3 2

Radius
Dorsal radiocarpal lig.
Scaphoid bone
Radial collateral lig.
Capitate
Trapezium bone
Capsule of 1st carpometacarpal joint
Trapezoid
1

Coronal section: dorsal view

Distal radioulnar joint
Meniscus
Pisiform bone
Hamate bone
Metacarpal bones
5 4 3 2 1

Articular disc of radiocarpal (wrist) joint
Lunate
Radiocarpal wrist joint
Scaphoid bone
Midcarpal joint
Trapezium bone
Carpometacarpal joint
Intermetacarpal joints

Flexor retinaculum removed: palmar view

Interosseous membrane
Palmar radiocarpal lig. [Radioscapholunate part / Radiocapitate part]
Radial collateral lig.
Tubercle of scaphoid
Tubercle of trapezium bone
Articular capsule of carpometacarpal joint of thumb
Capitate
Capitotriquetral lig.

Palmar radioulnar lig.
Ulnolunate part / Ulnotriquetral part] Palmar ulnocarpal lig.
Ulnar collateral lig.
Pisiform bone
Lunate
Hook of hamate bone

FIGURE 7.24 Wrist Joint Ligaments. (From *Netter's atlas of human anatomy*, ed 8, Plate 465; S-166.)

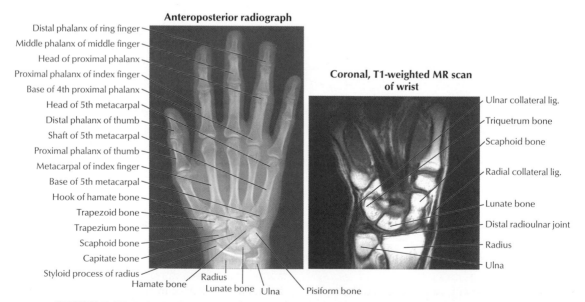

Anteroposterior radiograph

Distal phalanx of ring finger
Middle phalanx of middle finger
Head of proximal phalanx
Proximal phalanx of index finger
Base of 4th proximal phalanx
Head of 5th metacarpal
Distal phalanx of thumb
Shaft of 5th metacarpal
Proximal phalanx of thumb
Metacarpal of index finger
Base of 5th metacarpal
Hook of hamate bone
Trapezoid bone
Trapezium bone
Scaphoid bone
Capitate bone
Styloid process of radius
Hamate bone   Radius   Lunate bone   Ulna   Pisiform bone

Coronal, T1-weighted MR scan of wrist

Ulnar collateral lig.
Triquetrum bone
Scaphoid bone
Radial collateral lig.
Lunate bone
Distal radioulnar joint
Radius
Ulna

FIGURE 7.25 Radiographic Images of the Wrist and Hand. (Left image from *Netter's atlas of human anatomy*, ed 8, Plate 467; S-168; right image from Kelley LL, Petersen C: *Sectional anatomy for imaging professionals*, Philadelphia, 2007, Mosby.)

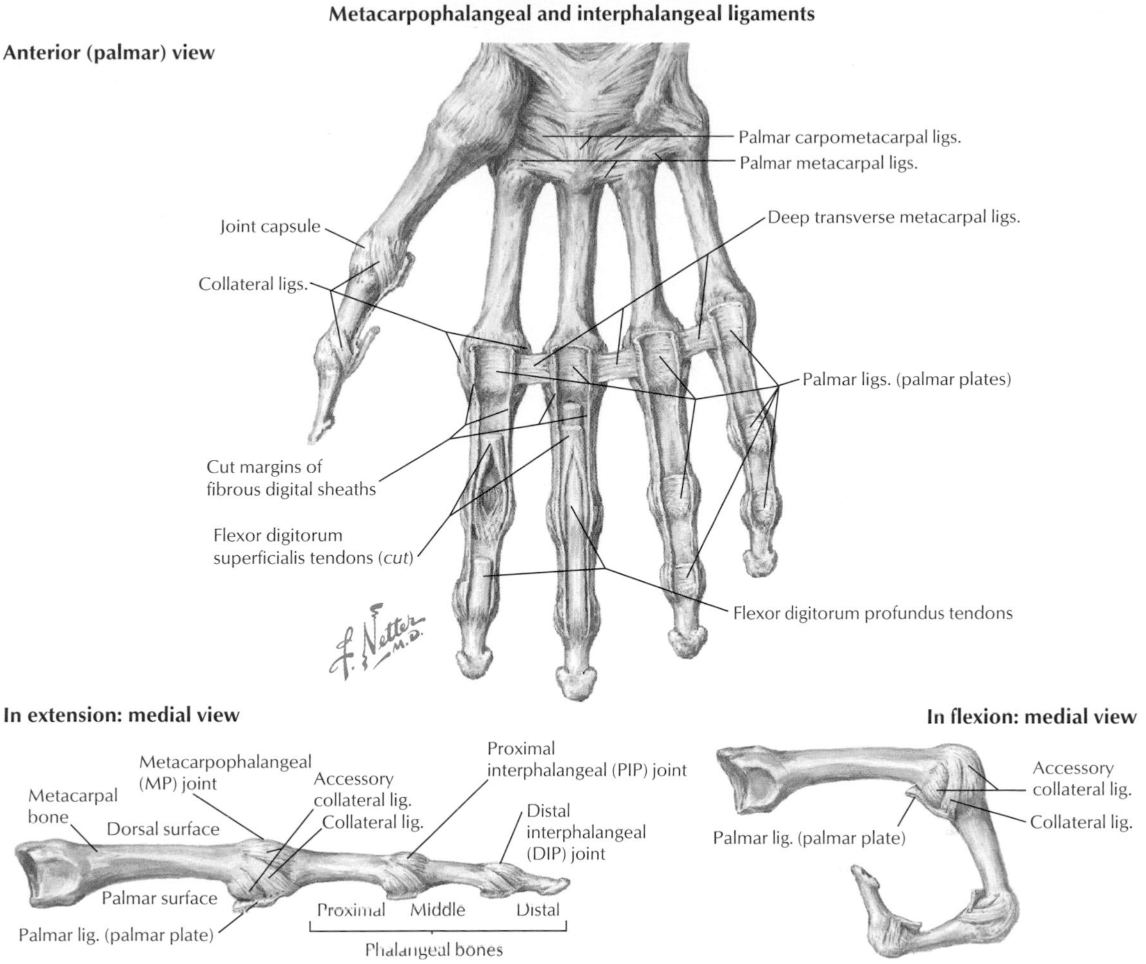

Metacarpophalangeal and interphalangeal ligaments

Anterior (palmar) view

Palmar carpometacarpal ligs.
Palmar metacarpal ligs.

Deep transverse metacarpal ligs.

Joint capsule

Collateral ligs.

Palmar ligs. (palmar plates)

Cut margins of
fibrous digital sheaths

Flexor digitorum
superficialis tendons (cut)

Flexor digitorum profundus tendons

In extension: medial view

In flexion: medial view

Metacarpophalangeal
(MP) joint

Accessory
collateral lig.

Proximal
interphalangeal (PIP) joint

Accessory
collateral lig.

Metacarpal
bone

Distal
interphalangeal
(DIP) joint

Collateral lig.

Dorsal surface

Collateral lig.

Palmar surface

Palmar lig. (palmar plate)

Palmar lig. (palmar plate)

Proximal   Middle   Distal

Phalangeal bones

FIGURE 7.26 Finger Joints and Ligaments. (From *Netter's atlas of human anatomy*, ed 8, Plate 468; S-169.)

powerful hand movements such as gripping objects (Fig. 7.30 and Table 7.16). The palm is covered with a thick layer of skin, which contains numerous sweat glands, and a tough fibrous palmar aponeurosis (shown in cross section in Fig. 7.32). The intrinsic hand muscles of the palm are divided into the thenar eminence or cone of muscles (thumb, first digit), the hypothenar eminence or cone of muscles (little finger, fifth digit), and the interosseous and lumbrical muscles. The **thenar eminence** is created by the following intrinsic muscles (all innervated by the *median nerve*):

- Flexor pollicis brevis.
- Abductor pollicis brevis.
- Opponens pollicis.

The **hypothenar eminence** is created by the following intrinsic muscles (all innervated by the *ulnar nerve*):

- Flexor digiti minimi brevis.

- Abductor digiti minimi.
- Opponens digiti minimi.

Although most intrinsic hand muscles are innervated by the *ulnar nerve*, the three thenar muscles and the two lateral lumbrical muscles (to the second and third digits) are innervated by the *median nerve*.

The blood supply to the hand is by the **radial** and **ulnar arteries,** which anastomose with each other through two **palmar arches** (a superficial arch largely from the ulnar artery and a deep arch largely from the radial artery) (Figs. 7.30 and 7.31; Table 7.17). Except for the thumb and lateral index finger, the remainder of the hand is supplied largely by the ulnar artery. Corresponding veins drain to the dorsum of the hand and collect in the cephalic (lateral) and basilic (medial) veins (see Fig. 7.2). Deeper veins parallel the arteries and throughout their course in the forearm and arm have connections with the

Finger movements

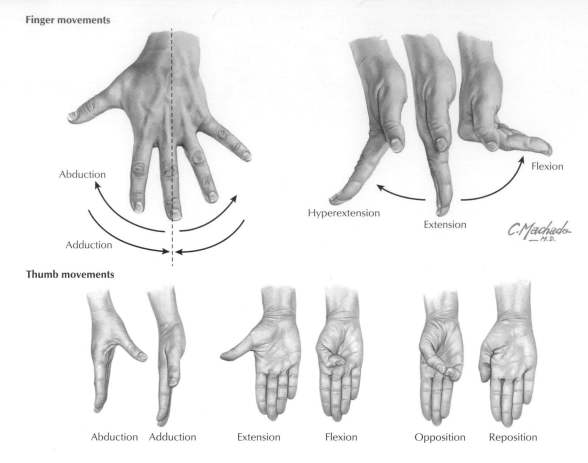

Abduction

Adduction

Hyperextension

Extension

Flexion

Thumb movements

Abduction   Adduction   Extension   Flexion   Opposition   Reposition

FIGURE 7.27 Finger and Thumb Movements.

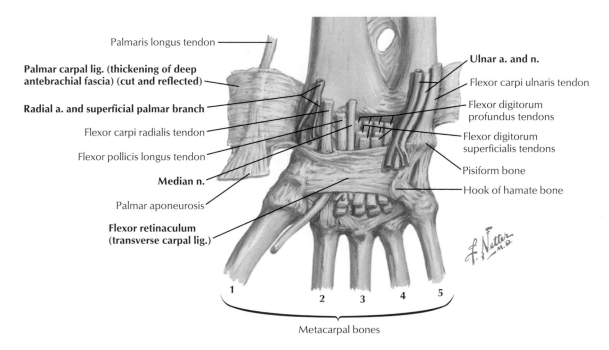

Palmaris longus tendon

Palmar carpal lig. (thickening of deep antebrachial fascia) (cut and reflected)

Radial a. and superficial palmar branch

Flexor carpi radialis tendon

Flexor pollicis longus tendon

Median n.

Palmar aponeurosis

Flexor retinaculum (transverse carpal lig.)

Ulnar a. and n.

Flexor carpi ulnaris tendon

Flexor digitorum profundus tendons

Flexor digitorum superficialis tendons

Pisiform bone

Hook of hamate bone

1   2   3   4   5

Metacarpal bones

FIGURE 7.28 Palmar View of Carpal Tunnel. (From *Netter's atlas of human anatomy,* ed 8, Plate 464; S-165.)

TABLE 7.15 Joints and Ligaments of the Wrist and Hand

LIGAMENT	ATTACHMENT	COMMENT
Radiocarpal (Biaxial Synovial Ellipsoid) Joint		
Capsule and disc	Surrounds joint; radius to scaphoid, lunate, and triquetrum	Provides little support; allows flexion, extension, abduction, adduction, and circumduction
Palmar (volar) radiocarpal ligaments	Radius to scaphoid, lunate, and triquetrum	Are strong and stabilizing
Dorsal radiocarpal	Radius to scaphoid, lunate, and triquetrum	Is weaker ligament
Radial collateral	Radius to scaphoid and triquetrum	Stabilizes proximal row of carpals
Distal Radioulnar (Uniaxial Synovial Pivot) Joint		
Capsule	Surrounds joint; ulnar head to ulnar notch of radius	Is thin superiorly; allows pronation and supination
Palmar and dorsal radio-ulnar	Extends transversely between the two bones	Articular disc binds bones together
Intercarpal (Synovial Plane) Joints		
Proximal row of carpals	Adjacent carpals	Permits gliding and sliding movements
Distal row of carpals	Adjacent carpals	Are united by anterior, posterior, and interosseous ligaments
Midcarpal (Synovial Plane) Joints		
Palmar (volar) intercarpal	Proximal and distal rows of carpals	Is location for one-third of wrist extension and two-thirds of flexion; permits gliding and sliding movements
Carpal collaterals	Scaphoid, lunate, and triquetrum to capitate and hamate	Stabilize distal row (ellipsoid synovial joint)
Carpometacarpal (CMC) (Plane Synovial) Joints (Except Thumb)		
Capsule	Carpals to metacarpals of digits 2-5	Surrounds joints; allows some gliding movement
Palmar and dorsal CMC	Carpals to metacarpals of digits 2-5	Dorsal ligament strongest
Interosseous CMC	Carpals to metacarpals of digits 2-5	
Thumb (Biaxial Saddle) Joint		
Same ligaments as CMC	Trapezium to 1st metacarpal	Allows flexion, extension, abduction, adduction, and circumduction
		Is common site for arthritis
Metacarpophalangeal (Biaxial Condyloid Synovial) Joint		
Capsule	Metacarpal to proximal phalanx	Surrounds joint; allows flexion, extension, abduction, adduction, and circumduction
Radial and ulnar collaterals	Metacarpal to proximal phalanx	Are tight in flexion and loose in extension
Palmar (volar) plate	Metacarpal to proximal phalanx	If broken digit, cast in flexion or ligament will shorten
Interphalangeal (Uniaxial Synovial Hinge) Joints		
Capsule	Adjacent phalanges	Surrounds joints; allows flexion and extension
Two collaterals	Adjacent phalanges	Are oriented obliquely
Palmar (volar) plate	Adjacent phalanges	Prevents hyperextension

Clinical Focus 7.13

Fracture of the Ulnar Shaft

Usually, a direct blow to or forced pronation of the forearm is the most common cause of a fracture of the shaft of the ulna. Fracture of the ulna with dislocation of the proximal radioulnar joint is termed a **Monteggia fracture.** The radial head usually dislocates anteriorly, but posterior, medial, or lateral dislocation also may occur. Such dislocations may put the posterior interosseous nerve (the deep branch of the radial nerve) at risk.

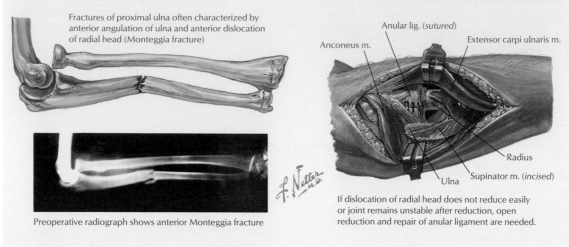

Fractures of proximal ulna often characterized by anterior angulation of ulna and anterior dislocation of radial head (Monteggia fracture)

Anular lig. (*sutured*)

Anconeus m.

Extensor carpi ulnaris m.

Radius

Ulna

Supinator m. (*incised*)

Preoperative radiograph shows anterior Monteggia fracture

If dislocation of radial head does not reduce easily or joint remains unstable after reduction, open reduction and repair of anular ligament are needed.

Clinical Focus 7.14

Distal Radial (Colles') Fracture

Fractures of the distal radius account for about 80% of forearm fractures in all age groups and often result from a fall on an outstretched hand. Colles' fracture is an extension-compression fracture of the distal radius that produces a typical *"dinner fork"* deformity.

Most commonly results from fall on outstretched extended hand

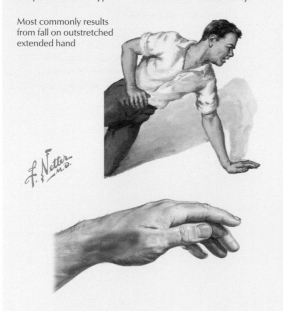

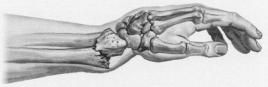

Lateral view of Colles' fracture demonstrates characteristic dinner fork deformity with dorsal and proximal displacement of distal fragment. Note dorsal instead of normal volar slope of articular surface of distal radius.

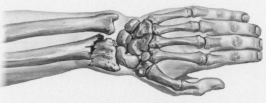

Dorsal view shows radial deviation of hand with ulnar prominence of styloid process of ulna.

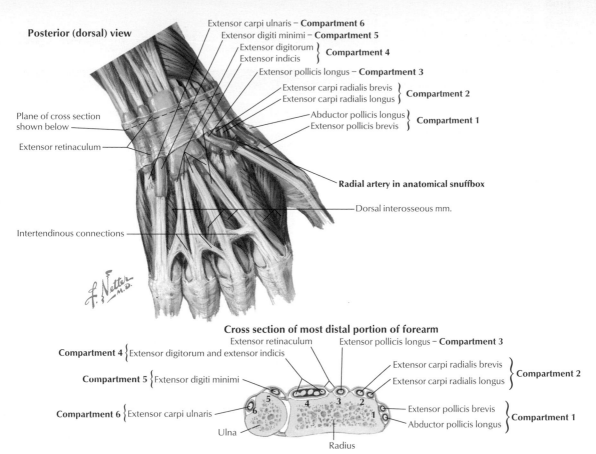

Posterior (dorsal) view

Extensor carpi ulnaris – **Compartment 6**
Extensor digiti minimi – **Compartment 5**
Extensor digitorum
Extensor indicis } **Compartment 4**
Extensor pollicis longus – **Compartment 3**
Extensor carpi radialis brevis
Extensor carpi radialis longus } **Compartment 2**
Abductor pollicis longus
Extensor pollicis brevis } **Compartment 1**

Plane of cross section shown below

Extensor retinaculum

Radial artery in anatomical snuffbox

Dorsal interosseous mm.

Intertendinous connections

Cross section of most distal portion of forearm
Extensor retinaculum   Extensor pollicis longus – **Compartment 3**
Compartment 4 { Extensor digitorum and extensor indicis
Compartment 5 { Extensor digiti minimi
Extensor carpi radialis brevis
Extensor carpi radialis longus } **Compartment 2**
Compartment 6 { Extensor carpi ulnaris
Extensor pollicis brevis
Abductor pollicis longus } **Compartment 1**
Ulna
Radius

FIGURE 7.29 Extensor Tendons and Sheaths of the Wrist. (From *Netter's atlas of human anatomy,* ed 8, Plate 480; S-260.)

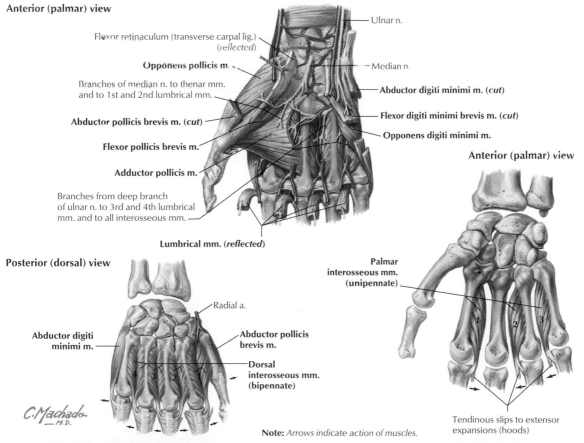

Anterior (palmar) view

Ulnar n.

Flexor retinaculum (transverse carpal lig.) (reflected)

Opponens pollicis m.

Median n.

Branches of median n. to thenar mm. and to 1st and 2nd lumbrical mm.

Abductor digiti minimi m. (*cut*)

Abductor pollicis brevis m. (*cut*)

Flexor digiti minimi brevis m. (*cut*)

Opponens digiti minimi m.

Flexor pollicis brevis m.

Anterior (palmar) view

Adductor pollicis m.

Branches from deep branch of ulnar n. to 3rd and 4th lumbrical mm. and to all interosseous mm.

Palmar interosseous mm. (unipennate)

Lumbrical mm. (*reflected*)

Posterior (dorsal) view

Radial a.

Abductor digiti minimi m.

Abductor pollicis brevis m.

Dorsal interosseous mm. (bipennate)

Tendinous slips to extensor expansions (hoods)

Note: *Arrows indicate action of muscles.*

FIGURE 7.30 Intrinsic Muscles of the Hand. (From *Netter's atlas of human anatomy,* ed 8, Plate 475; S-256.)

TABLE 7.16 Intrinsic Hand Muscles

MUSCLE	PROXIMAL ATTACHMENT	DISTAL ATTACHMENT	INNERVATION	MAIN ACTIONS
Abductor pollicis brevis	Flexor retinaculum and tubercles of scaphoid and trapezium	Base of proximal phalanx of thumb	Median nerve (recurrent branch) (C8-T1)	Abducts thumb
Flexor pollicis brevis	Flexor retinaculum and tubercle of trapezium	Lateral side of base of proximal phalanx of thumb	Median nerve (recurrent branch) (C8-T1)	Flexes proximal phalanx of thumb
Opponens pollicis	Flexor retinaculum and tubercle of trapezium	Lateral side of 1st metacarpal bone	Median nerve (recurrent branch) (C8-T1)	Opposes thumb toward center of palm and rotates it medially
Adductor pollicis	*Oblique head:* bases of 2nd and 3rd metacarpals and capitate *Transverse head:* anterior surface of body of 3rd metacarpal	Medial side of base of proximal phalanx of thumb	Ulnar nerve (deep branch) (C8-T1)	Adducts thumb toward middle digit
Abductor digiti minimi	Pisiform and tendon of flexor carpi ulnaris	Medial side of base of proximal phalanx of 5th digit	Ulnar nerve (deep branch) (C8-T1)	Abducts 5th digit
Flexor digiti minimi brevis	Hook of hamate and flexor retinaculum	Medial side of base of proximal phalanx of 5th digit	Ulnar nerve (deep branch) (C8-T1)	Flexes proximal phalanx of 5th digit
Opponens digiti minimi	Hook of hamate and flexor retinaculum	Palmar surface of 5th metacarpal	Ulnar nerve (deep branch) (C8-T1)	Draws 5th metacarpal anteriorly and rotates it, bringing 5th digit into opposition with thumb
Lumbricals 1 and 2	Lateral two tendons of flexor digitorum profundus	Lateral sides of extensor expansions of 2nd and 3rd digits	Median nerve (C8-T1)	Flex digits at MCP joints and extend IP joints
Lumbricals 3 and 4	Medial three tendons of flexor digitorum profundus	Lateral sides of extensor expansions of 4th and 5th digits	Ulnar nerve (deep branch) (C8-T1)	Flex digits at MCP joints and extend IP joints
Dorsal interossei	Adjacent sides of two metacarpals	Extensor expansions and bases of proximal phalanges of 2nd to 4th digits	Ulnar nerve (deep branch) (C8-T1)	Abduct digits; flex digits at MCP joints and extend IP joints
Palmar interossei	Sides of 2nd, 4th, and 5th metacarpal bones	Extensor expansions of digits and bases of proximal phalanges of 2nd, 4th, and 5th digits	Ulnar nerve (deep branch) (C8-T1)	Adduct digits; flex digits at MCP joints and extend IP joints

IP, Interphalangeal; *MCP*, metacarpophalangeal.
Variations in spinal nerve contributions to the innervation of muscles, their attachments, and their actions are common in human anatomy. Therefore, expect differences between texts and realize that anatomical variation is normal.

superficial veins. The upper limb veins possess *valves* to assist in venous return.

Palmar Spaces and Tendon Sheaths

As the long tendons pass through the hand toward the digits, they are surrounded by a **synovial sheath** and, in the digits, a **fibrous digital sheath** that binds them to the phalanges (Figs. 7.31 and 7.32; Table 7.18). Note from Fig. 7.32 that the synovial sheath of the fifth digit communicates with the common flexor sheath, while those of the second,

third, and fourth digits generally do not communicate with the other synovial sheaths. *Infections in the fifth digit* may "seed" the common flexor sheath, and vice versa, via this connection. Cross section of the palm shows that the long flexor tendons segregate out to their respective digits, creating *two potential spaces* (thenar and midpalmar) of the hand. These spaces can become infected and distended. The long flexor tendons (flexor digitorum superficialis and profundus tendons) course on the palmar side of the digits, with the

Palmar view: superficial

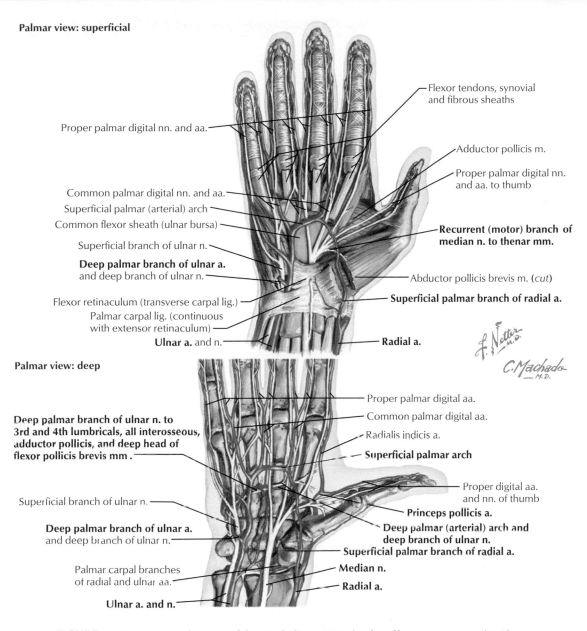

Proper palmar digital nn. and aa.

Flexor tendons, synovial and fibrous sheaths

Adductor pollicis m.

Proper palmar digital nn. and aa. to thumb

Common palmar digital nn. and aa.
Superficial palmar (arterial) arch
Common flexor sheath (ulnar bursa)
Superficial branch of ulnar n.
Deep palmar branch of ulnar a. and deep branch of ulnar n.

Recurrent (motor) branch of median n. to thenar mm.

Abductor pollicis brevis m. (*cut*)

Flexor retinaculum (transverse carpal lig.)
Palmar carpal lig. (continuous with extensor retinaculum)
Ulnar a. and n.

Superficial palmar branch of radial a.

Radial a.

Palmar view: deep

Deep palmar branch of ulnar n. to 3rd and 4th lumbricals, all interosseous, adductor pollicis, and deep head of flexor pollicis brevis mm .

Proper palmar digital aa.
Common palmar digital aa.
Radialis indicis a.
Superficial palmar arch

Superficial branch of ulnar n.

Proper digital aa. and nn. of thumb
Princeps pollicis a.

Deep palmar branch of ulnar a. and deep branch of ulnar n.

Deep palmar (arterial) arch and deep branch of ulnar n.
Superficial palmar branch of radial a.

Palmar carpal branches of radial and ulnar aa.

Median n.

Ulnar a. and n.

Radial a.

FIGURE 7.31 Arteries and Nerves of the Hand. (From *Netter's atlas of human anatomy,* ed 8, Plate 476; S-257.)

TABLE 7.17 Arteries of the Hand

ARTERY	COURSE	ARTERY	COURSE
Radial		*Ulnar*	
Superficial palmar branch	Forms superficial palmar arch with ulnar artery	Deep palmar branch	Forms deep palmar arch with radial artery
Princeps pollicis	Passes under flexor pollicis longus tendon, and divides into two proper digital arteries to thumb	Superficial palmar arch	Is formed by termination of ulnar artery; gives rise to three common digital arteries, each of which gives rise to two proper digital arteries
Radialis indicis	Passes to index finger on its lateral side		
Deep palmar arch	Is formed by terminal part of radial artery		

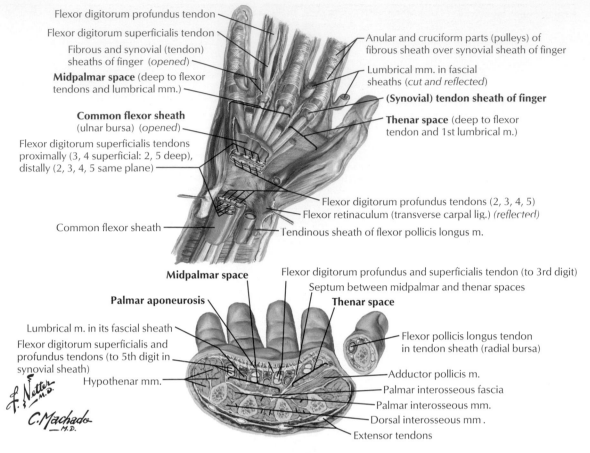

FIGURE 7.32 Bursae, Spaces, and Tendon Sheaths of the Hand. (From *Netter's atlas of human anatomy,* ed 8, Plate 473; S-254.)

TABLE 7.18 Palmar Spaces and Compartments

SPACE	COMMENT
Carpal tunnel	Osseofascial tunnel composed of carpal bones (carpal arch) and overlying flexor retinaculum; contains median nerve and nine tendons
Thenar eminence	Muscle compartment at base of thumb
Thenar space	Potential space just above adductor pollicis muscle
Hypothenar eminence	Muscle compartment at base of little finger
Central compartment	Compartment containing long flexor tendons and lumbrical muscles
Midpalmar space	Potential space deep to central compartment
Adductor compartment	Compartment containing adductor pollicis muscle
Synovial sheaths	Osseofibrous sheaths (tunnels) lined with synovium to facilitate sliding movements

superficialis tendon *splitting* to allow the profundus tendon to pass to the distal phalanx (Fig. 7.33). On the dorsum of the digits, the **extensor expansion (hood)** provides for insertion of the long extensor tendons and the insertion of the lumbrical and interosseous muscles. **Lumbricals** and **interossei muscles** flex the MCP joint and extend the PIP and DIP joints (see Table 7.16).

The extensor tendons of the thumb on the dorsum of the hand create the **anatomical snuffbox,** composed of the following tendons visible beneath the raised skin:

- Medially, the tendon of the **extensor pollicis longus muscle.**
- Laterally, the tendons of the **abductor pollicis longus** and **extensor pollicis brevis muscles.**

The "floor" of the snuffbox contains the **radial artery** (a pulse can be detected here when the artery is pressed against the underlying scaphoid bone) (Figs. 7.20 and 7.29) and the terminal end of the

Text continued on page 410

Clinical Focus 7.15

Median Nerve Compression and Carpal Tunnel Syndrome

Median nerve compression in the **carpal tunnel**, the most common compression neuropathy, is often linked to occupational repetitive movements related to wrist flexion and extension, holding the wrist in an awkward position, or strong gripping of objects. Long-term compression often leads to thenar atrophy and weakness of the thumb and index fingers, reflecting the loss of innervation to the muscles distal to the median nerve damage.

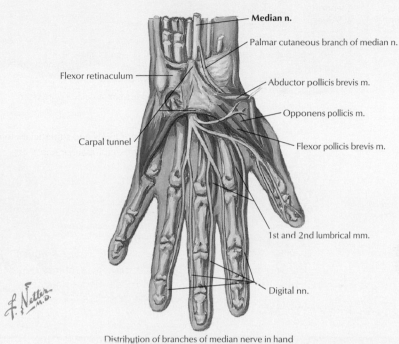

Median n.

Palmar cutaneous branch of median n.

Flexor retinaculum

Abductor pollicis brevis m.

Opponens pollicis m.

Carpal tunnel

Flexor pollicis brevis m.

1st and 2nd lumbrical mm.

Digital nn.

Distribution of branches of median nerve in hand

Flexor tendons in carpal tunnel   Ulnar n.

Flexor retinaculum (roof of carpal tunnel)

Median n. in carpal tunnel

Activities or medical conditions that increase contents and pressure within tunnel may result in nerve compression.

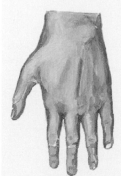

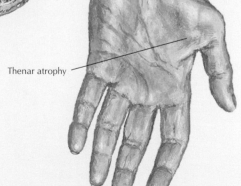

Thenar atrophy

Sensory distribution of median nerve

Long-term compression can result in thenar muscle weakness and atrophy

Clinical Focus 7.16

Fracture of the Scaphoid

The scaphoid bone is the *most frequently fractured carpal bone* and may be injured by falling on an extended wrist. Fracture of the middle third (waist) of the bone is most common. Pain and swelling in the "anatomical snuffbox" often occurs, and optimal healing depends on an adequate blood supply from the palmar carpal branch of the radial artery. Loss of the blood supply can lead to nonunion or avascular osteonecrosis.

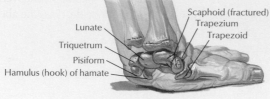

Lunate
Triquetrum
Pisiform
Hamulus (hook) of hamate

Scaphoid (fractured)
Trapezium
Trapezoid

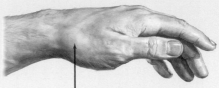

Usually caused by fall on outstretched hand with impact on thenar eminence

Clinical findings: pain, tenderness, and swelling in anatomical snuffbox

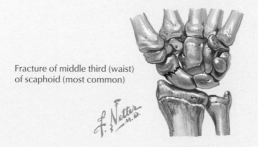

Fracture of middle third (waist) of scaphoid (most common)

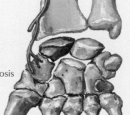

Because nutrient arteries only enter distal half of scaphoid, fracture often results in osteonecrosis of proximal fragment.

Clinical Focus 7.17

Allen's Test

The Allen's test is used to test the *vascular perfusion* distal to the wrist. The physician lightly places the thumbs on the patient's ulnar and radial arteries, and the patient makes a tight fist to "blanch" the palmar skin (squeeze the blood into the dorsal venous network). Then, while compressing the radial artery with the thumb, the physician releases the pressure on the ulnar artery and asks the patient to open the clenched fist. Normally the skin will turn pink immediately, indicating normal ulnar artery blood flow through the anastomotic palmar arches. The test is then repeated by occluding the ulnar artery to assess radial artery flow.

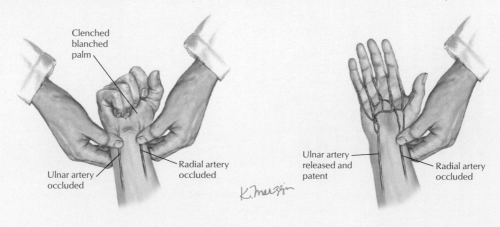

Clenched blanched palm

Ulnar artery occluded

Radial artery occluded

Ulnar artery released and patent

Radial artery occluded

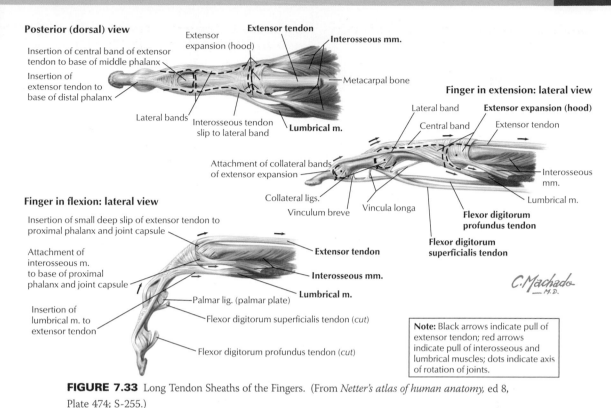

FIGURE 7.33 Long Tendon Sheaths of the Fingers. (From *Netter's atlas of human anatomy*, ed 8, Plate 474; S-255.)

Clinical Focus 7.18

De Quervain Tenosynovitis

In de Quervain tenosynovitis the **tendons of the abductor pollicis longus** and **extensor pollicis brevis muscles** pass through the same tendinous sheath on the dorsum of the wrist (first compartment in the extensor retinaculum). Excessive and repetitive use of the hands in a power grip or a twisting wringing action can cause friction and thickening of the sheath, leading to pain over the styloid process of the radius. This pain is mediated by the **superficial radial nerve** (sensory), and the pain can extend distally into the thumb and radiate up the lateral forearm.

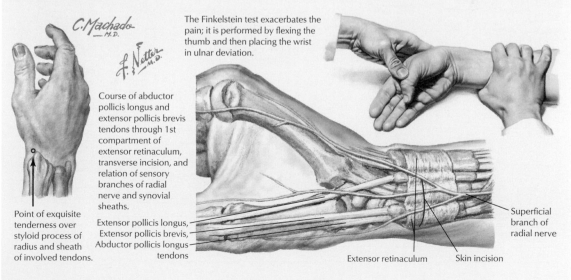

superficial radial nerve, which passes subcutaneously over this region.

8. UPPER LIMB MUSCLE SUMMARY

Table 7.19 summarizes the actions of major muscles on the joints. *The list is not exhaustive and highlights only major muscles responsible for each movement; the separate muscle tables provide more detail.* Most joints move because of the action of multiple muscles working on that joint, but this list only focuses on the more important muscles acting on that joint. For example, although the brachialis and biceps muscles are the major flexors of the forearm at the elbow, the brachioradialis and many of the forearm muscles originating from the medial and lateral epicondyles of the humerus also cross the elbow joint and have a weak flexor action on the elbow. However, this is not their primary action.

Clinical Focus 7.19

Proximal Interphalangeal Joint Dislocations

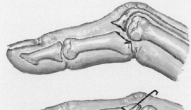

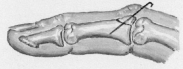

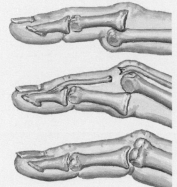

Dorsal dislocation (most common)

Palmar dislocation (uncommon)
Causes **boutonnière deformity.** Central slip of extensor tendon often torn, requiring open fixation, followed by dorsal splinting.

Rotational dislocation (rare)

Volar dislocation of middle phalanx with avulsion of central slip of extensor tendon, with or without bone fragment. Failure to recognize and properly treat this condition results in **boutonnière deformity** and severely restricted function.

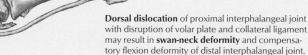

Dorsal dislocation of proximal interphalangeal joint with disruption of volar plate and collateral ligament may result in **swan-neck deformity** and compensatory flexion deformity of distal interphalangeal joint.

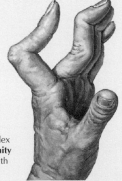

Boutonnière deformity of index finger with **swan-neck deformity** of other fingers in a patient with rheumatoid arthritis

Defect	Comment
Coach's finger	Dorsal dislocation of the joint; common
Boutonnière deformity	Dislocation or avulsion fracture of middle phalanx, with failure to treat causing deformity and chronic pain
Rotational	Rare dislocation with rotation of the metacarpal
Swan-neck deformity	Dorsal dislocation with disruption of palmar (volar) and collateral ligaments

Clinical Focus 7.20

Finger Injuries

Various traumatic finger injuries may occur, causing fractures, disruption of the flexor and extensor tendons, and torn ligaments. Each element must be carefully examined for normal function, including muscle groups, capillary refill (Allen's test; see Clinical Focus 7.17), and two-point sensory discrimination.

Mallet finger

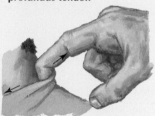

Usually caused by direct blow on extended distal phalanx, as in baseball, volleyball

Avulsion of flexor digitorum profundus tendon

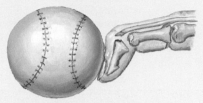

Caused by violent traction on flexed distal phalanx, as in catching on jersey of running football player

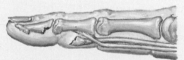

Flexor digitorum profundus tendon may be torn directly from distal phalanx or may avulse small or large bone fragment.

Fracture of metacarpals

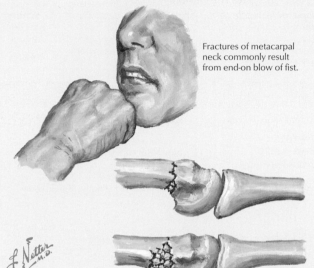

Fractures of metacarpal neck commonly result from end-on blow of fist.

In fractures of metacarpal neck, volar cortex often comminuted, resulting in marked instability after reduction, which often necessitates pinning

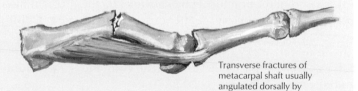

Transverse fractures of metacarpal shaft usually angulated dorsally by pull of interosseous muscles

Thumb injury other than fracture

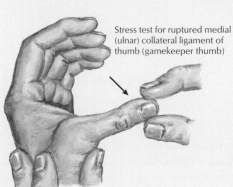

Stress test for ruptured medial (ulnar) collateral ligament of thumb (gamekeeper thumb)

Torn medial collateral lig.

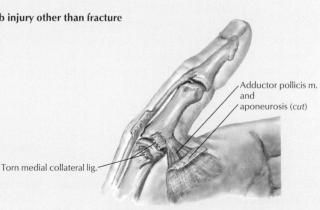

Adductor pollicis m. and aponeurosis (*cut*)

Ruptured medial collateral ligament of metacarpophalangeal joint of thumb

TABLE 7.19 Summary of Actions of Major Upper Limb Muscles*

Scapula

Elevate: levator scapulae, trapezius
Depress: pectoralis minor

Protrude: serratus anterior

Depress glenoid: rhomboids
Elevate glenoid: serratus anterior, trapezius
Retract: rhomboids, trapezius

Shoulder

Flex: pectoralis major, coracobrachialis
Extend: latissimus dorsi, teres major
Abduct: supraspinatus (initiates), deltoid

Adduct: pectoralis major, latissimus dorsi
Rotate medially: subscapularis, teres major, pectoralis major, latissimus dorsi
Rotate laterally: infraspinatus, teres minor

Elbow

Flex: brachialis, biceps

Extend: triceps, anconeus

Radioulnar

Pronate: pronators (teres and quadratus)

Supinate: supinator, biceps brachii

Wrist

Flex: flexor carpi radialis, ulnaris
Extend: all extensor carpi muscles
Abduct: flexor/extensor carpi radialis muscles

Adduct: flexor and extensor carpi ulnaris
Circumduct: combination of all movements

Metacarpophalangeal

Flex: interossei and lumbricals
Extend: extensor digitorum
Abduct: dorsal interossei

Adduct: palmar interossei
Circumduct: combination of all movements

Interphalangeal-Proximal

Flex: flexor digitorum superficialis

Extend: interossei and lumbricals

Interphalangeal-Distal

Flex: flexor digitorum profundus

Extend: interossei and lumbricals

*Accessory or secondary actions of muscles are detailed in the muscle tables.

9. UPPER LIMB ARTERY AND VEIN SUMMARY

Arteries of the Upper Limb

The **left subclavian artery** arises directly from the **aortic arch (1)**, while the **right subclavian artery (3)** arises from the **brachiocephalic trunk (2)**. The branches of both subclavian arteries are the same from that point on distally to the hand (Fig. 7.34). The **brachial artery (5)** bifurcates at the cubital fossa and gives rise to the **ulnar artery (6)** and **radial artery (7)**.

Major anastomoses occur between the subclavian artery and the **axillary artery (4)** around the branches supplying the muscles of the scapula. Likewise, a major anastomosis also occurs around the elbow between collateral arteries from the brachial artery and recurrent branches from the ulnar artery and radial artery. Carpal arteries at the wrist and palmar arches in the hand also participate in anastomoses.

Many of the major arteries also provide small arteries to muscles of the limb (these small branches are not listed) and to nutrient arteries to the adjacent bones (not named). **Arteriovenous (AV) anastomoses** are direct connections between small arteries and veins and usually are involved in cutaneous thermoregulation. They are numerous in the skin of the fingers, especially nail beds and fingertips.

The joints and their ligaments receive a rich blood supply provided by small articular branches of adjacent arteries. Major pulse points of the upper limb include the following:

- **Brachial pulse:** at the medial aspect of the midarm, where it may be pressed against the humerus.
- **Cubital pulse:** anterior to the elbow in the cubital fossa, where the brachial artery is felt just medial to the biceps brachii muscle tendon.
- **Radial pulse:** at the wrist, just lateral to the flexor carpi radialis muscle tendon; most common site to take a pulse.
- **Ulnar pulse:** at the wrist, just proximolateral to the pisiform carpal bone.

In the outline of arteries, major vessels often dissected in anatomy courses include the first-order arteries (in **bold** and numbered) and their second-order major branches. The third-order and fourth-order arteries are dissected only in more detailed anatomy courses.

Veins of the Upper Limb

The venous drainage begins largely on the dorsum of the hand, with venous blood returning proximally in both a superficial and a deep venous pattern. The **basilic vein (1)** and **cephalic vein (2)** drain into the **axillary vein (4)** in the shoulder. The deep venous drainage via the forearm ulnar and radial veins drains into the **brachial vein (3)**. Often these

1. **Aortic Arch**
2. **Brachiocephalic Trunk**
3. **Right/Left Subclavian Artery**
   Vertebral artery
   Internal thoracic artery
   Thyrocervical trunk
   Costocervical trunk
4. **Axillary Artery**
   Superior thoracic artery
   Thoracoacromial artery
   Lateral thoracic artery
   Subscapular artery
   Anterior humeral circumflex artery
   Posterior humeral circumflex artery
5. **Brachial Artery**
   Profunda brachii artery
      Radial collateral artery
      Medial collateral artery
   Superior ulnar collateral artery
   Inferior ulnar collateral artery
6. **Ulnar Artery**
   Ulnar recurrent artery
      Anterior ulnar recurrent artery
      Posterior ulnar recurrent artery
   Common interosseous artery
      Anterior interosseous artery
         Median artery
      Posterior interosseous artery
         Perforating branch
         Recurrent interosseous artery
   Dorsal carpal branch
   Palmar carpal branch
   Deep palmar branch
   Superficial palmar arch
   Common palmar digital arteries (3)
      Proper palmar digital arteries
7. **Radial Artery**
   Radial recurrent artery
   Palmar carpal branch
   Superficial palmar branch
   Dorsal carpal branch
      Dorsal carpal arch
      Dorsal metacarpal arteries
      Dorsal digital arteries
   Princeps pollicis artery
   Radialis indicis artery
   Deep palmar arch
      Palmar metacarpal arteries
      Perforating branches

*Direction of blood flow is from top (proximal) to bottom (distal).

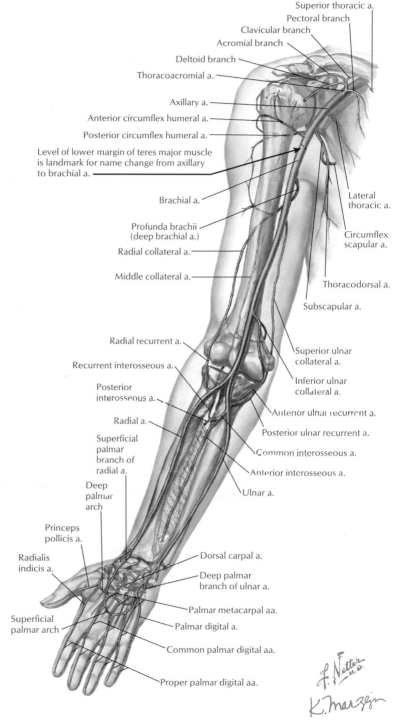

FIGURE 7.34 Arteries of Upper Limb.

Deep Veins

    Palmar metacarpal

    Deep venous arch

    Post. interosseous veins

    Ant. interosseous veins

Radial Vein(s)

Ulnar Vein(s)

3. Brachial Vein(s)

    Subscapular vein

    Circumflex scapular vein

        Thoracodorsal vein

        Post. circumflex scapular vein

        Ant. circumflex scapular vein

    Lateral thoracic vein

    Thoracoepigastric veins

    Areolar venous plexus (breast)

4. Axillary Vein

5. Subclavian Vein

6. Left and Right Brachiocephalic Veins

7. Superior Vena Cava

8. Heart (Right Atrium)

*Direction of blood flow is from distal
(hand) to proximal (heart).

Superficial Veins

    Palmar digital veins

    Superficial palmar arch

      Metacarpal/carpal tributaries

    Dorsal venous network of hand

Basilic vein of forearm

Cephalic vein of forearm

    Median vein of forearm

    Median cubital vein

1. Basilic Vein

    Thoracoacromial vein

2. Cephalic Vein

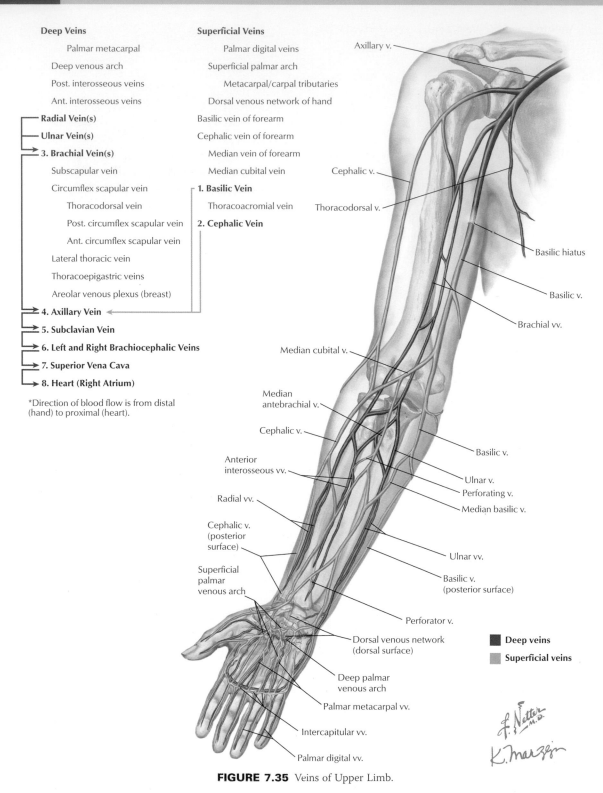

FIGURE 7.35 Veins of Upper Limb.

are multiple veins *(venae comitantes)* coursing with the single ulnar or radial artery (Fig. 7.35).

The **median cubital vein**, often coursing between the cephalic and basilic veins in the cubital fossa, is often accessed for venipuncture to withdraw a blood sample. Even the axillary vein usually consists of multiple veins surrounding the single axillary artery. The axillary vein(s) then drains into the **subclavian vein (5)** on each side (right and left). The subclavian vein(s) then drains into the **left** and **right brachiocephalic veins (6),** which drain into the **superior vena cava (7)** and then the **heart (right atrium) (8)** (see Fig. 3.28).

In the human body the venous system is the *compliance system,* and at rest about 65% of the blood resides in our low-pressure venous system. Veins generally are larger than their corresponding arteries and have thinner walls, and multiple veins often accompany a single artery; the body has many more veins than arteries, and veins are more variable in location than most arteries.

10. UPPER LIMB NERVE SUMMARY

Shoulder Region

Shoulder muscles are largely innervated by the **suprascapular** (C5, C6), **musculocutaneous** (C5, C6, C7) (which are largely elbow flexors, and an arm flexor/adductor for the coracobrachialis muscle), **long thoracic** (C5, C6, C7), **dorsal scapular, subscapular,** and **axillary nerves** (C5, C6); there may be some variability in spinal segment distribution to these nerves (Fig. 7.36). Table 7.20 lists some of the more common *neuropathies* associated with four of these six nerves.

Radial Nerve in the Arm and Forearm

The **radial nerve** (C5, C6, C7, C8, T1) innervates the muscles that extend the forearm at the elbow (posterior compartment arm muscles) and the skin of the posterior arm, via the inferior lateral and posterior cutaneous nerves of the arm (Fig. 7.37).

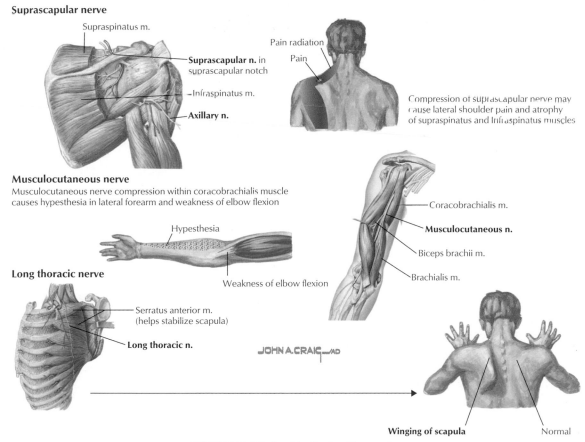

FIGURE 7.36 Shoulder Region Neuropathy.

TABLE 7.20 Shoulder Region Neuropathy (see Fig. 7.36)

INVOLVED NERVE	CONDITION	INVOLVED NERVE	CONDITION
Suprascapular	Posterolateral shoulder pain, which may radiate to arm and neck; weakness in shoulder rotation	Long thoracic	Injury at level of neck caused by stretching during lateral flexion of neck to opposite side; winged scapula
Musculocutaneous	Coracobrachialis compression and weakened flexion at the elbow, with hypesthesia of lateral forearm; weakened supination with elbow flexed	Axillary	Rare condition (quadrangular space syndrome) (not shown in Fig. 7.36); can produce weakness of deltoid muscle and abduction

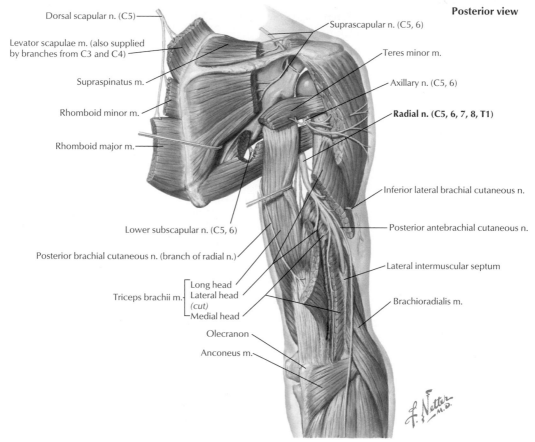

FIGURE 7.37 Radial Nerve Distribution in the Arm. (From *Netter's atlas of human anatomy,* ed 8, Plate 468; S-111.)

The radial nerve also innervates the extensor muscles of the wrist and fingers and the supinator muscle (posterior compartment forearm muscles). It also conveys cutaneous sensory information from the posterior forearm and the radial side of the dorsum of the hand. Pure **radial nerve sensation** (no overlap with other nerves) is tested on the skin overlying the *first dorsal interosseous* muscle (Fig. 7.38). The radial nerve is vulnerable in fractures of the humeral midshaft or by compression injuries of the arm. It also is

vulnerable to compression in the forearm because the deep branch of the radial nerve passes through the two heads of the supinator muscle. The superficial branch of the radial nerve is sensory and may be injured at the wrist (see Clinical Focus 7.21).

Median Nerve in Forearm and Hand

The **median nerve** (C6, C7, C8, T1) innervates all the muscles of the forearm anterior compartment (wrist and finger flexors and forearm pronators) except the flexor

Clinical Focus 7.21

Radial Nerve Compression

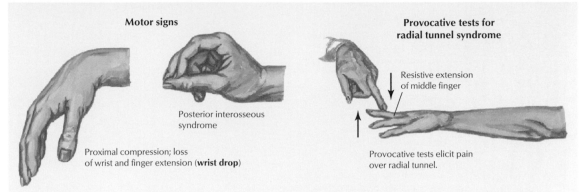

Motor signs

Posterior interosseous
syndrome

Proximal compression; loss
of wrist and finger extension (**wrist drop**)

Provocative tests for
radial tunnel syndrome

Resistive extension
of middle finger

Provocative tests elicit pain
over radial tunnel.

Sensory signs in radial tunnel syndrome

Pain and tenderness

Pain radiation

Paresthesia and
hypesthesias

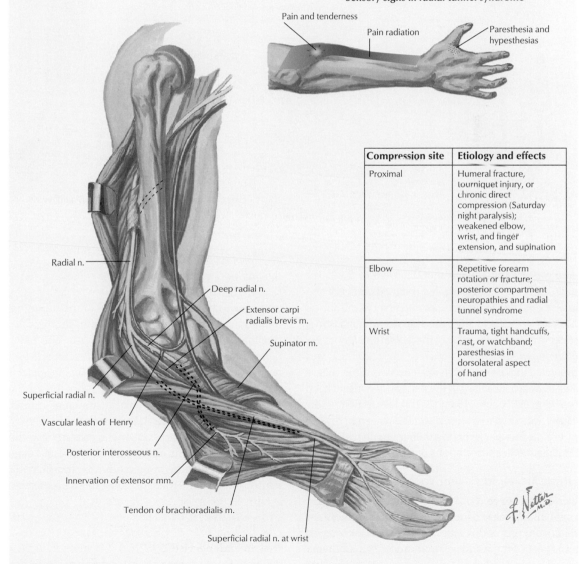

Radial n.

Deep radial n.

Extensor carpi
radialis brevis m.

Supinator m.

Superficial radial n.

Vascular leash of Henry

Posterior interosseous n.

Innervation of extensor mm.

Tendon of brachioradialis m.

Superficial radial n. at wrist

Compression site	Etiology and effects
Proximal	Humeral fracture, tourniquet injury, or chronic direct compression (Saturday night paralysis); weakened elbow, wrist, and finger extension, and supination
Elbow	Repetitive forearm rotation or fracture; posterior compartment neuropathies and radial tunnel syndrome
Wrist	Trauma, tight handcuffs, cast, or watchband; paresthesias in dorsolateral aspect of hand

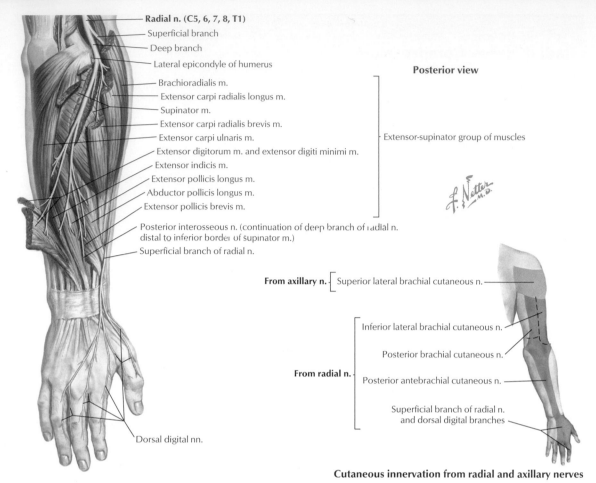

Radial n. (C5, 6, 7, 8, T1)
Superficial branch
Deep branch
Lateral epicondyle of humerus

Brachioradialis m.
Extensor carpi radialis longus m.
Supinator m.
Extensor carpi radialis brevis m.
Extensor carpi ulnaris m.
Extensor digitorum m. and extensor digiti minimi m.
Extensor indicis m.
Extensor pollicis longus m.
Abductor pollicis longus m.
Extensor pollicis brevis m.
Posterior interosseous n. (continuation of deep branch of radial n. distal to inferior border of supinator m.)
Superficial branch of radial n.

Posterior view

Extensor-supinator group of muscles

From axillary n. { Superior lateral brachial cutaneous n.

Inferior lateral brachial cutaneous n.
Posterior brachial cutaneous n.
From radial n. { Posterior antebrachial cutaneous n.
Superficial branch of radial n. and dorsal digital branches

Dorsal digital nn.

Cutaneous innervation from radial and axillary nerves

FIGURE 7.38 Radial Nerve Distribution in Forearm and Dorsal Hand. (From *Netter's atlas of human anatomy*, ed 8, Plate 489; S-112.)

carpi ulnaris muscle and the ulnar half of the flexor digitorum profundus muscle. The median nerve also innervates the thenar muscles and first two lumbrical muscles in the hand. Pure **median nerve sensation** is tested on the skin overlying the *palmar (volar) aspect of the tip of the index finger* (Fig. 7.39). Although well protected in the arm, the median nerve is more vulnerable to traumatic injury in the forearm, wrist, and hand (see Clinical Focus 7.15 and 7.22). Entrapment at the elbow and wrist may occur, and the recurrent branch of the median nerve on the thenar eminence may be damaged in deep lacerations of the palm.

Ulnar Nerve in Forearm and Hand

The **ulnar nerve** (C7, C8, T1) innervates the flexor carpi ulnaris muscle and the ulnar half of the flexor digitorum profundus muscle in the anterior forearm and most of the intrinsic hand muscles: hypothenar muscles, two lumbricals, adductor pollicis muscle, and all of the interossei muscles (palmar and dorsal). Pure **ulnar nerve sensation** is tested on the skin overlying

the *palmar (volar) aspect of the tip of the little finger* (Fig. 7.40). The ulnar nerve is vulnerable as it passes posterior to the medial epicondyle of the humerus; blunt trauma here can elicit the "I hit my funny bone" tingling sensation (Clinical Focus 7.23). The ulnar nerve is also vulnerable as it passes through the two heads of the flexor carpi ulnaris muscle and the cubital tunnel beneath the ulnar collateral ligament. At the wrist, the nerve is vulnerable in the ulnar tunnel, where it passes deep to the palmaris brevis muscle and palmar (volar) carpal ligament, just lateral to the pisiform bone (Clinical Focus 7.23). Clinical Focus 7.24 summarizes the more common compression neuropathies of the median, ulnar and radial nerves.

11. EMBRYOLOGY

Appendicular Skeleton

Along the embryonic axis, mesoderm derived from the sclerotome portion of the dermomyotome

Text continued on page 423

Anterior view

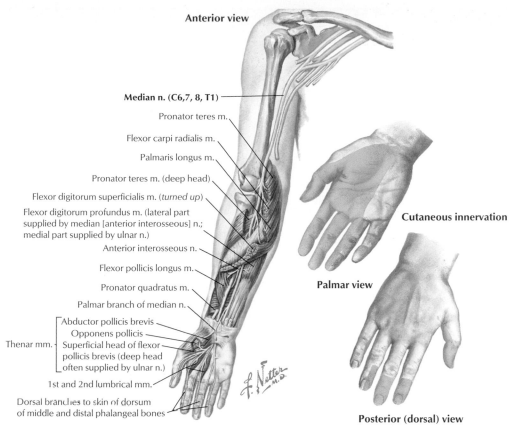

Median n. (C6,7, 8, T1)

Pronator teres m.

Flexor carpi radialis m.

Palmaris longus m.

Pronator teres m. (deep head)

Flexor digitorum superficialis m. (*turned up*)

Flexor digitorum profundus m. (lateral part supplied by median [anterior interosseous] n.; medial part supplied by ulnar n.)

Anterior interosseous n.

Flexor pollicis longus m.

Pronator quadratus m.

Palmar branch of median n.

Thenar mm. {
Abductor pollicis brevis
Opponens pollicis
Superficial head of flexor pollicis brevis (deep head often supplied by ulnar n.)
}

1st and 2nd lumbrical mm.

Dorsal branches to skin of dorsum of middle and distal phalangeal bones

Cutaneous innervation

Palmar view

Posterior (dorsal) view

FIGURE 7.39 Median Nerve Distribution in Forearm and Hand. (From *Netter's atlas of human anatomy*, ed 8, Plate 486; S-109.)

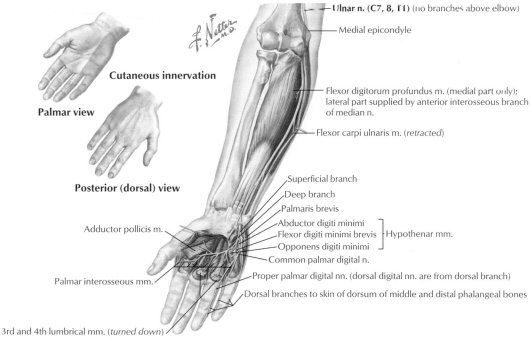

Ulnar n. (C7, 8, T1) (no branches above elbow)

Medial epicondyle

Flexor digitorum profundus m. (medial part only); lateral part supplied by anterior interosseous branch of median n.

Flexor carpi ulnaris m. (*retracted*)

Cutaneous innervation

Palmar view

Posterior (dorsal) view

Superficial branch

Deep branch

Palmaris brevis

Abductor digiti minimi

Flexor digiti minimi brevis } Hypothenar mm.

Opponens digiti minimi

Adductor pollicis m.

Common palmar digital n.

Palmar interosseous mm.

Proper palmar digital nn. (dorsal digital nn. are from dorsal branch)

Dorsal branches to skin of dorsum of middle and distal phalangeal bones

3rd and 4th lumbrical mm. (*turned down*)

FIGURE 7.40 Ulnar Nerve Distribution in Forearm and Hand. (From *Netter's atlas of human anatomy*, ed 8, Plate 487; S-110.)

Clinical Focus 7.22

Proximal Median Nerve Compression

Compression at the elbow is the second most common site of median nerve entrapment after the wrist (carpal tunnel). Repetitive forearm pronation and finger flexion, especially against resistance, can cause muscle hypertrophy and entrap the nerve.

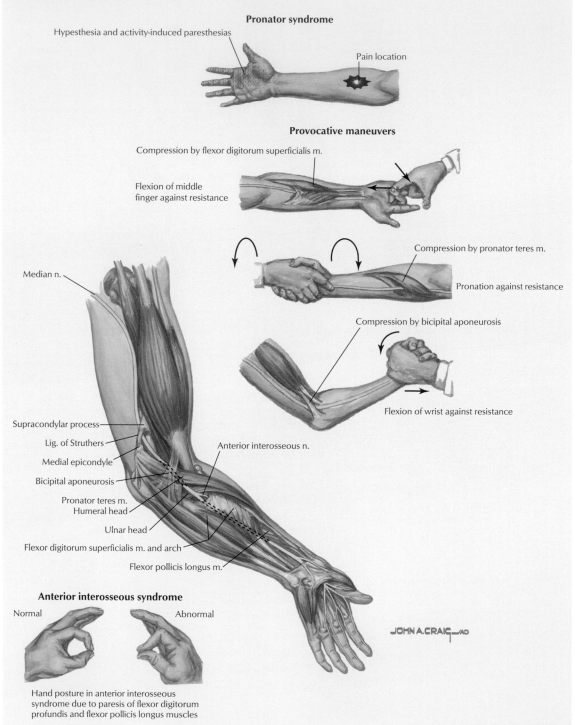

Pronator syndrome

Hypesthesia and activity-induced paresthesias

Pain location

Provocative maneuvers

Compression by flexor digitorum superficialis m.

Flexion of middle finger against resistance

Compression by pronator teres m.

Pronation against resistance

Compression by bicipital aponeurosis

Flexion of wrist against resistance

Median n.

Supracondylar process

Lig. of Struthers

Medial epicondyle

Bicipital aponeurosis

Pronator teres m.
Humeral head

Ulnar head

Flexor digitorum superficialis m. and arch

Flexor pollicis longus m.

Anterior interosseous n.

Anterior interosseous syndrome

Normal   Abnormal

JOHN A. CRAIG—AD

Hand posture in anterior interosseous syndrome due to paresis of flexor digitorum profundis and flexor pollicis longus muscles

Clinical Focus 7.23

Ulnar Tunnel Syndrome

The ulnar tunnel exists at the wrist where the ulnar nerve and artery pass deep to the palmaris brevis muscle and palmar (volar) carpal ligament, just lateral to the pisiform bone. Within the tunnel, the nerve divides into the superficial sensory and deep motor branches. Injury may result from trauma, ulnar artery thrombosis, fractures (hook of the hamate), dislocations (ulnar head, pisiform), arthritis, and repetitive movements. **Claw hand** may be present if the motor components are injured.

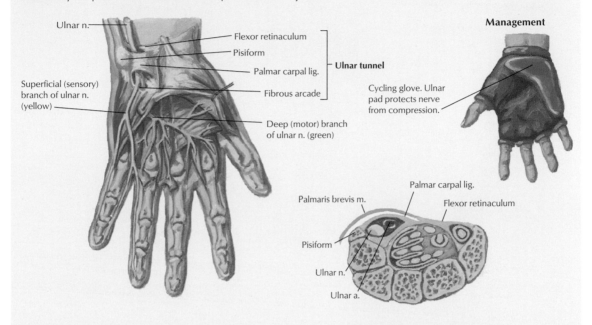

Ulnar n.

Flexor retinaculum

Pisiform

Palmar carpal lig.

Fibrous arcade

Ulnar tunnel

Superficial (sensory) branch of ulnar n. (yellow)

Deep (motor) branch of ulnar n. (green)

Management

Cycling glove. Ulnar pad protects nerve from compression.

Palmaris brevis m.

Palmar carpal lig.

Flexor retinaculum

Pisiform

Ulnar n.

Ulnar a.

Zones of nerve compression and clinical signs

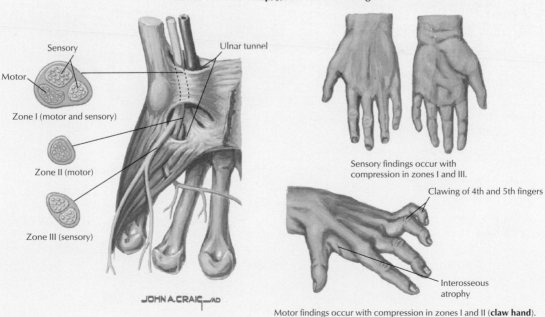

Sensory

Motor

Zone I (motor and sensory)

Zone II (motor)

Zone III (sensory)

Ulnar tunnel

Sensory findings occur with compression in zones I and III.

Clawing of 4th and 5th fingers

Interosseous atrophy

JOHN A. CRAIG—AD

Motor findings occur with compression in zones I and II (**claw hand**).

Clinical Focus 7.24

Clinical Evaluation of Compression Neuropathy

Compression injury to the **radial, median, and ulnar nerves** may occur at several sites along each of their courses down the arm and forearm. A review of the applied anatomy and clinical presentation of several common neuropathies is shown in this illustration. Refer to the muscle tables presented in this chapter for a review of the muscle actions and anticipated functional weaknesses.

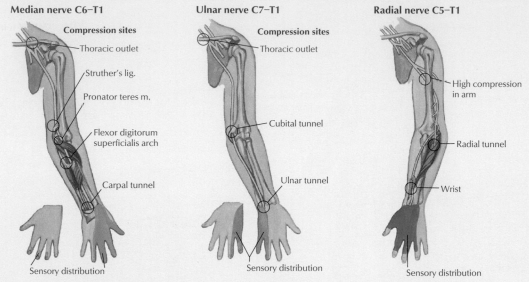

Median nerve C6–T1

Compression sites
Thoracic outlet
Struther's lig.
Pronator teres m.
Flexor digitorum superficialis arch
Carpal tunnel
Sensory distribution

Ulnar nerve C7–T1

Compression sites
Thoracic outlet
Cubital tunnel
Ulnar tunnel
Sensory distribution

Radial nerve C5–T1

High compression in arm
Radial tunnel
Wrist
Sensory distribution

Motor and sensory functions of each nerve assessed individually throughout entire upper extremity to delineate level of compression or entrapment

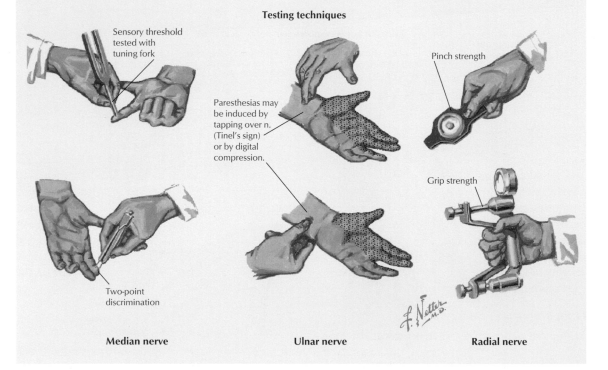

Testing techniques

Sensory threshold tested with tuning fork

Paresthesias may be induced by tapping over n. (Tinel's sign) or by digital compression.

Pinch strength

Grip strength

Two-point discrimination

Median nerve

Ulnar nerve

Radial nerve

Clinical Focus 7.25

Ulnar Nerve Compression in Cubital Tunnel

Cubital tunnel syndrome results from compression of the ulnar nerve as it passes beneath the ulnar collateral ligament and between the two heads of the flexor carpi ulnaris muscle. This syndrome is the second most common compression neuropathy after carpal tunnel syndrome. The tunnel space is significantly reduced with elbow flexion, which compresses and stretches the ulnar nerve. The nerve also may be injured by direct trauma to the subcutaneous portion as it passes around the medial epicondyle.

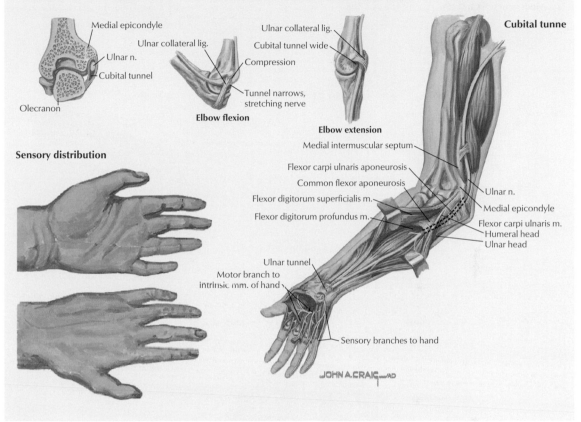

forms the axial skeleton and gives rise to the skull and spinal column (see Fig. 2.22 for more detailed development). The appendicular skeleton forms from mesenchyme that condenses to form hyaline cartilaginous precursors of limb bones. Upper (and lower) limb bones then develop by **endochondral ossification** from the cartilaginous precursors, *except the clavicle,* which develops largely by intramembranous ossification (Fig. 7.41).

Neuromuscular Development

Segmental somites give rise to myotomes that form collections of mesoderm dorsally called **epimeres** (which give rise to epaxial muscles). These epimeres are innervated by the posterior rami of the spinal nerves. The *epaxial muscles* form the intrinsic back muscles. Ventral mesodermal collections form the **hypomeres** (give rise to *hypaxial muscles*), which are innervated by the anterior rami of spinal nerves. Hypaxial muscles in the upper limbs divide into anterior (flexor) and posterior (extensor) muscles (Fig. 7.42). The terminal branches of the **brachial plexus** (axillary, musculocutaneous, radial, median, and ulnar nerves) then grow into the limb as the mesoderm develops, supplying the muscles of each compartment.

Limb Bud Rotation and Dermatomes

Initially, as the limb buds grow out from the embryonic trunk, the anterior muscle mass (future flexors) faces medially and the posterior mass (future extensors) faces laterally (Fig. 7.43). With continued

Chapter 7 Upper Limb

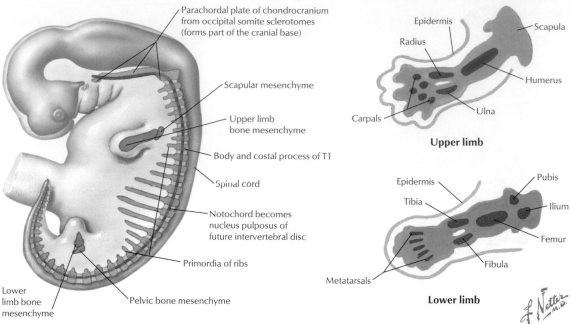

FIGURE 7.41 Development of the Appendicular Skeleton.

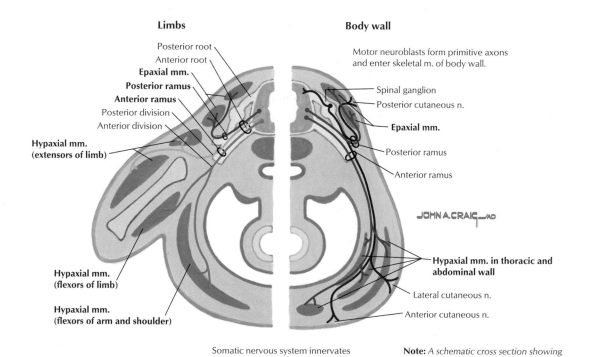

FIGURE 7.42 Neuromuscular Development.

growth and differentiation, the **upper limbs rotate 90 degrees laterally** so that in anatomical position, the anterior flexor muscle compartment faces anteriorly and the posterior extensor muscle compartment faces posteriorly. The **lower limbs rotate 90 degrees medially** and are thus 180 degrees out of phase with the upper limbs. (The elbow faces posteriorly, and the knee faces anteriorly.) Thus in the upper limbs the flexors of the shoulder, elbow, and wrist/fingers are positioned anteriorly, and extensor muscles of the same joints are aligned posteriorly.

Although the **dermatome** distribution on the trunk is fairly *linear* horizontally, on the limbs some *spiraling* occurs, especially noticeable on the lower limb (Fig. 7.44). The upper limb is more uniform, with dermatomes (C4-T2) that closely parallel the myotome innervation from the brachial plexus (C5-T1); a small contributing branch from C4 and T2 to the brachial plexus is normally observed. As noted previously, dermatome maps vary, and overlap of sensory innervation from the dermatome above and below is common.

Changes in position of limbs before birth

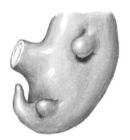
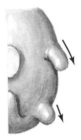

At 5 weeks. Upper and lower limbs have formed as finlike appendages pointing laterally and caudally.

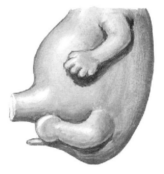
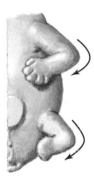

At 6 weeks. Limbs bend anteriorly, so elbows and knees point laterally, palms and soles face trunk.

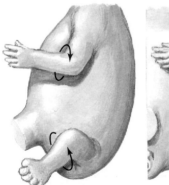
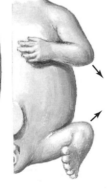

At 7 weeks. Upper and lower limbs have undergone 90 degrees of torsion about their long axes, but in opposite directions, so elbows point caudally and posteriorly, and the knees cranially and anteriorly.

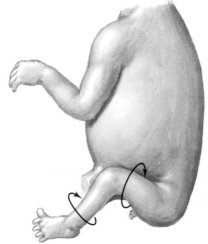
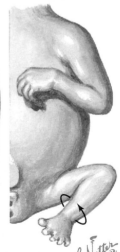

At 8 weeks. Torsion of lower limbs results in twisted or "barber pole" arrangement of their cutaneous innervation.

FIGURE 7.43 Limb Bud Rotation.

Changes in anterior dermatome pattern (cutaneous sensory nerve distribution) during limb development

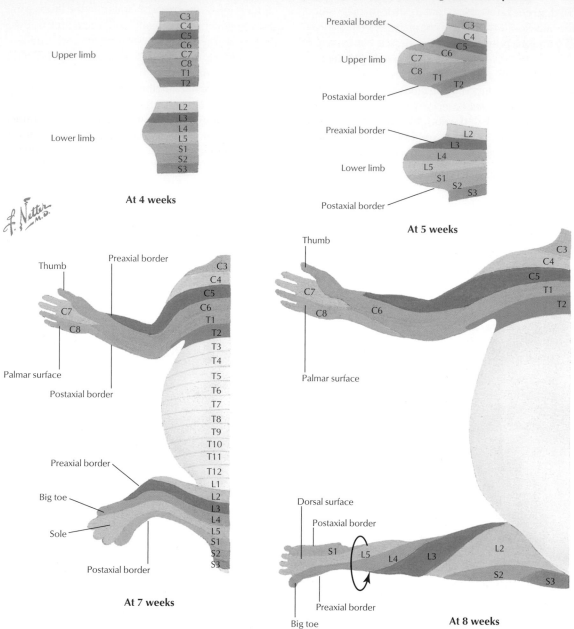

FIGURE 7.44 Limb Bud Rotation and Dermatome Patterns.

Clinical Focus

Available Online

7.26 Trigger Finger

7.27 Rheumatoid Arthritis

7.28 Central Venous Access

Additional figures available online (see inside front cover for details).

Challenge Yourself Questions

1. An elderly woman falls on her outstretched hand and fractures the surgical neck of her humerus. Several weeks later she presents with significant weakness in abduction of her arm and some weakened extension and flexion at the shoulder. Which of the following nerves is most likely injured?

   A. Accessory
   B. Axillary
   C. Radial
   D. Subscapular
   E. Thoracodorsal

2. Cancer spreading from the upper limb via the lymphatics passes into the axillary group of lymph nodes. Which of these axillary groups of nodes is most likely to receive this lymph first?

   A. Anterior (pectoral)
   B. Apical (subclavian)
   C. Central
   D. Lateral (brachial)
   E. Posterior (subscapular)

3. During a routine physical examination, the physician notes an absent biceps tendon reflex. Which spinal cord level is associated with this tendon reflex?

   A. C4-C5
   B. C5-C6
   C. C6-C7
   D. C7-C8
   E. C8-T1

4. A patient with a midshaft compound humeral fracture presents with bleeding and clinical signs of nerve entrapment. Which of the following nerves is most likely injured by the fracture?

   A. Axillary
   B. Median
   C. Musculocutaneous
   D. Radial
   E. Ulnar

5. A baseball pitcher delivers a 97-mph fastball to a batter and suddenly feels a sharp pain in his shoulder on release of the ball. The trainer examines the shoulder and concludes that the pitcher has a rotator cuff injury. Which muscle is most vulnerable and most likely torn by this type of injury?

   A. Infraspinatus
   B. Subscapularis
   C. Supraspinatus
   D. Teres major
   E. Teres minor

6. A fall on an outstretched hand results in swelling and pain on the lateral aspect of the wrist. Radiographic examination confirms a Colles' fracture. Which of the following bones is most likely fractured?

   A. Distal radius
   B. Distal ulna
   C. Lunate
   D. Scaphoid
   E. Trapezium

7. Following an assembly line worker's complaint of tingling pain in her wrist with muscle weakness and atrophy, her physician makes a diagnosis of carpal tunnel syndrome. Which of the following muscles is most likely to be atrophied?

   A. Adductor pollicis
   B. Dorsal interossei
   C. Flexor digitorum superficialis
   D. Lumbricals 3 and 4
   E. Thenar

8. A patient presents with numbness over his medial hand and atrophy of the hypothenar muscles after an injury several days ago over his medial humeral epicondyle. Which of the following nerves most likely was injured?

   A. Anterior interosseous
   B. Musculocutaneous
   C. Recurrent branch of median
   D. Superficial radial
   E. Ulnar

Multiple-choice and short-answer review questions available online; see inside front cover for details.

427

9. During your introductory course to clinical medicine, you are asked to take the radial pulse of your classmate. Which of the following muscle tendons can you use as a guide to locate the radial artery?

    A. Adductor pollicis longus
    B. Brachioradialis
    C. Flexor carpi radialis
    D. Flexor pollicis longus
    E. Palmaris longus

10. A football player has a complete fracture of his radius just proximal to the insertion of the pronator teres muscle. As a result of the actions of the muscles attached to the proximal and distal fragments of the radius, which of the following combinations accurately reflects the orientation of the proximal and distal radial fragments?

    A. Proximal extended, and distal pronated
    B. Proximal extended and pronated, and distal supinated
    C. Proximal flexed, and distal pronated
    D. Proximal flexed, and distal supinated
    E. Proximal flexed and supinated, and distal pronated

11. Intravenous fluid administered into the median cubital vein that enters the basilic vein would then most likely empty into which of the following veins?

    A. Axillary
    B. Brachial
    C. Cephalic
    D. Deep brachial
    E. Subclavian

12. A wrestler comes off the mat holding his right forearm flexed at the elbow and pronated, with his shoulder medially rotated and displaced inferiorly. Which of his bones is most likely broken?

    A. Clavicle
    B. Humerus
    C. Radius
    D. Scapula
    E. Ulna

13. A knife cut results in a horizontal laceration to the thoracic wall extending across the midaxillary and anterior axillary lines just above the level of the T4 dermatome. Which of the following patient presentations will the emergency department physician most likely observe on examining the patient?

    A. Tingling along anterolateral forearm
    B. Supinated forearm
    C. Weakened elbow extension
    D. Weakened elbow flexion
    E. Winged scapula

14. Which of the following tendons is most vulnerable to inflammation and sepsis in the shoulder joint?

    A. Glenoid labrum
    B. Infraspinatus
    C. Long head of biceps
    D. Long head of triceps
    E. Supraspinatus

15. Which of the following muscle-nerve combinations is tested when spreading the fingers against resistance?

    A. Abductor digiti minimi muscle and median nerve
    B. Abductor pollicis brevis muscle and radial nerve
    C. Abductor pollicis longus muscle and median nerve
    D. Dorsal interossei muscle and ulnar nerve
    E. Palmar interossei muscle and ulnar nerve

For each of the conditions described below (16-20), select the nerve from the list (A-K) that is most likely responsible for the condition or affected by it.

A. Axillary
B. Dorsal scapular
C. Long thoracic
D. Medial brachial cutaneous
E. Medial antebrachial cutaneous
F. Median
G. Musculocutaneous
H. Radial
I. Suprascapular
J. Thoracodorsal
K. Ulnar

_____ 16. A patient presents with a "claw hand" deformity.

_____ 17. When asked to make a fist, the patient is unable to flex the first three fingers into the palm, and the fourth and fifth fingers are partially flexed at the MCP and DIP joints.

_____ 18. Angina pectoris leads to referred pain, which radiates down the arm.

_____ 19. Despite injury to the radial nerve in the arm, a patient is still capable of supination of the forearm.

_____ 20. Dislocation of the shoulder places this nerve in jeopardy of injury.

21. Following a difficult forceps delivery, a newborn infant is examined by her pediatrician, who notes that her right upper limb is adducted and internally rotated. Which of the following components of her brachial plexus was most likely injured during the difficult delivery?

   A. Lateral cord
   B. Medial cord
   C. Posterior cord
   D. Roots of inferior trunk
   E. Roots of middle trunk
   F. Roots of superior trunk

22. During upper limb bud development, the limb myotomes give rise to collections of mesoderm that become the muscles of the shoulder, arm, forearm, and hand. Which of the following statements regarding this limb development is correct?

   A. The bones form by intramembranous ossification.
   B. The limb rotates 90 degrees medially.
   C. The muscles develop from epimeres.
   D. The muscles develop from hypomeres.
   E. The muscles are innervated by posterior rami.

23. A pulse may be taken at several locations on the upper limb. One such location is in the anatomical snuffbox, between the extensor pollicis brevis and longus tendons; at this location one may palpate the radial artery. In taking this pulse, the artery is pressed against which of the following bones?

   A. Capitate bone
   B. Scaphoid bone
   C. Trapezium bone
   D. Trapezoid bone
   E. Triquetrum bone

24. A football player has a dislocated shoulder. The trainer is able to reduce the dislocation, but the player still has significant pain over his dorsal shoulder and cannot abduct his arm in a normal manner. Which of the following muscles has most likely been injured by the dislocation?

   A. Coracobrachialis muscle
   B. Long head of the biceps muscle
   C. Long head of the triceps muscle
   D. Supraspinatus muscle
   E. Teres major muscle

25. A fracture of the first rib appears to have damaged the inferior trunk of the brachial plexus where it crosses the rib. Which of the following spinal nerve levels would most likely be affected by this injury?

   A. C4-C5
   B. C5-C6
   C. C6-C7
   D. C7-C8
   E. C8-T1

26. Cubital tunnel syndrome is the second most common compression neuropathy after carpal tunnel syndrome. Cubital tunnel syndrome occurs as which of the following nerves passes deep to a ligament and between the two heads of one of the flexor muscles of the wrist?

   A. Axillary nerve
   B. Median nerve
   C. Musculocutaneous nerve
   D. Radial nerve
   E. Ulnar nerve

27. A fracture of the clavicle results in some internal bleeding. Which of the following vessels is most likely the cause of the bleeding?

   A. Axillary vein
   B. Cephalic vein
   C. Internal jugular vein
   D. Internal thoracic vein
   E. Subclavian vein

28. An 81-year-old man presents with pain in his shoulder; it is especially acute upon abduction. Further examination reveals intramuscular inflammation that has spread over the head of the humerus. Which of the following structures is most likely inflamed?

   A. Biceps brachii tendon (long head)
   B. Glenoid cavity
   C. Glenoid labrum
   D. Infraspinatus muscle
   E. Subdeltoid bursa

29. A 34-year-old homemaker presents with pain over her dorsal wrist and the styloid process of the radius, probably as a result of repetitive movements. The pain is exacerbated by flexing the thumb and then placing the wrist in ulnar deviation (adduction of the wrist). Inflammation of which of the following muscle groups and their tendinous sheaths is most likely the cause of this condition?

A. Abductor pollicis longus and extensor pollicis brevis
B. Extensor carpi radialis longus and brevis
C. Extensor digitorum and extensor indicis
D. Extensor pollicis longus
E. Flexor pollicis longus and brevis

For each of the conditions described below (30-35), select the muscle from the list (A-K) that is most likely responsible for the condition or affected by it.

A. Biceps brachii
B. Brachialis
C. Brachioradialis
D. Flexor carpi radialis
E. Flexor carpi ulnaris
F. Flexor digitorum superficialis
G. Flexor pollicis longus
H. Palmaris longus
I. Pronator quadratus
J. Pronator teres
K. Supinator

_____ 30. Although innervated by the radial nerve, it is actually a flexor of the forearm at the elbow.

_____ 31. This muscle generally may not be the strongest flexor of the forearm at the elbow, but it is the strongest supinator of the hand.

_____ 32. This muscle's tendon has the highest rate of spontaneous rupture of any muscle tendon in the body!

_____ 33. The two heads of this muscle can compress the median nerve in the proximal forearm.

_____ 34. The tendon of this muscle may be used as a guide to find and take a radial artery pulse.

_____ 35. This is the deepest muscle in the forearm anterior muscle compartment innervated by the median nerve.

For each of the structures described below (36-37), select the label (A-H) from the radiograph of the hand and wrist that best matches the description.

Anteroposterior view

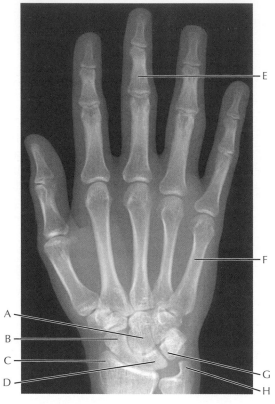

_____ 36. A fall on an outstretched hand often results in an extension-compression fracture and a "dinner fork deformity." Which labeled structure is fractured in this kind of injury?

_____ 37. A "round" carpal that articulates with the third metacarpal bone.

For each of the structures described below (38-40), select the label (A-H) from the radiograph of the shoulder joint that best matches the description.

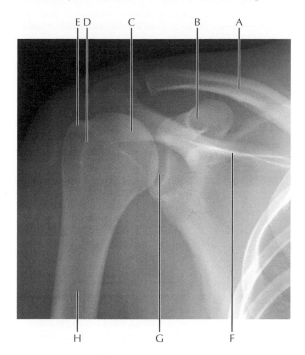

_____ 38. The most common type of shoulder dislocation results in the head of the humerus coming to lie just inferior to this structure.

_____ 39. Just above this bony feature lies the muscle that initiates abduction at the shoulder.

_____ 40. This bone is one of the first to begin to ossify (by intramembranous ossification), but it is usually the last one to fuse, at some time in the third decade of life.

Answers to Challenge Yourself Questions

1. **B.** Fractures of this portion of the humerus can place the axillary nerve in danger of injury. Her muscle weakness confirms that the deltoid muscle especially is weakened, and the deltoid and teres minor muscles are innervated by the axillary nerve.

2. **D.** Most of the lymph draining from the upper limb will collect initially into the lateral (brachial) group of axillary lymph nodes, coursing deeply along the neurovascular bundles of the arm.

3. **B.** The biceps tendon reflex tests the musculocutaneous nerve and especially the C5-C6 contribution. The triceps tendon reflex tests the C7-C8 spinal contributions of the radial nerve.

4. **D.** The radial nerve spirals around the posterior aspect of the midhumeral shaft and can be stretched or contused by a compound fracture of the humerus. This nerve innervates all the extensor muscles of the upper limb (posterior compartments of the arm and forearm).

5. **C.** The supraspinatus muscle is most often torn in rotator cuff injuries. Repeated abduction and flexion can cause the tendon to rub on the acromion and coracoacromial ligament, leading to tears or rupture.

6. **A.** The Colles' fracture (a fracture of the distal radius) presents with a classic dinner fork deformity with the dorsal and proximal displacement of the distal fragment. This is an extension-compression fracture.

7. **E.** The thenar muscles are located at the base of the thumb and are innervated by the median nerve, which passes through the carpal tunnel and is prone to injury in excessive repetitive movements at the wrist.

8. **E.** The ulnar nerve is subcutaneous as it passes around the medial epicondyle of the humerus. In this location, it is vulnerable to compression injury against the bone ("funny bone") or entrapment in the cubital tunnel (beneath the ulnar collateral ligament).

9. **C.** The radial pulse can be easily taken at the wrist where the radial artery lies just lateral to the tendon of the flexor carpi radialis muscle.

10. **E.** The proximal fragment will be flexed and supinated by the biceps brachii and supinator muscles, while the distal fragment will be pronated by the action of the pronator teres and pronator quadratus muscles.

11. **A.** The median cubital vein usually drains into the basilic vein, which then dives deeply and drains into the axillary vein.

12. **A.** Fractures of the clavicle are relatively common and occur most often in the middle third of the bone. The distal fragment is displaced downward by the weight of the shoulder and drawn medially by the action of the pectoralis major, teres major, and latissimus dorsi muscles.

13. **E.** This laceration probably severed the long thoracic nerve, which innervates the serratus anterior muscle. During muscle testing, the scapula will "wing" outwardly if this muscle is denervated.

14. **C.** The long head of the biceps tendon passes through the shoulder joint and attaches to the supraglenoid tubercle of the scapula. An infection in the joint could involve this tendon.

15. **D.** The dorsal interossei are innervated by the ulnar nerve and abduct the fingers (the little finger and thumb have their own abductors). This action is easily tested in a patient; dorsal interossei abduct the fingers (DAB) and palmar interossei adduct the fingers (PAD).

16. **K.** "Claw hand" is a typical deformity of the ulnar nerve. The last two digits may be hyperextended at the MCP joint (because of the unopposed action of the extensor digitorum muscle, which is innervated by the radial nerve), flexed at the PIP joint (because of the action of the flexor digitorum superficialis muscle, which is innervated by the median nerve), and extended at the DIP joint (because of the loss of action by the flexor digitorum profundus muscle, which is innervated by the ulnar nerve, and the action of the unopposed extensor expansion).

17. **F.** This suggests a lesion to the median nerve. The thenar muscles are affected, as are the long flexors of the digits (flexor digitorum superficialis muscle and profundus muscle to the index and middle fingers). Unopposed extension of the first three fingers occurs, and absence of flexion at the PIP joints of fingers 4 and 5 is evident. The thumb is adducted against the index finger. The position of the hand is that of a "papal" or "benediction" sign.

18. **D.** Referred pain from myocardial ischemia can be present along the medial aspect of the arm, usually on the left side, and is referred to this area by the medial brachial cutaneous nerve (T1). The intercostal brachial nerve (T2) may also contribute to this sensation.

19. **G.** While the supinator muscle is denervated (loss of radial nerve), the biceps brachii muscle is innervated by the musculocutaneous nerve and is a powerful supinator when the elbow is flexed.

20. **A.** The axillary nerve (innervates the deltoid and teres minor muscles) can be injured by shoulder dislocations. This nerve passes through the quadrangular space before innervating its two muscles.

21. **F.** Tension of the upper portion of the brachial plexus, specifically the superior trunk, can be injured by a forceps delivery. The adducted and internally rotated limb suggests an injury to the C5-C6 spinal roots known as Erb's palsy or Erb-Duchenne paralysis. Abduction, lateral rotation, and flexion of the arm may be weakened or lost.

22. **D.** Limb muscles develop from hypomeres (hypaxial muscles) and are innervated by the ventral rami of spinal nerves. The muscles derived from epimeres include the intrinsic back muscles (e.g., the erector spinae muscles) and are innervated by dorsal rami of the spinal nerve.

23. **B.** The radial pulse in the anatomical snuffbox may be palpated by pressing the artery against the underlying scaphoid tarsal. Most arterial pulses are felt by pressing the artery against an underlying bony structure.

24. **D.** The supraspinatus muscle is often injured by shoulder dislocation, which usually occurs in an anteroinferior direction. The supraspinatus muscle is critical for initiating the first 15 degrees of abduction at the shoulder before the deltoid muscle takes over.

25. **E.** The inferior trunk of the plexus crosses over the first rib, where it is vulnerable to injury. It arises from the C8 and T1 anterior rami of the spinal nerves.

26. **E.** The ulnar nerve passes under the ulnar collateral ligament at the elbow and then between the two heads of the flexor carpi ulnaris muscle. This injury is referred to as cubital tunnel syndrome and is not uncommon.

27. **E.** The most superficial of the listed structures to the clavicle is the subclavian vein, which passes between it and the first rib. The other vessels do not have this relationship. The subclavian artery also parallels the vein but lies on a deeper plane and is not one of the choices.

28. **E.** The subdeltoid bursa lies between the underlying supraspinatus tendon and the deltoid muscle, both of which are involved in abduction at the shoulder. Inflammation of these muscle tendons (neither is listed as an option) and the secondary inflammation of subdeltoid bursa is common (see Clinical Focus 7.5).

29. **A.** The tendons of the abductor pollicis longus and extensor pollicis brevis muscles pass through the same tendon sheath on the dorsum of the wrist. Repetitive movements (gripping or a twisting-wringing action) can lead to pain over the styloid process of the radius (de Quervain tenosynovitis; see Clinical Focus 7.18).

30. **C.** The brachialis muscle lies on the margin between the anterior and posterior compartment muscles of the forearm; it is considered along with the extensor/supinator muscles of the posterior compartment and is hence innervated by the radial nerve. It flexes the forearm at the elbow, especially when the forearm is in midpronation.

31. **A.** The biceps brachii muscle flexes the forearm at the elbow. It also is the "power supinator" when the elbow is flexed, but it does not supinate when the elbow is extended.

32. **A.** The biceps brachii tendon has the highest rate of spontaneous rupture of any muscle tendon in the body. Rupture of the long head of the biceps brachii tendon is the most common (see Clinical Focus 7.9).

33. **J.** The median nerve passes beneath the bicipital aponeurosis and then between the humeral and ulnar heads of the pronator teres muscle. This is the second most common site for median nerve compression after carpal tunnel compression at the wrist.

34. **D.** Making a slight fist will cause the flexor tendons of the wrist to become prominent under the skin. The tendon of the flexor carpi radialis muscle can then be used to locate the radial artery, which lies just lateral to this tendon. Be sure to feel the pulse with your index and/or middle finger, and not your thumb. If you use your thumb, you may be sensing you own pulse and not that of your patient!

35. **I.** The pronator quadratus muscle extends between the distal ulna and radius, is innervated by the median nerve, and is the deepest of the anterior compartment muscles of the forearm. It pronates the forearm and hand.

36. **C.** This is the description of a Colles' fracture, which is a fracture of the distal radius and styloid process. The distal fragment is displaced dorsally and proximally, giving the wrist and hand the appearance of a dinner fork (see Clinical Focus 7.14).

37. **A.** The capitate (round) carpal is in the distal row of carpals and articulates with the base of the middle (third) metacarpal.

38. **B.** Dislocation of the head of the humerus often happens in an anterior and slightly inferior direction, with the head coming to lie just beneath the coracoid process (a subcoracoid dislocation). When this happens, the axillary and/or musculocutaneous nerves may be injured.

39. **F.** The spine of the scapula separates the infra-spinous and supraspinous fossae. The supra-spinatus muscle lies superior to the spine and initiates abduction of the arm at the shoulder.

40. **A.** The clavicle is a bit unusual because it ossifies by intramembranous ossification, is one of the first bones to ossify, and is one of the last bones to fuse. All of the other bones of the appendicular skeleton ossify by endochondral bone formation. (There is some controversy regarding the scapula, which may ossify partly by the intramembranous process [the fossae] and partly by endochondral formation).

Head and Neck

1. INTRODUCTION

The head and neck area offers a unique challenge for students because of the density of small neurovascular structures; the complexity of its bony features, especially the skull; and the compactness of its anatomy. The head protects the brain, participates in communication and expresses our emotions, and houses the special senses (sight, sound, balance, smell, and taste). The neck connects the head to the thorax and is the conduit for visceral structures passing cranially or caudally within tightly partitioned fascial sleeves.

The anatomy of the head is best understood if you view it as a series of interconnected compartments, which include the following:

- **Cranium:** contains the brain and its meningeal coverings.
- **Orbits:** contain the eye and the muscles that move the eye.
- **Nasal cavities and paranasal sinuses:** form the uppermost part of the respiratory system.
- **Ears:** contain the apparatus for hearing and balance.
- **Oral cavity:** forms the proximal end of the digestive tract.

The anatomy of the neck is composed of a series of *concentric-like compartments* that provide a conduit for structures passing to the head or thorax, as follows:

- **Musculofascial:** superficial compartment encompassing the outer boundary of the neck.
- **Visceral:** anterocentral compartment that contains the upper respiratory (pharynx, larynx, trachea) and gastrointestinal (GI) tract (pharynx, esophagus), and the thyroid, parathyroid, and thymus glands.
- **Neurovascular:** two anterolateral compartments that contain the common carotid artery, internal jugular vein, and vagus nerve; all are contained within a fascial sleeve called the carotid sheath.
- **Prevertebral:** posterocentral compartment that contains the cervical vertebrae and the associated paravertebral cervical muscles.

2. SURFACE ANATOMY

The key surface features of the head and neck include the following (Fig. 8.1):

- **Glabella:** smooth prominence on the frontal bone above the root of the nose.
- **Zygomatic bone:** the cheekbone, which protrudes below the orbit and is vulnerable to fractures from facial trauma.
- **Ear (auricle or pinna):** skin-covered elastic cartilage with several consistent ridges, including the helix, antihelix, tragus, antitragus, and lobule.
- **Philtrum:** midline infranasal depression of the upper lip.
- **Nasolabial sulcus:** line between the nose and the corner of the lip.
- **Thyroid cartilage:** the laryngeal prominence ("Adam's apple").
- **Jugular (suprasternal) notch:** midline depression between the two sternal heads of the sternocleidomastoid muscle.

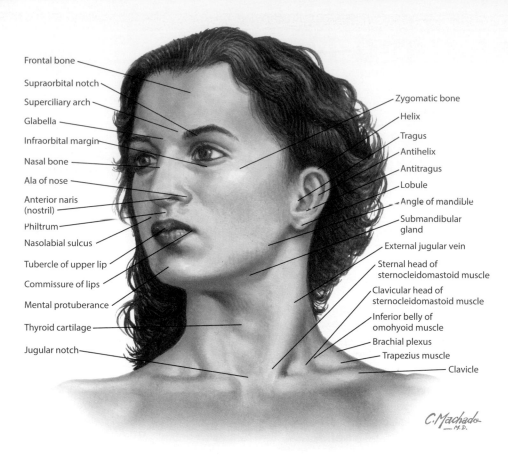

Frontal bone
Supraorbital notch
Superciliary arch
Glabella
Infraorbital margin
Nasal bone
Ala of nose
Anterior naris (nostril)
Philtrum
Nasolabial sulcus
Tubercle of upper lip
Commissure of lips
Mental protuberance
Thyroid cartilage
Jugular notch

Zygomatic bone
Helix
Tragus
Antihelix
Antitragus
Lobule
Angle of mandible
Submandibular gland
External jugular vein
Sternal head of sternocleidomastoid muscle
Clavicular head of sternocleidomastoid muscle
Inferior belly of omohyoid muscle
Brachial plexus
Trapezius muscle
Clavicle

FIGURE 8.1 Key Surface Anatomy Landmarks of the Head and Neck. (From *Netter's atlas of human anatomy*, ed 8, Plate 22; S-5.)

3. SKULL

The skull is composed of 22 bones (see Chapter 1, Fig. 1.5). Eight of these bones form the cranium (*neurocranium*, which contains the brain and meninges), and 14 of these form the face (*viscerocranium*). There are seven associated bones: the auditory ossicles (three in each middle ear) and the unpaired hyoid bone (Fig. 8.2 and Table 8.1). Using your atlas and dry bone specimens, note the complexity of the maxillary, temporal, and sphenoid bones. These bones are in close association with many of the cranial nerves and encase portions of many of our *special senses*—balance, hearing, smell, sight, and even taste—as the maxillae form a portion of the oral cavity.

Other features of the skull are noted as we review each region of the head. However, general external features include the following (Figs. 8.2 and 8.3 and Table 8.1):

- **Coronal suture:** region between the frontal bone and two parietal bones.
- **Sagittal suture:** region between the two parietal bones.
- **Lambdoid suture:** region between the occipital bone and the two parietal bones.
- **Nasion:** point at which the frontal and nasal bones meet.
- **Bregma:** point at which coronal and sagittal sutures meet.
- **Lambda:** point at which sagittal and lambdoid sutures meet.
- **Pterion:** point at which frontal, sphenoid, temporal, and parietal bones meet; the middle meningeal artery lies beneath this region.
- **Asterion:** point at which temporal, parietal, and occipital bones meet.
- **Inion:** the external occipital protuberance.

TABLE 8.1 Bones of the Skull

BONE	DESCRIPTION	BONE	DESCRIPTION
Frontal	Forms forehead, is thicker anteriorly, contains frontal sinuses	Temporal	Paired bones that form the lower portion of the lateral neurocranium and contain the middle and inner ear cavities, and the vestibular system for balance
Nasal	Paired bones that form the root of the nose		
Lacrimal	Small, paired bones that form part of the anteromedial wall of the orbit and contain the lacrimal sac	Sphenoid	Complex bone composed of a central body, and greater and lesser wings
Zygomatic	Paired cheekbones that form the inferolateral rim of the orbit and are frequently fractured by blunt trauma	Occipital	Forms the inferoposterior portion of the neurocranium
		Ethmoid	Forms the ethmoid sinuses, and contributes to the medial, lateral, and superior walls of the nasal cavity
Maxilla	Paired bones that form part of the cheek and contain 16 maxillary teeth		
Mandible	Lower jaw bone that contains 16 mandibular teeth	Inferior concha	Paired bones of the lateral nasal wall that form the inferior nasal concha
Parietal	Forms the superolateral portion of the neurocranium	Vomer	Forms the lower part of the nasal septum
		Palatine	Contributes to the lateral nasal wall, a small part of the nasal septum, and the hard palate

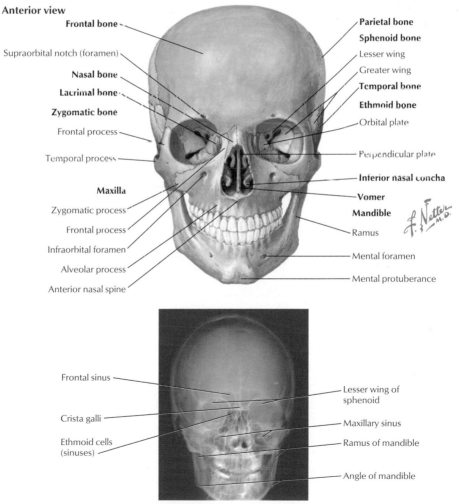

FIGURE 8.2 Anterior and Lateral Views of the Skull. (From *Netter's atlas of human anatomy*, ed 8, Plate 25; S-123.)

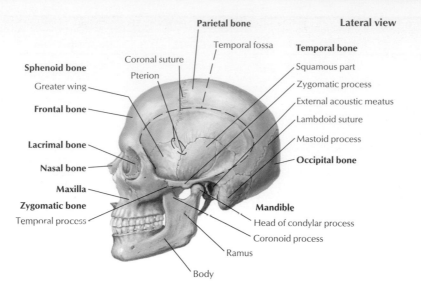

Lateral view

Parietal bone

Temporal fossa

Sphenoid bone
Greater wing
Pterion
Coronal suture

Frontal bone

Lacrimal bone

Nasal bone

Maxilla

Zygomatic bone
Temporal process

Temporal bone
Squamous part
Zygomatic process
External acoustic meatus
Lambdoid suture
Mastoid process

Occipital bone

Mandible
Head of condylar process
Coronoid process
Ramus

Body

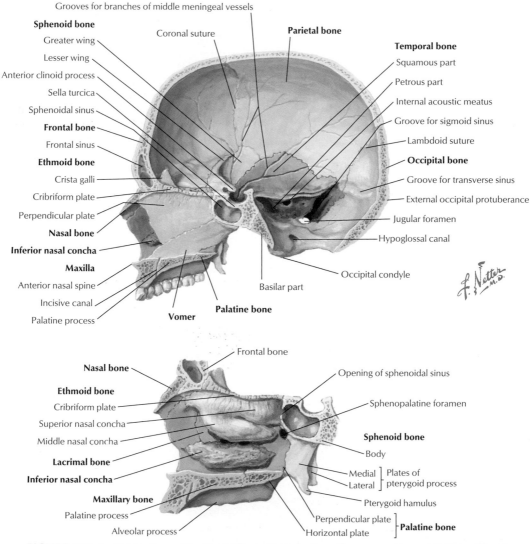

Grooves for branches of middle meningeal vessels

Sphenoid bone
Greater wing
Lesser wing
Anterior clinoid process
Sella turcica
Sphenoidal sinus

Frontal bone
Frontal sinus

Ethmoid bone
Crista galli
Cribriform plate
Perpendicular plate

Nasal bone

Inferior nasal concha

Maxilla
Anterior nasal spine
Incisive canal
Palatine process

Coronal suture

Parietal bone

Temporal bone
Squamous part
Petrous part
Internal acoustic meatus
Groove for sigmoid sinus
Lambdoid suture

Occipital bone
Groove for transverse sinus
External occipital protuberance
Jugular foramen
Hypoglossal canal

Occipital condyle

Basilar part

Vomer   Palatine bone

Frontal bone

Nasal bone

Ethmoid bone
Cribriform plate
Superior nasal concha
Middle nasal concha

Lacrimal bone

Inferior nasal concha

Maxillary bone
Palatine process
Alveolar process

Opening of sphenoidal sinus

Sphenopalatine foramen

Sphenoid bone
Body
Medial ⎤ Plates of
Lateral ⎦ pterygoid process
Pterygoid hamulus
Perpendicular plate ⎤ Palatine bone
Horizontal plate ⎦

FIGURE 8.3 Sagittal Sections of the Skull. (From *Netter's atlas of human anatomy,* ed 8, Plates 27 and 29; S-125 and S-129.)

Clinical Focus 8.1

Skull Fractures

Skull fractures may be classified as follows:

- **Linear:** presents with a distinct fracture line.
- **Comminuted:** presents with multiple fragments (depressed if driven inward; can compress or tear the underlying dura mater).
- **Diastasis:** fracture along a suture line.
- **Basilar:** fracture of the base of the skull.

Any fracture that communicates with a lacerated scalp, a paranasal sinus, or the middle ear is termed a **compound fracture.** Compound depressed fractures must be treated surgically.

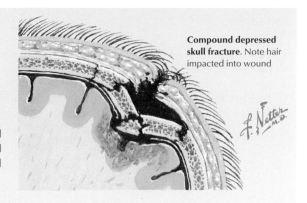

Compound depressed skull fracture. Note hair impacted into wound

Clinical Focus 8.2

Zygomatic Fractures

Trauma to the zygomatic bone (cheekbone) can disrupt the zygomatic complex and its articulations with the frontal, maxillary, temporal, sphenoid, and palatine bones. Often, *fractures involve suture lines with the frontal and maxillary bones,* resulting in displacement inferiorly, medially, and posteriorly. The typical clinical presentation is illustrated. Ipsilateral ocular and visual changes may include **diplopia** (double vision due to an upper outer gaze) and **hyphema** (blood in the anterior chamber of the eye), which requires immediate clinical attention.

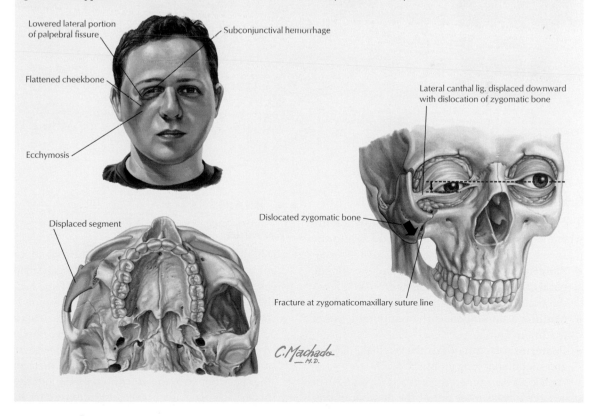

Lowered lateral portion of palpebral fissure

Subconjunctival hemorrhage

Flattened cheekbone

Ecchymosis

Lateral canthal lig. displaced downward with dislocation of zygomatic bone

Displaced segment

Dislocated zygomatic bone

Fracture at zygomaticomaxillary suture line

Midface Fractures

Midface fractures (of the maxilla, nasoorbital complex, and zygomatic bones) were classified by Le Fort as follows:

- **Le Fort I:** horizontal detachment of the maxilla at the level of the nasal floor.
- **Le Fort II:** pyramidal fracture that includes both maxillae and nasal bones, medial portions of both maxillary antra, infraorbital rims, orbits, and orbital floors.
- **Le Fort III:** includes Le Fort II and a fracture of both zygomatic bones; may cause airway problems, nasolacrimal apparatus obstruction, and cerebrospinal fluid leakage.

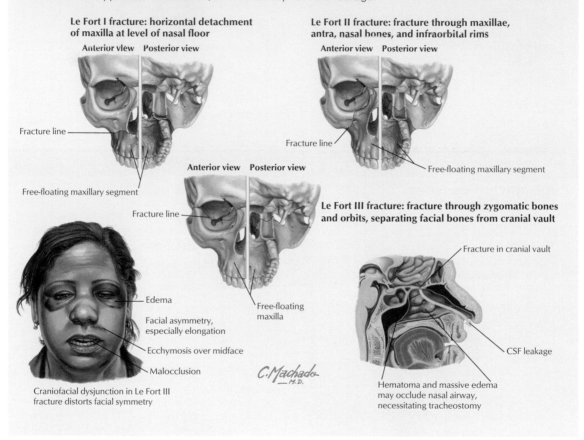

Le Fort I fracture: horizontal detachment of maxilla at level of nasal floor

Le Fort II fracture: fracture through maxillae, antra, nasal bones, and infraorbital rims

Le Fort III fracture: fracture through zygomatic bones and orbits, separating facial bones from cranial vault

Craniofacial dysjunction in Le Fort III fracture distorts facial symmetry

Hematoma and massive edema may occlude nasal airway, necessitating tracheostomy

Cranial Fossae

The cranial base is the floor of the neurocranium, which supports the brain, and is divided into the following three **cranial fossae** (Fig. 8.4):

- **Anterior:** the roof of the orbits and the midline nasal cavity; accommodates the frontal lobes of the brain.
- **Middle:** accommodates the temporal lobes of the brain.
- **Posterior:** accommodates the cerebellum, pons, and medulla oblongata of the brain.

Each fossa has numerous *foramina* (openings) for structures to pass in or out of the neurocranium.

4. BRAIN

Meninges

The brain and spinal cord are surrounded by three membranous connective tissue layers called the *meninges,* which include the following (Figs. 1.21 and 8.5):

- **Dura mater:** thick outermost meningeal layer that is richly innervated by sensory nerve fibers.
- **Arachnoid mater:** fine, weblike avascular membrane directly beneath the dural surface; the space between the arachnoid mater and the underlying pia mater is called the **subarachnoid**

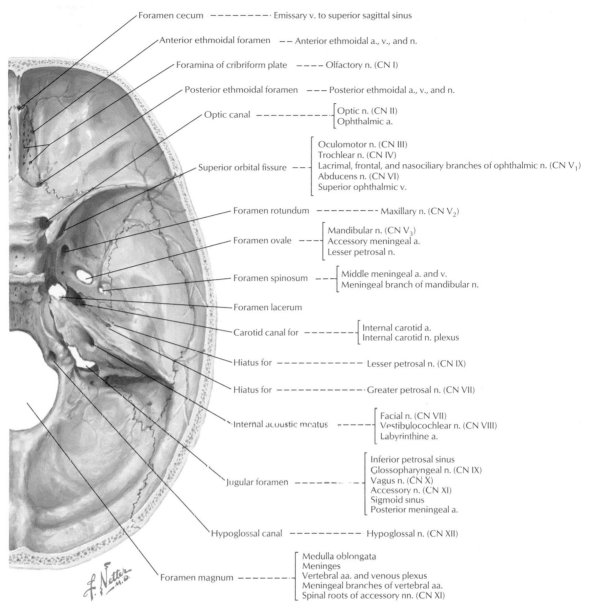

Foramen cecum ――――――― Emissary v. to superior sagittal sinus

Anterior ethmoidal foramen ―― Anterior ethmoidal a., v., and n.

Foramina of cribriform plate ―――― Olfactory n. (CN I)

Posterior ethmoidal foramen ――― Posterior ethmoidal a., v., and n.

Optic canal ―――――――
- Optic n. (CN II)
- Ophthalmic a.

Superior orbital fissure ――
- Oculomotor n. (CN III)
- Trochlear n. (CN IV)
- Lacrimal, frontal, and nasociliary branches of ophthalmic n. (CN V₁)
- Abducens n. (CN VI)
- Superior ophthalmic v.

Foramen rotundum ――――――― Maxillary n. (CN V₂)

Foramen ovale ―――
- Mandibular n. (CN V₃)
- Accessory meningeal a.
- Lesser petrosal n.

Foramen spinosum ―――
- Middle meningeal a. and v.
- Meningeal branch of mandibular n.

Foramen lacerum

Carotid canal for ―――――――
- Internal carotid a.
- Internal carotid n. plexus

Hiatus for ――――――――― Lesser petrosal n. (CN IX)

Hiatus for ――――――――― Greater petrosal n. (CN VII)

Internal acoustic meatus ――――――
- Facial n. (CN VII)
- Vestibulocochlear n. (CN VIII)
- Labyrinthine a.

Jugular foramen ―――――――
- Inferior petrosal sinus
- Glossopharyngeal n. (CN IX)
- Vagus n. (CN X)
- Accessory n. (CN XI)
- Sigmoid sinus
- Posterior meningeal a.

Hypoglossal canal ――――――――― Hypoglossal n. (CN XII)

Foramen magnum ―――――――
- Medulla oblongata
- Meninges
- Vertebral aa. and venous plexus
- Meningeal branches of vertebral aa.
- Spinal roots of accessory nn. (CN XI)

FIGURE 8.4 Superior Aspect of Cranial Base (Cranial Fossae). (From *Netter's atlas of human anatomy,* ed 8, Plate 34; S-134.)

space and contains cerebrospinal fluid, which bathes and protects the central nervous system (CNS).

- **Pia mater:** delicate membrane of connective tissue that intimately envelops the brain and spinal cord.

The cranial dura mater is distinguished from the dura mater covering the spinal cord by its two layers. An outer **periosteal layer** is attached to the inner aspect of the cranium and is supplied by the *meningeal arteries,* which lie on its surface between it and the bony skull. Imprints of these meningeal artery branches can be seen as depressions on the inner table of bone. This periosteal dura mater is continuous with the periosteum on the outer surface of the skull at the foramen magnum and where other intracranial foramina open onto the outer skull surface. The inner dural layer is termed the **meningeal layer** and is in close contact with the underlying arachnoid mater and is continuous with the spinal dura mater at the level of the foramen magnum.

The dura mater is richly innervated by meningeal sensory branches of the **trigeminal nerve** (fifth

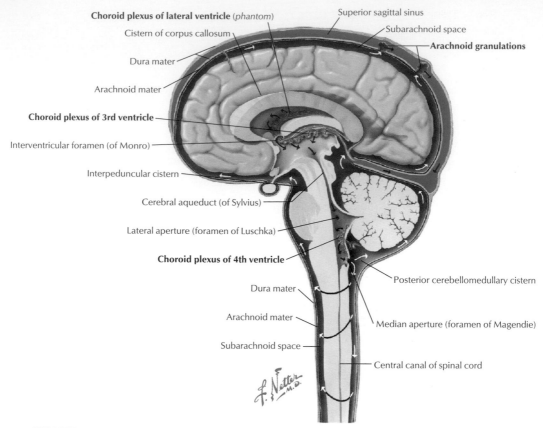

FIGURE 8.5 Central Nervous System Meninges, Cerebrospinal Fluid Circulation, and Arachnoid Granulations. (From *Netter's atlas of human anatomy,* ed 8, Plate 136; S-35.)

cranial nerve, CN V); the **vagus nerve** (CN X), specifically to the posterior cranial fossa; and the **upper cervical nerves**. A portion of the dura mater in the posterior cranial fossa also may receive some innervation from the *glossopharyngeal nerve* (CN IX), *accessory nerve* (CN XI), and *hypoglossal nerve* (CN XII). The arachnoid mater and pia mater lack sensory innervation. The periosteal dura mater and meningeal dura mater separate to form thick connective tissue folds or layers that separate various brain regions and lobes (Figs. 8.5–8.8):

- **Falx cerebri:** double layer of meningeal dura mater between the two cerebral hemispheres.
- **Falx cerebelli:** sickle-shaped layer of meningeal dura mater that projects between the two cerebellar hemispheres.
- **Tentorium cerebelli:** fold of meningeal dura mater that covers the cerebellum and supports the occipital lobes of the cerebral hemispheres.
- **Diaphragma sellae:** horizontal shelf of meningeal dura mater that forms the roof of the sella turcica covering the pituitary gland; the infundibulum passes through this dural shelf

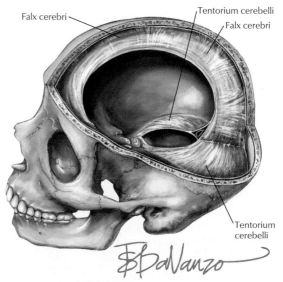

FIGURE 8.6 Dural Projections.

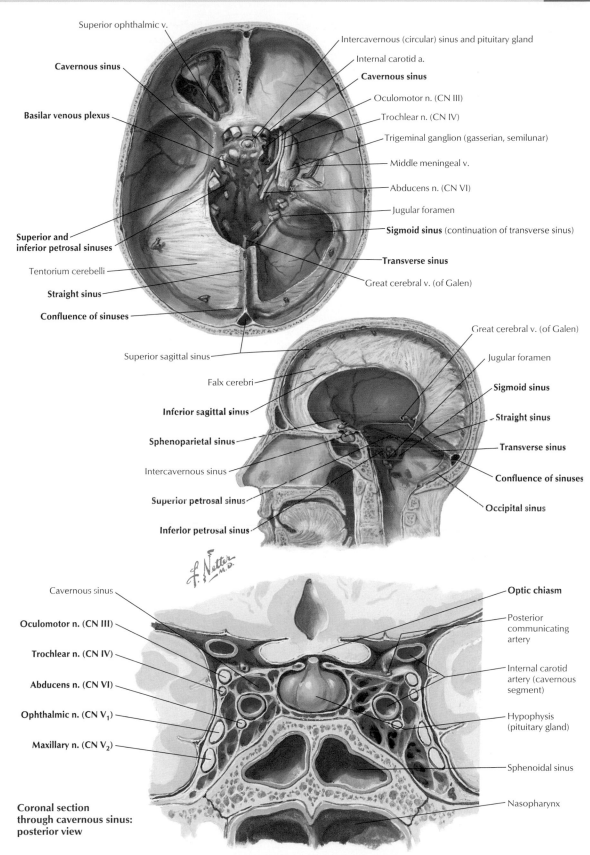

Superior ophthalmic v.

Intercavernous (circular) sinus and pituitary gland

Cavernous sinus

Internal carotid a.

Cavernous sinus

Oculomotor n. (CN III)

Basilar venous plexus

Trochlear n. (CN IV)

Trigeminal ganglion (gasserian, semilunar)

Middle meningeal v.

Abducens n. (CN VI)

Jugular foramen

Sigmoid sinus (continuation of transverse sinus)

Superior and inferior petrosal sinuses

Transverse sinus

Tentorium cerebelli

Great cerebral v. (of Galen)

Straight sinus

Confluence of sinuses

Superior sagittal sinus

Great cerebral v. (of Galen)

Jugular foramen

Falx cerebri

Sigmoid sinus

Inferior sagittal sinus

Straight sinus

Sphenoparietal sinus

Transverse sinus

Intercavernous sinus

Confluence of sinuses

Superior petrosal sinus

Occipital sinus

Inferior petrosal sinus

Cavernous sinus

Optic chiasm

Oculomotor n. (CN III)

Posterior communicating artery

Trochlear n. (CN IV)

Internal carotid artery (cavernous segment)

Abducens n. (CN VI)

Ophthalmic n. (CN V$_1$)

Hypophysis (pituitary gland)

Maxillary n. (CN V$_2$)

Sphenoidal sinus

Coronal section through cavernous sinus: posterior view

Nasopharynx

FIGURE 8.7 Dural Venous Sinuses. (From *Netter's atlas of human anatomy*, ed 8, Plates 130 and 131; S-29 and S-30.)

to connect the hypothalamus with the pituitary gland.

Dural Venous Sinuses

The dura mater also separates to form several large endothelial-lined venous channels between its **periosteal** and **meningeal layers;** these include the superior and inferior sagittal sinuses, straight sinus, confluence of sinuses, transverse, sigmoid, and cavernous sinuses, and several smaller dural sinuses (Table 8.2 and Fig. 8.7). These **dural venous sinuses** drain blood from the brain, largely posteriorly, and then largely into the *internal jugular veins.* These sinuses lack valves, however, so the direction of blood flow through the sinuses is pressure dependent. Of particular importance is the **cavernous venous sinus**

TABLE 8.2 Dural Venous Sinuses

SINUS	CHARACTERISTICS
Superior sagittal	Midline sinus along the convex superior border of the falx cerebri
Inferior sagittal	Midline sinus along the inferior free edge of the falx cerebri and joined by the great cerebral vein (of Galen)
Straight	Runs in the attachment of the falx cerebri and the tentorium cerebelli, and is formed by the inferior sagittal sinus and great cerebral vein
Confluence of sinuses	Meeting of superior and inferior sagittal sinuses, the straight sinus, and the occipital sinus
Transverse	Extends from the confluence of sinuses along the lateral edge of the tentorium cerebelli
Sigmoid	Continuation of the transverse sinus that passes inferomedially in an S-shaped pathway to the jugular foramen (becomes internal jugular vein)
Occipital	Runs in the falx cerebelli to the confluence of sinuses
Basilar	Network of venous channels on basilar part of the occipital bone, with connections to the petrosal sinuses; drains into vertebral venous plexus
Cavernous	Lies between dural layers on each side of the sella turcica; connects to the superior ophthalmic veins, pterygoid plexus of veins, sphenoparietal sinuses, petrosal sinuses, and basilar sinus
Sphenoparietal	Runs along the posterior edge of the lesser wing of the sphenoid bone and drains into the cavernous sinus
Emissary veins	Small veins connect the dural sinuses with the diploic veins in the bony skull, which are connected to scalp veins

(Fig. 8.7), which lies on either side of the sella turcica and has an anatomical relationship with the internal carotid artery and several cranial nerves, including CN III, CN IV, CN V_1, CN V_2, and CN VI. *Injury or inflammation in this region can affect some or all of these important structures.* Also, the optic chiasm lies just above this area, so CN II may be involved in any superior expansion of the cavernous sinus (e.g., pituitary tumor).

Subarachnoid Space

The **subarachnoid space** (between the arachnoid mater and pia mater) contains **cerebrospinal fluid** (CSF), which performs the following functions (Figs. 8.5 and 8.8):

- Supports and cushions the spinal cord and brain.
- Fulfills some functions normally provided by the lymphatic system by draining some CSF macromolecules into the meningeal dural lymphatics (the CNS glymphatic system).
- Occupies a volume of about 150 mL in the subarachnoid space.
- Is produced by **choroid plexuses** in the brain's ventricles.
- Is produced at a rate of about 500 to 700 mL/day.
- Is reabsorbed largely by the cranial arachnoid granulations and by microscopic arachnoid granulations feeding into venules along the length of the spinal cord.

The **arachnoid granulations** absorb most of the CSF and deliver it to the dural venous sinuses (see Figs. 8.5 and 8.8). These granulations are composed of convoluted aggregations of arachnoid mater that extend as "tufts" into the superior sagittal sinus and function as one-way valves for the clearance of CSF; the CSF crosses into the venous sinus, but venous blood cannot enter the subarachnoid space. Small, microscopic arachnoid cell herniations also occur along the *spinal cord,* where CSF (which circulates at a higher pressure than venous blood) is delivered directly into small spinal cord veins. The CSF circulating around the brain (and spinal cord) provides a protective cushion and buoyancy for the CNS, thus reducing the pressure of the brain on the vessels and nerves on its inferior surface. CSF also can serve as a fluid delivery system for certain chemical mediators (e.g., interleukins and prostaglandins), clears the CNS of metabolites directly or via the glymphatic system, and represents an internal paracrine communication system for certain CNS areas that are close to the ventricles.

Scalp, skull, meningeal, and cerebral blood vessels

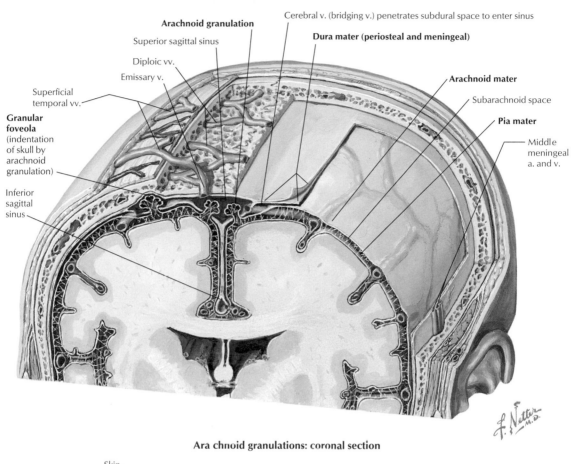

Ara chnoid granulations: coronal section

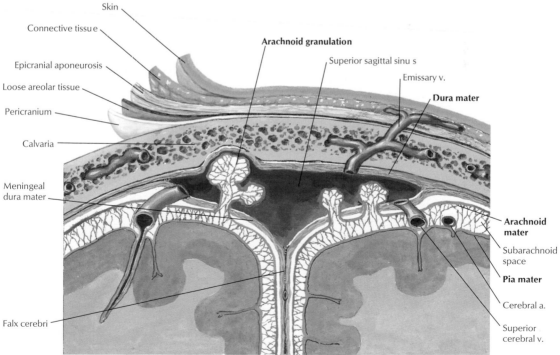

FIGURE 8.8 Relationship of Arachnoid Granulations and Venous Sinus. (From *Netter's atlas of human anatomy*, ed 8, Plates 127 and 129; S-26 and S-28.)

Clinical Focus 8.4

Hydrocephalus

Hydrocephalus is the accumulation of excess CSF within the brain's ventricular system. It is caused by overproduction or decreased absorption of CSF or by blockage of one of the passageways for CSF flow in the subarachnoid space.

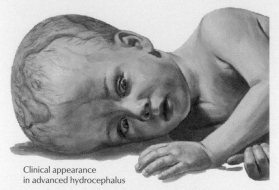

Clinical appearance
in advanced hydrocephalus

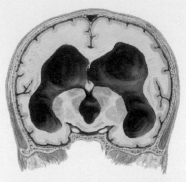

Section through brain showing marked
dilatation of lateral and 3rd ventricles

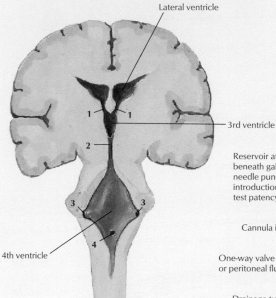

Lateral ventricle

3rd ventricle

4th ventricle

Potential lesion sites in obstructive hydrocephalus

1. Interventricular foramina (of Monro)
2. Cerebral aqueduct (of Sylvius)
3. Lateral apertures (of Luschka)
4. Median aperture (of Magendie)

Shunt procedure for hydrocephalus

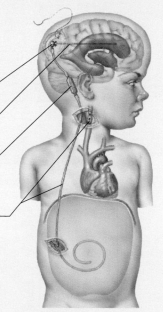

Reservoir at end of cannula implanted
beneath galea permits transcutaneous
needle puncture for withdrawal of CSF,
introduction of antibiotics, or dye to
test patency of shunt.

Cannula inserted into lateral ventricle

One-way valve to prevent reflux of blood
or peritoneal fluid and control CSF pressure

Drainage tube may be introduced into
internal jugular v. and thence into right
atrium via neck incision, or may be
continued subcutaneously to abdomen.

Type	Definition
Obstructive	Congenital stenosis of cerebral aqueduct (of Sylvius), or obstruction at other sites (illustrated) by tumors
Communicating	Obstruction outside the ventricular system, e.g., subarachnoid space (hemorrhage) or at arachnoid granulations
Normal pressure	Adult syndrome of progressive dementia, gait disorders, and urinary incontinence; computed tomography shows ventricular dilation and brain atrophy

Clinical Focus 8.5

Meningitis

Meningitis is a serious condition defined as an *inflammation of the arachnoid mater and pia mater.* It results most often from bacterial or aseptic causes. Aseptic causes include viral infections, drug reactions, and systemic diseases. Patients with meningitis usually present with the following symptoms:

- Headache
- Fever

- Seizures
- Painful stiff neck

Diagnosis is made by performing a lumbar puncture and examining the CSF.

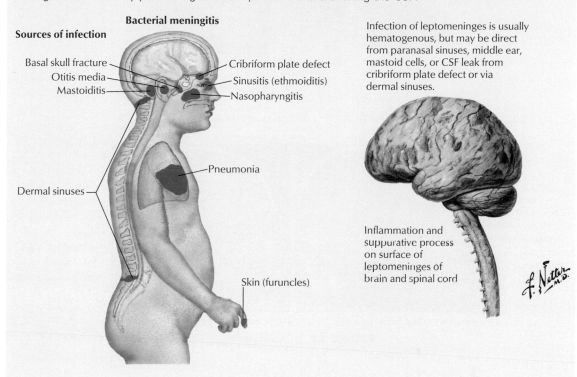

Bacterial meningitis

Sources of infection

Basal skull fracture
Otitis media
Mastoiditis

Cribriform plate defect
Sinusitis (ethmoiditis)
Nasopharyngitis

Infection of leptomeninges is usually hematogenous, but may be direct from paranasal sinuses, middle ear, mastoid cells, or CSF leak from cribriform plate defect or via dermal sinuses.

Pneumonia

Dermal sinuses

Skin (furuncles)

Inflammation and suppurative process on surface of leptomeninges of brain and spinal cord

Gross Anatomy of the Brain

The most notable feature of the human brain is its large **cerebral hemispheres** (Figs. 8.9 and 8.10). Several circumscribed regions of the cerebral cortex are associated with specific functions, and key surface landmarks of the typical human cerebrum are used to *divide the brain into lobes:* four or five, depending on classification, with the fifth lobe being either the insula or the limbic lobe. The lobes and their general functions are as follows:

- **Frontal:** mediates precise voluntary motor control, learned motor skills, planned movement, eye movement, expressive speech, personality, working memory, complex problem solving, emotions, judgment, socialization, olfaction, and drive.

- **Parietal:** affects sensory input, spatial discrimination, sensory representation and integration, taste, and receptive speech.
- **Occipital:** affects visual input and processing.
- **Temporal:** mediates auditory input and auditory memory integration, spoken language (dominant side), and body language (nondominant side).
- **Insula:** a fifth deep lobe that lies medial to the temporal lobe *(sometimes included as part of temporal lobe)*; influences vestibular function, some language, perception of visceral sensations (e.g., upset stomach), emotions, and limbic functions.
- **Limbic:** also sometimes considered a *fifth medial lobe* (cingulate cortex); influences emotions and some autonomic functions.

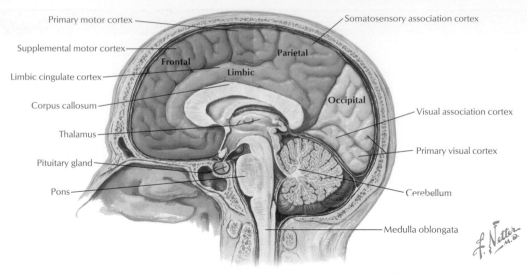

Primary motor cortex

Somatosensory association cortex

Supplemental motor cortex

Frontal

Parietal

Limbic cingulate cortex

Limbic

Corpus callosum

Occipital

Visual association cortex

Thalamus

Primary visual cortex

Pituitary gland

Pons

Cerebellum

Medulla oblongata

Medial aspect of the brain and brainstem

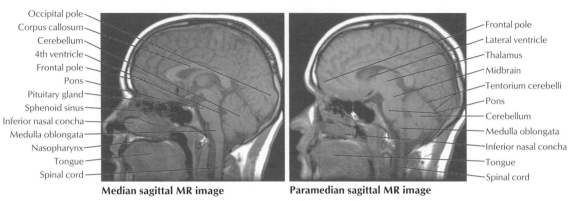

Occipital pole
Corpus callosum
Cerebellum
4th ventricle
Frontal pole
Pons
Pituitary gland
Sphenoid sinus
Inferior nasal concha
Medulla oblongata
Nasopharynx
Tongue
Spinal cord

Frontal pole
Lateral ventricle
Thalamus
Midbrain
Tentorium cerebelli
Pons
Cerebellum
Medulla oblongata
Inferior nasal concha
Tongue
Spinal cord

Median sagittal MR image   **Paramedian sagittal MR image**

FIGURE 8.9 Brain and Brainstem.

Other key areas of the brain include the following components (Fig. 8.9):

- **Thalamus:** gateway to the cortex; simplistically functions as an "executive secretary" to the cortex (relay center between cortical and subcortical areas).
- **Cerebellum:** coordinates smooth motor activities, and processes muscle position; possible role in behavior and cognition.
- **Brainstem:** includes the **midbrain, pons,** and **medulla oblongata;** conveys motor and sensory information from the body and autonomic and motor information from higher centers to peripheral targets.

Internally, the brain contains **four ventricles,** two lateral ventricles, and a central third and fourth ventricle (Fig. 8.11). **Cerebrospinal fluid,** produced by the choroid plexus (see Fig. 8.5), circulates through these ventricles and then enters the subarachnoid space through **two lateral apertures** (foramina of Luschka) or a **median aperture** (foramen of Magendie) in the fourth ventricle (Fig. 8.11).

Blood Supply to the Brain

Arteries supplying the brain arise largely from the following two pairs of arteries (Fig. 8.12 and Table 8.3):

- **Vertebrals:** these two arteries (right and left) arise from the *subclavian artery,* ascend through the transverse foramina of the C1-C6 vertebrae, and enter the foramen magnum of the skull.
- **Internal carotids:** these two arteries (right and left) arise from the *common carotid artery* in the lower neck, ascend superiorly in the neck, enter the carotid canal, and traverse the foramen lacerum to terminate as the *middle and anterior cerebral arteries,* which anastomose with the **arterial circle of Willis.**

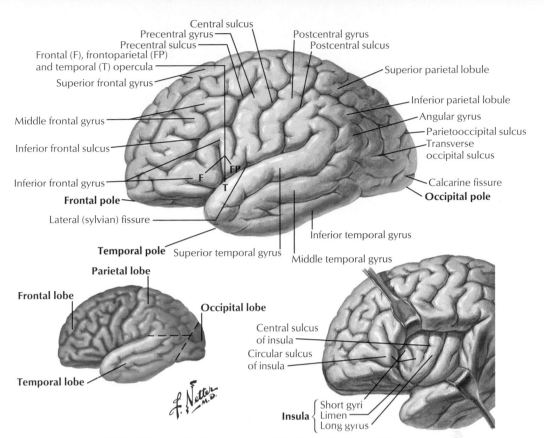

FIGURE 8.10 Surface Anatomy of the Forebrain: Lateral View.

Central sulcus
Precentral gyrus
Precentral sulcus
Frontal (F), frontoparietal (FP)
and temporal (T) opercula
Superior frontal gyrus
Middle frontal gyrus
Inferior frontal sulcus
Inferior frontal gyrus
Frontal pole
Lateral (sylvian) fissure
Temporal pole   Superior temporal gyrus
Postcentral gyrus
Postcentral sulcus
Superior parietal lobule
Inferior parietal lobule
Angular gyrus
Parietooccipital sulcus
Transverse occipital sulcus
Calcarine fissure
Occipital pole
Inferior temporal gyrus
Middle temporal gyrus

Parietal lobe
Frontal lobe
Temporal lobe
Occipital lobe

Central sulcus of insula
Circular sulcus of insula
Insula { Short gyri / Limen / Long gyrus

Clinical Focus 8.6

Subarachnoid Hemorrhage

Subarachnoid hemorrhage usually occurs from an arterial source and results in the collection of blood between the **arachnoid mater** and **pia mater**. The most common cause of subarachnoid hemorrhage is the rupture of a **saccular, or berry, aneurysm**.

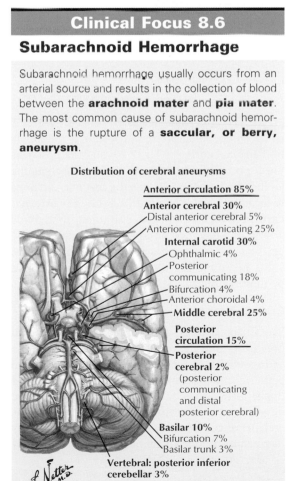

Distribution of cerebral aneurysms

Anterior circulation 85%

Anterior cerebral 30%
Distal anterior cerebral 5%
Anterior communicating 25%
Internal carotid 30%
Ophthalmic 4%
Posterior communicating 18%
Bifurcation 4%
Anterior choroidal 4%
Middle cerebral 25%

Posterior circulation 15%
Posterior cerebral 2%
(posterior communicating and distal posterior cerebral)

Basilar 10%
Bifurcation 7%
Basilar trunk 3%

Vertebral: posterior inferior cerebellar 3%

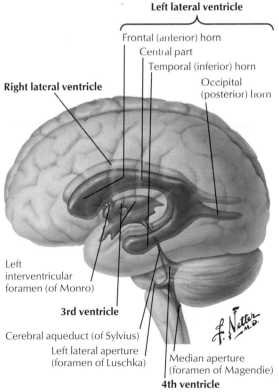

Left lateral ventricle
Frontal (anterior) horn
Central part
Temporal (inferior) horn
Occipital (posterior) horn
Right lateral ventricle

Left interventricular foramen (of Monro)
3rd ventricle
Cerebral aqueduct (of Sylvius)
Left lateral aperture (foramen of Luschka)
Median aperture (foramen of Magendie)
4th ventricle

FIGURE 8.11 Ventricular System of the Brain. (From *Netter's atlas of human anatomy*, ed 8, Plate 135; S-34.)

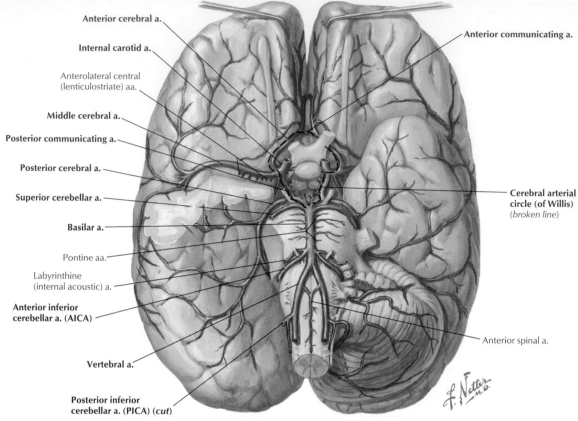

Anterior cerebral a.

Internal carotid a.

Anterolateral central (lenticulostriate) aa.

Middle cerebral a.

Posterior communicating a.

Posterior cerebral a.

Superior cerebellar a.

Basilar a.

Pontine aa.

Labyrinthine (internal acoustic) a.

Anterior inferior cerebellar a. (AICA)

Vertebral a.

Posterior inferior cerebellar a. (PICA) (cut)

Anterior communicating a.

Cerebral arterial circle (of Willis) (broken line)

Anterior spinal a.

FIGURE 8.12 Arterial Circle on Base of Brain. (From *Netter's atlas of human anatomy,* ed 8, Plate 166; S-44.)

TABLE 8.3 Blood Supply to the Brain

ARTERY	COURSE AND STRUCTURES SUPPLIED
Vertebral	From subclavian artery; supplies cerebellum
Posterior inferior cerebellar	From vertebral artery; supplies the posteroinferior cerebellum
Basilar	From both vertebrals; supplies brainstem, cerebellum, and cerebrum
Anterior inferior cerebellar	From basilar; supplies inferior cerebellum
Superior cerebellar	From basilar; supplies superior cerebellum
Posterior cerebral	From basilar; supplies inferior cerebrum and occipital lobe
Posterior communicating	Cerebral arterial circle (of Willis)
Internal carotid (IC)	From common carotid; supplies cerebral lobes and eye
Middle cerebral	From IC; supplies lateral aspect of cerebral hemispheres
Anterior communicating	Cerebral arterial circle (of Willis)
Anterior cerebral	From IC; supplies medial and superolateral cerebral hemispheres (except occipital lobe)

The **vertebral arteries** give rise to the anterior and posterior spinal arteries (a portion of the supply to the spinal cord; see Fig. 2.20) and the posterior inferior cerebellar arteries, and then join at about the level of the junction between the medulla and pons to form the **basilar artery** (Fig. 8.12). The **internal carotid arteries** each give rise to an ophthalmic artery, a posterior communicating artery, a middle cerebral artery, and an anterior cerebral artery. Table 8.3 summarizes the brain regions supplied by these vessels and their major branches.

Cranial Nerves

See Chapter 1 for an overview of the general organization of the nervous system.

In addition to the 31 pairs of spinal nerves, 12 pairs of cranial nerves arise from the brain and upper spinal cord (CN XI). As with the spinal nerves, cranial nerves are part of the peripheral nervous system and are identified both by name and by Roman numerals CN I to CN XII

Text continued on p. 457.

Clinical Focus 8.7

Epidural Hematomas

Epidural hematomas result most often from motor vehicle crashes, falls, and sports injuries. The blood collects between the *periosteal dura mater and bony cranium*. The source of the bleeding is usually arterial (85%); common locations include the frontal, temporal (middle meningeal artery is very susceptible, especially where it lies deep to the pterion), and occipital regions.

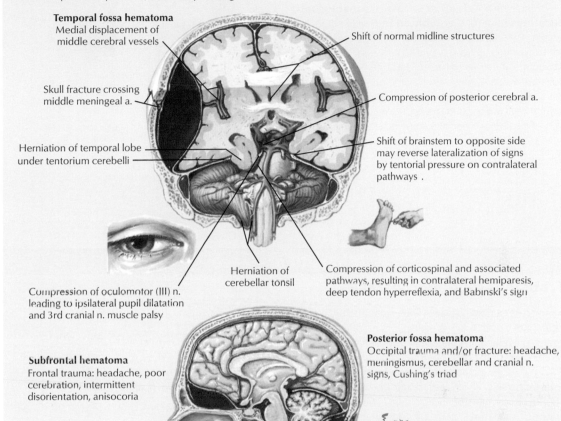

Temporal fossa hematoma
Medial displacement of middle cerebral vessels

Shift of normal midline structures

Skull fracture crossing middle meningeal a.

Compression of posterior cerebral a.

Herniation of temporal lobe under tentorium cerebelli

Shift of brainstem to opposite side may reverse lateralization of signs by tentorial pressure on contralateral pathways .

Herniation of cerebellar tonsil

Compression of oculomotor (III) n. leading to ipsilateral pupil dilatation and 3rd cranial n. muscle palsy

Compression of corticospinal and associated pathways, resulting in contralateral hemiparesis, deep tendon hyperreflexia, and Babinski's sign

Subfrontal hematoma
Frontal trauma: headache, poor cerebration, intermittent disorientation, anisocoria

Posterior fossa hematoma
Occipital trauma and/or fracture: headache, meningismus, cerebellar and cranial n. signs, Cushing's triad

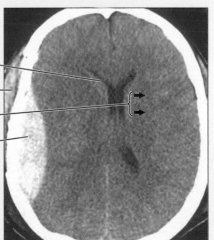

Compression of lateral ventricle

Scalp hematoma

Shift of midline structures

Epidural hematoma

Axial CT with a soft tissue (brain) window showing an acute epidural hematoma and scalp hematoma in a patient from a motor vehicle accident. Note the depression of the bony contour on the right. *(Reused with permission from Cochard LR. Netter's Introduction to Imaging, Elsevier, 2011, Fig. 8.39B.)*

Clinical Focus 8.8

Subdural Hematomas

Subdural hematomas are usually caused by an *acute venous hemorrhage of the cortical bridging veins* draining cortical blood into the superior sagittal sinus. Half are associated with skull fractures. In a subdural hematoma the blood collects between the **meningeal dura mater** and the **arachnoid mater** (a potential space). Clinical signs include a decreasing level of consciousness, ipsilateral pupillary dilation, headache, and contralateral hemiparesis. These hematomas may develop within 1 week after injury but often present with clinical signs within hours. Chronic subdural hematomas are most common in elderly persons and alcoholic patients who have some brain atrophy, which increases the space traversed by the bridging veins and renders the stretched vein susceptible to tearing.

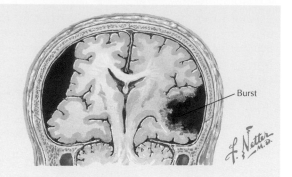

Burst

Section showing acute subdural hematoma on right side and subdural hematoma associated with temporal lobe intracerebral hematoma ("burst" temporal lobe) on left

Clinical Focus 8.9

Transient Ischemic Attack

A transient ischemic attack (TIA) is a temporary interruption of focal brain circulation that results in a neurologic deficit that lasts less than 24 hours, usually 15 minutes to 1 hour. The most common cause of TIA is embolic disease from the heart, carotid, or cerebral vessels, which may temporarily block a vessel. The onset of the deficit is abrupt, and recovery is gradual. The most common deficits include the following:

- Hemiparesis
- Hemisensory loss
- Aphasia
- Confusion
- Hemianopia
- Ataxia
- Vertigo

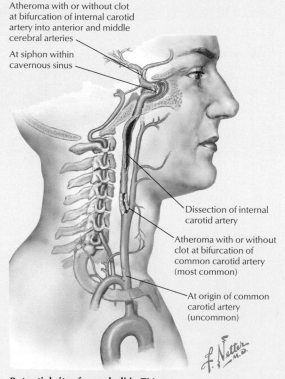

Atheroma with or without clot at bifurcation of internal carotid artery into anterior and middle cerebral arteries

At siphon within cavernous sinus

Dissection of internal carotid artery

Atheroma with or without clot at bifurcation of common carotid artery (most common)

At origin of common carotid artery (uncommon)

Potential sites for emboli in TIA

Clinical Focus 8.10

Stroke

Cerebrovascular accident (CVA) or stroke is a localized brain injury caused by a vascular episode that lasts more than 24 hours, whereas a transient ischemic attack (TIA) is a focal ischemic episode lasting less than 24 hours. Stroke is classified into the following two types:

- **Ischemic** (70-80%): infarction; thrombotic or embolic, resulting from atherosclerosis of the extracranial (usually carotid) and intracranial arteries or from underlying heart disease.
- **Hemorrhagic:** occurs when a cerebral vessel weakens and ruptures (subarachnoid or intracerebral hemorrhage), which causes intracranial bleeding, usually affecting a larger brain area.

Ischemic Stroke

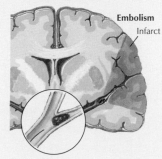

Embolism
Infarct

Clot fragment carried from heart or more proximal a.

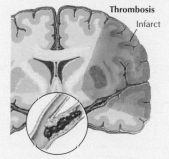

Thrombosis
Infarct

Clot in carotid a. extends directly to middle cerebral a.

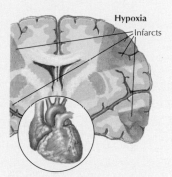

Hypoxia
Infarcts

Hypotension and poor cerebral perfusion: border zone infarcts, no vascular occlusion

Hemorrhagic Stroke

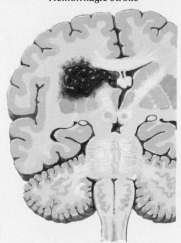

Intracerebral hemorrhage
(hypertensive)

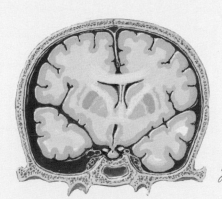

Subarachnoid hemorrhage
(ruptured aneurysm)

Carotid–Cavernous Sinus Fistula

More common than symptomatic intracavernous sinus aneurysms but less common than subarachnoid saccular (berry) aneurysms, carotid–cavernous sinus fistulas often result from trauma and are more common in men. These high-pressure (arterial) low-flow lesions are characterized by an orbital bruit, exophthalmos, chemosis, and extraocular muscle palsy *involving CN III, IV, and VI*. Blood collecting in the cavernous sinus drains by several venous pathways because the sinus has connections with other dural venous sinuses as well as with the ophthalmic veins and pterygoid plexus of veins in the infratemporal region.

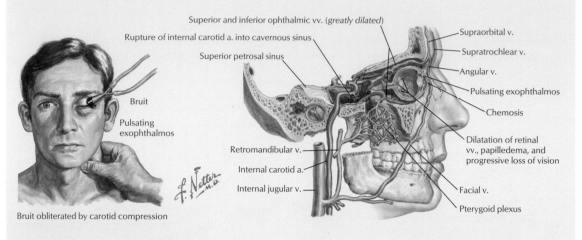

Collateral Circulation After Internal Carotid Artery Occlusion

If a major artery such as the internal carotid becomes occluded, extracranial and intracranial (circle of Willis) anastomoses may provide collateral routes of circulation. These routes are more likely to develop when occlusion is gradual, as in atherosclerosis, rather than acute, as in embolic obstruction.

Reversal of flow through ophthalmic artery

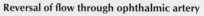

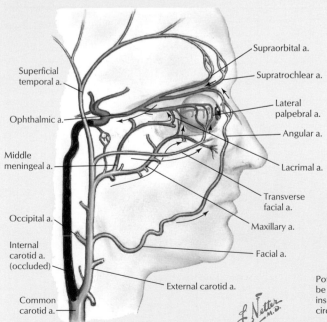

Via circle of Willis

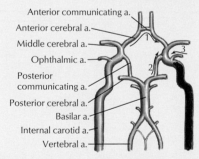

Circulation maintained by flow from:
1. Opposite internal carotid a. (anterior circulation)
2. Vertebrobasilar system (posterior circulation)
3. Ophthalmic a.

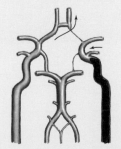

Potential collateral flow may be reduced by anomalous insufficiency of segments of circle of Willis.

Clinical Focus 8.13

Vascular (Multiinfarct) Dementia

Dementia is an *acquired neurologic syndrome* that presents with multiple cognitive deficits. By definition, dementia includes short-term memory impairment, behavioral disturbance, and/or difficulties with daily functioning and independence. Dementia can be classified as degenerative, vascular, alcoholic, or human immunodeficiency virus (HIV) related. Vascular dementias are caused by anoxic damage from small infarcts and account for about 15% to 20% of dementia cases. Multiinfarct dementia is associated with heart disease, diabetes mellitus, hypertension, and inflammatory diseases.

Clinical characteristics

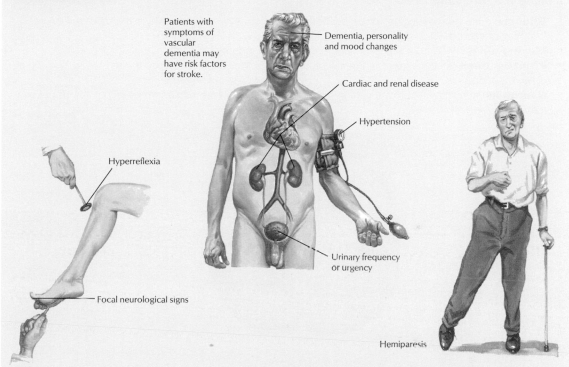

Patients with symptoms of vascular dementia may have risk factors for stroke.

Dementia, personality and mood changes

Cardiac and renal disease

Hypertension

Hyperreflexia

Urinary frequency or urgency

Focal neurological signs

Hemiparesis

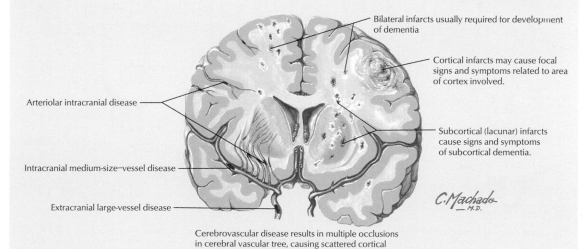

Bilateral infarcts usually required for development of dementia

Cortical infarcts may cause focal signs and symptoms related to area of cortex involved.

Arteriolar intracranial disease

Subcortical (lacunar) infarcts cause signs and symptoms of subcortical dementia.

Intracranial medium-size–vessel disease

Extracranial large-vessel disease

C. Machado — M.D.

Cerebrovascular disease results in multiple occlusions in cerebral vascular tree, causing scattered cortical and subcortical infarcts.

Clinical Focus 8.14

Brain Tumors

Clinical signs and symptoms of brain tumors depend on the location and the degree to which intracranial pressure (ICP) is elevated. Slow-growing tumors in relatively silent areas (e.g., frontal lobes) may go undetected and can become quite large before symptoms occur. Small tumors in key brain areas can lead to seizures, hemiparesis, or aphasia. Increased ICP can initiate broader damage by compressing critical brain structures. Early symptoms of increased ICP include malaise, headache, nausea, papilledema, and less often abducens nerve palsy and Parinaud's syndrome. Classic signs of hydrocephalus are loss of upward gaze, downward ocular deviation ("setting sun" syndrome), lid retraction, and light-near dissociation of pupils. **Primary tumors include the following**:

- **Gliomas:** arise from astrocytes or oligodendrocytes; glioblastoma multiforme is the most malignant form (astrocytic series).
- **Meningiomas:** arise from the arachnoid mater and can extend into the brain.
- **Pituitary tumors:** can expand in the sella turcica and affect CN II, III, IV, V_1, V_2, and VI; about 15% of primary tumors.
- **Neuromas:** acoustic neuroma, a benign tumor of CN VIII, is a common example; about 7% of primary tumors.

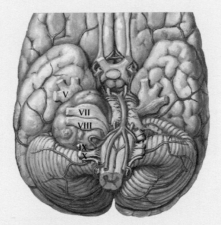

Large acoustic neuroma filling
cerebellopontine angle, distorting
brainstem and cranial nerves
V, VII, VIII, IX, X

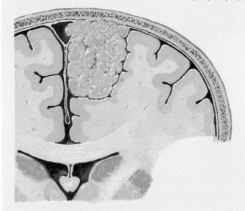

Meningioma invading superior sagittal sinus

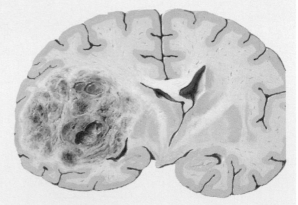

Large, hemispheric glioblastoma multiforme
with central areas of necrosis. Brain distorted
to opposite side.

Clinical Focus 8.15

Metastatic Brain Tumors

Metastatic brain tumors are *more common* than primary brain tumors. Most spread via the bloodstream, with cells seeded between the white matter (fiber tract pathways) and gray matter (cortical neurons). Some tumors metastasize directly from head and neck cancers or through Batson's vertebral venous plexus. Presentation often includes headache (50%), seizures (25%), and elevated intracranial pressure.

Common primary sources

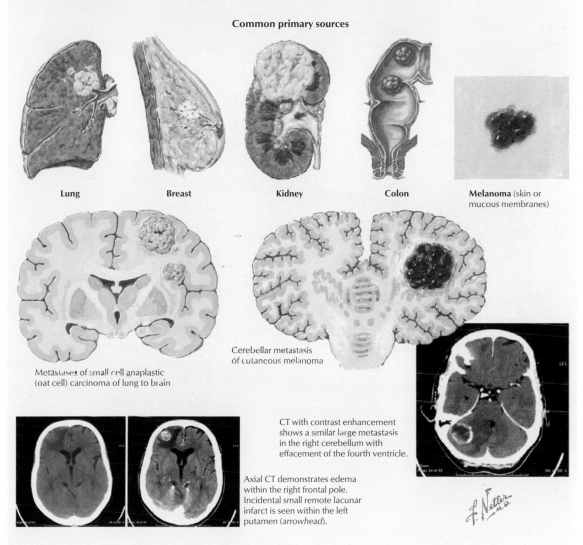

Lung   Breast   Kidney   Colon   Melanoma (skin or mucous membranes)

Metastases of small cell anaplastic (oat cell) carcinoma of lung to brain

Cerebellar metastasis of cutaneous melanoma

CT with contrast enhancement shows a similar large metastasis in the right cerebellum with effacement of the fourth ventricle.

Axial CT demonstrates edema within the right frontal pole. Incidental small remote lacunar infarct is seen within the left putamen (*arrowhead*).

(Fig. 8.13). Cranial nerves are somewhat unique and may contain the following multiple functional components:

- **General (G):** same general functions as spinal nerves.
- **Special (S):** functions found only in cranial nerves (special senses of vision, hearing, and balance, and the sensations of smell and taste).
- **Afferent (A)** or **efferent (E):** sensory or motor functions, respectively.
- **Somatic (S)** or **visceral (V):** related to skin and skeletal muscle innervation (**somatic**), or to smooth muscle, cardiac muscle, and glands (**visceral**).

By convention, each cranial nerve is classified as either general (G) or special (S), and then somatic (S) or visceral (V), and finally as afferent (A) or

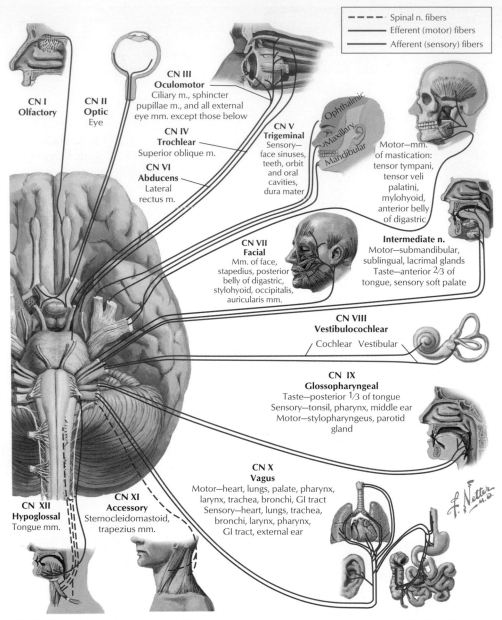

FIGURE 8.13 Overview of Cranial Nerves. (From *Netter's atlas of human anatomy*, ed 8, Plate 145; S-53.)

efferent (E). For example, a cranial nerve that is classified GVE (general visceral efferent) means it contains motor fibers to visceral structures, such as parasympathetic fibers in the vagus nerve.

In general, cranial nerves are described as follows (Table 8.4):

- **CN I** and **II:** arise from the forebrain; are really *tracts* of the brain for the special senses of smell and sight, respectively; they are *brain extensions* surrounded by all three meningeal coverings, with CSF in the subarachnoid space—but still are classified as cranial nerves.
- **CN III, IV,** and **VI:** move the extraocular skeletal muscles of the eyeball.

- **CN V:** has three divisions; V_1 and V_2 are sensory, and V_3 is both sensory and motor.
- **CN VII, IX,** and **X:** are both motor and sensory.
- **CN VIII:** is the special sense of hearing and balance, but unlike CN I and II, is not a brain tract.
- **CN XI** and **XII:** are motor to skeletal muscle.
- **CN III, VII, IX,** and **X:** also contain parasympathetic (visceral) fibers of origin, although many of these autonomic fibers "jump" onto branches of CN V to reach their targets, because the branches of CN V pass almost everywhere in the head.

TABLE 8.4 Functional Components of the Cranial Nerves

CRANIAL NERVE	FUNCTIONAL COMPONENT
I Olfactory nerve	SSA (Special sense of smell)
II Optic nerve	SSA (Special sense of sight)
III Oculomotor nerve	GSE (Motor to extraocular muscles)
	GVE (Parasympathetic to smooth muscle in eye)
IV Trochlear nerve	GSE (Motor to one extraocular muscle)
V Trigeminal nerve	GSA (Sensory to face, orbit, nose, and anterior tongue)
	SVE (Motor to skeletal muscles)
VI Abducens nerve	GSE (Motor to one extraocular muscle)
VII Facial nerve	GSA (Sensory to skin of ear)
	SVA (Special sense of taste to anterior tongue)
	GVE (Motor to salivary, nasal, and lacrimal glands)
	SVE (Motor to facial muscles)
VIII Vestibulocochlear nerve	SSA (Special sense of hearing and balance)
IX Glossopharyngeal nerve	GSA (Sensory to posterior tongue)
	SVA (Special sense of taste—posterior tongue)
	GVA (Sensory from middle ear, pharynx, carotid body, and sinus)
	GVE (Motor to parotid gland)
	SVE (Motor to one muscle of pharynx)
X Vagus nerve	GSA (Sensory external ear)
	SVA (Special sense of taste—epiglottis)
	GVA (Sensory from pharynx, larynx, and thoracic and abdominal organs)
	GVE (Motor to thoracic and abdominal organs)
	SVE (Motor to muscles of pharynx/larynx)
XI Accessory nerve	GSE (Motor to two muscles)
XII Hypoglossal nerve	GSE (Motor to tongue muscles)

Rather than describe each cranial nerve and all its branches in detail at this time, we will review each nerve anatomically and clinically as we encounter it in the various regions of the head and neck. *It may be helpful to refer back to this section each time you are introduced to a new region and its cranial nerve innervation.* Autonomic components of the cranial nerves (parasympathetics) and their autonomic ganglia are summarized in Fig. 1.26 and Table 1.4. All of the cranial nerves and their components also are summarized at the end of this chapter.

5. SCALP AND FACE

Layers of the Scalp

The layers of the **SCALP** include the following (Fig. 8.8):
- **S**kin.
- **C**onnective tissue that contains a rich supply of blood vessels of the scalp; *lacerations of the scalp bleed profusely* because this dense connective tissue layer often holds the vessels open and prevents their retraction into the tissue.
- **A**poneurosis (galea aponeurotica) of the epicranial muscles (frontalis and occipitalis).
- **L**oose connective tissue deep to the aponeurosis, which contains emissary veins that communicate with the cranial diploë and dural sinuses within the cranium.
- **P**eriosteum (pericranium) on the surface of the bony skull.

The *loose connective tissue layer* allows the skin to move over the skull when one rubs the head and also allows infections to spread through this layer (Fig. 8.8). Small **emissary veins** communicate with this layer and can pass infections intracranially.

Muscles of Facial Expression

The muscles of facial expression are skeletal muscles that lie in the *subcutaneous tissue* of the face. They are all innervated by the **terminal motor branches of the facial nerve (CN VII)**, and most originate from the underlying facial skeleton but insert into the skin or facial cartilages (Fig. 8.14). Table 8.5 summarizes several of the major facial muscles, which are derived from the second branchial embryonic arch (see Embryology) and are often referred to as *branchial (branchiomeric) muscles.* These muscles are skeletal muscles, but their derivation from the branchial arches means they are innervated by cranial nerves rather than spinal nerves.

Innervation of the facial muscles is by the five terminal branches of CN VII. The facial nerve enters the internal acoustic meatus of the skull, passes through the facial canal in the petrous portion of the temporal bone, and then descends to emerge from the **stylomastoid foramen.** CN VII then passes through the parotid salivary gland, and its terminal branches are distributed over the face and neck (Fig. 8.15). The five terminal motor (branchial motor) branches are as follows:
- **Temporal.**
- **Zygomatic.**

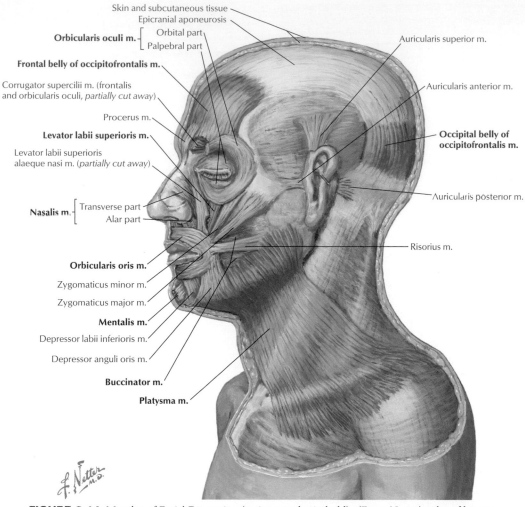

FIGURE 8.14 Muscles of Facial Expression (major muscles in bold). (From *Netter's atlas of human anatomy*, ed 8, Plate 48; S-184.)

TABLE 8.5 Summary of Major Facial Muscles

MUSCLE	ORIGIN ATTACHMENT	INSERTION ATTACHMENT	MAIN ACTIONS
Frontal belly of occipitofrontalis	Epicranial aponeurosis	Skin of forehead, epicranial aponeurosis	Elevates eyebrows and forehead; wrinkles forehead
Orbicularis oculi	Medial orbital margin, medial palpebral ligament, and lacrimal bone	Skin around margin of orbit; tarsal plates of eyelids	Closes eyelids; orbital part forcefully and palpebral part for blinking
Nasalis	Superior part of canine ridge of maxilla	Nasal cartilages	Draws ala of nose toward septum to compress opening
Orbicularis oris	Median plane of maxilla superiorly and mandible inferiorly; other fibers from deep surface of skin	Mucous membrane of lips	Closes and protrudes lips (e.g., purses them during whistling)
Levator labii superioris	Frontal process of maxilla and infraorbital region	Skin of upper lip and alar cartilage	Elevates lip, dilates nostril, raises angle of mouth
Platysma	Superficial fascia of deltoid and pectoral regions	Mandible, skin of cheek, angle of mouth, and orbicularis oris	Depresses mandible and tenses skin of lower face and neck
Mentalis	Incisive fossa of mandible	Skin of chin	Elevates and protrudes lower lip and wrinkles chin
Buccinator	Mandible, pterygomandibular raphe, and alveolar processes of maxilla and mandible	Angle of mouth	Presses cheek against molar teeth, thereby aiding chewing, expels air

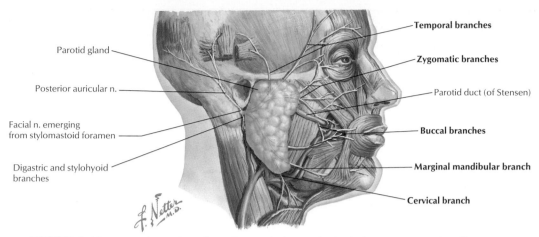

FIGURE 8.15 Terminal Branches of Facial Nerve and Parotid Gland. (From *Netter's atlas of human anatomy*, ed 8, Plate 71; S-64.)

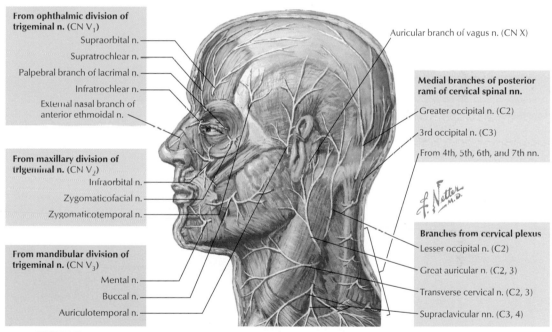

FIGURE 8.16 Cutaneous Nerves of the Face and Neck. (From *Netter's atlas of human anatomy*, ed 8, Plate 23; S-185.)

- **Buccal.**
- **Marginal mandibular.**
- **Cervical.**

The sensory innervation of the face is by the **three divisions of the trigeminal nerve** (CN V), with some contributions by the cervical plexus. Fig. 8.16 lists the specific nerves for each division. All the sensory neurons in CN V reside in the **trigeminal (semilunar, gasserian) ganglion.** The trigeminal nerve is divided as follows:

- **Ophthalmic (CN V$_1$) division:** exits the skull via the superior orbital fissure.

- **Maxillary (CN V$_2$) division:** exits the skull via the foramen rotundum.
- **Mandibular (CN V$_3$) division:** exits the skull via the foramen ovale.

The blood supply to and venous drainage from the face includes the following vessels (Fig. 8.17):

- **Facial artery:** arises from the external carotid artery.
- **Superficial temporal artery:** one of the two terminal branches of the external carotid artery.

Clinical Focus 8.16

Trigeminal Neuralgia

Trigeminal neuralgia (or *tic douloureux*) is a neurologic condition characterized by episodes of brief, intense facial pain over one of the three areas of distribution of CN V. The pain is so intense that the patient winces, which produces a facial muscle tic.

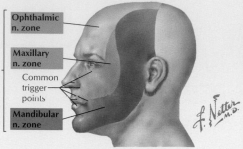

Zones of skin innervation of trigeminal nerve divisions, where pain may occur in trigeminal neuralgia

Ophthalmic n. zone

Maxillary n. zone

Common trigger points

Mandibular n. zone

Characteristic	Description
Etiology	Uncertain; possibly vascular compression of trigeminal sensory ganglion by superior cerebellar artery
Presentation	Recurrent, lancinating, burning pain, usually affecting CN V_2 or CN V_3 unilaterally (<6% involve CN V_1), usually in a person older than 50 years
Triggers	Touch; draft of cool air

Clinical Focus 8.17

Herpes Zoster (Shingles)

Herpes zoster, or shingles, is the most common infection of the peripheral nervous system (PNS). It is an acute neuralgia confined to the dermatome distribution of a specific spinal or cranial sensory nerve root.

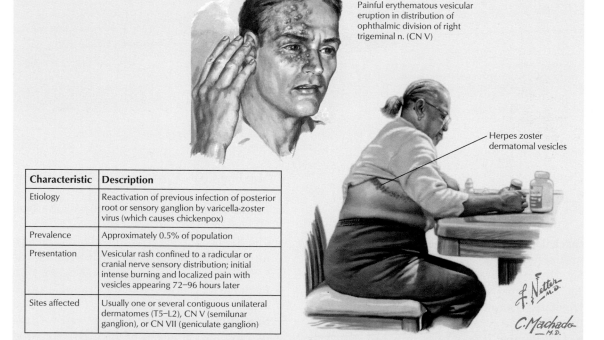

Painful erythematous vesicular eruption in distribution of ophthalmic division of right trigeminal n. (CN V)

Herpes zoster dermatomal vesicles

Characteristic	Description
Etiology	Reactivation of previous infection of posterior root or sensory ganglion by varicella-zoster virus (which causes chickenpox)
Prevalence	Approximately 0.5% of population
Presentation	Vesicular rash confined to a radicular or cranial nerve sensory distribution; initial intense burning and localized pain with vesicles appearing 72–96 hours later
Sites affected	Usually one or several contiguous unilateral dermatomes (T5–L2), CN V (semilunar ganglion), or CN VII (geniculate ganglion)

Clinical Focus 8.18

Facial Nerve (Bell's) Palsy

Acute, unilateral idiopathic facial palsy is the most common cause of facial muscle weakness and cranial neuropathy. Facial nerve palsy also may be caused by herpes simplex virus (HSV) infection. Manifestations associated with lesions at various points along the path of CN VII are illustrated.

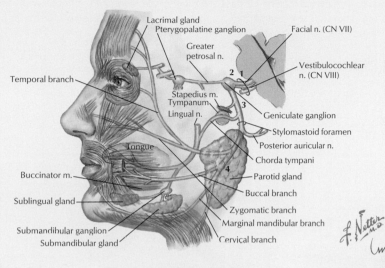

Hyperacusis

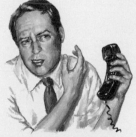

This may be early or initial symptom of a peripheral CN VII nerve palsy: patient holds phone away from ear because of painful sensitivity to sound. Loss of taste also may occur on affected side.

Left Peripheral (CN VII) Facial Weakness

Attempt to close eye results in eyeball rolling superiorly, exposing sclera (Bell's phenomenon) but no closure of the lid per se.

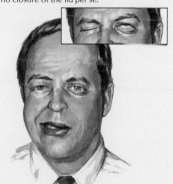

Patient unable to wrinkle forehead; eyelid droops very slightly; cannot show teeth at all on affected side in attempt to smile; and lower lip droops slightly.

Left Central (CN VII) Facial Weakness

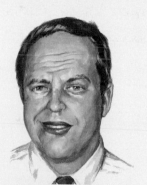

Incomplete smile with very subtle flattening of affected nasolabial fold; relative preservation of brow and forehead movement.

Sites of lesions and their manifestations (sites numbered in top image)

1. Intracranial and/or internal auditory meatus
   All symptoms of 2, 3, and 4, plus deafness due to involvement of vestibulocochlear nerve (CN VIII).

2. Geniculate ganglion
   All symptoms of 3 and 4, plus pain behind ear. Herpes of tympanum and of external auditory meatus may occur.

3. Facial canal
   All symptoms of 4, plus loss of taste in anterior tongue and decreased salivation on affected side due to chorda tympani involvement. Hyperacusis due to effect on nerve branch to stapedius muscle.

4. Below stylomastoid foramen (parotid gland tumor, trauma)
   Facial paralysis (mouth draws to opposite side; on affected side, patient unable to close eye or wrinkle forehead; food collects between teeth and cheek due to paralysis of buccinator muscle).

Clinical Focus 8.19

Tetanus

The PNS motor unit is vulnerable to three bacteria-produced toxins: tetanospasmin (motor neuron), diphtheria toxin (peripheral nerve), and botulin (neuromuscular junction). The hearty spore of *Clostridium tetani* is commonly found in soil, dust, and feces and can enter the body through wounds, blisters, burns, skin ulcers, insect bites, and surgical procedures. Symptoms include restlessness, low-grade fever, and stiffness or soreness. Eventually, nuchal rigidity, trismus (lockjaw), dysphagia, laryngospasm, and acute, massive muscle spasms can occur. Prophylaxis (immunization) is the best management.

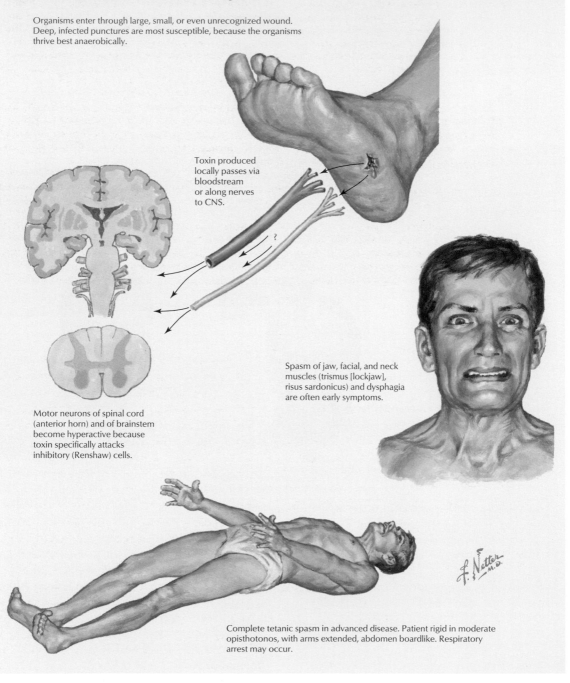

Organisms enter through large, small, or even unrecognized wound. Deep, infected punctures are most susceptible, because the organisms thrive best anaerobically.

Toxin produced locally passes via bloodstream or along nerves to CNS.

Motor neurons of spinal cord (anterior horn) and of brainstem become hyperactive because toxin specifically attacks inhibitory (Renshaw) cells.

Spasm of jaw, facial, and neck muscles (trismus [lockjaw], risus sardonicus) and dysphagia are often early symptoms.

Complete tetanic spasm in advanced disease. Patient rigid in moderate opisthotonos, with arms extended, abdomen boardlike. Respiratory arrest may occur.

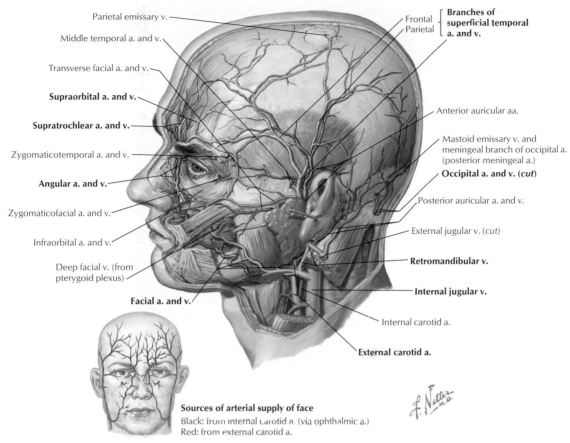

Parietal emissary v.
Middle temporal a. and v.
Transverse facial a. and v.
Supraorbital a. and v.
Supratrochlear a. and v.
Zygomaticotemporal a. and v.
Angular a. and v.
Zygomaticofacial a. and v.
Infraorbital a. and v.
Deep facial v. (from pterygoid plexus)
Facial a. and v.

Frontal ⎫ **Branches of**
Parietal ⎬ **superficial temporal**
        ⎭ **a. and v.**

Anterior auricular aa.
Mastoid emissary v. and meningeal branch of occipital a. (posterior meningeal a.)
Occipital a. and v. (*cut*)
Posterior auricular a. and v.
External jugular v. (*cut*)
Retromandibular v.
Internal jugular v.
Internal carotid a.
External carotid a.

Sources of arterial supply of face
Black: from internal carotid a. (via ophthalmic a.)
Red: from external carotid a.

FIGURE 8.17 Arteries and Veins of the Face. (From *Netter's atlas of human anatomy,* ed 8, Plate 16; S-343.)

- **Ophthalmic artery**: arises from the internal carotid artery and distributes its terminal branches over the forehead.
- **Facial vein:** drains into the internal jugular vein, directly or as a common facial vein.
- **Retromandibular vein:** formed by the union of the maxillary and superficial temporal veins; ultimately drains into the external and/or the internal jugular vein.
- **Ophthalmic veins:** tributaries from the forehead drain into superior and inferior ophthalmic veins in the orbit (and also anastomose with the facial vein) and then posteriorly into the cavernous dural sinus and/or the pterygoid plexus of veins in the infratemporal region (see Fig. 8.32).

6. ORBIT AND EYE

Bony Orbit

The bones contributing to the orbit include the following (Fig. 8.18):

- **Frontal** (orbital surface).
- **Maxilla** (orbital surface).
- **Zygomatic** (orbital surface).
- **Sphenoid.**
- **Palatine** (orbital plate).
- **Ethmoid** (orbital plate).
- **Lacrimal.**

The back of the orbit has three large openings that include the following:

- **Superior orbital fissure:** CN III, IV, VI, and V_1 (frontal, lacrimal, and nasociliary nerves) pass through the fissure along with the ophthalmic vein.
- **Inferior orbital fissure:** CN V_2 and infraorbital vessels pass through this fissure.
- **Optic canal:** CN II and the ophthalmic artery pass through this canal.

The periosteum of the orbital bones is a distinct layer of connective tissue called the **periorbita.** It is continuous with the pericranium (periosteum) covering the skull and, where the orbit communicates with the cranial cavity (e.g., superior orbital fissure),

Right orbit: frontal and slightly lateral view

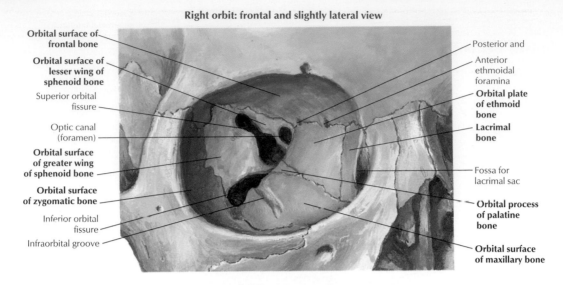

Orbital surface of frontal bone
Orbital surface of lesser wing of sphenoid bone
Superior orbital fissure
Optic canal (foramen)
Orbital surface of greater wing of sphenoid bone
Orbital surface of zygomatic bone
Inferior orbital fissure
Infraorbital groove

Posterior and
Anterior ethmoidal foramina
Orbital plate of ethmoid bone
Lacrimal bone
Fossa for lacrimal sac
Orbital process of palatine bone
Orbital surface of maxillary bone

Muscle attachments and nerves and vessels entering right orbit

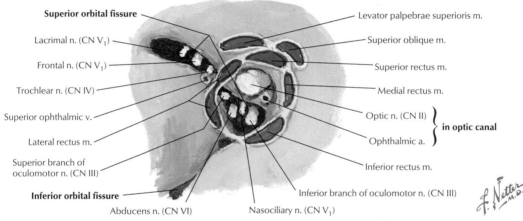

Superior orbital fissure
Lacrimal n. (CN V₁)
Frontal n. (CN V₁)
Trochlear n. (CN IV)
Superior ophthalmic v.
Lateral rectus m.
Superior branch of oculomotor n. (CN III)
Inferior orbital fissure
Abducens n. (CN VI)
Nasociliary n. (CN V₁)
Inferior branch of oculomotor n. (CN III)
Inferior rectus m.
Ophthalmic a.
Optic n. (CN II) } in optic canal
Medial rectus m.
Superior rectus m.
Superior oblique m.
Levator palpebrae superioris m.

FIGURE 8.18 Bony Orbit and Its Openings. (From *Netter's atlas of human anatomy*, ed 8, Plates 25 and BP 27; S-123 and S-BP7.)

the periorbita is continuous with the *periosteal layer of the dura mater.*

Eyelids and Lacrimal Apparatus

The eyelids protect the eyeballs and keep the corneas moist. Each eyelid contains a **tarsal plate** of dense connective tissue; **tarsal glands** that secrete an oily mixture into the tears; modified **sebaceous glands** associated with each eyelash; **apocrine glands** (modified sweat glands); **accessory lacrimal glands** along the inner surface of the upper eyelid; and in the superior eyelid only, a small slip of **smooth muscle (superior tarsal [Müller's] muscle)**, which attaches to the tarsal plate along with the **levator palpebrae superioris muscle** (Fig. 8.19). The tears contain albumins, lactoferrin, lysozyme, lipids, metabolites, and electrolytes. The

lacrimal glands *secrete continuously,* and as one blinks, the tears are evenly spread across the conjunctiva and cornea. Tears not only keep the eye surface moist but also possess antimicrobial properties. The lacrimal apparatus includes the following structures (Fig. 8.19):

- **Lacrimal glands:** secrete tears; innervated by the facial nerve postganglionic parasympathetic fibers.
- **Lacrimal ducts:** excretory ducts of the glands.
- **Lacrimal canaliculi:** collect tears into openings on the medial aspect of each lid called the puncta, and convey them to the lacrimal sacs.
- **Lacrimal sacs:** collect tears and release them into the nasolacrimal duct when one blinks (contraction of the orbicularis oculi muscle).

Clinical Focus 8.20

Orbital Blow-Out Fracture

A massive zygomaticomaxillary complex fracture or a direct blow to the front of the orbit (e.g., by baseball or fist) may cause a rapid increase in intraorbital pressure resulting in a blow-out fracture of the *thin orbital floor*. In severe comminuted fractures of the orbital floor, the orbital soft tissues may herniate into the underlying maxillary paranasal sinus. Clinical signs include diplopia, infraorbital nerve paresthesia, enophthalmos, edema, and ecchymosis.

Clinical findings

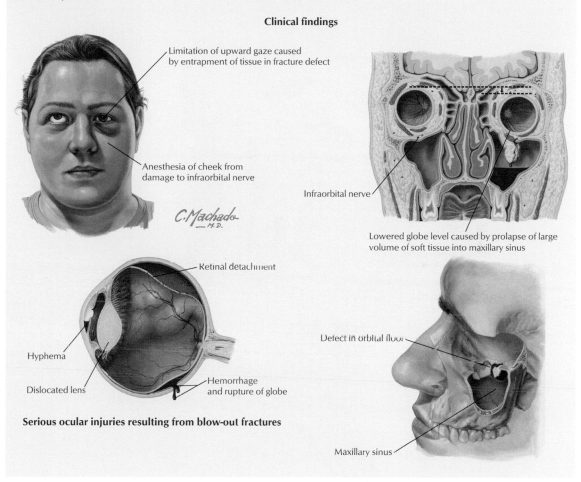

Limitation of upward gaze caused by entrapment of tissue in fracture defect

Anesthesia of cheek from damage to infraorbital nerve

C. Machado — M.D.

Infraorbital nerve

Lowered globe level caused by prolapse of large volume of soft tissue into maxillary sinus

Retinal detachment

Hyphema

Dislocated lens

Hemorrhage and rupture of globe

Defect in orbital floor

Maxillary sinus

Serious ocular injuries resulting from blow-out fractures

- **Nasolacrimal ducts:** convey tears from lacrimal sacs to the inferior meatus of the nasal cavity.

The lacrimal glands receive secretomotor parasympathetic fibers from the facial nerve (CN VII) that originate in the **superior salivatory nucleus.** These preganglionic parasympathetic fibers travel in the greater petrosal nerve and in the nerve of the pterygoid canal (vidian nerve), and the fibers then synapse in the **pterygopalatine ganglion.** Postganglionic parasympathetic fibers travel through the maxillary nerve (CN V_2), zygomatic nerve, and lacrimal nerve (CN V_1) to the lacrimal gland (see Figs. 8.72 and 8.73). Some of the postganglionic sympathetic nerves from the **superior cervical ganglion (SCG)** pass from the internal carotid plexus and form the deep petrosal nerve, join the greater petrosal nerve, and form the **nerve of the pterygoid canal**. These postganglionic sympathetic fibers (largely **vasomotor** in function) then follow the same course up to the lacrimal glands. The sensory innervation of the lacrimal gland is through the ophthalmic division of the trigeminal nerve (via the lacrimal branch).

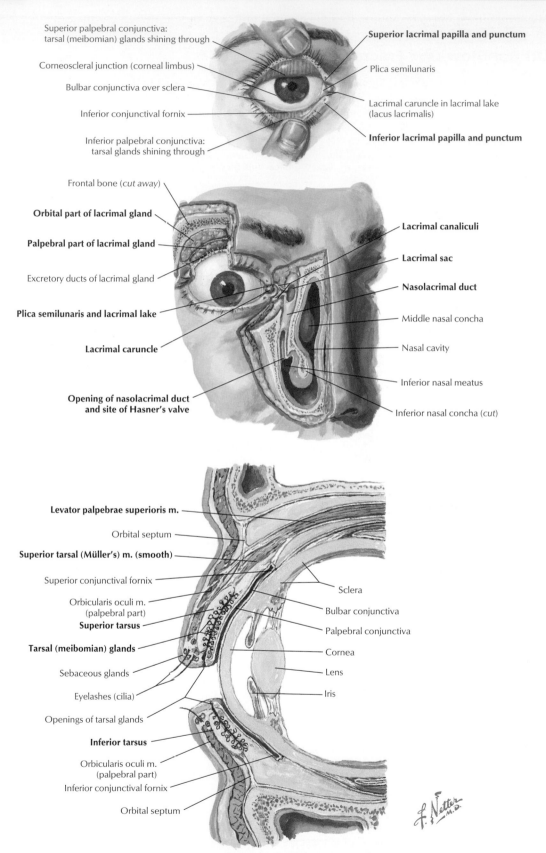

Superior palpebral conjunctiva: tarsal (meibomian) glands shining through

Corneoscleral junction (corneal limbus)

Bulbar conjunctiva over sclera

Inferior conjunctival fornix

Inferior palpebral conjunctiva: tarsal glands shining through

Superior lacrimal papilla and punctum

Plica semilunaris

Lacrimal caruncle in lacrimal lake (lacus lacrimalis)

Inferior lacrimal papilla and punctum

Frontal bone (*cut away*)

Orbital part of lacrimal gland

Palpebral part of lacrimal gland

Excretory ducts of lacrimal gland

Plica semilunaris and lacrimal lake

Lacrimal caruncle

Opening of nasolacrimal duct and site of Hasner's valve

Lacrimal canaliculi

Lacrimal sac

Nasolacrimal duct

Middle nasal concha

Nasal cavity

Inferior nasal meatus

Inferior nasal concha (*cut*)

Levator palpebrae superioris m.

Orbital septum

Superior tarsal (Müller's) m. (smooth)

Superior conjunctival fornix

Orbicularis oculi m. (palpebral part)

Superior tarsus

Tarsal (meibomian) glands

Sebaceous glands

Eyelashes (cilia)

Openings of tarsal glands

Inferior tarsus

Orbicularis oculi m. (palpebral part)

Inferior conjunctival fornix

Orbital septum

Sclera

Bulbar conjunctiva

Palpebral conjunctiva

Cornea

Lens

Iris

FIGURE 8.19 Eyelids and Lacrimal Apparatus. (From *Netter's atlas of human anatomy,* ed 8, Plates 110 and 111; S-82 and S-83.)

Clinical Focus 8.21

Clinical Testing of the Extraocular Muscles

Because extraocular muscles act as synergists and antagonists and may be responsible for multiple movements (see Table 8.6), it is difficult to test each muscle individually. However, the generalist physician can check extraocular muscle (or nerve) impairment by assessing the ability of individual muscles to elevate or depress the globe with the eye abducted or adducted, **thereby aligning the globe with the *pull* (line of contraction) of the muscle.** Generally, intorsion and extorsion are too difficult to assess in a routine eye examination. The examiner can use an **H pattern** to assess how each eye tracks movement of an object (the tester's finger). For example, when the finger is held up and to the right of the patient's eyes, the patient must primarily use the superior rectus (SR) muscle of the right eye and the inferior oblique (IO) muscle of the left eye to focus on the finger. Pure abduction is done by the lateral rectus muscle, and pure adduction is done by the medial rectus muscle. In all other cases, two muscles elevate the eye (SR and IO, with minimal intorsion or extorsion) and two muscles depress the eye (inferior rectus and superior oblique muscles, with minimal intorsion or extorsion) in abduction and adduction, respectively. At the end of this test, the examiner can bring the finger directly to the midline to test convergence (medial rectus muscles of both eyes). If an eye movement disorder is detected by this method, a clinical specialist may be consulted for further evaluation.

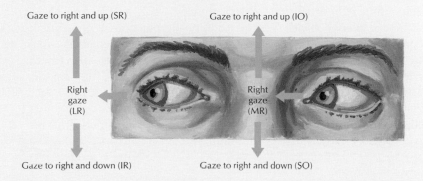

Gaze to right and up (SR)   Gaze to right and up (IO)

Right gaze (LR)   Right gaze (MR)

Gaze to right and down (IR)   Gaze to right and down (SO)

RIGHT EYE	LEFT EYE
Right gaze: Lateral rectus (CN VI) Right gaze-up: Superior rectus (CN III) Right gaze-down: Inferior rectus (CN III)	Right gaze: Medial rectus (CN III) Right gaze-up: Inferior oblique (CN III) Right gaze-down: Superior oblique (CN IV)

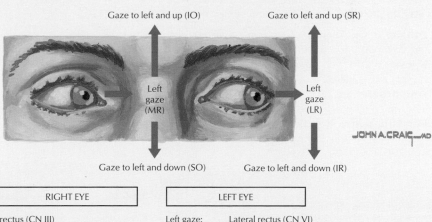

Gaze to left and up (IO)   Gaze to left and up (SR)

Left gaze (MR)   Left gaze (LR)

Gaze to left and down (SO)   Gaze to left and down (IR)

JOHN A.CRAIG—MD

RIGHT EYE	LEFT EYE
Left gaze: Medial rectus (CN III) Left gaze-up: Inferior oblique (CN III) Left gaze-down: Superior oblique (CN IV)	Left gaze: Lateral rectus (CN VI) Left gaze-up: Superior rectus (CN III) Left gaze-down: Inferior rectus (CN III)

Six cardinal positions of gaze place each eye in the field of action of a single extraocular muscle, and allow testing of the action of each muscle and its innervation.

Muscles

The orbital muscles include **six extraocular skeletal muscles** that move the eyeball and one skeletal muscle that elevates the upper eyelid (Fig. 8.20 and Table 8.6). In addition to the movements of elevation, depression, abduction, and adduction, the superior rectus and superior oblique muscles medially rotate *(intorsion)* the eyeball, and the inferior rectus and inferior oblique muscles laterally rotate *(extorsion)* the eyeball. The actions of the extraocular muscles detailed in Table 8.6 reflect their **"anatomical" actions;** because of how the muscles insert into the globe, any single action of the eye often involves multiple muscles contracting at the same time. For example, two muscles elevate the eyeball (superior rectus and inferior oblique muscles), and three muscles abduct the eyeball (lateral rectus, superior oblique, and inferior oblique muscles). Clinically, one needs to "isolate" the multiple actions of the muscles so that an individual muscle's action can be assessed (e.g., elevation or depression; see Clinical Focus 8.21). Therefore, it is important for clinicians to understand how to *"clinically assess"* the individual extraocular muscles, because this is how one will diagnose extraocular muscle weakness and/or nerve lesions (CN III, CN IV, and CN VI) (Clinical Focus 8.21).

The **levator palpebrae superioris muscle** elevates the upper eyelid and, from its distal inferior surface, has a small amount of smooth muscle **(superior tarsal muscle)** connecting it to the tarsal plate (Fig. 8.19, *bottom* image). This smooth muscle is innervated by postganglionic sympathetic fibers from the superior cervical ganglion. The interruption of this sympathetic pathway can lead to a moderate or **partial ptosis,** or drooping, of the upper eyelid ipsilaterally. Interruption of the innervation of the levator palpebrae superioris from CN III, on the other hand, can lead to a *significant ptosis.*

Nerves in the Orbit

Three cranial nerves innervate the extraocular skeletal muscles (CN III, CN IV, and CN VI) (Table 8.6). Additionally, one cranial nerve mediates the special sense of sight (CN II), and one cranial nerve conveys general sensory information from the orbit and eye (CN V_1) (Fig. 8.21). The major branches of the **ophthalmic nerve** (CN V_1) include the following:

- **Frontal:** runs on the superior aspect of the levator palpebrae superioris muscle and ends

---

Clinical Focus 8.22

Horner's Syndrome

Horner's syndrome occurs when there is a lesion somewhere along the pathway of the **sympathetic fibers** traveling to the head, usually from the sympathetic trunk distally. The cardinal signs are as follows:

- **Ptosis:** partial drooping of the upper eyelid on the affected side caused by paralysis of the superior tarsal smooth muscle in the free edge of the levator palpebrae superioris muscle.
- **Miosis:** pupillary constriction on the affected side caused by the paralysis of the pupillary dilator smooth muscle in the iris.
- **Anhidrosis:** loss of sweating on the affected side of the head caused by loss of sweat gland innervation by the sympathetic fibers.
- **Flushed, warm dry skin:** vasodilation of the subcutaneous arteries on the affected side caused by a lack of sympathetic vasoconstriction tone and sweat gland innervation.

Interruption of the sympathetic fibers outside the brain causes ipsilateral ptosis, anhidrosis, and miosis without abnormal ocular mobility.

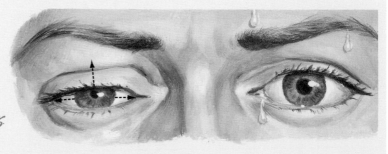

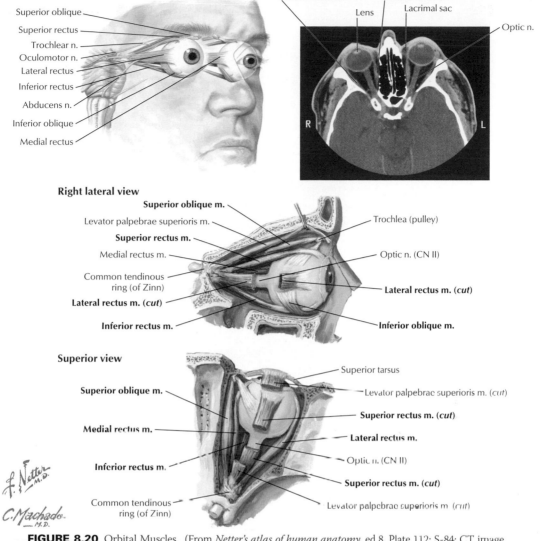

FIGURE 8.20 Orbital Muscles. (From *Netter's atlas of human anatomy,* ed 8, Plate 112; S-84; CT image from Kelley LL, Petersen C: *Sectional anatomy for imaging professionals,* Philadelphia, 2007, Mosby.)

TABLE 8.6 Summary of Orbital Muscles

MUSCLE	ORIGIN ATTACHMENT	INSERTION ATTACHMENT	INNERVATION	MAIN ACTIONS
Levator palpebrae superioris	Lesser wing of sphenoid bone, anterosuperior optic canal	Tarsal plate and skin of upper eyelid	Oculomotor nerve	Elevates upper eyelid
Superior rectus	Common tendinous ring	Superior aspect of eyeball, posterior to the corneoscleral junction	Oculomotor nerve	Elevates, adducts, and rotates eyeball medially
Inferior rectus	Common tendinous ring	Inferior aspect of eyeball, posterior to corneoscleral junction	Oculomotor nerve	Depresses, adducts, and rotates eyeball laterally
Medial rectus	Common tendinous ring	Medial aspect of eyeball, posterior to corneoscleral junction	Oculomotor nerve	Adducts eyeball
Lateral rectus	Common tendinous ring	Lateral aspect of eyeball, posterior to corneoscleral junction	Abducens nerve	Abducts eyeball
Superior oblique	Body of sphenoid bone (above optic canal)	Passes through trochlea and inserts into sclera	Trochlear nerve	Medially rotates, depresses, and abducts eyeball
Inferior oblique	Anterior floor of orbit	Sclera deep to lateral rectus muscle	Oculomotor nerve	Laterally rotates and elevates and abducts eyeball

Variations in spinal nerve contributions to the innervation of muscles, their attachments, and their actions are common in human anatomy. Therefore, expect differences between texts and realize that anatomical variation is normal.

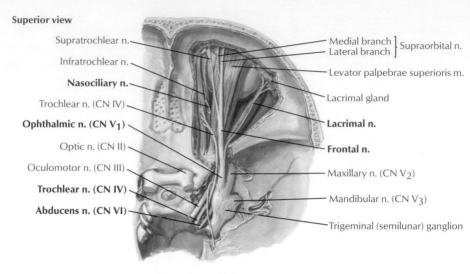

Superior view

Supratrochlear n.
Infratrochlear n.
Nasociliary n.
Trochlear n. (CN IV)
Ophthalmic n. (CN V₁)
Optic n. (CN II)
Oculomotor n. (CN III)
Trochlear n. (CN IV)
Abducens n. (CN VI)

Medial branch ⎤
Lateral branch ⎦ Supraorbital n.
Levator palpebrae superioris m.
Lacrimal gland
Lacrimal n.
Frontal n.
Maxillary n. (CN V₂)
Mandibular n. (CN V₃)
Trigeminal (semilunar) ganglion

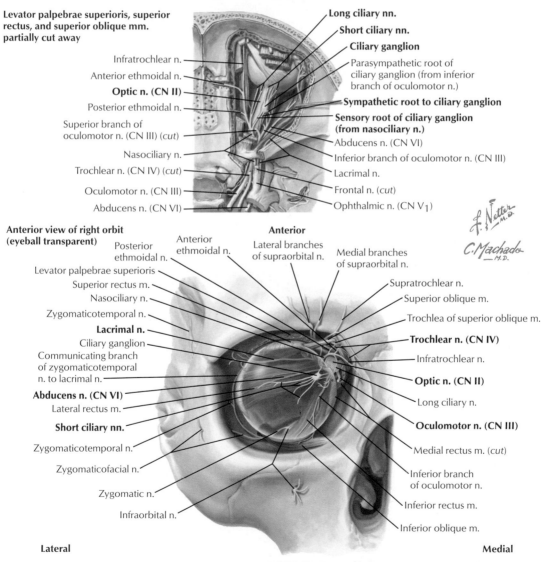

Levator palpebrae superioris, superior
rectus, and superior oblique mm.
partially cut away

Infratrochlear n.
Anterior ethmoidal n.
Optic n. (CN II)
Posterior ethmoidal n.
Superior branch of
oculomotor n. (CN III) (cut)
Nasociliary n.
Trochlear n. (CN IV) (cut)
Oculomotor n. (CN III)
Abducens n. (CN VI)

Long ciliary nn.
Short ciliary nn.
Ciliary ganglion
Parasympathetic root of
ciliary ganglion (from inferior
branch of oculomotor n.)
Sympathetic root to ciliary ganglion
**Sensory root of ciliary ganglion
(from nasociliary n.)**
Abducens n. (CN VI)
Inferior branch of oculomotor n. (CN III)
Lacrimal n.
Frontal n. (cut)
Ophthalmic n. (CN V₁)

Anterior view of right orbit
(eyeball transparent)

Posterior
ethmoidal n.
Levator palpebrae superioris
Superior rectus m.
Nasociliary n.
Zygomaticotemporal n.
Lacrimal n.
Ciliary ganglion
Communicating branch
of zygomaticotemporal
n. to lacrimal n.
Abducens n. (CN VI)
Lateral rectus m.
Short ciliary nn.
Zygomaticotemporal n.
Zygomaticofacial n.
Zygomatic n.
Infraorbital n.

Anterior
ethmoidal n.

Anterior

Lateral branches
of supraorbital n.

Medial branches
of supraorbital n.

Supratrochlear n.
Superior oblique m.
Trochlea of superior oblique m.
Trochlear n. (CN IV)
Infratrochlear n.
Optic n. (CN II)
Long ciliary n.
Oculomotor n. (CN III)
Medial rectus m. (cut)
Inferior branch
of oculomotor n.
Inferior rectus m.
Inferior oblique m.

Lateral

Medial

FIGURE 8.21 Nerves of the Orbit. (From *Netter's atlas of human anatomy*, ed 8, Plates 113 and 114; S-85 and S-86.)

as the **supratrochlear** and **supraorbital nerves;** sensory to forehead, scalp, frontal sinus, and upper eyelid.

- **Lacrimal:** courses laterally on the superior aspect of the lateral rectus muscle to the lacrimal gland; sensory to conjunctiva and skin of the upper eyelid, and the lacrimal gland.
- **Nasociliary:** gives rise to short and long ciliary nerves, posterior and anterior ethmoidal nerves, and infratrochlear nerve; sensory to iris and cornea, sphenoid and ethmoid sinuses, lower eyelid, lacrimal sac, and skin of the anterior nose.

The **optic nerve** (CN II) is actually a brain tract that conveys sensory information from the retina, via the ganglion cell axons, to the brain (see Fig. 8.13). The optic nerve is covered by the same three meningeal layers as the rest of the CNS, and the retina is really our "window" into the brain (see Clinical Focus 8.25).

In addition to supplying five of the seven skeletal muscles in the orbit (see Table 8.6), the **oculomotor nerve** (CN III) also provides **parasympathetic** fibers, which exhibit the following features (see Figs. 8.69 and 8.71):

- Preganglionic parasympathetic fibers arise centrally from the **nucleus of Edinger-Westphal** (accessory oculomotor nucleus) and course along CN III and its inferior division to synapse in the **ciliary ganglion** on postganglionic parasympathetic neurons.
- Postganglionic parasympathetic fibers then course via **short ciliary nerves** to the eyeball.
- These postganglionic fibers innervate the **sphincter muscle of the pupil** (sphincter pupillae) and the **ciliary muscle** for accommodation of the lens.

Sympathetic innervation to the eyeball is arranged as follows (see Figs. 8.69–8.71):

- Preganglionic sympathetic nerve fibers arise from the **upper thoracic intermediolateral cell column** of the spinal cord (T1-T2) and send preganglionic fibers into the sympathetic trunk, where these fibers ascend to synapse in the **superior cervical ganglion** (SCG).
- Postganglionic sympathetic fibers course along the internal carotid artery, enter the orbit on the ophthalmic artery and ophthalmic nerve, and pass through the ciliary ganglion or along the **long and short ciliary nerves** to the eyeball.
- These postganglionic fibers innervate the **dilator muscle of the pupil** (dilator pupillae) and the

superior tarsal muscle by joining the oculomotor nerve to the upper eyelid.

Eyeball (Globe)

The human eyeball measures about 25 mm in diameter, is tethered in the bony orbit by six extraocular muscles that move the globe, and is cushioned by fat that surrounds the posterior two-thirds of the globe (Fig. 8.22). The outer fibrous white coat of the eyeball is the **sclera** and is continuous anteriorly with the **transparent cornea.** A middle vascular layer called the **choroid** is continuous anteriorly with the *ciliary body, ciliary process, and iris.* It provides oxygen and nutrients to the underlying retina. The inner layer is the optically receptive **retina** posteriorly and an anterior nonvisual retinal extension that lines the internal surface of the ciliary body and iris (Table 8.7).

The large chamber behind the lens is the **vitreous chamber** (body) and is filled with a gel-like substance called the **vitreous humor,** which helps cushion and protect the fragile retina during rapid eye movements (see Fig. 8.22).

The chamber between the cornea and the iris is the **anterior chamber;** the space between the iris and lens is the **posterior chamber.** Both chambers are filled with **aqueous humor,** which is produced by the **ciliary body** and circulates from the posterior chamber, through the pupil, and into the anterior chamber, where it is absorbed by the trabecular meshwork into the **scleral venous sinus** (canal of Schlemm) at the angle of the cornea and iris.

Retina

The retina consists of the optic or **neural retina,** which is sensitive to light, and the **nonvisual retina,** which lines the internal surface of the ciliary body and iris. The junction separating the neural from the nonvisual retina is called the **ora serrata** (see Fig. 8.22).

The neural retina is composed of an outer **retinal pigmented epithelium** lying adjacent to the vascular choroid and a photosensitive region consisting of photoreceptive cells: **rods** are more sensitive to light and are the receptors for low-light conditions (gray tones); **cones** are less sensitive to low light but are very sensitive to red, green, and blue regions of the visual spectrum. Interspersed layers of conducting and association neurons and supporting cells lie more internally in the retina, closer to the vitreous body.

The axons of ganglion cells ultimately convey the photosensory information to the **optic disc,**

Clinical Focus 8.23

Eyelid Infections and Conjunctival Disorders

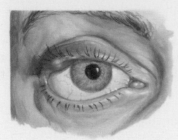

Acute meibomianitis

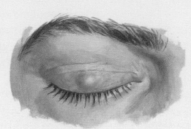

Chalazion

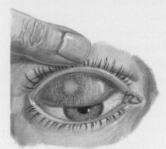

Chalazion; lid everted

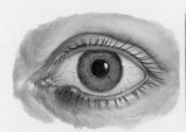

Hordeolum (sty) of lower lid

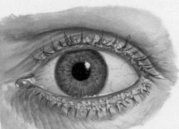

Blepharitis

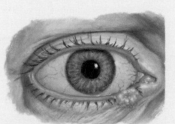

Carcinoma of lower lid

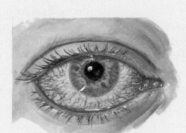

Conjunctivitis

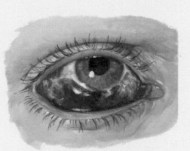

Subconjunctival hemorrhage

Condition	Description
Meibomianitis	Inflammation of meibomian (tarsal) glands
Chalazion	Cyst formation in meibomian gland
Hordeolum (sty)	Infection of sebaceous gland at base of eyelash follicle
Blepharitis	Inflammation of eyelash margin (scaly or ulcerated)
Conjunctival hyperemia (bloodshot eye)	Dilated, congested conjunctival vessels caused by local irritants (e.g., dust, smoke) (not illustrated)
Conjunctivitis (pink eye)	Common inflammation; result of injection of conjunctival vessels caused by allergy, infection, or external irritant
Subconjunctival hemorrhage	Painless, homogeneous red area; result of rupture of subconjunctival capillaries

where the axons course in the optic nerve and are relayed centrally. The optic disc is our "blind spot" because no cones or rods are present in this region of the retina.

The **fovea centralis** of the macula is the *central focusing area* and most sensitive portion of the retina. This region is thin because most of the other layers of the retina are absent. Here the photoreceptor layer consists *only of cones,* specialized for color vision and acute discrimination.

Accommodation of the Lens

The **ciliary body** contains smooth muscle arranged in a circular fashion like a **sphincter** (see Fig. 8.22). When relaxed, it pulls a set of zonular fibers attached to the elastic lens taut and *flattens the lens* for viewing objects at some distance from the eye. When focusing on near objects, the sphincter-like ciliary muscle (parasympathetically innervated by CN III) contracts and constricts closer to the lens, *relaxing the zonular fibers* and allowing the

TABLE 8.7 Features of the Eyeball

STRUCTURE	DEFINITION	STRUCTURE	DEFINITION
Sclera	Outer fibrous layer of eyeball	Refractive media	Light rays focused by the cornea, aqueous humor, lens, and vitreous humor
Cornea	Transparent part of outer layer; very sensitive to pain		
Choroid	Vascular middle layer of eyeball	Retina	Optically receptive part of optic nerve (optic retina); contains rods (dim light vision) and cones (color vision)
Conjunctiva	Thin membrane that lines the inner aspect of the eyelids and reflects onto the sclera, ending at the scleral-corneal junction	Macula lutea	Yellowish region of retina lateral to the optic disc that contains the fovea centralis
Ciliary body	Vascular and muscular extension of choroid anteriorly	Fovea centralis	Area of macula with the most acute vision; contains only cones and is the center of the visual axis (ideal focus point)
Ciliary process	Radiating pigmented ridge on ciliary body; secretes aqueous humor that fills posterior and anterior chambers		
Iris	Contractile diaphragm with central aperture (pupil)	Optic disc	Nonreceptive area (blind spot) where retinal ganglion cell nerve axons leave the retina in the optic nerve and pass to the brain
Lens	Transparent lens supported in capsule by zonular fibers		

Clinical Focus 8.24

Papilledema

The optic nerve is a tract of the brain and is therefore surrounded by the three meningeal layers that cover the CNS. The subarachnoid space extends along the nerve to the point where it attaches to the posterior aspect of the eyeball. If intracranial pressure is increased, this pressure also compresses the optic nerve and its venous return through the retinal veins. This results in edema of the optic disc, which can be detected by ophthalmoscopic examination (see Fig. 8.22).

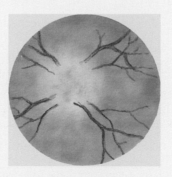

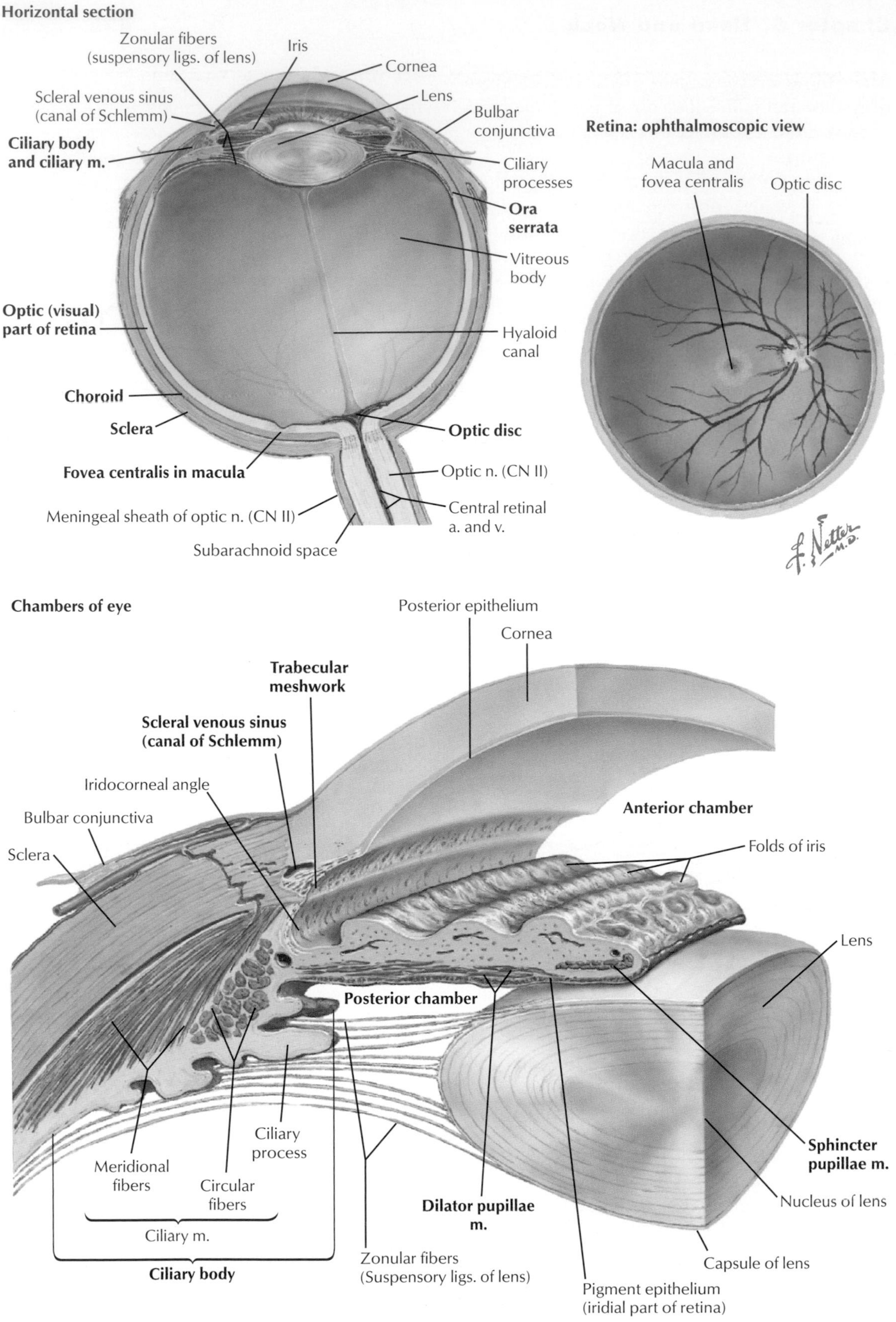

Horizontal section

Zonular fibers
(suspensory ligs. of lens)
Iris
Cornea
Scleral venous sinus
(canal of Schlemm)
Lens
**Ciliary body
and ciliary m.**
Bulbar
conjunctiva
Ciliary
processes
**Ora
serrata**
Vitreous
body
**Optic (visual)
part of retina**
Hyaloid
canal
Choroid
Sclera
Optic disc
Fovea centralis in macula
Optic n. (CN II)
Meningeal sheath of optic n. (CN II)
Central retinal
a. and v.
Subarachnoid space

Retina: ophthalmoscopic view

Macula and
fovea centralis
Optic disc

Chambers of eye

Posterior epithelium
Cornea
**Trabecular
meshwork**
**Scleral venous sinus
(canal of Schlemm)**
Iridocorneal angle
Anterior chamber
Bulbar conjunctiva
Sclera
Folds of iris
Lens
Posterior chamber
Meridional
fibers
Circular
fibers
Ciliary
process
**Dilator pupillae
m.**
Zonular fibers
(Suspensory ligs. of lens)
Pigment epithelium
(iridial part of retina)
**Sphincter
pupillae m.**
Nucleus of lens
Capsule of lens
Ciliary m.
Ciliary body

Note: For clarity, only single plane of zonular fibers shown; actually, fibers surround entire circumference of lens.

FIGURE 8.22 Eyeball and Retina. (From *Netter's atlas of human anatomy*, ed 8, Plates 116, 117, and 119; S-88, S-89, and S-91.)

Clinical Focus 8.25

Diabetic Retinopathy

Diabetic retinopathy develops in almost all patients with type 1 diabetes mellitus (DM) and in 50% to 80% of patients with type 2 DM of 20 years' duration or more. Retinopathy can progress rapidly in pregnant women with type 1 DM. Diabetic retinopathy is the number-one cause of blindness in middle-aged individuals and the fourth leading cause of blindness overall in the United States.

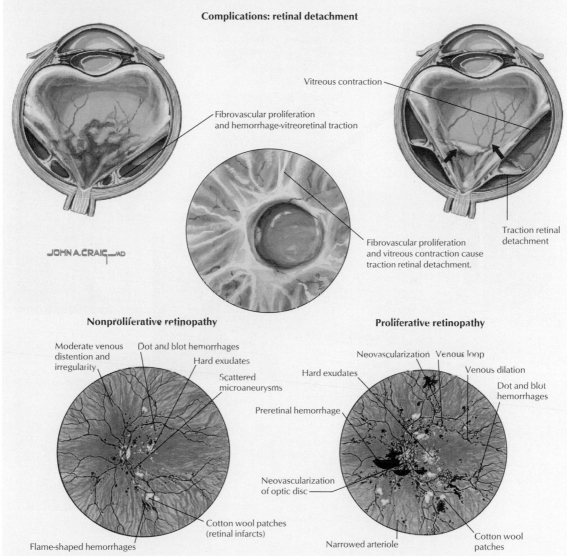

Complications: retinal detachment

Vitreous contraction

Fibrovascular proliferation and hemorrhage-vitreoretinal traction

Fibrovascular proliferation and vitreous contraction cause traction retinal detachment.

Traction retinal detachment

JOHN A. CRAIG—AD

Nonproliferative retinopathy

Moderate venous distention and irregularity

Dot and blot hemorrhages

Hard exudates

Scattered microaneurysms

Flame-shaped hemorrhages

Cotton wool patches (retinal infarcts)

Proliferative retinopathy

Neovascularization   Venous loop

Hard exudates

Venous dilation

Dot and blot hemorrhages

Preretinal hemorrhage

Neovascularization of optic disc

Narrowed arteriole

Cotton wool patches

Characteristic	Description
Etiology	Hyperglycemia through an interaction of hemodynamic, biochemical, and hormonal mechanisms leading to capillary endothelial cell damage (retinal hemorrhages, venous distention, microaneurysms, edema, and microangiopathy)
Types	Nonproliferative and proliferative (abnormal neovascularization and fibrosis)
Complications	Vitreous hemorrhage, retinal edema, retinal detachment

Clinical Focus 8.26

Glaucoma

Glaucoma is an optic neuropathy that can lead to visual field deficits and is often associated with elevated intraocular pressure (IOP).

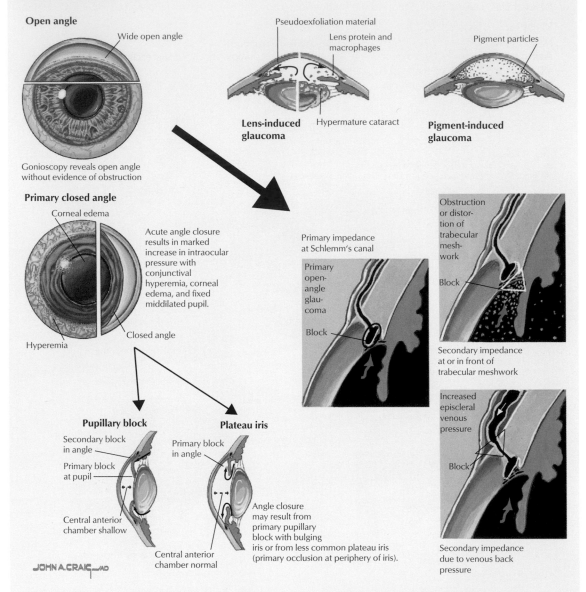

Open angle

Wide open angle

Gonioscopy reveals open angle without evidence of obstruction

Pseudoexfoliation material

Lens protein and macrophages

Lens-induced glaucoma

Hypermature cataract

Pigment particles

Pigment-induced glaucoma

Primary closed angle

Corneal edema

Hyperemia

Closed angle

Acute angle closure results in marked increase in intraocular pressure with conjunctival hyperemia, corneal edema, and fixed middilated pupil.

Primary impedance at Schlemm's canal

Primary open-angle glaucoma

Block

Obstruction or distortion of trabecular meshwork

Block

Secondary impedance at or in front of trabecular meshwork

Pupillary block

Secondary block in angle

Primary block at pupil

Central anterior chamber shallow

Plateau iris

Primary block in angle

Central anterior chamber normal

Angle closure may result from primary pupillary block with bulging iris or from less common plateau iris (primary occlusion at periphery of iris).

Increased episcleral venous pressure

Block

Secondary impedance due to venous back pressure

JOHN A. CRAIG—AD

Characteristic	Description
Etiology	Usually increased resistance to outflow of aqueous humor, which leads to increased IOP (reference range, 10–21 mm Hg)
Types	Primary open-angle glaucoma (POAG) most common; closed angle (iris blocks trabecular meshwork)
Risk factors	African-American, family history, age, increased IOP
POAG pathogenesis	Blocked canal of Schlemm (angle is normal) or from obstruction or malfunction of anterior segment angle
Closed-angle pathogenesis	Age-related anatomical changes that block angle or secondary to diseases that pull iris over angle

Clinical Focus 8.27

Ocular Refractive Disorders

Ametropia is the aberrant focusing of light rays on a site other than the optimal site on the retina (macula). Optically, the cornea, lens, and axial length of the eyeball must be in precise balance to achieve sharp focus on the macula. Common disorders include the following:

- **Myopia:** nearsightedness; 80% of ametropias (see close objects better)
- **Hyperopia:** farsightedness; age-related occurrence (see distant objects better)
- **Astigmatism:** nonspherical cornea causes focusing at multiple locations instead of at a single point; affects 25% to 40% of the U.S. population.
- **Presbyopia:** age-related progressive loss of accommodative ability (lens is less flexible); see distant objects better than close objects, e.g., trouble reading small type.

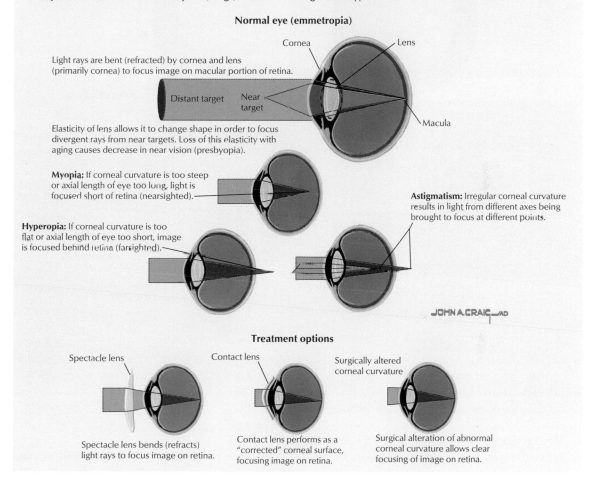

Normal eye (emmetropia)

Cornea   Lens

Light rays are bent (refracted) by cornea and lens (primarily cornea) to focus image on macular portion of retina.

Distant target   Near target

Macula

Elasticity of lens allows it to change shape in order to focus divergent rays from near targets. Loss of this elasticity with aging causes decrease in near vision (presbyopia).

Myopia: If corneal curvature is too steep or axial length of eye too long, light is focused short of retina (nearsighted).

Astigmatism: Irregular corneal curvature results in light from different axes being brought to focus at different points.

Hyperopia: If corneal curvature is too flat or axial length of eye too short, image is focused behind retina (farsighted).

JOHN A.CRAIG—MD

Treatment options

Spectacle lens   Contact lens   Surgically altered corneal curvature

Spectacle lens bends (refracts) light rays to focus image on retina.

Contact lens performs as a "corrected" corneal surface, focusing image on retina.

Surgical alteration of abnormal corneal curvature allows clear focusing of image on retina.

elastic lens to round up for *accommodation* (near vision).

Blood Supply to the Orbit and Eye

The **ophthalmic artery** arises from the internal carotid artery just as it exits the cavernous sinus, and it supplies the orbit and eye by the following branches (Fig. 8.23):

- **Central artery of the retina:** travels in the optic nerve; occlusion leads to blindness.
- **Short and long posterior ciliary arteries**: pierce the sclera and supply the ciliary body, iris, and choroid.

Clinical Focus 8.28

Cataract

A cataract is an opacity, or cloudy area, in the crystalline lens. Risk factors for cataracts include age, smoking, alcohol use, sun exposure, low educational status, diabetes, and systemic steroid use. Treatment is most often surgical, involving lens removal (patient becomes extremely farsighted); vision is corrected with glasses, contact lenses, or implanted plastic lens (intraocular lens).

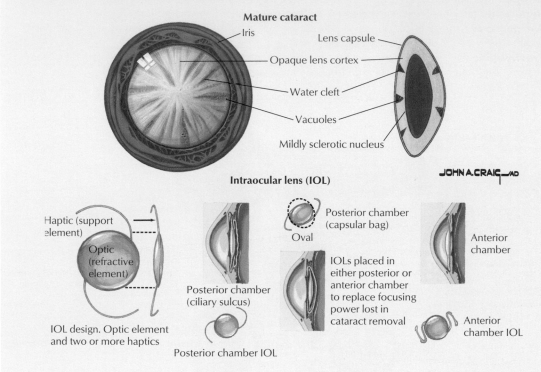

- **Lacrimal arteries:** supply the lacrimal gland, conjunctiva, and eyelids.
- **Ethmoidal arteries:** supply the ethmoid and frontal sinuses, nasal cavity, and external anterior nose.
- **Medial palpebrae arteries:** supply the eyelids.
- **Muscular arteries**: supply skeletal muscles of the orbit and smooth muscles of the eyeball.
- **Dorsal nasal arteries:** supply the lateral nose and lacrimal sac.
- **Supraorbital artery:** passes through the supraorbital notch and supplies the forehead and scalp.
- **Supratrochlear artery:** supplies the forehead and scalp.

The venous drainage is by the **superior and inferior ophthalmic veins,** with connections to the cavernous sinus posteriorly (principal drainage),

the pterygoid plexus of veins in the infratemporal fossa inferiorly, and the facial vein anteriorly (see Fig. 8.23).

7. EAR

The human ear consists of the following three parts (Fig. 8.24):

- **External:** the auricle (pinna), external acoustic meatus (conducts sound waves to the eardrum), and **tympanic membrane** (eardrum).
- **Middle:** the air-filled tympanic cavity between the eardrum and labyrinthine wall, which contains the three middle ear ossicles—**malleus, incus,** and **stapes**—and the stapedius and tensor tympani muscles; communicates posteriorly with the mastoid antrum and anteriorly with the auditory (pharyngotympanic, eustachian) tube.

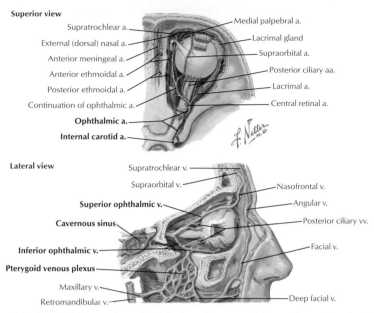

Superior view

Supratrochlear a.

External (dorsal) nasal a.

Anterior meningeal a.

Anterior ethmoidal a.

Posterior ethmoidal a.

Continuation of ophthalmic a.

Ophthalmic a.

Internal carotid a.

Medial palpebral a.

Lacrimal gland

Supraorbital a.

Posterior ciliary aa.

Lacrimal a.

Central retinal a.

Lateral view

Supratrochlear v.

Supraorbital v.

Superior ophthalmic v.

Cavernous sinus

Inferior ophthalmic v.

Pterygoid venous plexus

Maxillary v.

Retromandibular v.

Nasofrontal v.

Angular v.

Posterior ciliary vv.

Facial v.

Deep facial v.

FIGURE 8.23 Branches of Ophthalmic Artery and Veins. (From *Netter's atlas of human anatomy,* ed 8, Plate 115; S-87.)

Clinical Focus 8.29

Pupillary Light Reflex

Bright light stimulation causes a pupillary constriction response that is mediated by optic nerve (CN II) afferents (from the retina) responding to the light stimulus and evoking a **bilateral efferent response** in the nucleus of Edinger-Westphal preganglionic parasympathetic fibers. These fibers synapse in the ciliary ganglion and send postganglionic fibers to the pupillary constrictor muscle of each iris, which constricts the pupils symmetrically and bilaterally, limiting the light's effect on the retina.

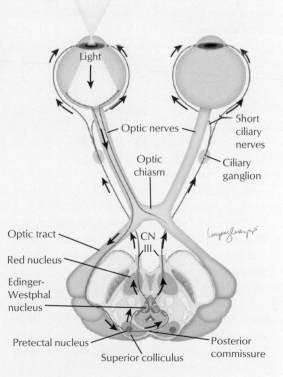

Light

Optic nerves

Optic chiasm

Short ciliary nerves

Ciliary ganglion

Optic tract

Red nucleus

Edinger-Westphal nucleus

Pretectal nucleus

CN III

Superior colliculus

Posterior commissure

- **Internal (inner):** contains the acoustic apparatus (cochlea) and vestibular apparatus (for balance), and includes the vestibule with the utricle and saccule and the three semicircular canals.

External Ear

The **auricle** is composed of skin and elastic cartilage and helps funnel sound waves into the external acoustic meatus. It is innervated by auricular branches from CN V_3, VII, and X and by the lesser occipital (C2) and greater auricular (C2-3) nerves from the cervical plexus in the neck. The **external acoustic meatus** is about 2.5 cm long and is composed of cartilage (lateral third) and bone. Its lining of skin contains hairs and modified sweat glands *(ceruminous glands)* that secrete earwax that protects the skin. It is innervated mostly by CN V_3 and CN X, with minor contributions from CN VII (concha of the auricle) and CN IX. The **tympanic membrane** lies at an oblique angle (Fig. 8.24), sloping medially from posterosuperior to anteroinferior, and is attached on its medial side to the handle of the **malleus,** which creates a depression in its middle called the *umbo.* Because of its oblique position and the umbo, the tympanic membrane gives off a reflection of light when viewed with an otoscope (the **cone of light**). Its external surface is innervated primarily by CN V_3 (auriculotemporal nerve) and a small auricular branch of CN X. Its internal surface is innervated by CN IX.

Middle Ear

The middle ear cavity resembles a box with six sides and is air filled and lined with a mucous membrane. Its boundaries include the following (Fig. 8.25):
- *Roof:* **tegmen tympani,** a layer of bone that is part of the petrous portion of the temporal bone.
- *Floor:* **jugular fossa,** a thin layer of bone separating the middle ear from the internal jugular vein.
- *Posterior wall:* an incomplete wall with a small aperture (aditus ad antrum) leading to the **mastoid air cells.**
- *Anterior wall:* an incomplete wall with a thin, bony lower portion separating the cavity from the internal carotid artery (in the carotid canal) and superiorly an opening for the **auditory** (pharyngotympanic; eustachian) **tube** and tensor tympani muscle.
- *Lateral wall:* the **tympanic membrane** and **epitympanic recess** above the eardrum; the

chorda tympani branch of CN VII passes through the cavity.
- *Medial wall:* the **labyrinthine wall** exhibiting superiorly a prominence of the lateral semicircular canal and a second prominence for CN VII; the **oval** (fenestra vestibuli) **window** for the base of the **stapes;** a promontory (basal turn of the cochlea), with the tympanic nerve plexus (CN IX) on its surface; and most inferiorly the **round** (fenestra cochlea) **window** covered with a membrane.

Vibrations of the eardrum cause the three middle ear ossicles to vibrate, which causes the base of the stapes to vibrate against the **oval window** and thus initiates a wave action within the fluid-filled **scala vestibuli** (filled with **perilymph**) and **scala tympani** of the cochlea (described in the next section). The **stapedius** (smallest skeletal muscle in the body) and **tensor tympani muscles** dampen excessive vibrations in the stapes (stapedius) and eardrum (tensor) in response to loud noises (Fig. 8.25).

The innervation of the middle ear is via the tympanic branch of CN IX to the **tympanic plexus** lying beneath the mucosa of the promontory on the medial wall of the middle ear. The **lesser petrosal preganglionic parasympathetic nerve** arises from this plexus, passes through the petrous portion of the temporal bone, runs in a hiatus just inferior to the greater petrosal nerve, and courses to the foramen ovale, where it synapses in the **otic ganglion.** The postganglionic parasympathetic fibers of the otic ganglion innervate the parotid salivary gland through the auriculotemporal branch of CN V_3 (see Temporal Region).

Internal Ear

The internal ear houses the special senses of hearing and balance and comprises the following two elements (Figs. 8.24 and 8.26):
- **Bony labyrinth:** includes the vestibule, the three semicircular canals, and the cochlea, which are all housed within the temporal bone and filled with **perilymph.**
- **Membranous labyrinth:** is suspended within the perilymph of the bony labyrinth and is filled with **endolymph**; consists of the **cochlear duct** (the organ of hearing) and the **utricle, saccule,** and **semicircular ducts** (the organs of balance).

Vibrations of the middle ear ossicles and the base plate of the stapes on the oval window initiate a wave action within the perilymph-filled scala vestibuli

Frontal section

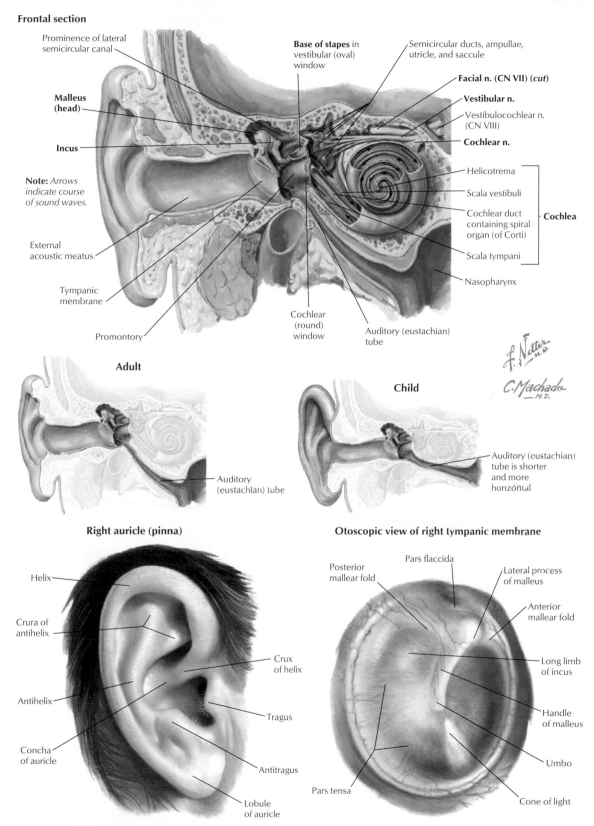

Prominence of lateral semicircular canal

Base of stapes in vestibular (oval) window

Semicircular ducts, ampullae, utricle, and saccule

Facial n. (CN VII) (*cut*)

Malleus (head)

Vestibular n.

Vestibulocochlear n. (CN VIII)

Incus

Cochlear n.

Note: *Arrows indicate course of sound waves.*

Helicotrema

Scala vestibuli

Cochlear duct containing spiral organ (of Corti)

Cochlea

External acoustic meatus

Scala tympani

Tympanic membrane

Nasopharynx

Promontory

Cochlear (round) window

Auditory (eustachian) tube

Adult

Child

Auditory (eustachian) tube

Auditory (eustachian) tube is shorter and more horizontal

Right auricle (pinna)

Otoscopic view of right tympanic membrane

Helix

Posterior mallear fold

Pars flaccida

Lateral process of malleus

Crura of antihelix

Anterior mallear fold

Crux of helix

Long limb of incus

Antihelix

Tragus

Handle of malleus

Concha of auricle

Antitragus

Umbo

Pars tensa

Cone of light

Lobule of auricle

FIGURE 8.24 General Anatomy of Right Ear. (From *Netter's atlas of human anatomy*, ed 8, Plates 121 and 122; S-93 and S-94.)

Membranous wall

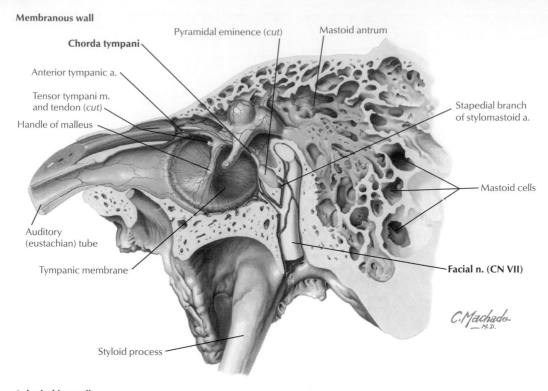

Pyramidal eminence (*cut*)

Mastoid antrum

Chorda tympani

Anterior tympanic a.

Tensor tympani m. and tendon (*cut*)

Handle of malleus

Stapedial branch of stylomastoid a.

Mastoid cells

Auditory (eustachian) tube

Tympanic membrane

Mastoid cells

Facial n. (CN VII)

Styloid process

C. Machado
_M.D.

Labyrinthine wall

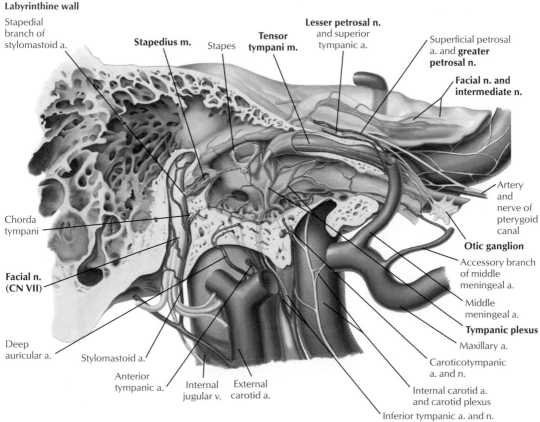

Stapedial branch of stylomastoid a.

Stapedius m.

Stapes

Tensor tympani m.

Lesser petrosal n. and superior tympanic a.

Superficial petrosal a. and **greater petrosal n.**

Facial n. and intermediate n.

Chorda tympani

Facial n. (CN VII)

Deep auricular a.

Stylomastoid a.

Anterior tympanic a.

Internal jugular v.

External carotid a.

Artery and nerve of pterygoid canal

Otic ganglion

Accessory branch of middle meningeal a.

Middle meningeal a.

Tympanic plexus

Maxillary a.

Caroticotympanic a. and n.

Internal carotid a. and carotid plexus

Inferior tympanic a. and n.

FIGURE 8.25   Walls of Right Middle Ear.   (From *Netter's atlas of human anatomy*, ed 8, Plate 123; S-95.)

Clinical Focus 8.30

Acute Otitis Externa and Otitis Media

Acute otitis externa (swimmer's ear) involves inflammation or bacterial infection of the external acoustic meatus, usually because the protective earwax has been washed from the ear. **Otitis media** is an inflammation of the middle ear and is common in children younger than 15 years because the auditory tube is short and relatively horizontal at this age, which limits drainage by gravity and provides a route for infection from the nasopharynx. When viewed with an otoscope, the normal translucent appearance of the tympanic membrane is gone, the eardrum is erythematous and bulging, and the cone of light is absent.

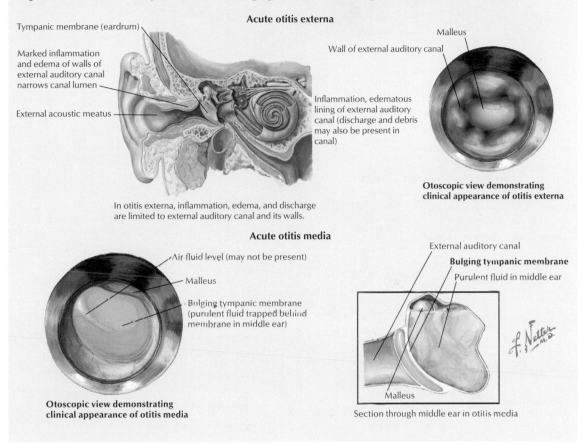

Acute otitis externa

Tympanic membrane (eardrum)

Marked inflammation and edema of walls of external auditory canal narrows canal lumen

External acoustic meatus

Wall of external auditory canal

Inflammation, edematous lining of external auditory canal (discharge and debris may also be present in canal)

Malleus

Otoscopic view demonstrating clinical appearance of otitis externa

In otitis externa, inflammation, edema, and discharge are limited to external auditory canal and its walls.

Acute otitis media

Air fluid level (may not be present)

Malleus

Bulging tympanic membrane (purulent fluid trapped behind membrane in middle ear)

External auditory canal

Bulging tympanic membrane

Purulent fluid in middle ear

Malleus

Otoscopic view demonstrating clinical appearance of otitis media

Section through middle ear in otitis media

and scala tympani of the cochlea (see Fig. 8.24, *top* image). This wave action causes the deflection and depolarization of tiny hair cells within the **organ of Corti** (membranous labyrinth). This stimulates action potentials in the afferent axons of the spiral ganglion cells that are conveyed centrally to the brain through the **vestibulocochlear nerve (CN VIII)**, with final processing in the auditory cortex of the *temporal lobe.*

A similar mechanism of depolarization also occurs in the endolymph of the vestibular system (hair cells and a single kinocilium), where the receptors for equilibrium comprise the following two functional components:

- **Static:** a special receptor called the **macula** resides in each **utricle** and **saccule;** participate in positioning of the head and linear acceleration, as well as gravity and low-frequency vibrations (saccule only).
- **Dynamic:** a special receptor called the **crista ampullaris** resides in the ampulla of each semicircular canal (anterior, lateral, and posterior canals); these receptors participate in angular (rotational) movements of the head.

Vestibular afferents passing back to the CNS provide input to help modulate and coordinate muscle movement, tone, and posture, as well as regulate head and neck movements and coordinate

Right membranous labyrinth with nerves: posteromedial view

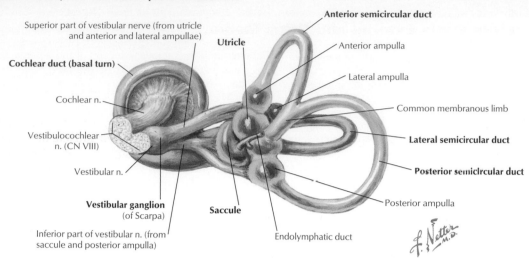

Bony and membranous labyrinths: schema

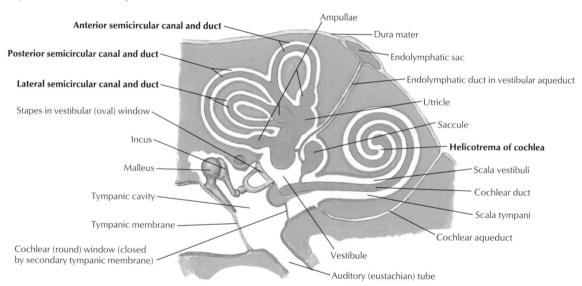

FIGURE 8.26 Structures of Right Internal Ear. (From *Netter's atlas of human anatomy*, ed 8, Plates 124 and 125; S-96 and S-97.)

eye movements. The neuronal cell bodies of these vestibular afferents reside within the **vestibular ganglion** in the internal acoustic meatus (Fig. 8.26, *top image*).

8. TEMPORAL REGION

The temporal region includes the temporal bone region and infratemporal fossa, and focuses on the muscles of mastication, the mandibular division of the trigeminal nerve (CN V₃), and the two terminal branches of the external carotid artery—the

maxillary and superficial temporal arteries. The **temporal fossa** lies superior to the zygomatic arch, and the **infratemporal fossa** is a wedge-shaped area inferior and deep to the zygomatic arch. The lateral wall of this fossa is formed by the mandibular ramus.

Muscles of Mastication

The muscles of mastication provide a coordinated set of movements that facilitate biting and chewing (grinding action of lower jaw). These muscles participate in movements of elevation, retrusion (retraction), and protrusion of the mandible. Embryologically, the muscles are derived from the first branchial arch, and all are innervated by CN V_3 (Fig. 8.27 and Table 8.8).

The **temporomandibular joint** (TMJ) is the articulation between the condylar process of the mandible and the squamous portion of the temporal bone (mandibular fossa) (Figs. 8.28 and 8.29 and Table 8.9). The TMJ is a modified hinge-type synovial joint. Unlike most synovial joints, the TMJ surfaces are covered with fibrous cartilage rather than hyaline cartilage and the joint cavity is divided by a **fibrocartilaginous articular disc.**

Parotid Gland

The parotid gland is the largest of the three pairs of salivary glands and occupies the retromandibular space between the mandibular ramus and mastoid process (see Figs. 8.15 and 8.17). It is encased within the parotid sheath, a tough extension of the deep cervical fascia. The **parotid duct** courses medially across the medial border of the masseter muscle and then dives deeply into the buccal fat pad, piercing the **buccinator muscle** of the cheek and opening in the mouth just lateral to the **second maxillary (upper) molar.** As noted previously, the terminal portion of the facial nerve to the face

Clinical Focus 8.31

Cochlear Implant

Two million Americans have profound bilateral deafness. A cochlear implant consists of a speech processor and implanted electrodes. An external microphone detects sound, which is converted by the processor into electrical signals transmitted to the cochlear implant and vestibulocochlear nerve.

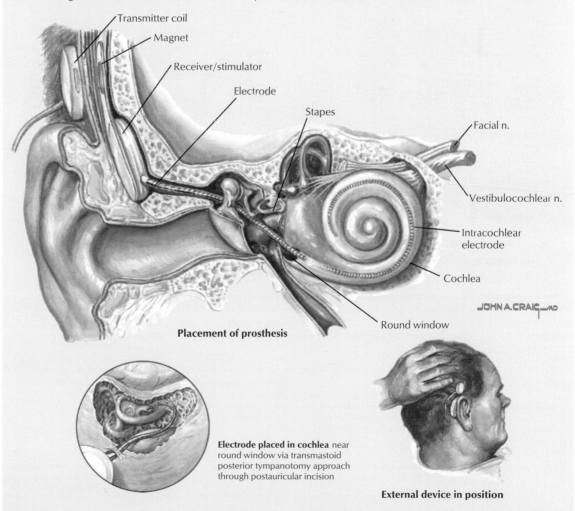

Transmitter coil
Magnet
Receiver/stimulator
Electrode
Stapes
Facial n.
Vestibulocochlear n.
Intracochlear electrode
Cochlea
Round window

Placement of prosthesis

JOHN A.CRAIG—MD

Electrode placed in cochlea near round window via transmastoid posterior tympanotomy approach through postauricular incision

External device in position

Clinical Focus 8.32

Mandibular Dislocation

Temporomandibular joint dislocation (subluxation) occurs when the mandibular condyle moves anterior to the articular eminence and the mouth has the appearance of being wide open. TMJ dislocation can be quite painful and can occur from a variety of actions, including a large yawn. Once the ligaments are stretched, subsequent dislocations may occur more frequently.

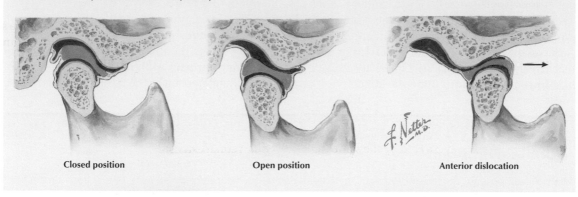

Closed position   Open position   Anterior dislocation

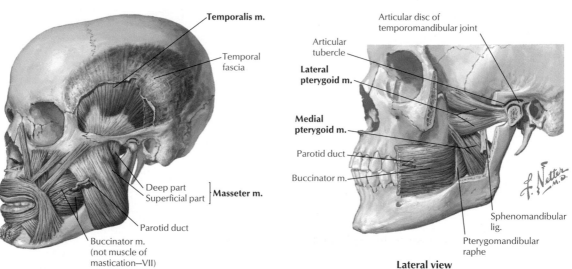

FIGURE 8.27 Muscles of Mastication. (From *Netter's atlas of human anatomy*, ed 8, Plates 72 and 73; S-186 and S-187.)

TABLE 8.8 Summary of the Muscles of Mastication

MUSCLE	ORIGIN ATTACHMENT	INSERTION ATTACHMENT	MAIN ACTIONS
Temporalis*	Floor of temporal fossa and deep temporal fascia	Ramus of mandible and coronoid process	Elevates mandible; posterior fibers retract mandible
Masseter	Zygomatic arch	Ramus of mandible and coronoid process	Elevates and protrudes mandible; deep fibers retract mandible
Lateral pterygoid	*Superior head*: infratemporal surface of greater wing of sphenoid *Inferior head*: lateral pterygoid plate	Pterygoid fovea, capsule of TMJ, articular disc	Acting together, protrude mandible; acting alone and alternately, produces side-to-side movements
Medial pterygoid	*Deep head*: medial surface of lateral pterygoid plate and palatine bone *Superficial head*: tuberosity of maxilla	Medial surface of ramus and angle of mandible inferior to mandibular foramen	Elevates mandible; acting together, protrude mandible; acting alone, protrudes side of jaw; acting alternately, produces grinding motion

*All innervated by CN V₃.

Mandible of adult: anterolateral superior view

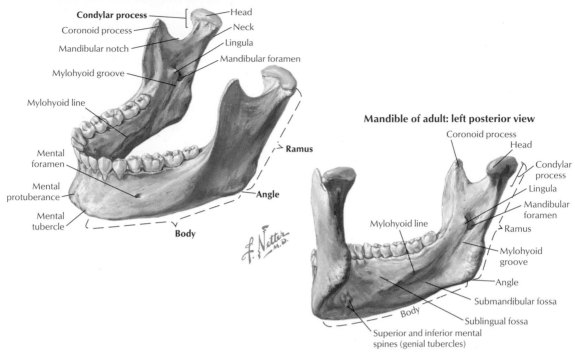

Condylar process — Head
Coronoid process — Neck
Mandibular notch — Lingula
Mylohyoid groove — Mandibular foramen
Mylohyoid line
Mental foramen
Mental protuberance
Mental tubercle
Body
Ramus
Angle

Mandible of adult: left posterior view

Coronoid process
Head
Condylar process
Lingula
Mandibular foramen
Mylohyoid line
Ramus
Mylohyoid groove
Angle
Submandibular fossa
Sublingual fossa
Body
Superior and inferior mental spines (genial tubercles)

FIGURE 8.28 Mandible. (From *Netter's atlas of human anatomy,* ed 8, Plate 39; S-135.)

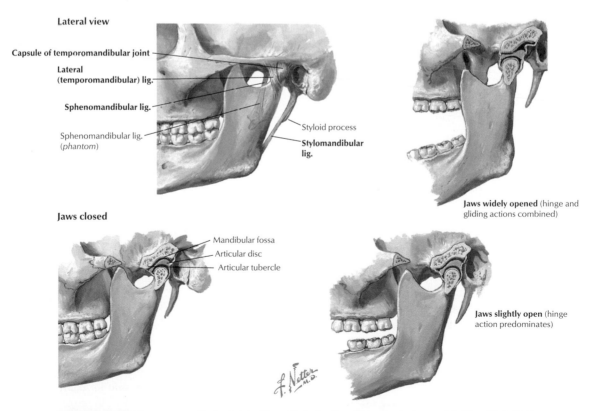

Lateral view

Capsule of temporomandibular joint
Lateral (temporomandibular) lig.
Sphenomandibular lig.
Sphenomandibular lig. (*phantom*)
Styloid process
Stylomandibular lig.

Jaws widely opened (hinge and gliding actions combined)

Jaws closed
Mandibular fossa
Articular disc
Articular tubercle

Jaws slightly open (hinge action predominates)

FIGURE 8.29 Temporomandibular Joint. (From *Netter's atlas of human anatomy,* ed 8, Plate 42; S-136.)

TABLE 8.9 Features of the TMJ

LIGAMENT	ATTACHMENT	COMMENT
Capsule	Temporal fossa and tubercle to mandibular head	Permits side-to-side motion, protrusion, and retraction
Lateral (TMJ)	Temporal to mandible	Thickened fibrous band of capsule
Articular disc	Between temporal bone and mandible	Divides joint into two synovial compartments
Stylomandibular	Styloid process to posterior ramus and angle of jaw	Limits anterior protrusion of mandible
Sphenomandibular	Spine of sphenoid to lingula of mandible	May act as a pivot by providing tension during opening and closing

Clinical Focus 8.33

Mandibular Fractures

Because of its vulnerable location, the mandible is the second most fractured facial bone, after the nasal bone. The mandible's U shape renders it liable to multiple fractures (more than 50%). The most common sites are the cuspid (canine tooth) area and the third molar area. Oozing blood from the mandible collects in loose tissues of the mouth floor (ecchymosis) and is virtually pathognomonic of a fracture.

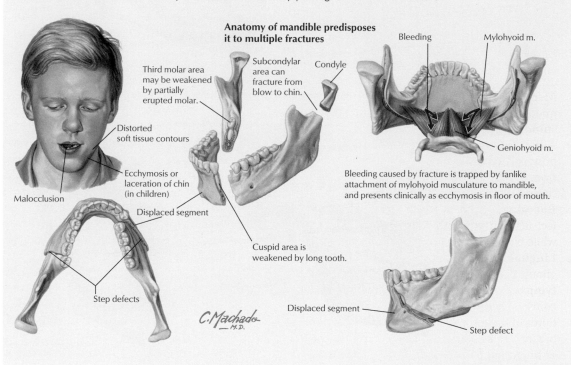

exits the stylomastoid foramen and passes through the parotid gland to distribute to the muscles of facial expression (Fig. 8.15). The parotid gland is innervated by secretomotor parasympathetic fibers from the glossopharyngeal nerve (CN IX), which we will review in the next section (see Figs. 8.13 and 8.75).

Infratemporal Fossa

The wedge-shaped infratemporal fossa is the space inferior to the zygomatic arch, medial to the

mandibular ramus and posterior to the maxilla. CN V₃, the largest division of CN V, exits the **foramen ovale,** which is located in the roof of the fossa, and its branches in this region include the following (Fig. 8.30):

- **Muscular:** small motor nerves to the four muscles of mastication, and to the tensor veli palatini, mylohyoid, anterior belly of the digastric, and tensor tympani (in middle ear) muscles; embryologically, derived from the first branchial arch (see Embryology).

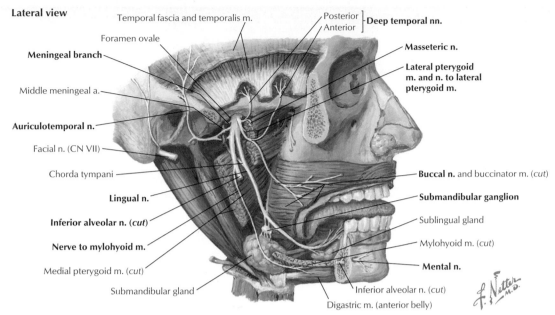

FIGURE 8.30 Infratemporal Fossa and Mandibular Nerve (CN V₃). (From *Netter's atlas of human anatomy,* ed 8, Plate 77; S-62.)

- **Meningeal:** small nerve that accompanies the middle meningeal artery through the **foramen spinosum;** sensory to the dura mater.
- **Auriculotemporal:** this nerve conveys CN IX postganglionic parasympathetic secretory fibers from the **otic ganglion** to the parotid gland, sensory to the auricle and temple.
- **Buccal:** this nerve is sensory to the cheek (you feel it when you bite your cheek accidentally while chewing your food).
- **Lingual:** this nerve conveys CN VII preganglionic parasympathetics of the **chorda tympani** to the **submandibular ganglion,** and conveys taste fibers from the anterior two-thirds of the tongue to the **geniculate ganglion** of CN VII; sensory to the anterior two-thirds of the tongue. These sensory fibers have their cell bodies in the sensory trigeminal ganglion of CN V.
- **Inferior alveolar:** this nerve passes into the **mandibular canal** and is sensory to the mandibular teeth and gums via inferior dental and gingival branches and to the chin via the mental branch from the inferior alveolar nerve. The **mylohyoid branch** that leaves the inferior alveolar nerve before it enters the mandibular canal courses in the mylohyoid groove of the medial mandible and innervates the mylohyoid muscle and anterior belly of the digastric muscle.

Parasympathetic preganglionic fibers from the glossopharyngeal nerve (CN IX) **(inferior salivatory nucleus)** run through the middle ear tympanic plexus. Arising from this plexus is the **lesser petrosal nerve,** which conveys these preganglionic parasympathetic fibers to the **otic ganglion,** which is located on the medial aspect of CN V₃ as it exits the foramen ovale (see Figs. 8.72 and 8.75). The preganglionic fibers synapse in the otic ganglion, and the secretomotor postganglionic parasympathetic fibers then join the **auriculotemporal nerve** (a branch of CN V₃) and terminate in the *parotid gland.*

Additionally, parasympathetic preganglionic fibers from CN VII **(superior salivatory nucleus)** pass through the middle ear and exit through a small fissure (petrotympanic fissure) in the temporal bone as the **chorda tympani nerve,** to join the lingual branch of CN V₃ and pass to the **submandibular ganglion,** where the preganglionic parasympathetic fibers synapse (see Figs. 8.72 and 8.73). Secretomotor postganglionic parasympathetic fibers then innervate the submandibular and sublingual salivary glands.

Vascular Supply

The **external carotid artery** terminates as the superficial temporal and maxillary arteries (see Fig. 8.17 and Table 8.16). The **superficial temporal artery** supplies the scalp and upper face via its transverse facial branch. The **maxillary artery** supplies the infratemporal region, nasal cavities,

Rhinosinusitis

Rhinosinusitis is an inflammation of the paranasal sinuses (usually the *ethmoid and maxillary sinuses*) and the nasal cavity. Physical examination of the paranasal sinuses is usually sufficient to make the diagnosis, although a CT of the sinus may help in difficult cases.

Characteristic	Description
Etiology	Respiratory viral infection or bacterial infection (often secondary); deviation of nasal septum
Pathogenesis	Obstruction of discharge of normal sinus secretions compromises normal sterility of sinuses
Signs and symptoms	Nasal congestion, facial pain and/or pressure, purulent discharge, fever, headache, painful maxillary teeth, halitosis

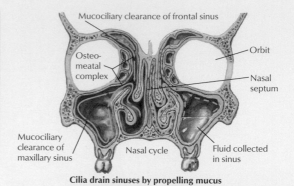

Mucociliary clearance of frontal sinus

Osteo-meatal complex

Orbit

Nasal septum

Mucociliary clearance of maxillary sinus

Nasal cycle

Fluid collected in sinus

Cilia drain sinuses by propelling mucus toward natural ostia (mucociliary clearance)

Sinuses palpated to elicit localized pain or tenderness

Eyes examined to reveal swelling of eyelids or signs of intraorbital spread

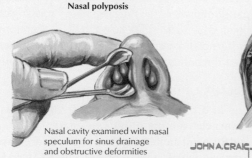

Neck examined for cervical lymphadenopathy

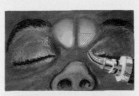

Transillumination of frontal and maxillary sinuses in darkened room. May reveal pooling of sinus secretions (green).

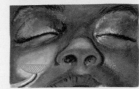

Polyp in middle meatus

Antral choanal polyp obstructs ostium of maxillary sinus

Nasal polyposis

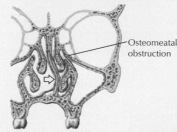

Osteomeatal obstruction

Deviation of nasal septum

Ears examined for middle ear infection and eustachian (auditory) tube involvement

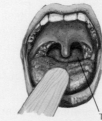

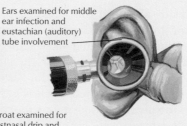

Nasal cavity examined with nasal speculum for sinus drainage and obstructive deformities

JOHN A. CRAIG—AD

Throat examined for postnasal drip and tonsillar hypertrophy

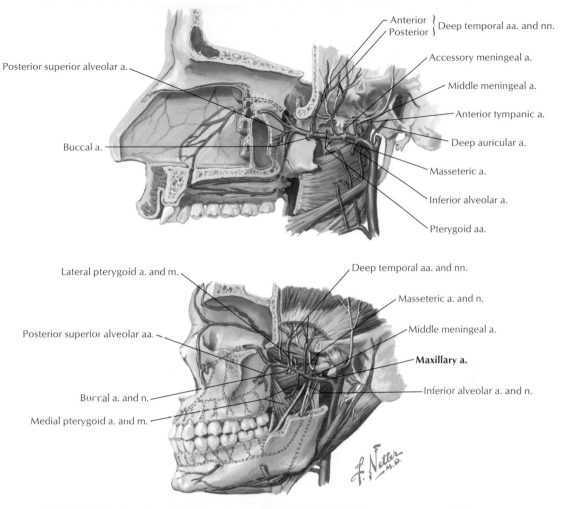

FIGURE 8.31 Branches of Maxillary Artery. (From *Netter's atlas of human anatomy*, ed 8, Plate 74; S-189.)

palate, and maxillary teeth (Fig. 8.31). For descriptive purposes, the maxillary artery is divided into the following three parts:

- **Retromandibular:** arteries enter foramina and supply the dura mater, mandibular teeth and gums, ear, and chin.
- **Pterygoid:** branches supply muscles of mastication and buccinator muscle.
- **Pterygopalatine:** branches enter foramina and supply the maxillary teeth and gums, orbital floor, nose, paranasal sinuses, palate, auditory tube, and superior pharynx.

Major branches of the **maxillary artery** include the inferior alveolar and middle meningeal branches from the first *(retromandibular)* part, branches to the muscles of mastication from the second *(pterygoid)* part, and the superior alveolar, infraorbital, greater palatine, and sphenopalatine branches from

the third *(pterygopalatine)* part (Figs. 8.31, 8.64, and 8.67 for a complete list of all its branches). The terminal portion of the maxillary artery (often referred to by clinicians as the "internal maxillary artery") passes into the **pterygopalatine fossa** (see Fig. 8.31) to gain access to the nasal cavity and nasopharynx. Here it is joined by the maxillary nerve (CN V_2) and its branches.

The infratemporal fossa is largely drained by **veins of the pterygoid plexus** (Fig. 8.32), which have extensive anastomoses with *dural, ophthalmic, and facial veins.* Tributaries from each of the areas supplied by the branches of the maxillary artery ultimately drain into the pterygoid venous plexus and/or its principal anastomotic veins (for a more extensive list of these veins, see Figs. 8.65 and 8.68). These veins are valveless, so flow can go in either direction based on gravity and pressure.

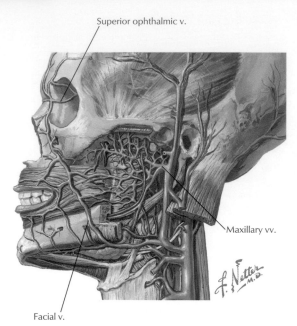

FIGURE 8.32 Pterygoid Plexus of Veins in Infratemporal Fossa. (From *Netter's atlas of human anatomy,* ed 8, Plate 84: S-328.)

9. PARANASAL SINUSES AND NASAL CAVITY

Paranasal Sinuses

The four paired paranasal sinuses are the frontal, ethmoid, maxillary, and sphenoid sinuses, named for the bones in which they reside (Fig. 8.33). The paranasal sinuses surround the nose and orbits and are lined with respiratory epithelium (pseudostratified columnar epithelium with cilia). The sinuses lighten the weight of the facial skeleton, assist in warming and humidifying inspired air, add resonance to the voice, and drain mucus secretions into the nasal cavities. Sneezing and blowing the nose, as well as gravity and the action of epithelial cilia, help to drain the paranasal sinuses of mucus.

The innervation, blood supply, and drainage of the paranasal sinuses include the following (see Figs. 8.31 to 8.33, 8.35, 8.37, and 8.38):

- **Frontal sinus:** sensory innervation from CN V_1 (supraorbital nerve); the blood supply is from the *anterior ethmoidal arteries* (from the ophthalmic

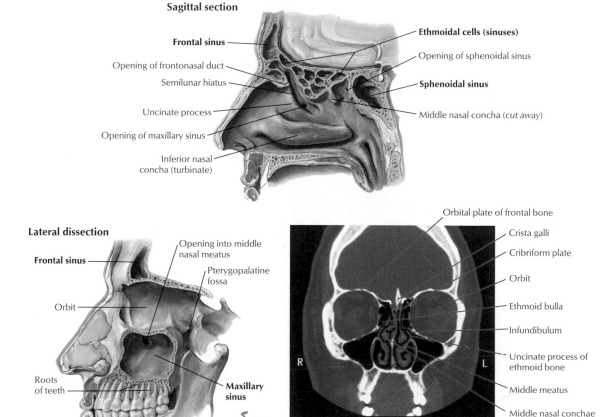

FIGURE 8.33 Paranasal Sinuses. (From *Netter's atlas of human anatomy,* ed 8, Plate 67; S-369; CT image from Kelley LL, Petersen C: *Sectional anatomy for imaging professionals,* Philadelphia, 2007, Mosby.)

artery); the frontal sinus drains via the frontonasal duct into the **semilunaris hiatus** (middle meatus; the recess beneath the middle concha).

- **Ethmoid sinus:** sensory innervation from CN V_1 (nasociliary nerve's ethmoidal branches) and CN V_2 (orbital branches); blood supply from the *ethmoidal arteries* (from the ophthalmic artery); the anterior ethmoid sinus drains into the **semilunaris hiatus** (middle meatus; the recess beneath the middle concha); the middle ethmoid sinus drains into the **ethmoid bulla** (middle meatus); and the posterior ethmoid sinus drains into the **superior meatus** (recess beneath the superior concha).
- **Sphenoid sinus:** sensory innervation from CN V_2 (orbital branches); the blood supply is from the *pharyngeal arteries* (from the maxillary artery); the sphenoid sinus drains into the **sphenoethmoidal recess** above the superior concha.
- **Maxillary sinus:** sensory innervation from CN V_2 (infraorbital and alveolar branches); the blood supply is from the *infraorbital and alveolar arteries* (from the maxillary artery); the maxillary sinus drains into the **semilunar hiatus** (middle meatus; the recess beneath the middle concha).

Note also that the **nasolacrimal duct** drains tears into the **inferior meatus,** which is located beneath the inferior concha; thus your nose "runs" when you cry.

External Nose

The upper portion of the external nose is formed by the paired nasal bones, which are continuous with the forehead (frontal bone) and are flanked laterally by the maxillae. The inferior two-thirds of the external nose is *cartilaginous* and formed by lateral processes of the septal cartilage, a midline septal cartilage, a major alar cartilage (tip of the nose), and several small, minor alar cartilages (Fig. 8.34).

Nasal Cavities

Air entering the nose passes through the following areas (Fig. 8.35):
- **Nares:** anterior apertures or nostrils.
- **Vestibule:** dilated portion of the nose inside each aperture; region is covered with a highly vascular epithelium with hair.
- **Respiratory region:** nasal cavity proper, lined with a *highly vascularized respiratory epithelial* covering and three bony conchae, which increase the surface area for filtering, warming, and humidifying inspired air. The inferior nasal concha is a separate bone, but the middle and

Anterolateral view

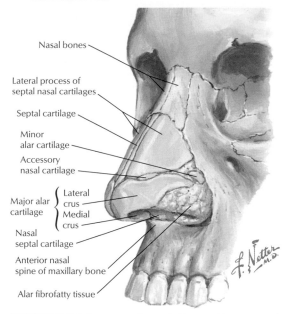

Nasal bones

Lateral process of septal nasal cartilages

Septal cartilage

Minor alar cartilage

Accessory nasal cartilage

Major alar cartilage
{ Lateral crus
{ Medial crus

Nasal septal cartilage

Anterior nasal spine of maxillary bone

Alar fibrofatty tissue

FIGURE 8.34 Structure of External Nose. (From *Netter's atlas of human anatomy,* ed 8, Plate 59; S-122.)

superior nasal conchae are parts of the ethmoid bone (Fig. 8.36). These bony conchae are covered by respiratory epithelium and, therefore, are sometimes called **turbinates** by clinicians.
- **Olfactory region:** small, apical region of the nasal cavity where the olfactory receptors reside.
- **Choanae:** pair of posterior apertures where the nasal cavity communicates with the **nasopharynx.**

Bones of the nasal cavity include the following (Fig. 8.36):
- **Ethmoid:** unpaired bone that contains the ethmoid cells (sinuses); contributes to the roof and the lateral and medial walls of the nasal cavity.
- **Sphenoid:** unpaired bone that contains the sphenoid sinus; forms the posterior part of the nasal cavity.
- **Frontal:** unpaired bone that contains the frontal sinus; forms part of the roof and septum of the cavity.
- **Vomer:** unpaired bone that contributes to the septum.
- **Nasal:** paired bones that form part of the anterior roof and lateral wall.
- **Maxilla:** paired bones that form the floor, septum, and lateral walls of the cavity.
- **Palatine:** paired bones that form the floor, septum, and lateral walls of the cavity.
- **Lacrimal:** bone that forms part of the lateral wall of the nasal cavity.

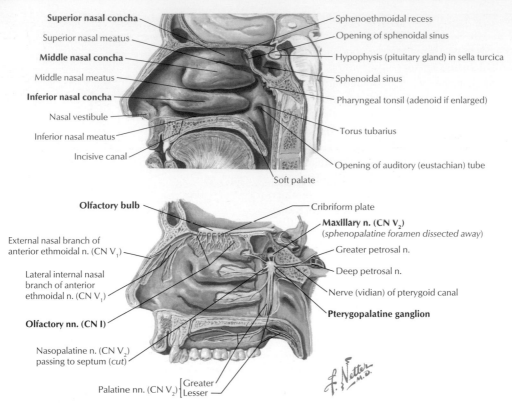

Superior nasal concha — Sphenoethmoidal recess
Superior nasal meatus — Opening of sphenoidal sinus
Middle nasal concha — Hypophysis (pituitary gland) in sella turcica
Middle nasal meatus — Sphenoidal sinus
Inferior nasal concha — Pharyngeal tonsil (adenoid if enlarged)
Nasal vestibule — Torus tubarius
Inferior nasal meatus —
Incisive canal — Opening of auditory (eustachian) tube
Soft palate

Olfactory bulb — Cribriform plate
Maxillary n. (CN V₂)
(*sphenopalatine foramen dissected away*)
External nasal branch of — Greater petrosal n.
anterior ethmoidal n. (CN V₁)
Deep petrosal n.
Lateral internal nasal
branch of anterior — Nerve (vidian) of pterygoid canal
ethmoidal n. (CN V₁)
Pterygopalatine ganglion
Olfactory nn. (CN I)
Nasopalatine n. (CN V₂)
passing to septum (*cut*)
Palatine nn. (CN V₂) {Greater / Lesser

FIGURE 8.35 Lateral Wall of Nasal Cavity. (From *Netter's atlas of human anatomy*, ed 8, Plates 61 and 64; S-361 and S-364.)

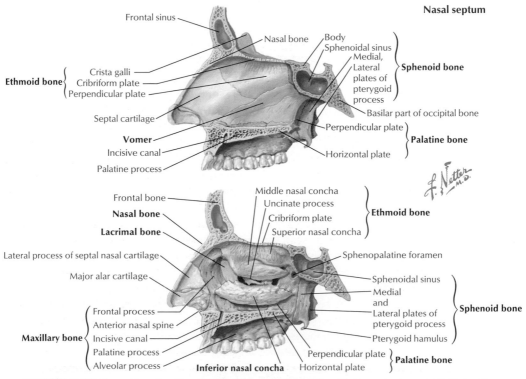

Nasal septum
Frontal sinus —
Nasal bone — Body
Sphenoidal sinus
Medial,
Lateral
plates of
Ethmoid bone {Crista galli / Cribriform plate / Perpendicular plate — pterygoid
process — Sphenoid bone
Septal cartilage — Basilar part of occipital bone
Vomer — Perpendicular plate
Incisive canal — Horizontal plate — Palatine bone
Palatine process —

Frontal bone — Middle nasal concha
Nasal bone — Uncinate process
Lacrimal bone — Cribriform plate — Ethmoid bone
Superior nasal concha
Lateral process of septal nasal cartilage — Sphenopalatine foramen
Major alar cartilage — Sphenoidal sinus
Medial
and
Frontal process — Lateral plates of
Anterior nasal spine — pterygoid process — Sphenoid bone
Maxillary bone {Incisive canal — Pterygoid hamulus
Palatine process — Perpendicular plate } Palatine bone
Alveolar process — Inferior nasal concha — Horizontal plate

FIGURE 8.36 Bones Forming Nasal Cavity. (From *Netter's atlas of human anatomy*, ed 8, Plates 62 and 63; S-360 and S-362.)

Clinical Focus 8.35

Nosebleed

A nosebleed, or **epistaxis,** is a common occurrence and often involves the richly vascularized region of the vestibule and the anteroinferior aspect of the nasal septum *(Kiesselbach's area)*. Nosebleeds usually result from trauma to the septal branch of the superior labial artery from the facial artery.

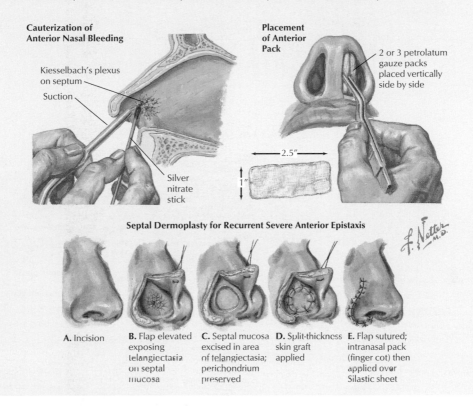

Cauterization of Anterior Nasal Bleeding

Kiesselbach's plexus on septum

Suction

Silver nitrate stick

Placement of Anterior Pack

2 or 3 petrolatum gauze packs placed vertically side by side

2.5"

1"

Septal Dermoplasty for Recurrent Severe Anterior Epistaxis

A. Incision

B. Flap elevated exposing telangiectasia on septal mucosa

C. Septal mucosa excised in area of telangiectasia; perichondrium preserved

D. Split-thickness skin graft applied

E. Flap sutured; intranasal pack (finger cot) then applied over Silastic sheet

- **Inferior nasal concha:** paired bones that form part of the lateral wall.

Blood Supply and Innervation

Blood supply to the nasal cavities originates from the following major arteries (Fig. 8.37):
- **Ophthalmic:** provides anterior and posterior ethmoidal arteries
- **Maxillary:** sphenopalatine artery (terminal branch of the maxillary artery) and its septal branches, and the greater palatine arteries
- **Facial:** provides lateral nasal and septal branches, as well as the superior labial artery

Corresponding veins drain the floor, lateral walls, and nasal septum, with most of the venous return passing into the **pterygoid plexus of veins** (Fig. 8.32 and 8.37). Some venous drainage also passes into the facial vein anteriorly and into the inferior ophthalmic veins superiorly.

The innervation of the nasal cavity includes the following (Fig. 8.38; see also Fig. 8.73):
- **Olfactory:** CN I olfactory receptors (special sense of smell) in the olfactory epithelium convey axons that pass from the upper part of the nasal cavity, through the **cribriform plate,** and synapse in the olfactory bulbs. The olfactory bulbs are actually brain tracts surrounded by the three meningeal layers of the CNS, not unlike CN II.
- **Ophthalmic:** CN V_1 general afferents are conveyed by the anterior and posterior ethmoidal nerves of the nasociliary nerve in the orbit to the trigeminal (sensory) ganglion.
- **Maxillary:** CN V_2 general afferents are conveyed to the trigeminal (sensory) ganglion via small nasal branches and by the nasopalatine nerve on the septum.
- **Sympathetics:** comprised largely of postganglionic sympathetic vasomotor fibers from the

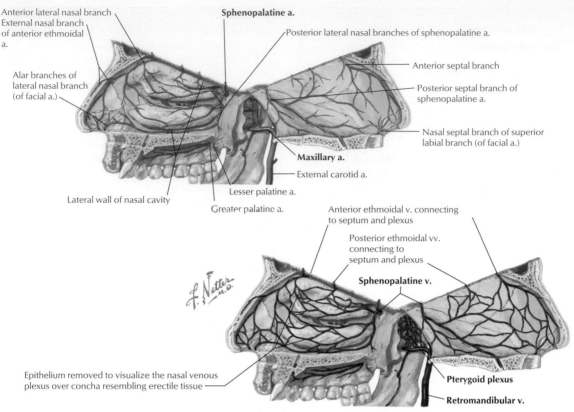

Anterior lateral nasal branch
External nasal branch of anterior ethmoidal a.

Sphenopalatine a.

Posterior lateral nasal branches of sphenopalatine a.

Anterior septal branch

Alar branches of lateral nasal branch (of facial a.)

Posterior septal branch of sphenopalatine a.

Nasal septal branch of superior labial branch (of facial a.)

Maxillary a.

External carotid a.

Lateral wall of nasal cavity

Lesser palatine a.

Greater palatine a.

Anterior ethmoidal v. connecting to septum and plexus

Posterior ethmoidal vv. connecting to septum and plexus

Sphenopalatine v.

Epithelium removed to visualize the nasal venous plexus over concha resembling erectile tissue

Pterygoid plexus

Retromandibular v.

FIGURE 8.37 Arterial Supply and Venous Drainage of Nasal Cavity (septum hinged open).

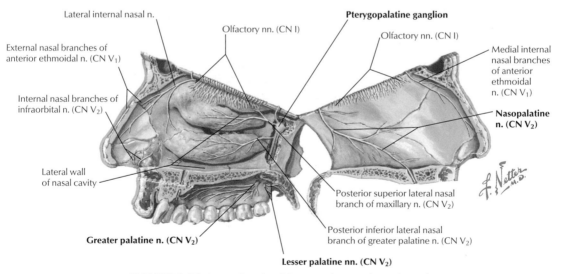

Lateral internal nasal n.

Olfactory nn. (CN I)

Pterygopalatine ganglion

Olfactory nn. (CN I)

External nasal branches of anterior ethmoidal n. (CN V$_1$)

Medial internal nasal branches of anterior ethmoidal n. (CN V$_1$)

Internal nasal branches of infraorbital n. (CN V$_2$)

Nasopalatine n. (CN V$_2$)

Lateral wall of nasal cavity

Posterior superior lateral nasal branch of maxillary n. (CN V$_2$)

Greater palatine n. (CN V$_2$)

Posterior inferior lateral nasal branch of greater palatine n. (CN V$_2$)

Lesser palatine nn. (CN V$_2$)

FIGURE 8.38 Nerve Supply of the Nose (septum hinged open).

superior cervical ganglion that reach the nose by traveling on blood vessels and existing nerves (mostly CN V$_2$); other fibers also may course via the **deep petrosal nerve** (postganglionic sympathetic fibers on the internal carotid artery), which joins the greater petrosal nerve to become

the **nerve of the pterygoid canal** (vidian nerve), and may be distributed with branches of CN V$_2$ within the nasal cavity.

- **Parasympathetics:** preganglionic secretomotor fibers to the mucosal glands of the nose and paranasal sinuses come from the **superior**

salivatory nucleus of CN VII and travel via the greater petrosal nerve and the nerve of the pterygoid canal; the fibers synapse in the **pterygopalatine ganglion;** postganglionic parasympathetic fibers then are distributed on existing nerves of CN V₂ to the nasal mucosa (Fig. 8.73).

10. ORAL CAVITY

The mouth consists of an **oral vestibule,** the space between the teeth and lips or cheeks, and the **oral cavity proper,** internal to the teeth and gums. Features of the oral cavity proper include the palate (hard and soft), teeth, gums (gingivae), tongue, and salivary glands

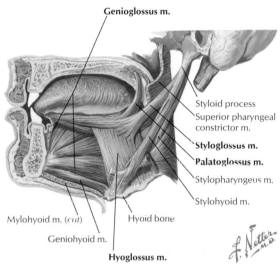

Genioglossus m.

Styloid process
Superior pharyngeal constrictor m.
Styloglossus m.
Palatoglossus m.
Stylopharyngeus m.
Stylohyoid m.

Mylohyoid m. (cut)   Hyoid bone
Geniohyoid m.
Hyoglossus m.

FIGURE 8.39 Tongue and Extrinsic Muscles. (From *Netter's atlas of human anatomy,* ed 8, Plate 88; S-401.)

(see Figs. 8.39, 8.42, and 8.45). The mucosa of the hard palate, cheeks, tongue, and lips contain numerous minor salivary glands that secrete directly into the oral cavity. Paired collections of lymphoid tissue called the **palatine tonsils** lie between the *palatoglossal and palatopharyngeal folds* (which contain small skeletal muscles of the same name) and "guard" the entrance into the oropharynx (Fig. 8.40). Unless the palatine tonsils have been removed surgically, they usually atrophy significantly as people age.

Muscles

The tongue is a strong muscular organ (gram for gram, one of the strongest muscles in the body) consisting of **intrinsic** skeletal muscle arranged in four different planes, all innervated by the hypoglossal nerve, CN XII:

- Superior longitudinal muscle fibers
- Inferior longitudinal muscle fibers
- Transverse muscle fibers
- Vertical muscle fibers

Additionally, three extrinsic skeletal muscles originate outside the tongue and insert into it (Fig. 8.39 and Table 8.10). The **genioglossus muscle** depresses and protrudes the tongue. The **hyoglossus** and **styloglossus muscles** retract the tongue during swallowing, pushing the bolus of food up against the palate as it is pushed posteriorly into the oropharynx (see Fig. 8.59). The **palatoglossus muscle** (elevates tongue) can be considered both a muscle of the tongue and a muscle of the palate. Because it is innervated by the vagus nerve rather than the hypoglossal nerve, the palatoglossus may be grouped with the muscles of the palate.

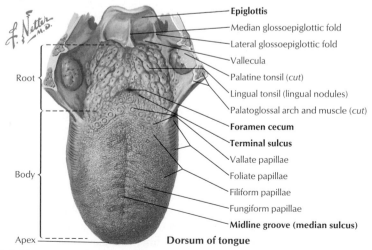

Epiglottis
Median glossoepiglottic fold
Lateral glossoepiglottic fold
Vallecula
Palatine tonsil (*cut*)
Lingual tonsil (lingual nodules)
Palatoglossal arch and muscle (*cut*)
Foramen cecum
Terminal sulcus
Vallate papillae
Foliate papillae
Filiform papillae
Fungiform papillae
Midline groove (median sulcus)

Root

Body

Apex

Dorsum of tongue

FIGURE 8.40 Dorsum of Tongue. (From *Netter's atlas of human anatomy,* ed 8, Plate 89; S-402.)

TABLE 8.10 Extrinsic Tongue Muscles

MUSCLE	ORIGIN ATTACHMENT	INSERTION ATTACHMENT	INNERVATION	MAIN ACTIONS
Genioglossus	Mental spine of mandible	Dorsum of tongue and hyoid bone	Hypoglossal nerve	Depresses and protrudes tongue
Hyoglossus	Body and greater horn of hyoid bone	Lateral and inferior aspect of tongue	Hypoglossal nerve	Depresses and retracts tongue
Styloglossus	Styloid process and stylohyoid ligament	Lateral and inferior aspect of tongue	Hypoglossal nerve	Retracts tongue and draws it up for swallowing
Palatoglossus	Palatine aponeurosis of soft palate	Lateral aspect of tongue	Vagus nerve and pharyngeal plexus	Elevates posterior tongue, depresses palate

Variations in spinal nerve contributions to the innervation of muscles, their attachments, and their actions are common in human anatomy. Therefore, expect differences between texts and realize that anatomical variation is normal.

The surface of the tongue is characterized by small lingual papillae, divided into four types (Fig. 8.40):

- **Filiform:** numerous slender projections that lack taste buds; give the tongue its rough or furry feel.
- **Fungiform:** larger mushroom-shaped papillae (may appear as red caps, especially if irritated by hot foods) scattered on the dorsum of the tongue's surface; possess taste buds and are difficult to see grossly.
- **Circumvallate:** larger papillae that lie in a row just anterior to the sulcus terminalis; possess taste buds.
- **Foliate:** lie along the sides of the tongue and are *rudimentary in humans;* possess taste buds.

The tongue receives its blood supply largely by the **lingual artery** (from the external carotid artery) and is innervated by the following five cranial nerves (Fig. 8.41):

- **Trigeminal:** via **lingual nerve,** a branch of the mandibular nerve; provides general sensation to the anterior two-thirds of the tongue.
- **Facial:** via **chorda tympani nerve**, which joins the lingual nerve; provides taste on the anterior two-thirds of the tongue.
- **Glossopharyngeal:** general sensation and taste on the posterior third of the tongue.
- **Vagus:** via the internal branch of the superior laryngeal nerve, for general sensation and taste on the base of the tongue at the epiglottic region.
- **Hypoglossal:** motor to the intrinsic and extrinsic tongue muscles, except the palatoglossus muscle, which is considered a muscle of the palate (and is innervated by the vagus nerve CN X).

Teeth and Gums (Gingivae)

The **maxillary teeth** (upper jaw) number 16 in adults: 4 incisors, 2 canines, 4 premolars (bicuspids), and 6 molars (tricuspids). The **mandibular teeth** (lower jaw) also have 16 teeth of the same name, for a total of 32 adult teeth (Figs. 8.41 and 8.42). The third set of molars are the last to erupt and are commonly referred to as the "wisdom teeth." Children possess 20 deciduous teeth (4 incisors, 2 canines, and 4 molars in each jaw), which usually have erupted by the third year of life. The central mandibular incisors usually are the first deciduous teeth to erupt at about the sixth or seventh month of age.

The maxillary teeth (gums) receive sensory innervation by the anterior, middle, and posterior superior alveolar nerves from **CN V_2** and the mandibular teeth by the inferior alveolar nerve (CN V_3) (Fig. 8.41).

The maxillary buccal (side facing the cheek) gingivae (gums) receive sensory innervation by the same nerves from CN V_2 as the maxillary teeth, but the lingual (side facing the tongue) gingivae are innervated by the greater palatine and nasopalatine nerves of CN V_2. The mandibular buccal gingivae receive sensory innervation by the buccal and mental nerves from CN V_3 and the lingual gingivae from the lingual nerve (CN V_3).

The blood to the maxillary teeth comes from the **anterior superior alveolar artery** (a branch of the infraorbital branch of the maxillary artery) and **posterior superior alveolar artery** (a branch of the maxillary artery). The blood supply to the mandibular teeth comes from the **inferior alveolar artery** (branch of the maxillary artery) (Fig. 8.31). The venous drainage is from corresponding veins, most of which drain into the pterygoid plexus of veins in the infratemporal fossa (Fig. 8.32).

Salivary Glands

Whereas there are thousands of microscopic minor salivary glands in the oral and lingual mucosa, there also are three pairs of larger salivary glands (Figs. 8.43 and 8.44 and Table 8.11). Saliva contains water, mucins, α-amylase for initial digestion of carbohydrates, lysozyme to control bacterial flora, bicarbonate ions for buffering, antibodies, and the calcium and phosphate essential for healthy teeth. We produce about 1.2 L of saliva each day. As summarized in

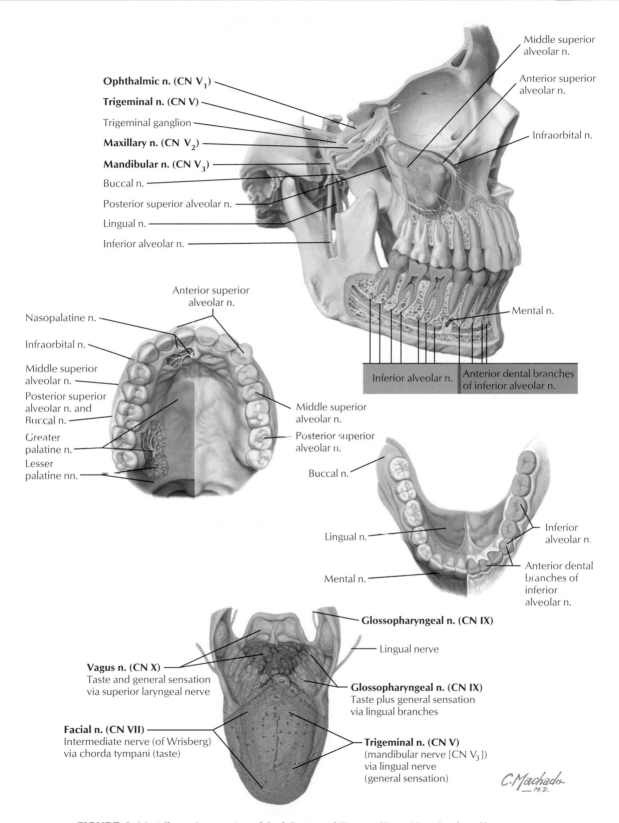

FIGURE 8.41 Afferent Innervation of Oral Cavity and Tongue. (From *Netter's atlas of human anatomy*, ed 8, Plate 84; S-406.)

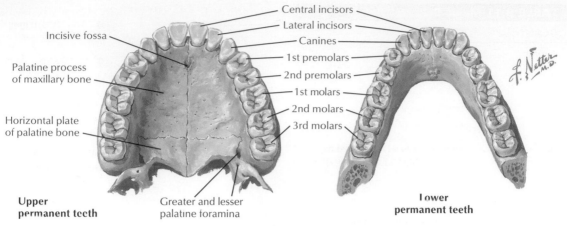

Central incisors

Lateral incisors

Canines

1st premolars

2nd premolars

1st molars

2nd molars

3rd molars

Incisive fossa

Palatine process
of maxillary bone

Horizontal plate
of palatine bone

**Upper
permanent teeth**

Greater and lesser
palatine foramina

**Lower
permanent teeth**

FIGURE 8.42 Teeth. (From *Netter's atlas of human anatomy*, ed 8, Plate 40; S-404.)

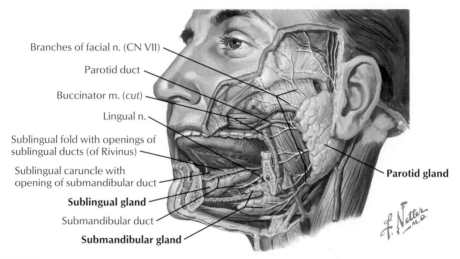

Branches of facial n. (CN VII)

Parotid duct

Buccinator m. (*cut*)

Lingual n.

Sublingual fold with openings of
sublingual ducts (of Rivinus)

Sublingual caruncle with
opening of submandibular duct

Sublingual gland

Submandibular duct

Submandibular gland

Parotid gland

FIGURE 8.43 Major Salivary Glands. (From *Netter's atlas of human anatomy*, ed 8, Plate 70; S-396.)

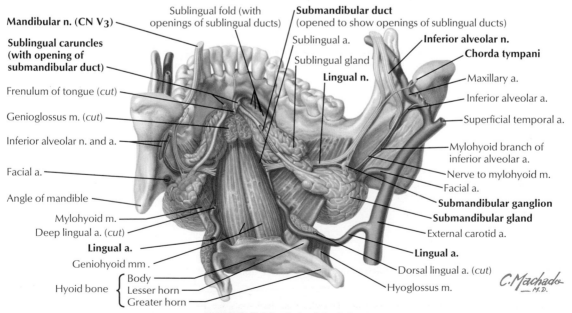

Mandibular n. (CN V₃)

**Sublingual caruncles
(with opening of
submandibular duct)**

Frenulum of tongue (*cut*)

Genioglossus m. (*cut*)

Inferior alveolar n. and a.

Facial a.

Angle of mandible

Mylohyoid m.

Deep lingual a. (*cut*)

Lingual a.

Geniohyoid mm.

Hyoid bone { Body
Lesser horn
Greater horn

Sublingual fold (with
openings of sublingual ducts)

Sublingual a.

Sublingual gland

Lingual n.

Submandibular duct
(opened to show openings of sublingual ducts)

Inferior alveolar n.

Chorda tympani

Maxillary a.

Inferior alveolar a.

Superficial temporal a.

Mylohyoid branch of
inferior alveolar a.

Nerve to mylohyoid m.

Facial a.

Submandibular ganglion

Submandibular gland

External carotid a.

Lingual a.

Dorsal lingual a. (*cut*)

Hyoglossus m.

FIGURE 8.44 Floor of Oral Cavity.

TABLE 8.11 Major Salivary Glands

GLAND	TYPE AND INNERVATION
Parotid	Serous gland innervated by CN IX parasympathetics that course via lesser petrosal nerve (CN IX), synapsing in otic ganglion, with postganglionics conveyed to the gland in auriculotemporal nerve (branch of CN V_3); secretes via **parotid** (Stensen's) **duct**
Submandibular	Seromucous gland innervated by CN VII parasympathetics that course to the gland via chorda tympani branch of CN VII and join lingual nerve to synapse in submandibular ganglion (branch of CN V_3); secretes via **submandibular** (Wharton's) **duct**
Sublingual	Largely mucous gland innervated by CN VII parasympathetics coursing similar to those supplying submandibular gland above; secretes via many **small ducts in sublingual fold**

Table 8.11, the three pairs of salivary glands are innervated by *parasympathetic nerve fibers* from CN VII (submandibular and sublingual glands) and CN IX (parotid gland).

Palate

The palate forms the floor of the nasal cavity and the roof of the oral cavity. The palate is divided as follows (Figs. 8.42, 8.45, and 8.46):

- **Hard palate:** bony anterior two-thirds of the palate; formed by the palatal process of the maxilla and horizontal process of the palatine bone (Fig. 8.42); covered by a thick mucosa that overlies numerous mucus-secreting palatal glands (Fig. 8.45).
- **Soft palate:** posterior third of the palate (Figs. 8.45 and 8.46). It is composed of a mucosa and mucus-secreting palatal glands, with five muscles that contribute to the soft palate and its movements; closes off the nasopharynx during swallowing.

Sensory innervation of the hard palate is largely via the **nasopalatine** and **greater palatine nerves** (CN V_2), whereas sensory innervation of the soft palate is largely through the **lesser palatine nerves** (CN V_2) (Fig. 8.45). The muscles of the soft palate (Fig. 8.46) and their actions are summarized in Table 8.12.

11. NECK

The neck is divided descriptively into two major triangles. Each triangle contains key structures used as landmarks by anatomists and physicians operating in this area. The neck is a vertical conduit for structures entering or leaving the head. It is tightly bound in several fascial layers that divide the neck into descriptive compartments. The two major triangles of the neck are as follows (Fig. 8.47):

- **Posterior Triangle:** bounded by the posterior border of the sternocleidomastoid muscle (SCM), anterior border of the trapezius muscle, and middle third of the clavicle.
- **Anterior Triangle:** bounded by the anterior border of the SCM, inferior border of mandible,

TABLE 8.12 Muscles of the Soft Palate

MUSCLE	ORIGIN ATTACHMENT	INSERTION ATTACHMENT	INNERVATION	MAIN ACTIONS
Levator veli palatini	Auditory tube and temporal bone	Palatine aponeurosis	Vagus nerve via pharyngeal plexus	Elevates soft palate during swallowing
Tensor veli palatini	Scaphoid fossa of medial pterygoid plate, spine of sphenoid, and auditory tube	Palatine aponeurosis	Mandibular nerve	Tenses soft palate and opens auditory tube during swallowing and yawning
Palatoglossus	Palatine aponeurosis of soft palate	Side of tongue	Vagus nerve via pharyngeal plexus	Elevates posterior tongue, depresses palate
Palatopharyngeus	Hard palate and palatine aponeurosis	Lateral wall of pharynx	Vagus nerve via pharyngeal plexus	Tenses soft palate; pulls walls of pharynx superiorly, anteriorly, and medially during swallowing
Musculus uvulae	Nasal spine and palatine aponeurosis	Mucosa of uvula	Vagus nerve via pharyngeal plexus	Shortens, elevates, and retracts uvula

Variations in spinal nerve contributions to the innervation of muscles, their attachments, and their actions are common in human anatomy. Therefore, expect differences between texts and realize that anatomical variation is normal.

Anterior view

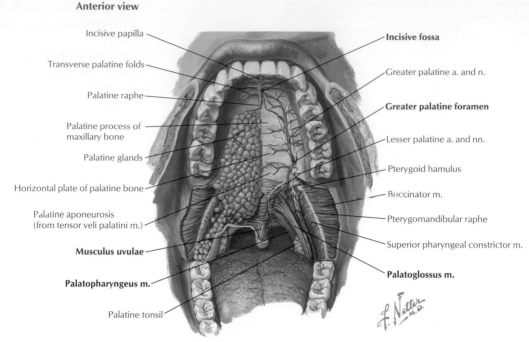

Incisive papilla

Transverse palatine folds

Palatine raphe

Palatine process of maxillary bone

Palatine glands

Horizontal plate of palatine bone

Palatine aponeurosis (from tensor veli palatini m.)

Musculus uvulae

Palatopharyngeus m.

Palatine tonsil

Incisive fossa

Greater palatine a. and n.

Greater palatine foramen

Lesser palatine a. and nn.

Pterygoid hamulus

Buccinator m.

Pterygomandibular raphe

Superior pharyngeal constrictor m.

Palatoglossus m.

FIGURE 8.45 Oral Cavity With Partial Dissection of Palate. (From *Netter's atlas of human anatomy,* ed 8, Plate 85; S-398.)

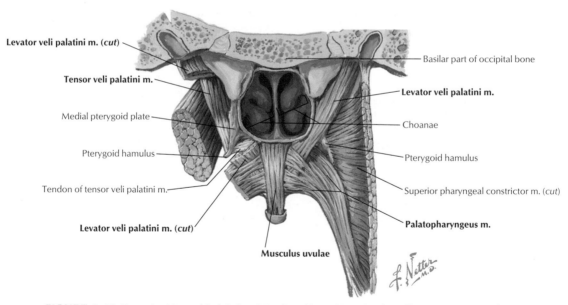

Levator veli palatini m. (*cut*)

Tensor veli palatini m.

Medial pterygoid plate

Pterygoid hamulus

Tendon of tensor veli palatini m.

Levator veli palatini m. (*cut*)

Musculus uvulae

Basilar part of occipital bone

Levator veli palatini m.

Choanae

Pterygoid hamulus

Superior pharyngeal constrictor m. (*cut*)

Palatopharyngeus m.

FIGURE 8.46 Posterior View of Soft Palate Muscles. (From *Netter's atlas of human anatomy,* ed 8, Plate 85; S-398.)

and midline of the neck; also subdivided into the following triangles:

- Submandibular.
- Carotid.
- Muscular.
- Submental.

The neck is surrounded by a sleeve of **superficial cervical fascia** that lies deep to the skin and invests the platysma muscle (a muscle of facial expression). A second sleeve of **deep cervical fascia** tightly invests the neck structures and is divided into the following three layers (Fig. 8.48):

Clinical Focus 8.36

Common Oral Lesions

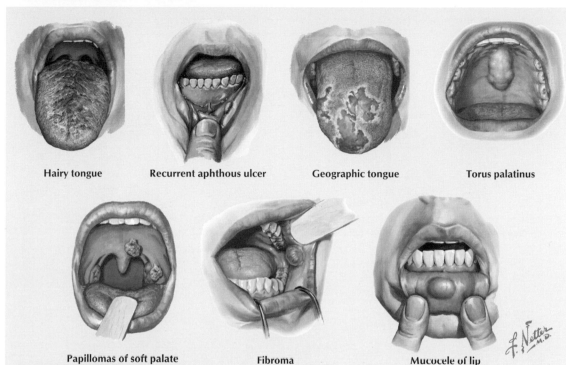

Hairy tongue	Recurrent aphthous ulcer	Geographic tongue	Torus palatinus

Papillomas of soft palate and anterior pillar	Fibroma	Mucocele of lip

Lesion	Description
Recurrent aphthous ulcer (canker sore)	Common; etiology uncertain (nutrition, hormonal, bacterial or viral infection, genetic [Crohn's disease])
Viral stomatitis	Herpes simplex; occurs on lip, gums, tongue, and hard palate; heals spontaneously in 10–14 days
Oral candidiasis (oral thrush)	Most common fungal infection (30–60% of healthy adults); white, plaquelike lesions with hemorrhagic underlying mucosa
Hairy tongue	Benign condition caused by accumulation of keratin and bacteria on filiform papillae of tongue
Geographic tongue	Benign condition; etiology unknown; area of atrophied filiform papillae; sensitivity to some foods and liquids
Torus palatinus	Benign smooth, hard lesions on midline hard palate
Oral papilloma	Infection with strains of human papillomavirus; pedunculated, cauliflowerlike squamous epithelial masses that can be excised
Fibroma	Soft lesions at sites of chronic trauma that lead to inflammation and fibrous hyperplasia
Mucocele	Salivary extrusion from a minor salivary gland into surrounding tissue, usually lower lip; may burst and recur

- **Superficial** investing: surrounds the neck and invests the trapezius and SCM muscles (*red fascia*, Fig. 8.48).
- **Pretracheal** (visceral): limited to the anterior neck; invests the infrahyoid muscles, thyroid gland, trachea, and esophagus; posteriorly called the **buccopharyngeal fascia** because it covers the buccinator and pharyngeal constrictor muscles (*purple, blue,* and *green* fasciae, Fig. 8.48).

Inferiorly, the buccopharyngeal fascia separates the pharynx and esophagus from the prevertebral layer.

- **Prevertebral:** tubular sheath that invests the prevertebral muscles and vertebral column; includes the **alar fascia** anteriorly (*orange* fascia, Fig. 8.48).

The **carotid sheath** blends with these three fascial layers but is distinct and contains the

Clinical Focus 8.37

Cancer of the Oral Cavity

Squamous cell carcinoma (SCC) accounts for more than 90% of cancers in this region, so the information here focuses on SCC. All these lesions may present with palpable submental, submandibular, and upper cervical lymph nodes.

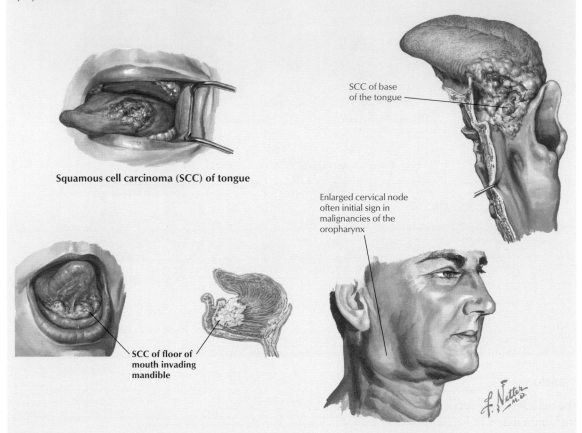

Squamous cell carcinoma (SCC) of tongue

SCC of base of the tongue

Enlarged cervical node often initial sign in malignancies of the oropharynx

SCC of floor of mouth invading mandible

Type and site of lesion	Presentation	Risk factors
Premalignant		
Erythroplasia	Red, raised lesion or a smooth, atrophic red lesion	Alcohol, tobacco use (synergistic effect)
Leukoplakia	White patchy mucosa	Alcohol, tobacco use
Malignant		
Lip SCC (90% lower lip)	Nonhealing, crusting ulcerative lesion or scaly, hyperkeratotic lesion at vermilion border of lip	Ultraviolet (sun) exposure
Tongue SCC	Anterolateral tongue; nonhealing ulcer; exophytic lesion	Alcohol, tobacco use
Floor of mouth	Anterior tongue; may infiltrate mandible; trismus if muscles of mastication involved	Alcohol, tobacco use
Oropharynx SCC	Ulcerative or infiltrating mucosal lesions; pain; dysphagia	Alcohol, tobacco use

common **carotid artery, internal jugular vein,** and **vagus nerve** (*dark blue-green* fascial sheath in Fig. 8.48, *top* cross-sectional image).

The investing fascia is not limited to the neck but extends superiorly to the hyoid bone and envelops the **submandibular salivary gland.** As it courses along the inferior margin of the mandible, the investing fascia also envelops the **parotid salivary gland** and then extends to the mastoid process and zygomatic arch.

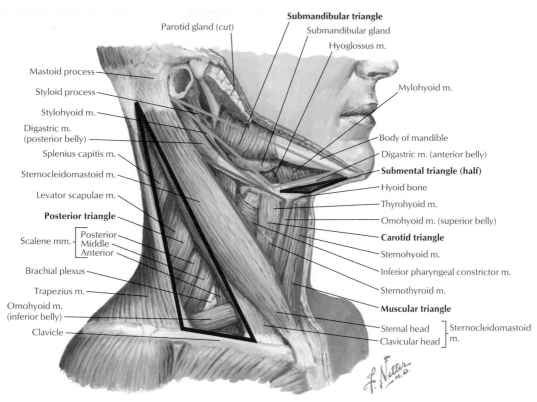

FIGURE 8.47 Triangles of the Neck.

Muscles

The muscles of the anterior and posterior triangles are summarized in Fig. 8.49 and Table 8.13. The **suprahyoid muscles** raise the hyoid bone toward a stabilized mandible during swallowing. The **infrahyoid muscles** depress the hyoid bone and larynx during swallowing and vocalization.

Cervical Plexus

The accessory nerve (CN XI) exits the jugular foramen and crosses the posterior triangle, innervating the SCM and trapezius muscles (Fig. 8.50). However, the **cervical plexus**, composed of the **anterior rami of C1-C4,** innervates most of the neck muscles and provides sensory innervation to the anterior and lateral neck (Table 8.14). Additional innervation includes:

- The **mylohyoid nerve** (a branch of CN V$_3$) innervates the mylohyoid muscle and anterior belly of the digastric muscle beneath the chin.
- The **facial nerve** (CN VII) innervates the platysma muscle through its cervical branch.

- The **glossopharyngeal nerve** (CN IX) supplies the carotid body and sinus (visceral sensory).
- The **vagus nerve** (CN X) supplies the larynx through its superior and recurrent (inferior) laryngeal nerves.
- The **hypoglossal nerve** (CN XII) loops through the neck around the external carotid artery to innervate the tongue (Fig. 8.52).

Blood Supply

The arterial supply to the neck is by the **subclavian artery** (Fig. 8.51 and Table 8.15) and some of the branches of the **external carotid artery,** a branch of the common carotid artery (Fig. 8.51 and Table 8.16). The subclavian *artery* is divided for descriptive purposes into *three parts:* Part 1 lies medial, Part 2 lies posterior, and Part 3 lies lateral to the anterior scalene muscle (Fig. 8.50). Of the branches of the *subclavian artery* listed in Table 8.15, the vertebral artery and the thyrocervical trunk and its branches are the primary blood supply to the neck. Of the branches of the *external carotid artery* listed in Table 8.16, the

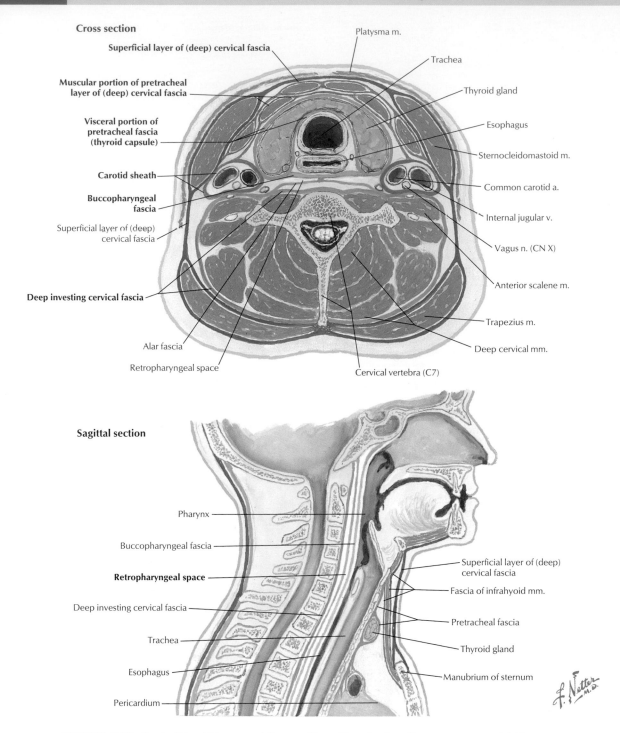

FIGURE 8.48 Cervical Fascial Layers and Spaces. (From *Netter's atlas of human anatomy*, ed 8, Plate 51; S-196.)

superior thyroid, the ascending pharyngeal, and the lingual branches also contribute to the blood supply of the neck.

The venous drainage of the neck is highly variable, but most of the blood ultimately drains into **tributaries of the external and internal jugular veins** (Figs. 8.53 and 8.54). The external jugular vein is formed by the *posterior auricular and posterior branches of the retromandibular veins,* while the internal jugular vein begins at the jugular

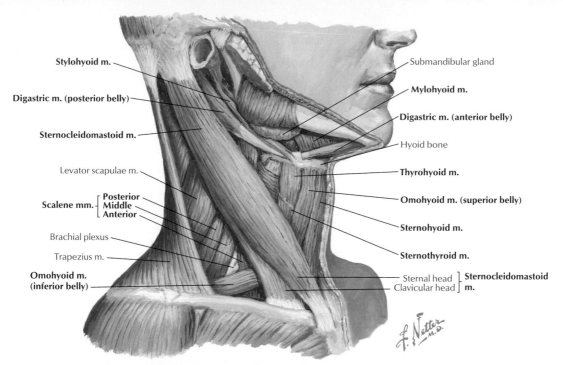

FIGURE 8.49 Muscles of the Neck. (From *Netter's atlas of human anatomy*, ed 8, Plate 54; S-192.)

TABLE 8.13 Muscles of the Neck

MUSCLE	ORIGIN ATTACHMENT	INSERTION ATTACHMENT	INNERVATION	MAIN ACTIONS
Sternocleidomastoid	*Sternal head:* manubrium *Clavicular head:* medial third of clavicle	Mastoid process and lateral half of superior nuchal line of occipital bone	Spinal root of cranial nerve CN XI and C2-C3 (sensory)	Tilts head to one side, i.e., laterally flexes and rotates head so face is turned superiorly toward opposite side; acting together, muscles flex neck
Posterior scalene	Posterior tubercles of transverse processes of C4-C6	2nd rib	C5-C8	Flexes neck laterally; elevates 2nd rib
Middle scalene	Posterior tubercles of transverse processes of C2-C7	1st rib	C3-C7	Flexes neck laterally; elevates 1st rib
Anterior scalene	Anterior tubercles of transverse processes of C3-C6	1st rib	C5-C8	Flexes neck laterally; elevates 1st rib
Digastric	*Anterior belly:* digastric fossa of mandible *Posterior belly:* mastoid notch	Intermediate tendon to hyoid bone	*Anterior belly:* mylohyoid nerve, a branch of inferior alveolar nerve *Posterior belly:* facial nerve	Depresses mandible; raises hyoid bone and steadies it during swallowing and speaking
Sternohyoid	Manubrium of sternum and medial end of clavicle	Body of hyoid bone	C1-C3 from ansa cervicalis	Depresses hyoid bone and larynx after swallowing
Sternothyroid	Posterior surface of manubrium, 1st costal cartilage	Oblique line of thyroid lamina	C2 and C3 from ansa cervicalis	Depresses larynx and thyroid cartilage after swallowing
Thyrohyoid	Oblique line of thyroid cartilage	Body and greater horn of hyoid bone	C1 via hypoglossal nerve	Depresses hyoid bone and elevates larynx when hyoid bone is fixed
Omohyoid	Superior border of scapula near suprascapular notch	Inferior border of hyoid bone	C1-C3 from ansa cervicalis	Depresses and fixes hyoid bone
Mylohyoid	Mylohyoid line of mandible	Raphe and body of hyoid bone	Mylohyoid nerve, a branch of inferior alveolar nerve of CN V₃	Elevates hyoid bone, floor of mouth, and tongue during swallowing and depresses mandible
Stylohyoid	Styloid process	Body of hyoid bone	Facial nerve	Elevates and retracts hyoid bone

Variations in spinal nerve contributions to the innervation of muscles, their attachments, and their actions are common in human anatomy. Therefore, expect differences between texts and realize that anatomical variation is normal.

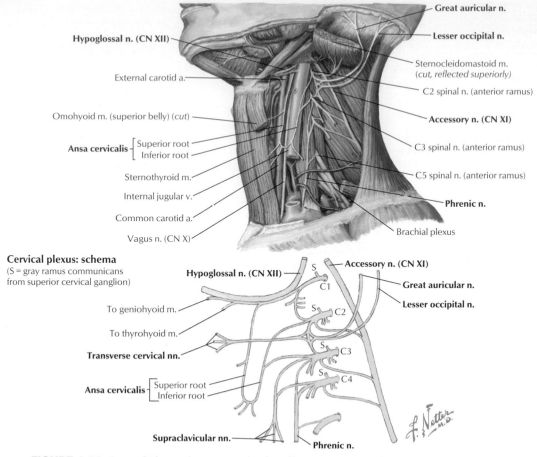

FIGURE 8.50 Cervical Plexus. (From *Netter's atlas of human anatomy,* ed 8, Plate 56 and 57; S-194 and S-195.)

TABLE 8.14 Cervical Plexus

NERVE	INNERVATION	NERVE	INNERVATION
C1	Travels with cranial nerve CN XII to innervate geniohyoid and thyrohyoid muscles	Supraclavicular	From C3 to C4, are anterior, middle, and posterior sensory branches to skin over clavicle and shoulder region
Ansa cervicalis	Is C1-C3 loop that sends motor branches to infrahyoid muscles	Phrenic	From C3 to C5, is motor and sensory nerve to diaphragm
Lesser occipital	From C2, is sensory to neck and scalp posterior to ear	Motor branches	Are small twigs that supply scalene, levator scapulae, and prevertebral muscles
Great auricular	From C2 to C3, is sensory over parotid gland and posterior ear		
Transverse cervical	From C2 to C3, is sensory to anterior triangle of neck		

foramen as a continuation of the *sigmoid dural sinus* (the much smaller inferior petrosal sinus also ends at this point).

The **thoracic lymphatic duct** ascends through the thorax just anterior to the vertebral bodies, enters the root of the neck by passing posterior to the left carotid sheath, and loops inferiorly to empty into the junction between the left subclavian vein and left internal jugular vein (see Fig. 1.16 and 3.12). The smaller **right lymphatic duct** collects lymph from the right side of the head, neck, thorax, and right upper limb and drains

TABLE 8.15 Branches of the Subclavian Artery

BRANCH	COURSE
Part 1	
Vertebral	Ascends through C6 to C1 transverse foramina and enters foramen magnum
Internal thoracic	Descends parasternally to anastomose with superior epigastric artery
Thyrocervical trunk	Gives rise to inferior thyroid, transverse cervical, and suprascapular arteries
Part 2	
Costocervical trunk	Gives rise to deep cervical and superior intercostal arteries
Part 3	
Dorsal scapular	Is inconstant; may also arise from transverse cervical artery

it into the corresponding junction of the right subclavian vein and right internal jugular vein (see Figs. 1.16 and 3.12).

Thyroid and Parathyroid Glands

The **thyroid gland** lies at the C5-T1 vertebral level, anterior to the trachea, and is a ductless endocrine gland that weighs about 20 grams (Figs. 8.48, 8.53, 8.54; Tables 1.5 and 8.17). The thyroid gland has two lateral lobes connected by an **isthmus** that lies anterior to the second to fourth tracheal cartilaginous rings. It is enveloped in the visceral layer of the pretracheal fascia (*blue* fascia in Fig. 8.48). In about 50% of cases, a **pyramidal lobe** may extend superiorly from the isthmus, demarcating the *embryonic migratory pathway* of the thyroid from the base of the tongue (see Clinical Focus 8.46). The thyroid gland secretes

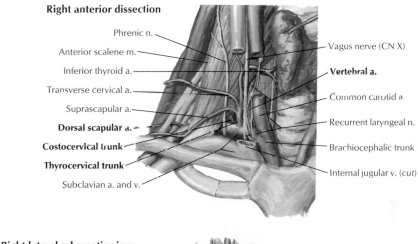

Right anterior dissection

Phrenic n.
Anterior scalene m.
Inferior thyroid a.
Transverse cervical a.
Suprascapular a.
Dorsal scapular a.
Costocervical trunk
Thyrocervical trunk
Subclavian a. and v.

Vagus nerve (CN X)
Vertebral a.
Common carotid a.
Recurrent laryngeal n.
Brachiocephalic trunk
Internal jugular v. (*cut*)

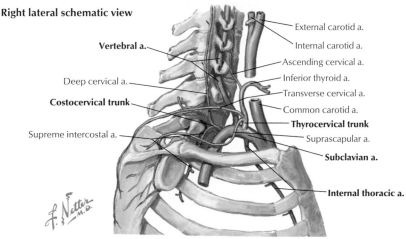

Right lateral schematic view

Vertebral a.
Deep cervical a.
Costocervical trunk
Supreme intercostal a.

External carotid a.
Internal carotid a.
Ascending cervical a.
Inferior thyroid a.
Transverse cervical a.
Common carotid a.
Thyrocervical trunk
Suprascapular a.
Subclavian a.
Internal thoracic a.

FIGURE 8.51 Subclavian Artery and Branches. (From *Netter's atlas of human anatomy,* ed 8, Plates 57 and BP 24; S-195 and S-BP 49.)

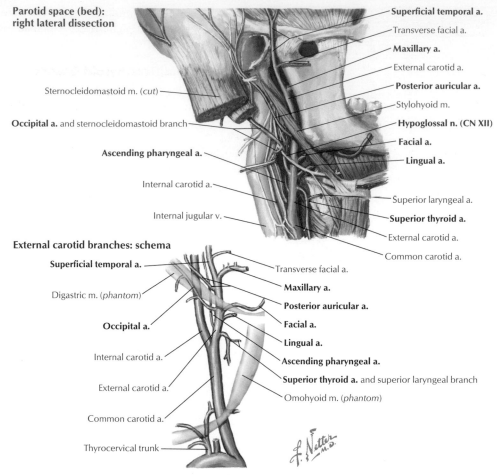

Parotid space (bed):
right lateral dissection

Superficial temporal a.
Transverse facial a.
Maxillary a.
External carotid a.
Posterior auricular a.
Stylohyoid m.
Sternocleidomastoid m. (*cut*)
Hypoglossal n. (CN XII)
Occipital a. and sternocleidomastoid branch
Facial a.
Ascending pharyngeal a.
Lingual a.
Internal carotid a.
Superior laryngeal a.
Internal jugular v.
Superior thyroid a.
External carotid a.
Common carotid a.

External carotid branches: schema

Superficial temporal a.
Transverse facial a.
Maxillary a.
Digastric m. (*phantom*)
Posterior auricular a.
Occipital a.
Facial a.
Lingual a.
Internal carotid a.
Ascending pharyngeal a.
External carotid a.
Superior thyroid a. and superior laryngeal branch
Common carotid a.
Omohyoid m. (*phantom*)
Thyrocervical trunk

FIGURE 8.52 External Carotid Artery and Branches. (From *Netter's atlas of human anatomy*, ed 8, Plate 58; S-324.)

TABLE 8.16 Branches of the External Carotid Artery	
BRANCH	**COURSE AND STRUCTURES SUPPLIED**
Superior thyroid	Supplies thyroid gland, larynx, and infrahyoid muscles
Ascending pharyngeal	Supplies pharyngeal region, middle ear, meninges, and prevertebral muscles
Lingual	Passes deep to hyoglossus muscle to supply the tongue
Facial	Courses over the mandible and supplies the face
Occipital	Supplies SCM and anastomoses with costocervical trunk
Posterior auricular	Supplies region posterior to ear
Maxillary	Passes into infratemporal fossa (described later)
Superficial temporal	Supplies face, temporalis muscle, and lateral scalp

thyroxine (T_4), triiodothyronine (T_3), and calcitonin and performs the following functions:

- Increases the metabolic rate of tissues.
- Increases the consumption of oxygen.
- Increases the heart rate, ventilation, and renal function.
- Is required for growth hormone production and is important in CNS growth.
- Increases the deposition of calcium and phosphate in bones (via the hormone calcitonin).

The **parathyroid glands** are paired superior and inferior glands (number and location can vary significantly) located on the posterior aspect of the thyroid gland (see Fig. 8.54). The parathyroid glands secrete parathyroid hormone (PTH) in response to low calcium levels in the bloodstream and perform the following functions:

- Cause the resorption and release of calcium from bone; 99% of the body's calcium is stored in bone.
- Cause the resorption of calcium by the kidney.

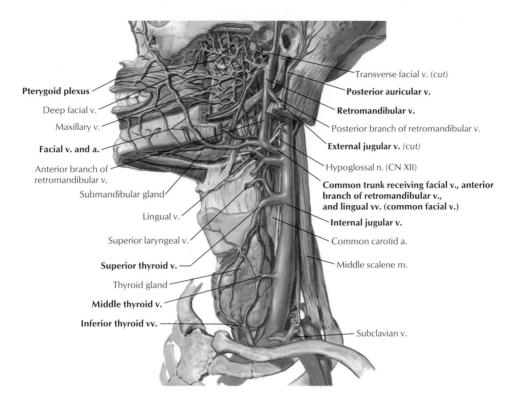

Pterygoid plexus

Deep facial v.

Maxillary v.

Facial v. and a.

Anterior branch of
retromandibular v.

Submandibular gland

Lingual v.

Superior laryngeal v.

Superior thyroid v.

Thyroid gland

Middle thyroid v.

Inferior thyroid vv.

Transverse facial v. (cut)

Posterior auricular v.

Retromandibular v.

Posterior branch of retromandibular v.

External jugular v. (cut)

Hypoglossal n. (CN XII)

Common trunk receiving facial v., anterior
branch of retromandibular v.,
and lingual vv. (common facial v.)

Internal jugular v.

Common carotid a.

Middle scalene m.

Subclavian v.

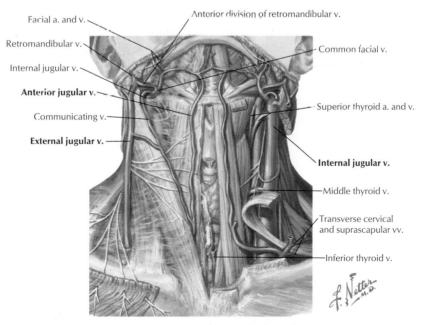

Facial a. and v.

Retromandibular v.

Internal jugular v.

Anterior jugular v.

Communicating v.

External jugular v.

Anterior division of retromandibular v.

Common facial v.

Superior thyroid a. and v.

Internal jugular v.

Middle thyroid v.

Transverse cervical
and suprascapular vv.

Inferior thyroid v.

FIGURE 8.53 External and Internal Jugular Veins. (From *Netter's atlas of human anatomy*, ed 8, Plates 50 and 100; S-328 and S-329.)

- Alter vitamin D metabolism, critical for calcium absorption from the GI tract.

Prevertebral Muscles

A group of deep neck flexor muscles called the *prevertebral muscles* lie surrounded by the prevertebral fascia adjacent to the bodies of the

cervical and upper thoracic vertebrae (Fig. 8.55 and Table 8.18). Generally, these muscles stabilize the cervical vertebrae and flex the neck. Additionally, the **scalene muscles** (posterior, middle, and anterior muscles) help elevate the rib cage and laterally flex the neck (see Table 8.13). The anterior rami of the nerves forming the **cervical plexus** (C1-C4) and **brachial plexus** (C5-T1) pass laterally between the anterior and middle scalene muscles. The **phrenic nerve** (anterior rami of C3-C5), which innervates the respiratory diaphragm, emerges from between the middle and *anterior scalene muscles* and can usually be found lying on the anterior surface of the anterior scalene muscle as it descends to enter the thoracic cavity (see Figs. 3.14, 8.50, and 8.51).

TABLE 8.17 Features of the Thyroid Gland	
STRUCTURE	CHARACTERISTICS
Lobes	Right and left, with a thin isthmus joining them
Blood supply	Superior and inferior thyroid arteries
Venous drainage	Superior, middle, and inferior thyroid veins
Pyramidal lobe	Variable (50% of time) superior extension of thyroid tissue

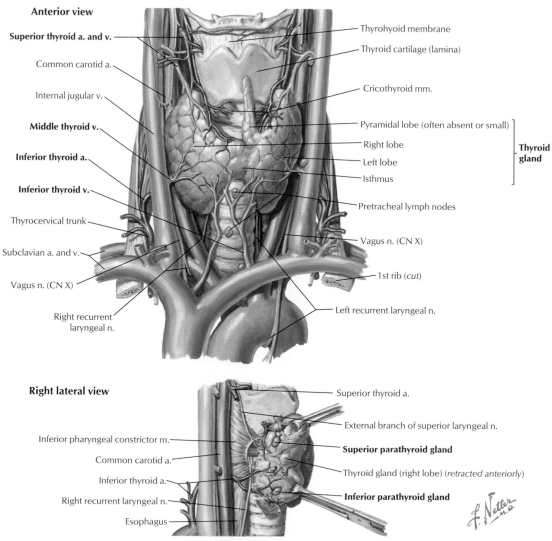

FIGURE 8.54 Thyroid and Parathyroid Glands and Blood Supply. (From *Netter's atlas of human anatomy*, ed 8, Plates 103 and 105; S-525 and S-527.)

Clinical Focus 8.38

Hyperthyroidism With Diffuse Goiter (Graves' Disease)

Graves' disease is the most common cause of hyperthyroidism in patients younger than 40. Excess synthesis and release of thyroid hormone (T_3 and T_4) result in **thyrotoxicosis,** which upregulates tissue metabolism and leads to symptoms, indicating increased metabolism. Besides Graves' disease, hyperthyroidism can be caused by benign growth of the thyroid gland, benign growth of the anterior pituitary gland, thyroiditis, the ingestion of excessive amounts of thyroid hormones and iodine, and tumors of the ovaries.

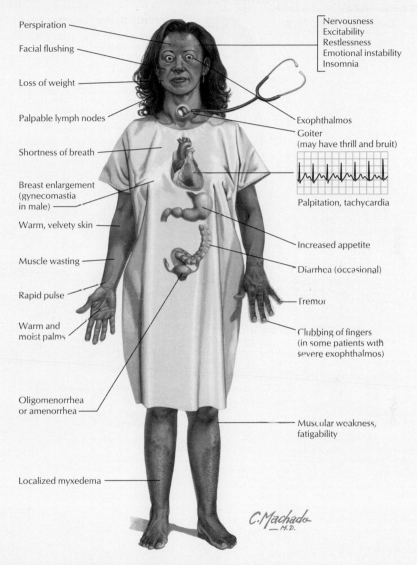

Perspiration
Facial flushing
Loss of weight
Palpable lymph nodes
Shortness of breath
Breast enlargement (gynecomastia in male)
Warm, velvety skin
Muscle wasting
Rapid pulse
Warm and moist palms
Oligomenorrhea or amenorrhea
Localized myxedema

Nervousness
Excitability
Restlessness
Emotional instability
Insomnia

Exophthalmos
Goiter (may have thrill and bruit)
Palpitation, tachycardia
Increased appetite
Diarrhea (occasional)
Tremor
Clubbing of fingers (in some patients with severe exophthalmos)
Muscular weakness, fatigability

C. Machado M.D.

Characteristic	Description
Etiology	Autoimmune disease with antibodies directed against thyroid-stimulating hormone (TSH) receptor, stimulating release of hormone or increasing thyroid epithelial cell activity; familial predisposition
Prevalence	Seven times more common in women than in men; peak incidence between 20 and 40 years of age
Signs	Thyrotoxicosis (hyperfunctional state), lid lag, exophthalmos (infiltrative increase in retrobulbar connective tissue and extraocular muscles), pretibial myxedema (thickened skin on leg); most common cause of endogenous hyperthyroidism

Clinical Focus 8.39

Primary Hypothyroidism

Primary hypothyroidism is a disease in which the thyroid gland produces inadequate amounts of thyroid hormone to meet the body's needs. Thyroid-stimulating hormone (TSH) levels are elevated. In addition to the autoimmune form of the disease, hypothyroidism also may occur from thyroidectomy and radiation-related damage.

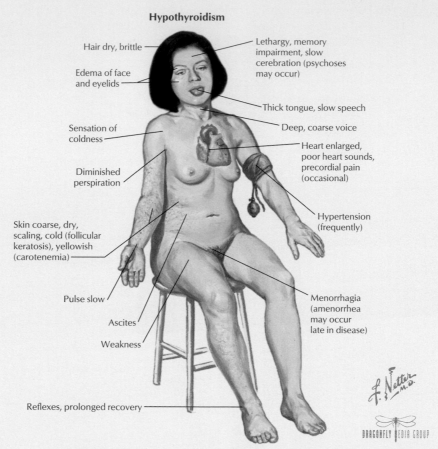

Hypothyroidism

Hair dry, brittle

Edema of face and eyelids

Sensation of coldness

Diminished perspiration

Skin coarse, dry, scaling, cold (follicular keratosis), yellowish (carotenemia)

Pulse slow

Ascites

Weakness

Reflexes, prolonged recovery

Lethargy, memory impairment, slow cerebration (psychoses may occur)

Thick tongue, slow speech

Deep, coarse voice

Heart enlarged, poor heart sounds, precordial pain (occasional)

Hypertension (frequently)

Menorrhagia (amenorrhea may occur late in disease)

Characteristic	Description
Etiology	Surgical ablation (thyroidectomy), radiation damage, Hashimoto's thyroiditis (autoimmune inflammatory disorder), idiopathic causes
Prevalence	More common in women than in men; can occur in any age group; congenital cases about 1 in 5000 births
Signs and symptoms	Myxedema (clinical manifestations illustrated)

12. PHARYNX

The **pharynx** (throat), a fibromuscular tube, connects the nasal and oral cavities of the head with the larynx and esophagus in the neck (Figs. 8.56–8.58). It extends from the base of the skull to the cricoid cartilage, where it is continuous with the esophagus. The pharynx is subdivided as follows:

- **Nasopharynx:** lies posterior to the nasal cavity above the soft palate.
- **Oropharynx:** extends from the soft palate to the superior tip of the epiglottis; it is the region that lies posterior to the oral cavity.
- **Laryngopharynx:** extends from the tip of the epiglottis to the inferior aspect of the cricoid cartilage; also known clinically as the *hypopharynx*.

Clinical Focus 8.40

Manifestations of Primary Hyperparathyroidism

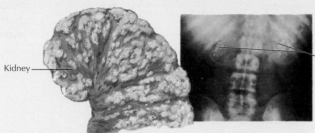

Kidney

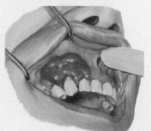

Nephrocalcinosis

Nephrocalcinosis

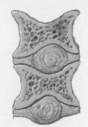

"Codfishing" of vertebrae

Nephrolithiasis

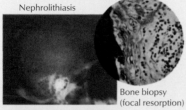

Bone biopsy (focal resorption)

"Salt and pepper" skull

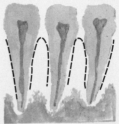

Absence of lamina dura (broken line indicates normal contour)

Epulis (giant cell tumor)

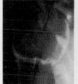

Bone rare-faction; cysts, fractures

Subperiosteal resorption

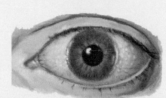

Limbus keratopathy

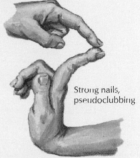

Strong nails, pseudoclubbing

Increased flexibility of joints

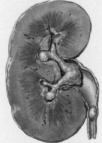

Nephrolithiasis

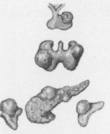

Multiple adenomas (pituitary, thyroid, pancreas, adrenals)

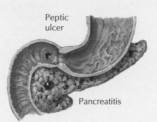

Peptic ulcer

Pancreatitis

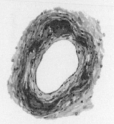

Calcium deposits in blood vessels; hypertension; heart failure

Characteristic	Description
Etiology	Hypertrophy of parathyroid glands (>85% are solitary benign adenomas), which leads to secretion of excess parathyroid hormone that causes increased calcium levels
Presentation	Mild or nonspecific symptoms including fatigue, constipation, polyuria, polydipsia, depression, skeletal pain, and nausea
Prevalence	Approximately 100,000 new cases/year in the United States; 2:1 prevalence in women, which increases with age
Management	Surgical removal of parathyroid glands

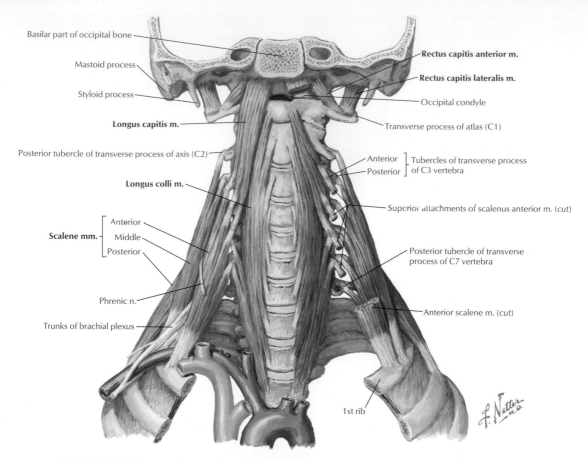

Basilar part of occipital bone

Mastoid process

Styloid process

Longus capitis m.

Posterior tubercle of transverse process of axis (C2)

Longus colli m.

Scalene mm. — Anterior / Middle / Posterior

Phrenic n.

Trunks of brachial plexus

Rectus capitis anterior m.

Rectus capitis lateralis m.

Occipital condyle

Transverse process of atlas (C1)

Anterior / Posterior — Tubercles of transverse process of C3 vertebra

Superior attachments of scalenus anterior m. (*cut*)

Posterior tubercle of transverse process of C7 vertebra

Anterior scalene m. (*cut*)

1st rib

FIGURE 8.55 Prevertebral Muscles. (From *Netter's atlas of human anatomy*, ed 8, Plate 55; S-193)

TABLE 8.18 Prevertebral Muscles

MUSCLE	ORIGIN ATTACHMENT	INSERTION ATTACHMENT	INNERVATION	MAIN ACTIONS
Longus colli	Body of T1-T3 with attachments to bodies of C4-C7 and transverse processes of C3-C5 vertebrae	Anterior tubercle of C1 (atlas), transverse processes of C3-C6, and bodies of C2-C4 vertebrae	C2-C8 spinal nerves	Flexes cervical vertebrae; allows slight rotation
Longus capitis	Anterior tubercles of C3-C6 transverse processes	Basilar part of occipital bone	C1-C3 spinal nerves	Flexes head
Rectus capitis anterior	Lateral mass of C1 (atlas)	Base of occipital bone, anterior to occipital condyle	C1-C2 spinal nerves	Flexes head
Rectus capitis lateralis	Transverse process of C1 (atlas)	Jugular process of occipital bone	C1-C2 spinal nerves	Flexes laterally and helps stabilize head

Variations in spinal nerve contributions to the innervation of muscles, their attachments, and their actions are common in human anatomy. Therefore, expect differences between texts and realize that anatomical variation is normal.

The muscles (pharyngeal constrictors) of the pharynx participate in *swallowing* (deglutition) and contract serially from superior to inferior to move a bolus of food from the oropharynx and laryngopharynx into the proximal esophagus (Figs. 8.56–8.59; Table 8.19).

The blood supply to the pharynx is via branches of the **thyrocervical trunk** (subclavian artery), especially the ascending cervical artery (see Fig. 8.51 and Table 8.15) and the **external carotid artery** (principally its superior thyroid, facial, ascending pharyngeal, and maxillary branches) (see Figs. 8.52,

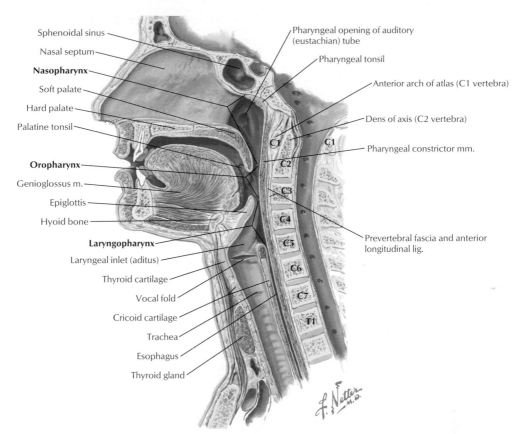

FIGURE 8.56 Subdivisions of the Pharynx. (From *Netter's atlas of human anatomy,* ed 8, Plate 95; S-372.)

Labels for Figure 8.56:
- Sphenoidal sinus
- Nasal septum
- **Nasopharynx**
- Soft palate
- Hard palate
- Palatine tonsil
- **Oropharynx**
- Genioglossus m.
- Epiglottis
- Hyoid bone
- **Laryngopharynx**
- Laryngeal inlet (aditus)
- Thyroid cartilage
- Vocal fold
- Cricoid cartilage
- Trachea
- Esophagus
- Thyroid gland
- Pharyngeal opening of auditory (eustachian) tube
- Pharyngeal tonsil
- Anterior arch of atlas (C1 vertebra)
- Dens of axis (C2 vertebra)
- Pharyngeal constrictor mm.
- Prevertebral fascia and anterior longitudinal lig.
- C1, C2, C3, C4, C5, C6, C7, T1

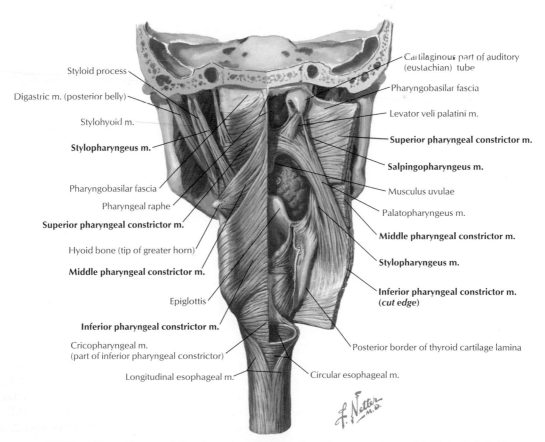

FIGURE 8.57 Pharyngeal Muscles. (From *Netter's atlas of human anatomy,* ed 8, Plate 92; S-409.)

Labels for Figure 8.57:
- Styloid process
- Digastric m. (posterior belly)
- Stylohyoid m.
- **Stylopharyngeus m.**
- Pharyngobasilar fascia
- Pharyngeal raphe
- **Superior pharyngeal constrictor m.**
- Hyoid bone (tip of greater horn)
- **Middle pharyngeal constrictor m.**
- Epiglottis
- **Inferior pharyngeal constrictor m.**
- Cricopharyngeal m. (part of inferior pharyngeal constrictor)
- Longitudinal esophageal m.
- Cartilaginous part of auditory (eustachian) tube
- Pharyngobasilar fascia
- Levator veli palatini m.
- **Superior pharyngeal constrictor m.**
- **Salpingopharyngeus m.**
- Musculus uvulae
- Palatopharyngeus m.
- **Middle pharyngeal constrictor m.**
- **Stylopharyngeus m.**
- **Inferior pharyngeal constrictor m.** (*cut edge*)
- Posterior border of thyroid cartilage lamina
- Circular esophageal m.

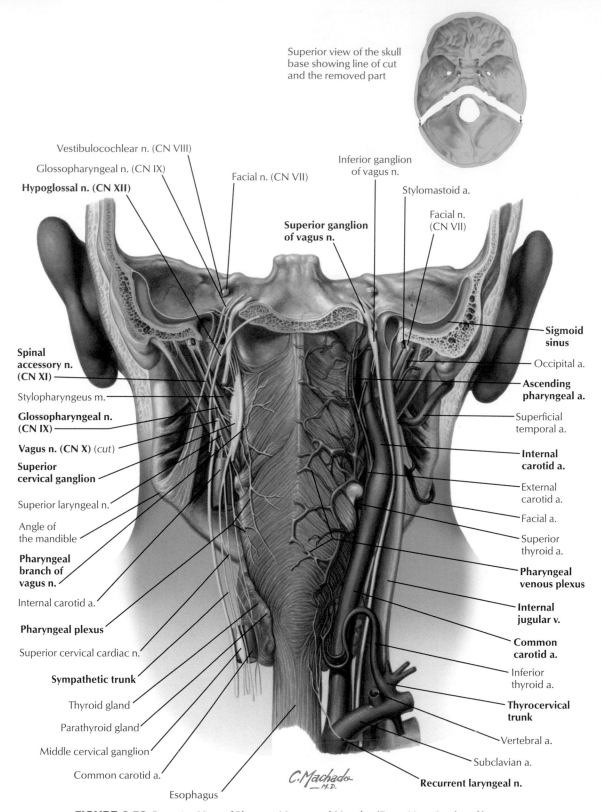

Superior view of the skull
base showing line of cut
and the removed part

Vestibulocochlear n. (CN VIII)

Glossopharyngeal n. (CN IX)

Hypoglossal n. (CN XII)

Facial n. (CN VII)

Inferior ganglion
of vagus n.

Stylomastoid a.

Facial n.
(CN VII)

**Superior ganglion
of vagus n.**

**Spinal
accessory n.
(CN XI)**

Stylopharyngeus m.

**Glossopharyngeal n.
(CN IX)**

Vagus n. (CN X) *(cut)*

**Superior
cervical ganglion**

Superior laryngeal n.

Angle of
the mandible

**Pharyngeal
branch of
vagus n.**

Internal carotid a.

Pharyngeal plexus

Superior cervical cardiac n.

Sympathetic trunk

Thyroid gland

Parathyroid gland

Middle cervical ganglion

Common carotid a.

Esophagus

**Sigmoid
sinus**

Occipital a.

**Ascending
pharyngeal a.**

Superficial
temporal a.

**Internal
carotid a.**

External
carotid a.

Facial a.

Superior
thyroid a.

**Pharyngeal
venous plexus**

**Internal
jugular v.**

**Common
carotid a.**

Inferior
thyroid a.

**Thyrocervical
trunk**

Vertebral a.

Subclavian a.

Recurrent laryngeal n.

C.Machado
_M.D._

FIGURE 8.58 Posterior View of Pharynx: Nerves and Vessels. (From *Netter's atlas of human
anatomy,* ed 8, Plate 91; S-72.)

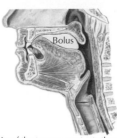

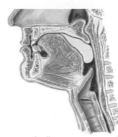

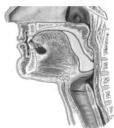

A. The tip of the tongue contacts the anterior part of palate while the bolus is pushed posteriorly in a groove between tongue and palate. The soft palate is drawn upward as a bulge forms in the upper part of posterior pharyngeal wall (Passavant's ridge) and approaches the rising soft palate.

B. As tongue gradually presses more of its dorsal surface against the hard palate, the bolus is pushed posteriorly into the oropharynx. The soft palate is drawn superiorly to contact Passavant's ridge and closes off the nasopharynx. A receptive space is created in the oropharynx as the root of the tongue moves slightly anteriorly. The stylopharyngeus and upper pharyngeal constrictor mm. contract to raise the pharyngeal wall over the bolus.

C. When the bolus has reached the vallecula, the hyoid and larynx move superiorly and anteriorly, while the epiglottis is tipped inferiorly. A "stripping wave" on the posterior pharyngeal wall moves inferiorly.

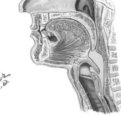

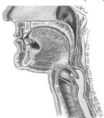

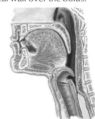

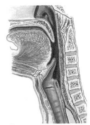

D. The soft palate is pulled inferiorly and approximated to the root of tongue by contraction of the palatopharyngeus and pressure of the descending "stripping wave." The oropharyngeal cavity is closed by contraction of upper pharyngeal constrictors. Relaxation of the cricopharyngeus permits entry of the bolus into the esophagus. A trickle of food may enter the laryngeal aditus.

E. "Stripping wave" reaches vallecula and presses out the last of the bolus. The cricopharyngeus remains relaxed and the bolus has largely passed into the esophagus.

F. "Stripping wave" passes the pharynx, and the epiglottis begins to turn superiorly as the hyoid and larynx descend. Communication with the nasopharynx is reestablished.

G. All structures of the pharynx return to their resting positions as the "stripping wave" passes into the esophagus, pushing the bolus before it.

FIGURE 8.59 Deglutition (swallowing).

TABLE 8.19 Pharyngeal Muscles

MUSCLE	ORIGIN ATTACHMENT	INSERTION ATTACHMENT	INNERVATION	MAIN ACTIONS
Superior pharyngeal constrictor	Hamulus, pterygomandibular raphe, mylohyoid line of mandible	Median raphe of pharynx	Vagus via pharyngeal plexus	Constricts wall of pharynx during swallowing
Middle pharyngeal constrictor	Stylohyoid ligament and horns of hyoid bone	Median raphe of pharynx	Vagus via pharyngeal plexus	Constricts wall of pharynx during swallowing
Inferior pharyngeal constrictor	Oblique line of thyroid cartilage, and cricoid cartilage	Median raphe of pharynx	Vagus via pharyngeal plexus	Constricts wall of pharynx during swallowing
Salpingopharyngeus	Auditory (pharyngotympanic) tube	Side of wall of pharynx	Vagus via pharyngeal plexus	Elevates pharynx and larynx during swallowing and speaking
Stylopharyngeus	Medial aspect of styloid process	Pharyngeal wall and posterior border of thyroid cartilage	Glossopharyngeal nerve	Elevates pharynx and larynx during swallowing and speaking

Variations in spinal nerve contributions to the innervation of muscles, their attachments, and their actions are common in human anatomy. Therefore, expect differences between texts and realize that anatomical variation is normal.

8.58 and Table 8.16). **Venous drainage** is via the pharyngeal venous plexus, the pterygoid plexus of veins, and the facial, lingual, and superior thyroid veins, all of which drain primarily into the internal jugular vein (see Figs. 8.53 and 8.58).

The **sensory innervation** of the nasopharynx is by the pharyngeal branch of CN V_2; sensory innervation to the oropharynx is by CN IX; and sensory innervation of the laryngopharynx is by CN X. The **motor innervation** is by CN X and its pharyngeal plexus, except the stylopharyngeus muscle, which is innervated by CN IX (Figs. 8.58, 8.75–8.76).

Swallowing, or **deglutition,** includes the following sequence of events (Fig. 8.59):

- The tongue pushes the bolus of food up against the hard palate.
- The soft palate elevates to close off the nasopharynx.
- The tongue pushes the bolus back into the oropharynx.
- As the bolus reaches the epiglottis, the larynx elevates and the tip of the epiglottis tips downward over the laryngeal opening (aditus).
- Contractions of the pharyngeal constrictors squeeze the bolus into two streams that pass on either side of the epiglottis and down along the piriform recesses and into the upper esophagus.
- The soft palate pulls downward to assist in moving the bolus around the epiglottis.
- The laryngeal vestibular folds (the rima vestibuli is the space between the vestibular folds) and rima glottidis (space between the vocal folds) close to protect the larynx.
- Once the bolus is in the esophagus, all structures return to their starting positions.

The superior openings into the pharynx (nasal and oral cavities) are "guarded" by a ring of lymphoid tissue in the mucosa that composes **Waldeyer's tonsillar ring** and includes the following (Fig. 8.60):

- **Tubal tonsils:** diffuse lymphoid tissue adjacent to the opening of the auditory tube; this tissue may be continuous with the pharyngeal tonsils.
- **Pharyngeal tonsils:** lie in the posterior wall and roof of the nasopharynx; called **adenoids** when enlarged.
- **Palatine tonsils:** guard the oropharynx and lie between the *palatoglossal and palatopharyngeal folds;* receive a rich blood supply from branches of facial, lingual, ascending pharyngeal, and maxillary arteries of the external carotid.
- **Lingual tonsils:** collection of lymphoid nodules on the posterior third of the tongue.

Collections of lymphoid tissue in the pharyngeal mucosa also can be found coursing down in lateral bands, demarcated by the salpingopharyngeal folds, to the level of the epiglottis.

The **"gag reflex"** can be elicited by touching the posterior portion of the tongue. Sensation is conveyed by the afferent branches of CN IX, and the soft palate is elevated by the efferent action of the vagus nerve (CN X). Should an object (food or foreign object) gain access to the vestibule of the larynx, a very powerful gag reflex would be elicited by the vagus nerve in an effort to protect the vocal folds and avoid aspiration into the trachea.

13. LARYNX

The **larynx** (voice box) is a musculoligamentous and cartilaginous structure that lies at the C3-C6 vertebral level, just superior to the trachea. It

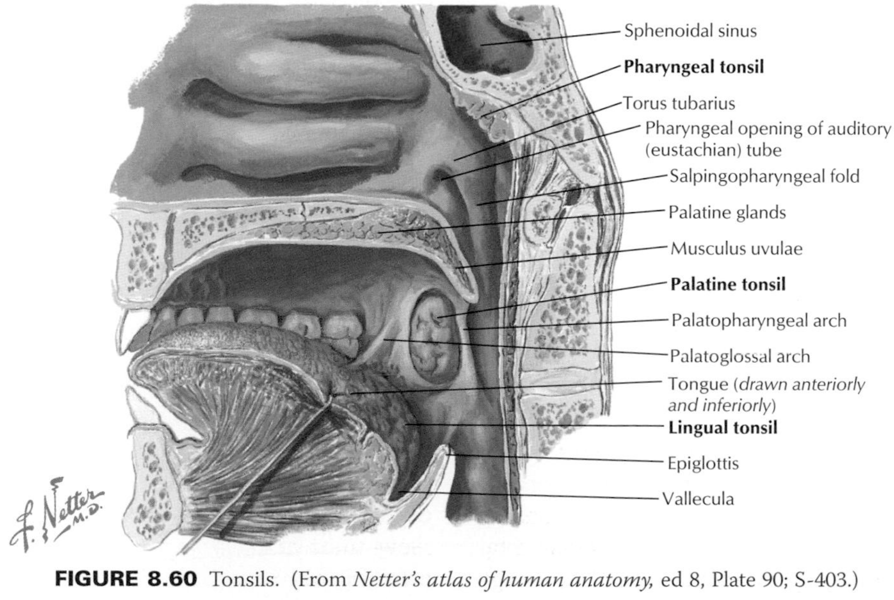

Medial view
Median (sagittal) section

- Sphenoidal sinus
- **Pharyngeal tonsil**
- Torus tubarius
- Pharyngeal opening of auditory (eustachian) tube
- Salpingopharyngeal fold
- Palatine glands
- Musculus uvulae
- **Palatine tonsil**
- Palatopharyngeal arch
- Palatoglossal arch
- Tongue (*drawn anteriorly and inferiorly*)
- **Lingual tonsil**
- Epiglottis
- Vallecula

FIGURE 8.60 Tonsils. (From *Netter's atlas of human anatomy,* ed 8, Plate 90; S-403.)

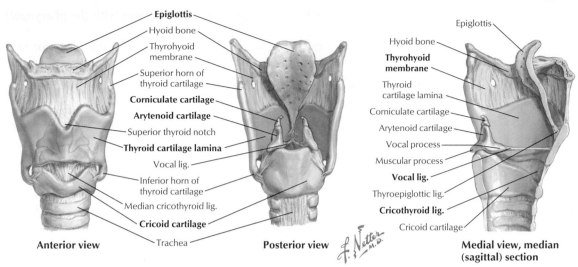

Epiglottis
Hyoid bone
Thyrohyoid membrane
Superior horn of thyroid cartilage
Corniculate cartilage
Arytenoid cartilage
Superior thyroid notch
Thyroid cartilage lamina
Vocal lig.
Inferior horn of thyroid cartilage
Median cricothyroid lig.
Cricoid cartilage
Trachea

Anterior view   **Posterior view**

Epiglottis
Hyoid bone
Thyrohyoid membrane
Thyroid cartilage lamina
Corniculate cartilage
Arytenoid cartilage
Vocal process
Muscular process
Vocal lig.
Thyroepiglottic lig.
Cricothyroid lig.
Cricoid cartilage

Medial view, median (sagittal) section

FIGURE 8.61 Laryngeal Cartilages, Ligaments, and Membranes. (From *Netter's atlas of human anatomy,* ed 8, Plate 106; S-375.)

TABLE 8.20 Laryngeal Cartilages	
CARTILAGE	**DESCRIPTION**
Thyroid	Two hyaline laminae and laryngeal prominence (Adam's apple)
Cricoid	Signet ring–shaped hyaline cartilage just inferior to thyroid
Epiglottis	Spoon-shaped elastic plate attached to thyroid cartilage
Arytenoid	Paired pyramidal cartilages that rotate on cricoid cartilage
Corniculate	Paired cartilages that lie on apex of arytenoid cartilages
Cuneiform	Paired cartilages in aryepiglottic folds that have no articulations

functions both as a sphincter to close off the airway and as a "reed instrument" to produce sound. Its framework consists of nine cartilages joined by ligaments and membranes (Fig. 8.61 and Table 8.20).

The intrinsic skeletal muscles of the larynx attach to the laryngeal cartilages and act largely to adjust the tension on the vocal folds (ligaments, cords); to open or close the **rima glottidis** (space between the vocal folds); and to open or close the **rima vestibuli,** which is the space between the vestibular folds (false folds) (Fig. 8.62). The opening or closing of the rima vestibuli by the vestibular (false) folds is important during swallowing, preventing aspiration into the trachea, but also slightly adjusting the size of the vestibule (region above the vestibular folds) during phonation, which enhances the quality of the sound. All these muscles are innervated by the **recurrent laryngeal branch of CN X,** except

the cricothyroid muscle, which is innervated by the external branch of the **superior laryngeal nerve (CN X).** Sensation above the vocal folds is conveyed by the *superior laryngeal nerve* of CN X and by the *recurrent laryngeal nerve* below the vocal folds.

The vocal folds (vocal ligaments covered with mucosa) control phonation as a reed might function in an instrument. Vibrations of the folds produce sounds as air passes through the rima glottidis (the space between the vocal folds). The **posterior cricoarytenoid muscles** are important because they are the *only laryngeal muscles* that abduct the vocal folds and maintain the opening of the rima glottidis (Figs. 8.62–8.63). The vestibular folds have a primarily protective function but can slightly alter the quality of sound.

Rotation of the arytenoid cartilages moves the vocal folds medially *(adduction)* by the action of the lateral cricoarytenoid muscle and the transverse and oblique arytenoid muscles. This action narrows the space between the vocal folds (rima glottidis), and the air rushing through the rima glottidis vibrates the vocal folds and their mucosal lining (higher tones) (Fig. 8.63). Lateral movement *(abduction)* of the arytenoid cartilages widens the rima glottidis, producing lower tones. The vocal folds also can be lengthened *(increased tension* on the vocal ligaments), producing a higher pitch, or shortened *(relaxation* of the ligaments), producing a lower pitch, by the cricothyroid joint, a synovial joint that allows the thyroid cartilage to be tilted anteriorly. The **cricothyroid muscles** tilt it anteriorly, increasing

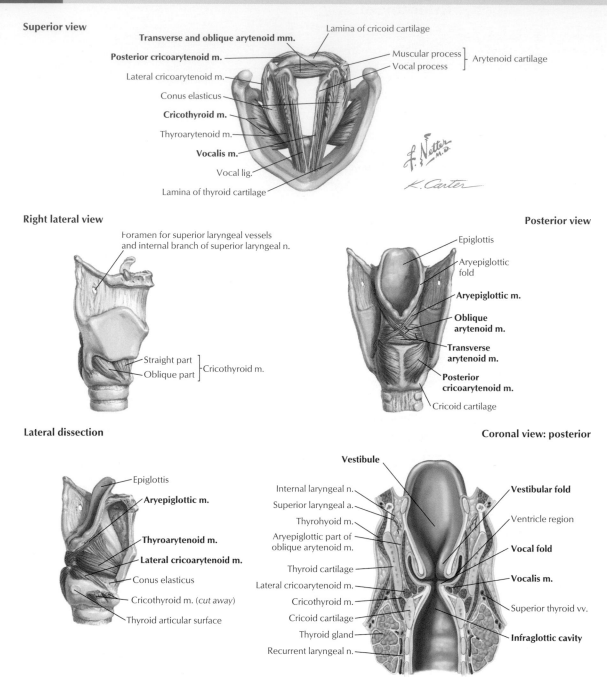

FIGURE 8.62 Muscles of the Larynx. (From *Netter's atlas of human anatomy*, ed 8, Plates 107 and 108; S-376 and S-378.)

the tension, and the **thyroarytenoid muscles** tilt the thyroid cartilage back into position to relax the vocal ligaments. As males reach puberty, the thyroid cartilage enlarges and the vocal ligaments become longer and thicker, leading to a deeper sound in the voice. The quality of each person's voice also is influenced by the shape of the oral and pharyngeal spaces, nose and paranasal sinuses, tongue and lips, and soft palate.

The arterial supply to the larynx is by the **superior laryngeal artery,** a branch of the superior thyroid artery off the external carotid artery, and by the **inferior laryngeal artery,** a branch of the inferior thyroid artery off the thyrocervical trunk of the subclavian artery (Figs. 8.51 and 8.52). The venous drainage is by laryngeal veins that drain into the superior and inferior thyroid veins (Figs. 8.53 and 8.54).

Clinical Focus 8.41

Emergency Airway: Cricothyrotomy

When all other methods of establishing an airway have been exhausted or determined to be unsuitable, an incision can be made through the skin and the underlying cricothyroid membrane to gain access to the trachea. The site of the incision can be judged by locating the thyroid notch and sliding your finger inferiorly until the space between the thyroid and cricoid cartilages is palpated (about one fingerbreadth inferior to the thyroid notch). If the patient has a midline pyramidal lobe arising from the thyroid gland, this procedure may lacerate that tissue and cause significant bleeding.

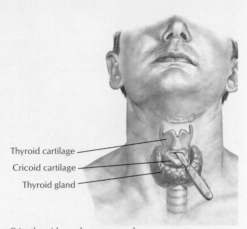

Thyroid cartilage
Cricoid cartilage
Thyroid gland

Cricothyroid membrane identified by palpating for transverse indentation between thyroid cartilage and cricoid cartilage

Cricothyroid membrane opened with scalpel, knife, or other sharp instrument that may be at hand. Opening may be enlarged by twisting instrument and patency preserved by inserting rubber tubing or any other suitable object available

F. Netter M.D.

Clinical Focus 8.42

Manifestations of Hoarseness

Hoarseness can be caused by any condition that results in improper vibration or coaptation of the vocal folds.

Inflammation of the larynx

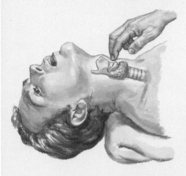

Acute laryngitis

Subglottic inflammation and swelling in inflammatory croup

Edematous vocal cords in chronic laryngitis

Lesions of the vocal cords

Pedunculated papilloma at anterior commissure

Sessile polyp

Subglottic polyp

Hyperkeratosis of right cord

Cancer of the larynx

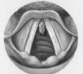

Carcinoma involving anterior commissure

Extensive carcinoma of right vocal cord involving arytenoid region

F. Netter M.D.

Node in neck often initial sign in carcinoma of the extrinsic larynx

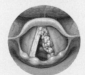

Condition	Description
Acute laryngitis	Inflammation and edema caused by smoking, gastroesophageal reflux disease, chronic rhinosinusitis, cough, voice overuse, myxedema, infection
Stiffness	Caused by surgical scarring or inflammation
Mass lesion	Caused by nodule, cyst, granuloma, neoplasm, fungal infection
Paralysis or paresis	Occurs after viral infection, recurrent laryngeal nerve lesion, or stroke; can have congenital causes or be iatrogenic

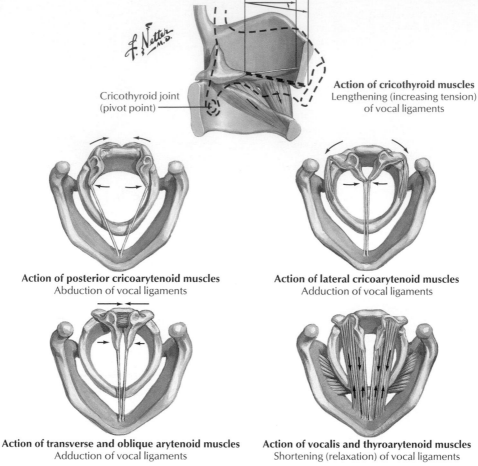

Cricothyroid joint
(pivot point)

Action of cricothyroid muscles
Lengthening (increasing tension)
of vocal ligaments

Action of posterior cricoarytenoid muscles
Abduction of vocal ligaments

Action of lateral cricoarytenoid muscles
Adduction of vocal ligaments

Action of transverse and oblique arytenoid muscles
Adduction of vocal ligaments

Action of vocalis and thyroarytenoid muscles
Shortening (relaxation) of vocal ligaments

FIGURE 8.63 Action of Intrinsic Muscles of Larynx. (From *Netter's atlas of human anatomy*, ed 8, Plate 109; S-377.)

14. HEAD AND NECK VASCULAR AND LYMPHATIC SUMMARY

Arteries of the head and neck largely include branches derived from the following major vessels (Fig. 8.64):

- **Subclavian artery:** supplies the lower neck (thyrocervical and costocervical trunks), thyroid gland, thoracic wall, shoulder, upper back, and the brain via paired vertebral arteries.
- **External carotid artery:** supplies the thyroid gland, larynx, pharynx, neck, oral cavity, face, nasal cavity, meninges, and temporal and infratemporal regions via its eight primary branches.
- **Internal carotid artery:** supplies the brain, orbit, eyeball, lacrimal glands, forehead, and ethmoid sinuses.

The venous drainage of the head and neck ultimately collects in the following major veins

(numerous variations and anastomoses exist between these veins) (Fig. 8.65):

- **Retromandibular vein:** receives tributaries from the temporal and infratemporal regions (pterygoid plexus), orbit, nasal cavity, pharynx, and oral cavity.
- **Internal jugular vein:** drains the brain (dural venous sinuses), face, thyroid gland, and neck.
- **External jugular vein:** drains the superficial neck, lower neck and shoulder, and upper back (often communicates with the retromandibular vein) (Fig. 8.53).

Lymph nodes and vessels of the head and neck tend to follow the venous drainage, with most of the lymph ultimately collecting in the **deep cervical lymphatic chain** (jugulodigastric and juguloomohyoid nodes), which courses along the internal jugular veins (Fig. 8.66). Superficial cervical nodes drain the superficial structures of the neck along lymphatic vessels that parallel the *external jugular*

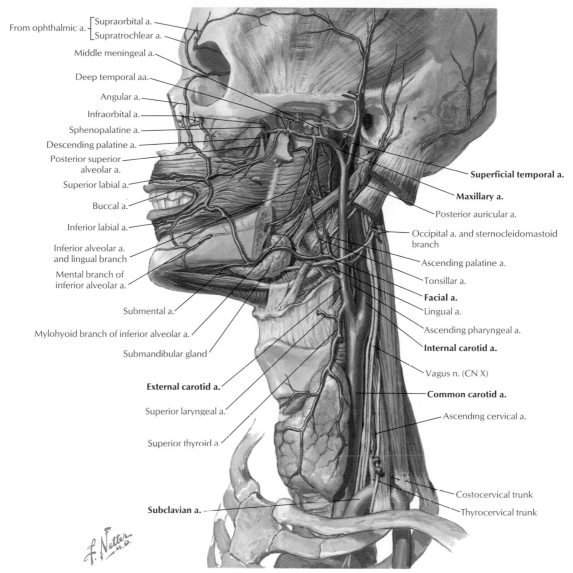

From ophthalmic a. — [Supraorbital a.
                     [Supratrochlear a.
Middle meningeal a.
Deep temporal aa.
Angular a.
Infraorbital a.
Sphenopalatine a.
Descending palatine a.
Posterior superior alveolar a.
Superior labial a.
Buccal a.
Inferior labial a.
Inferior alveolar a. and lingual branch
Mental branch of inferior alveolar a.
Submental a.
Mylohyoid branch of inferior alveolar a.
Submandibular gland
External carotid a.
Superior laryngeal a.
Superior thyroid a.
Subclavian a.

Superficial temporal a.
Maxillary a.
Posterior auricular a.
Occipital a. and sternocleidomastoid branch
Ascending palatine a.
Tonsillar a.
Facial a.
Lingual a.
Ascending pharyngeal a.
Internal carotid a.
Vagus n. (CN X)
Common carotid a.
Ascending cervical a.
Costocervical trunk
Thyrocervical trunk

FIGURE 8.64 Major Arteries of the Head and Neck. (From *Netter's atlas of human anatomy*, ed 8, Plate 99; S-323.)

vein. The right side of the head and neck drains into the right lymphatic duct, and the left side of the head and neck drains into the thoracic duct (see Fig. 1.16).

15. HEAD AND NECK ARTERIOVENOUS SUMMARY

Arteries of the Head and Neck (see **Figs. 8.64 and 8.67**)

After the **ascending aorta (1)** gives rise to the two coronary arteries, it forms the **aortic arch (2),** which gives rise to three branches: the **brachiocephalic artery (3),** the **left common carotid artery,** and

the **left subclavian artery** (Fig. 8.67). The brachiocephalic artery is short and gives rise to the **right common carotid artery (4)** and the **right subclavian artery (7).**

The common carotid artery, *on both the right and left sides,* ascends in the neck and divides into the **internal carotid artery (5),** which passes superiorly to become intracranial (giving off only several very small branches as it ascends in the neck), and the **external carotid artery (6).**

The external carotid artery (*again on both sides*) gives rise to eight major branches to the neck, face, and occipital region and terminates as the **superficial temporal artery** on the lateral aspect of the head

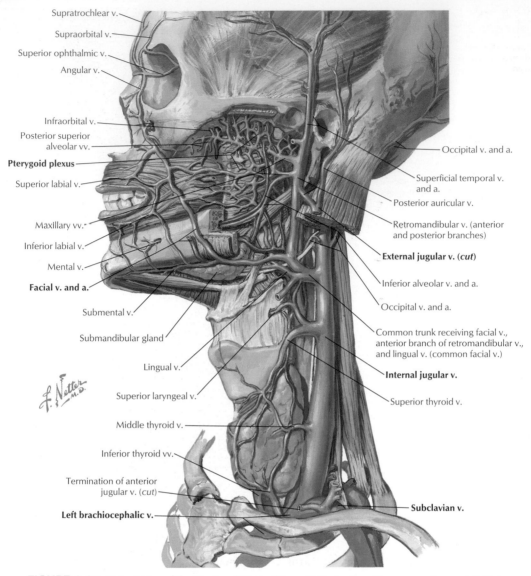

Supratrochlear v.
Supraorbital v.
Superior ophthalmic v.
Angular v.

Infraorbital v.
Posterior superior alveolar vv.
Pterygoid plexus
Superior labial v.

Maxillary vv.
Inferior labial v.
Mental v.
Facial v. and a.

Submental v.

Submandibular gland

Lingual v.

Superior laryngeal v.

Middle thyroid v.

Inferior thyroid vv.

Termination of anterior jugular v. (*cut*)

Left brachiocephalic v.

Occipital v. and a.
Superficial temporal v. and a.
Posterior auricular v.
Retromandibular v. (anterior and posterior branches)
External jugular v. (*cut*)
Inferior alveolar v. and a.
Occipital v. and a.
Common trunk receiving facial v., anterior branch of retromandibular v., and lingual v. (common facial v.)
Internal jugular v.
Superior thyroid v.

Subclavian v.

FIGURE 8.65 Major Veins of the Head and Neck. (From *Netter's atlas of human anatomy,* ed 8, Plate 100; S-328.)

and as the **maxillary artery**, which then passes into the infratemporal region. The **maxillary artery** itself gives off about 15 additional branches to the infratemporal region and its muscles, meninges, mandible, maxilla, orbit, palate, and nasal cavities.

The **subclavian artery (7)** *(on both sides)* gives off four major branches: one to the posterior brain and cervical spinal cord (vertebral artery), an artery to the thorax (internal thoracic artery), and branches to the neck and shoulder region, via its thyrocervical and costocervical trunks.

The subclavian artery then becomes the **axillary artery**(*both sides*) after crossing the first rib (see Figs. 7.14 and 7.34).

A rich vascular supply is given to the brain by the **two vertebral** and **two internal carotid arteries** (see Fig. 8.12 and Table 8.3). The infratemporal fossa, upper jaw, orbital floor, nasal cavity and paranasal sinuses, palate, auditory tube, and superior pharynx receive a rich blood supply by way of the maxillary artery (Fig. 8.31). The neck and the thyroid and parathyroid endocrine glands (superior and inferior thyroid arteries) receive blood from the external carotid artery and branches of the subclavian arteries (Fig. 8.51 and Table 8.15). A rich vascular anastomosis also exists around the shoulder joint and scapula by the branches of the subclavian and axillary arteries (see Figs. 7.7 and 7.8).

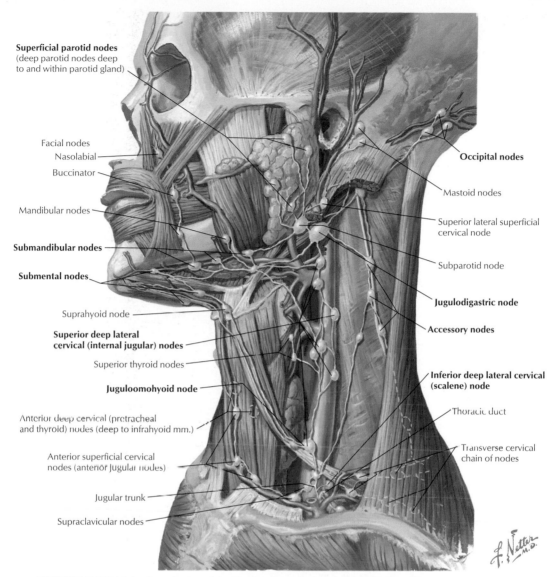

FIGURE 8.66 Major Lymphatics of the Head and Neck. (From *Netter's atlas of human anatomy*, ed 8, Plate 101; S-344.)

Veins of the Head and Neck

The veins of the head and neck have numerous interconnections (Fig. 8.68). The dural venous sinuses converge at the sigmoid dural sinus to form the **superior bulb of the jugular vein (1)** at the jugular foramen (CN IX, X, and XI also exit the skull here). Note that the veins outlined below are bilateral *(right and left veins)* and can often communicate across the midline of the face and neck. The **internal jugular vein (2)** *(both sides)* then descends within the carotid sheath and receives numerous tributaries from the head and face; one major tributary is the **retromandibular vein (3),** which itself receives

tributaries from the head and facial regions (listed separately in the outline). The retromandibular vein communicates directly not only with the internal jugular vein but also with the **anterior jugular vein** and **external jugular vein(s),** which are in the superficial fascia. Both the internal jugular vein and the tributaries of the retromandibular vein and external jugular vein drain inferiorly to join the **subclavian vein (4)** *(both sides).* The subclavian vein and internal jugular vein unite to form the **brachiocephalic vein (5)** on the right and left sides. The brachiocephalic veins receive small tributaries from the superior mediastinum, including the

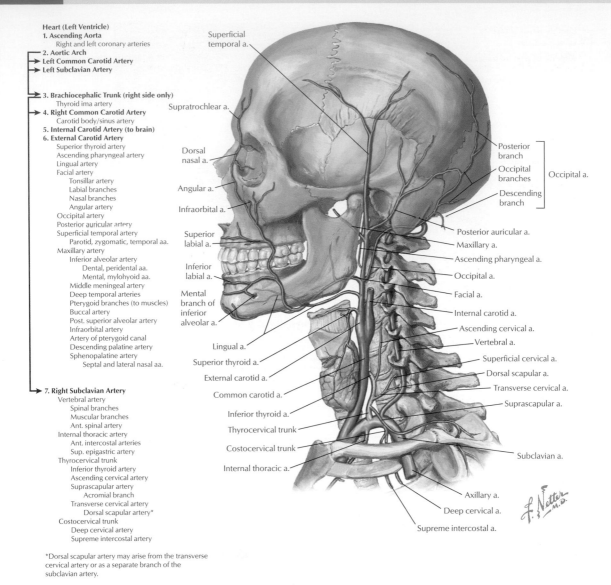

Heart (Left Ventricle)
1. **Ascending Aorta**
    Right and left coronary arteries
2. **Aortic Arch**
→ **Left Common Carotid Artery**
→ **Left Subclavian Artery**

→ 3. **Brachiocephalic Trunk (right side only)**
    Thyroid ima artery
→ 4. **Right Common Carotid Artery**
    Carotid body/sinus artery
5. **Internal Carotid Artery (to brain)**
6. **External Carotid Artery**
    Superior thyroid artery
    Ascending pharyngeal artery
    Lingual artery
    Facial artery
        Tonsillar artery
        Labial branches
        Nasal branches
        Angular artery
    Occipital artery
    Posterior auricular artery
    Superficial temporal artery
        Parotid, zygomatic, temporal aa.
    Maxillary artery
        Inferior alveolar artery
            Dental, peridental aa.
            Mental, mylohyoid aa.
        Middle meningeal artery
        Deep temporal arteries
        Pterygoid branches (to muscles)
        Buccal artery
        Post. superior alveolar artery
        Infraorbital artery
        Artery of pterygoid canal
        Descending palatine artery
        Sphenopalatine artery
            Septal and lateral nasal aa.

→ 7. **Right Subclavian Artery**
    Vertebral artery
        Spinal branches
        Muscular branches
        Ant. spinal artery
    Internal thoracic artery
        Ant. intercostal arteries
        Sup. epigastric artery
    Thyrocervical trunk
        Inferior thyroid artery
        Ascending cervical artery
        Suprascapular artery
            Acromial branch
        Transverse cervical artery
            Dorsal scapular artery*
    Costocervical trunk
        Deep cervical artery
        Supreme intercostal artery

*Dorsal scapular artery may arise from the transverse
cervical artery or as a separate branch of the
subclavian artery.

FIGURE 8.67 Arteries of the Head and Neck.

inferior thyroid, vertebral, intercostal, pericardial, laryngeal, esophageal, and bronchial veins. The left and right brachiocephalic veins then join to form the **superior vena cava (6)** on the right aspect of the superior mediastinum, and the SVC then drains into the **right atrium of the heart (7).**

Variations and interconnections are common, especially with the smaller veins. The **ophthalmic veins** of the orbit drain into the **(1)** cavernous sinus posteriorly and intracranially, **(2)** into the facial veins externally on the face, and **(3)** into the infratemporal fossa and the pterygoid plexus of veins. Ultimately, these veins and their tributaries drain into the retromandibular vein and internal jugular vein (see Fig. 8.68). A rich venous

anastomosis also exits in the neck as three pairs of veins drain the thyroid/parathyroid endocrine glands (superior, middle, and inferior thyroid veins) (Figs. 8.65 and 8.68).

16. CRANIAL NERVE SUMMARY

Autonomic Innervation

The autonomic distribution to the head involves *preganglionic parasympathetic axons* that arise from neurons in the CNS and synapse in peripheral ganglia (Fig. 8.69). *Postganglionic parasympathetic axons* then arise from neurons in these peripheral ganglia and course to their respective targets (smooth muscle and glands). Except for the parasympathetic

Confluence of Sinuses*
Transverse Sinus
Sigmoid Sinus
1. Superior Bulb of Jugular Vein

Vein of cochlear aqueduct
Pharyngeal veins
Meningeal veins
Lingual vein
Superior laryngeal vein
Superior thyroid vein
Middle thyroid vein
2. Internal Jugular Veins

Superficial temporal vein
Middle temporal vein
Pterygoid plexus of veins
(meningeal, deep temporal,
parotid, articular, tympanic,
inf. ophthalmic veins)
Transverse facial vein
Posterior auricular vein
Maxillary veins
Facial vein
(ophthalmic, nasal, labial, parotid vv.)
3. Retromandibular Vein

Transverse cervical vein
Suprascapular vein
Anterior jugular vein
External jugular vein

4. Subclavian Vein

Vertebral vein
Inferior thyroid vein
Supreme intercostal vein
Internal thoracic veins
Pericardial veins
5. Brachiocephalic Vein
6. Superior Vena Cava
7. Right Atrium of Heart

*Distal (dural sinuses) to Heart (right atrium)

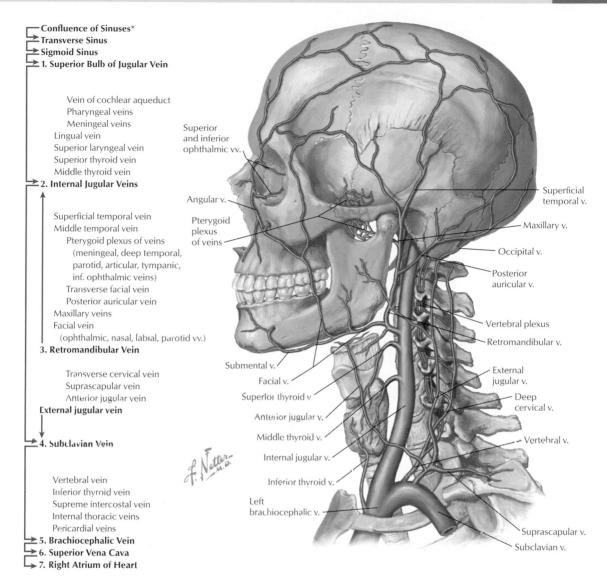

Superior and inferior ophthalmic vv.

Angular v.

Pterygoid plexus of veins

Superficial temporal v.

Maxillary v.

Occipital v.

Posterior auricular v.

Vertebral plexus

Retromandibular v.

Submental v.

Facial v.

Superior thyroid v.

Anterior jugular v.

Middle thyroid v.

Internal jugular v.

Inferior thyroid v.

Left brachiocephalic v.

External jugular v.

Deep cervical v.

Vertebral v.

Suprascapular v.

Subclavian v.

FIGURE 8.68 Veins of the Head and Neck.

fibers to the eye (constrictor of the pupil and ciliary muscle for accommodation) and parotid salivary gland, *all* the other preganglionic parasympathetics arise from the **superior salivatory nucleus** of the facial nerve (CN VII) via the intermediate portion *(intermediate nerve)* of the facial nerve. These preganglionic fibers then course either in the **greater petrosal nerve** to the pterygopalatine ganglion or via the **chorda tympani nerve** and lingual nerve (from CN V$_3$) to the submandibular ganglion. The *vagus nerve* (not shown in Fig. 8.69) provides parasympathetic innervation to the neck, thorax, and upper two-thirds of the abdominal viscera, but none to the head region (see Fig. 4.30).

Preganglionic sympathetic fibers from the upper thoracic spinal cord levels (T1-T2) ascend via the sympathetic trunk and synapse in the **superior cervical ganglion (SCG)** (Fig. 8.70). *Postganglionic axons* from the SCG then course along blood vessels or existing nerves to reach their targets, mainly vasomotor smooth muscle, skin sweat and sebaceous glands, and the smooth muscle of the dilator of the pupil and the superior tarsal muscle in the upper eyelid (Figs. 8.69–8.71).

Cranial Nerves

We reviewed the general components of the cranial nerves earlier in this chapter (see Fig. 8.13; Table 8.4),

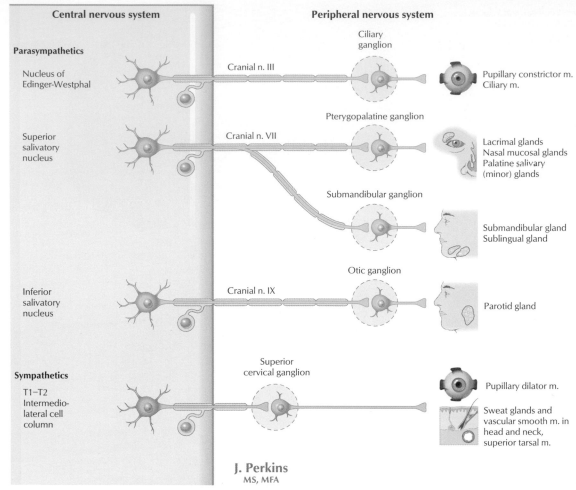

FIGURE 8.69 Autonomic Distribution to the Head.

so we will focus this summary selectively on the more complex cranial nerves (Table 8.21).

Oculomotor, Trochlear, and Abducens Nerves

The **oculomotor nerve (CN III)** innervates five skeletal (branchiomeric) muscles in the orbit (general somatic efferents; see Table 8.6) and conveys parasympathetic preganglionic fibers from the **accessory oculomotor (Edinger-Westphal) nucleus** to the **ciliary ganglion**, where they synapse on the postganglionic neurons. Postganglionic parasympathetic fibers then course via **short ciliary nerves** to the eyeball (these postganglionic fibers mediate pupillary constriction and accommodation of the lens by their action on the ciliary smooth muscle). The **trochlear nerve (CN IV)** innervates the superior oblique muscle, and the **abducens nerve (CN VI)** innervates the lateral rectus muscle (Fig. 8.71; Table 8.21).

Trigeminal Nerve

The **trigeminal nerve (CN V),** the *major sensory nerve of the head,* conveys general somatic afferents centrally to the **trigeminal sensory ganglion** (also called the semilunar or gasserian ganglion by clinicians) via its ophthalmic (CN V$_1$), maxillary (CN V$_2$), and mandibular (CN V$_3$) divisions (Fig. 8.72). Its mandibular division also innervates skeletal (branchiomeric) muscles derived from the **first embryonic branchial arch** (see Embryology). Because of the extensive distribution of CN V, most of the parasympathetic fibers from CN III, VII, and IX course with branches of CN V to reach their targets (smooth muscle and glands) (Figs. 8.69 and 8.72). These targets include:

- **Lacrimal gland:** preganglionic parasympathetics from the superior salivatory nucleus of CN VII travel in the **greater petrosal nerve** to synapse in the **pterygopalatine ganglion** and send

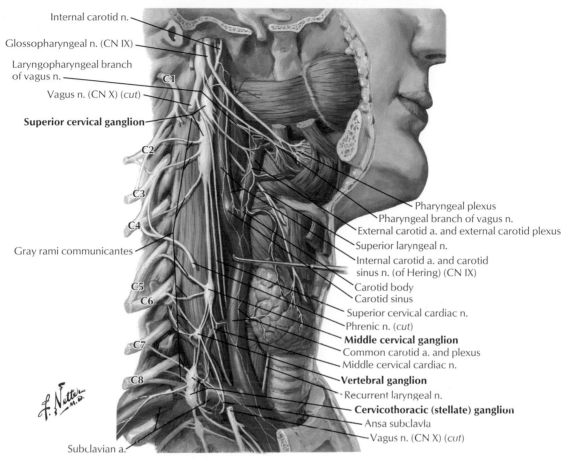

Internal carotid n.
Glossopharyngeal n. (CN IX)
Laryngopharyngeal branch of vagus n.
Vagus n. (CN X) (*cut*)
Superior cervical ganglion
C1
C2
C3
C4
Gray rami communicantes
C5
C6
C7
C8
Subclavian a.

Pharyngeal plexus
Pharyngeal branch of vagus n.
External carotid a. and external carotid plexus
Superior laryngeal n.
Internal carotid a. and carotid sinus n. (of Hering) (CN IX)
Carotid body
Carotid sinus
Superior cervical cardiac n.
Phrenic n. (*cut*)
Middle cervical ganglion
Common carotid a. and plexus
Middle cervical cardiac n.
Vertebral ganglion
Recurrent laryngeal n.
Cervicothoracic (stellate) ganglion
Ansa subclavia
Vagus n. (CN X) (*cut*)

FIGURE 8.70 Sympathetic Ganglia and Nerves to the Head. (From *Netter's atlas of human anatomy*, ed 8, Plate 157; S-76.)

postganglionic fibers via CN V$_2$ (the zygomatic nerve) to the distal portion of the lacrimal nerve (CN V$_1$) and then to the gland (Figs. 8.69, 8.72, and 8.73).

- **Submandibular and sublingual salivary glands:** preganglionic parasympathetics from the superior salivatory nucleus of CN VII travel via the **chorda tympani** nerve to the lingual nerve of CN V$_3$ and synapse in the **submandibular ganglion**. Postganglionic fibers then innervate the submandibular and sublingual salivary glands, as well as minor salivary and mucous glands of the mandibular gingiva (Figs. 8.69, 8.72, and 8.73).
- **Nasal glands:** preganglionic parasympathetics from the superior salivatory nucleus of CN VII travel in the **greater petrosal nerve** to synapse in the **pterygopalatine ganglion** and send postganglionic fibers throughout the nasal cavity, paranasal sinuses, palate, and upper nasopharynx

to innervate glands in these regions (Figs. 8.38, 8.69, 8.73, and 8.74).

Facial Nerve

The **facial nerve (CN VII),** the *major motor nerve of the head,* conveys general somatic efferents to skeletal (branchiomeric) muscles derived from the **second embryonic branchial arch.** Additionally, CN VII sends preganglionic parasympathetic fibers from the **superior salivatory nucleus** to the **pterygopalatine ganglia** via the greater petrosal nerve and the nerve of the pterygoid canal, and to the **submandibular ganglia** via the chorda tympani and lingual nerves (see description above for CN V) (Fig. 8.73). The facial nerve also conveys special visceral afferents from taste receptors on the anterior two-thirds of the tongue along the chorda tympani to the **geniculate sensory ganglion** of CN VII (Figs. 8.73 and 8.74).

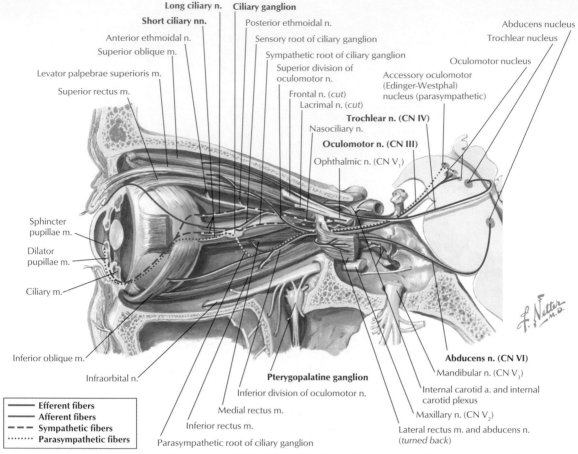

Long ciliary n. Ciliary ganglion

Short ciliary nn.

Posterior ethmoidal n.

Anterior ethmoidal n.

Sensory root of ciliary ganglion

Superior oblique m.

Sympathetic root of ciliary ganglion

Levator palpebrae superioris m.

Superior division of oculomotor n.

Superior rectus m.

Frontal n. (cut)

Lacrimal n. (cut)

Abducens nucleus

Trochlear nucleus

Oculomotor nucleus

Accessory oculomotor (Edinger-Westphal) nucleus (parasympathetic)

Trochlear n. (CN IV)

Nasociliary n.

Oculomotor n. (CN III)

Ophthalmic n. (CN V₁)

Sphincter pupillae m.

Dilator pupillae m.

Ciliary m.

Inferior oblique m.

Infraorbital n.

Pterygopalatine ganglion

Inferior division of oculomotor n.

Medial rectus m.

Inferior rectus m.

Parasympathetic root of ciliary ganglion

Abducens n. (CN VI)

Mandibular n. (CN V₃)

Internal carotid a. and internal carotid plexus

Maxillary n. (CN V₂)

Lateral rectus m. and abducens n. (turned back)

——— Efferent fibers
——— Afferent fibers
– – – Sympathetic fibers
········· Parasympathetic fibers

FIGURE 8.71 Pathway Summary for CN III, IV, and VI. (From *Netter's atlas of human anatomy*, ed 8, Plate 148; S-58.)

Glossopharyngeal Nerve

The **glossopharyngeal nerve (CN IX)** innervates the stylopharyngeus muscle (derived from the **third embryonic branchial arch**) and sends preganglionic parasympathetics from the **inferior salivatory nucleus** via the **lesser petrosal nerve** to the **otic ganglion**, where these fibers synapse on the postganglionic neurons (Figs. 8.69 and 8.75). Postganglionic fibers then course via the auriculotemporal branch of CN V₃ to the **parotid gland.** CN IX also conveys *special visceral afferents* from taste receptors on the posterior third of the tongue to the sensory ganglia of CN IX. General visceral afferents also return from the *carotid sinus* (baroreceptors) and *carotid body* (chemoreceptors), and general somatic afferents return from the posterior tongue, palatine tonsils, pharynx, and middle ear (Fig. 8.75).

Vagus Nerve

The **vagus nerve (CN X)** innervates the pharyngeal and laryngeal (branchiomeric) muscles of the **fourth**

embryonic branchial arch via its superior laryngeal nerve and the **sixth embryonic branchial arch** via the recurrent (inferior) laryngeal nerve. CN X also sends preganglionic parasympathetic fibers from its **dorsal nucleus** to smooth muscle and glands of the neck, thorax (including cardiac muscle of the heart), and proximal two-thirds of the abdominal GI tract, with its fibers synapsing in **terminal ganglia** in or near the structures innervated (Figs. 1.26 and 8.76). *Vagal afferents* arise from visceral structures of the same thoracic and GI regions and from aortic baroreceptors and chemoreceptors that course to the brainstem. These sensory nerve cell bodies reside in the **inferior (nodose) ganglion** of the vagus nerve (Fig. 8.76). Special sensory fibers from taste buds on the epiglottis and general somatic afferents arising from skin around the ear, larynx, external acoustic meatus, and posterior dura mater also travel in the vagus nerve (Fig. 8.76). Sensory nerve cell bodies of those afferents from the ear and dura mater only reside in the *superior ganglion* of the vagus nerve; all other vagal afferents have

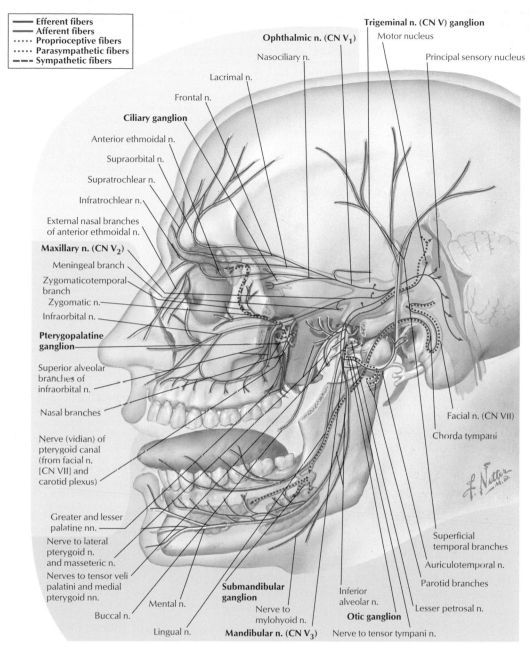

Efferent fibers
Afferent fibers
····· **Proprioceptive fibers**
····· **Parasympathetic fibers**
--- **Sympathetic fibers**

Trigeminal n. (CN V) ganglion
Motor nucleus
Principal sensory nucleus

Ophthalmic n. (CN V₁)
Nasociliary n.
Lacrimal n.
Frontal n.
Ciliary ganglion
Anterior ethmoidal n.
Supraorbital n.
Supratrochlear n.
Infratrochlear n.
External nasal branches of anterior ethmoidal n.
Maxillary n. (CN V₂)
Meningeal branch
Zygomaticotemporal branch
Zygomatic n.
Infraorbital n.
Pterygopalatine ganglion
Superior alveolar branches of infraorbital n.
Nasal branches
Nerve (vidian) of pterygoid canal (from facial n. [CN VII] and carotid plexus)
Greater and lesser palatine nn.
Nerve to lateral pterygoid n. and masseteric n.
Nerves to tensor veli palatini and medial pterygoid nn.
Mental n.
Buccal n.
Lingual n.
Submandibular ganglion
Nerve to mylohyoid n.
Mandibular n. (CN V₃)
Inferior alveolar n.
Otic ganglion
Nerve to tensor tympani n.
Facial n. (CN VII)
Chorda tympani
Superficial temporal branches
Auriculotemporal n.
Parotid branches
Lesser petrosal n.

f. Netter M.D.

FIGURE 8.72 Pathway Summary for CN V. (From *Netter's atlas of human anatomy,* ed 8, Plate 149; S-59.)

their cell bodies in the *larger inferior ganglion* of CN X.

17. EMBRYOLOGY

Brain Development

The cranial end of the neural tube begins to expand into definitive swellings and characteristic flexures during the fourth week of development, giving rise to the **forebrain, midbrain,** and **hindbrain** (Fig. 8.77). By the fifth week, these three divisions subdivide into five regions that ultimately give rise to the definitive brain structures.

Cranial Nerve Development

The 12 pairs of cranial nerves develop from cranial to caudal (except for CN XI, which arises from the brainstem and upper cervical spinal cord) as direct

TABLE 8.21 Cranial Nerve Clinical Summary

CRANIAL NERVE	FIBER TYPE	CRANIAL EXIT	LESION SITE	CLINICAL DEFICIT/ FINDINGS
Olfactory	Special sensory	Cribriform plate of ethmoid	Fracture of cribriform plate	Anosmia (loss of smell), cerebrospinal rhinorrhea
Optic	Special sensory	Optic canal	Fracture of optic canal, eye trauma, optic pathway lesion	Pupillary constriction, altered light reflex, visual field deficits, blindness
Oculomotor	Somatic motor Visceral motor	Superior orbital fissure	Pressure on nerve, cavernous sinus pathology, fracture	Dilated pupil, ptosis, absent pupillary reflex, eye directed down and out, diplopia, difficulty with lens accommodation
Trochlear	Somatic motor	Superior orbital fissure	Orbital fracture, cavernous sinus pathology, stretched	Cannot look down and in, diplopia
Trigeminal	General sensory (all 3 divisions) Branchial motor (V_3 only)	Superior orbital fissure (V_1) Foramen rotundum (V_2) Foramen ovale (V_3)	Fracture, herpes zoster, cavernous sinus pathology, orbital floor fracture, compression, mandibular fracture	Loss of sensation over face, jaws, anterior head, nasal cavity, and most of the dura mater, loss of muscles of mastication and sensation over anterior two-thirds of tongue (V_3), absent corneal reflex (V_1)
Abducens	Somatic motor	Superior orbital fissure	Fracture, cavernous sinus pathology	Cannot abduct eye, diplopia
Facial	General sensory Special sensory Branchial motor Visceral motor	Internal acoustic meatus, facial canal, stylomastoid foramen	Fracture of temporal bone, Bell's palsy, laceration over parotid region	Ipsilateral facial muscle paralysis (Bell's palsy), loss of taste at anterior two-thirds of tongue, dry eye (lacrimal gland), diminished salivation (submandibular and sublingual glands), dry nose and palate
Vestibulocochlear	Special sensory	Internal acoustic meatus	Tumor, fracture of temporal bone	Unilateral hearing loss, tinnitus, vertigo
Glossopharyngeal	Special sensory General sensory Visceral sensory Branchial motor Visceral motor	Jugular foramen	Brainstem lesion, neck laceration	Loss of taste on posterior one-third of tongue, diminished gag reflex, decreased pharynx sensation, decreased parotid salivation, diminished chemoreceptor and baroreceptor reflex
Vagus	Special sensory General sensory Visceral sensory Branchial motor Visceral motor	Jugular foramen	Brainstem lesion, neck laceration	Hoarseness or loss of vocalization, deviated soft palate, uvula deviated to normal side, dysphagia, diminished baroreceptor and chemoreceptor reflexes, loss of sensation over occipital dura mater, cardiopulmonary disturbances, decreased bowel sounds, altered peristalsis
Accessory	Somatic motor	Jugular foramen	Neck laceration	Paralysis of sternocleidomastoid and trapezius muscles, drooping shoulder
Hypoglossal	Somatic motor	Hypoglossal canal	Basal skull fracture, neck laceration, trauma to floor of mouth	Ipsilateral atrophy of tongue, protruded tongue deviates to affected side, altered speech (dysarthria)

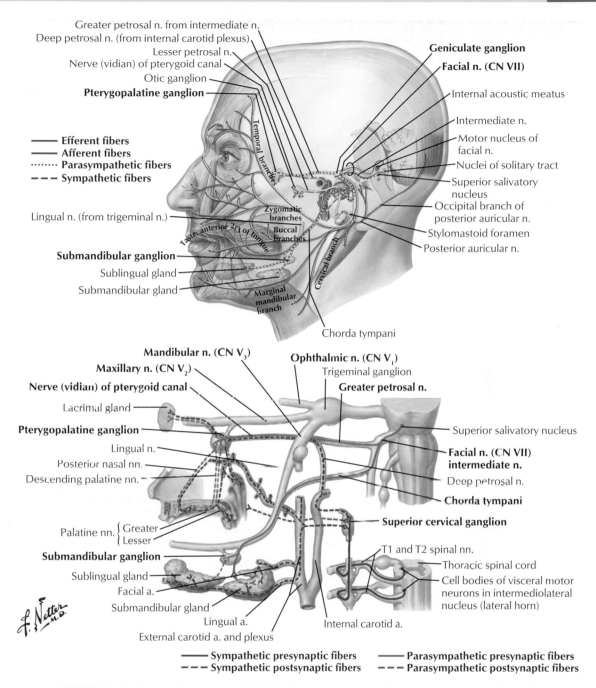

Efferent fibers
Afferent fibers
Parasympathetic fibers
Sympathetic fibers

Greater petrosal n. from intermediate n.
Deep petrosal n. (from internal carotid plexus)
Lesser petrosal n.
Nerve (vidian) of pterygoid canal
Otic ganglion
Pterygopalatine ganglion

Geniculate ganglion
Facial n. (CN VII)
Internal acoustic meatus
Intermediate n.
Motor nucleus of facial n.
Nuclei of solitary tract
Superior salivatory nucleus
Occipital branch of posterior auricular n.
Stylomastoid foramen
Posterior auricular n.

Temporal branches
Zygomatic branches
Buccal branches
Cervical branch

Lingual n. (from trigeminal n.)
Taste: anterior 2/3 of tongue
Submandibular ganglion
Sublingual gland
Submandibular gland
Marginal mandibular branch
Chorda tympani

Mandibular n. (CN V₃)
Maxillary n. (CN V₂)
Nerve (vidian) of pterygoid canal
Lacrimal gland
Pterygopalatine ganglion
Lingual n.
Posterior nasal nn.
Descending palatine nn.
Palatine nn. { Greater / Lesser
Submandibular ganglion
Sublingual gland
Facial a.
Submandibular gland
Lingual a.
External carotid a. and plexus

Ophthalmic n. (CN V₁)
Trigeminal ganglion
Greater petrosal n.
Superior salivatory nucleus
Facial n. (CN VII) intermediate n.
Deep petrosal n.
Chorda tympani
Superior cervical ganglion
T1 and T2 spinal nn.
Thoracic spinal cord
Cell bodies of visceral motor neurons in intermediolateral nucleus (lateral horn)
Internal carotid a.

Sympathetic presynaptic fibers
Sympathetic postsynaptic fibers
Parasympathetic presynaptic fibers
Parasympathetic postsynaptic fibers

FIGURE 8.73 Pathway Summary for CN VII. (From *Netter's atlas of human anatomy*, ed 8, Plates 150 and 160; S-65 and S-79.)

extensions of the neural tube (CN I and II), or as peripheral nerve outgrowths to surface placodes, somitomeres (head somites), and pharyngeal arches. Consequently, the cranial nerves innervate the structures and tissues derived from these targets (Figs. 8.77 and 8.78). The accessory nerve (CN XI) is unique in that it innervates two muscles derived

from cervical somites, the trapezius and sterno-cleidomastoid muscles.

Pharyngeal Arch and Pouch Development

Pharyngeal arches develop from the *human ancestral gill (branchial) arch system* as an

Clinical Focus 8.43

Nerve Lesions (CN X and CN XII)

A lesion of the **vagus nerve** is easily detected by asking the patient to say "ah." If the nerve is intact, the soft palate and uvula will elevate symmetrically. If the vagus nerve has a lesion on one side, the elevation will be asymmetrical, with the palate and uvula deviating away from the lesioned side.

A lesion of the **hypoglossal nerve** peripherally (lower motor neuron) will cause the tongue to deviate toward the side of the lesioned nerve when the patient is asked to stick out the tongue. The ipsilateral tongue will also show evidence of muscle atrophy.

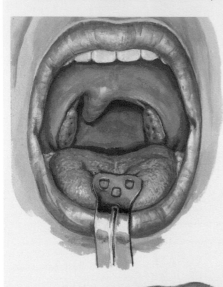

Uvular paralysis: uvula drawn to nonparalyzed side when patient says "A-AH"

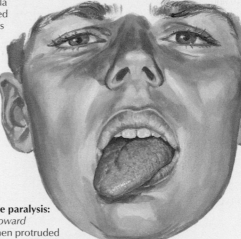

Hypoglossal nerve paralysis: tongue deviates *toward* paralyzed side when protruded

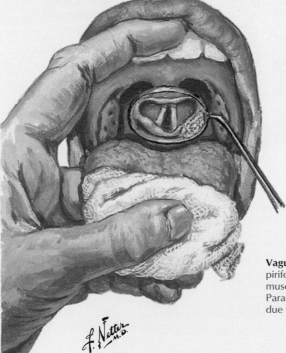

Vagus nerve paralysis: accumulation of saliva in piriform fossa on affected side due to cricopharyngeal muscle paralysis and inability to swallow. Paramedian vocal cord with poor or no movement due to paralysis.

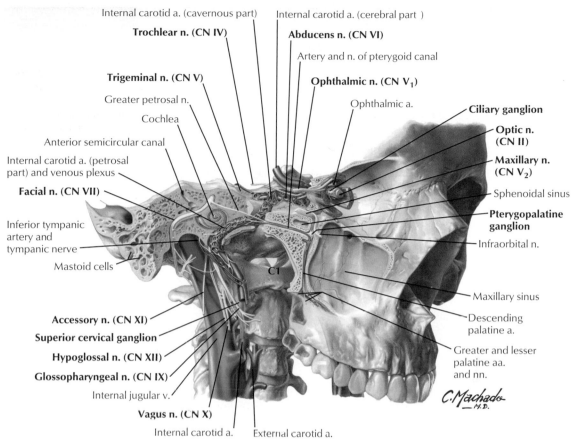

Internal carotid a. (cavernous part)   Internal carotid a. (cerebral part)

Trochlear n. (CN IV)   Abducens n. (CN VI)

                                              Artery and n. of pterygoid canal

Trigeminal n. (CN V)   Ophthalmic n. (CN V₁)

Greater petrosal n.   Ophthalmic a.   Ciliary ganglion

Cochlea   Optic n.
                                                                              (CN II)
Anterior semicircular canal
                                                                              Maxillary n.
Internal carotid a. (petrosal   (CN V₂)
part) and venous plexus
                                                                              Sphenoidal sinus
Facial n. (CN VII)
                                                                              Pterygopalatine
                                                                              ganglion
Inferior tympanic
artery and   Infraorbital n.
tympanic nerve

Mastoid cells   C1

                                                                              Maxillary sinus

Accessory n. (CN XI)   Descending
                                                                              palatine a.
Superior cervical ganglion
                                                                              Greater and lesser
Hypoglossal n. (CN XII)   palatine aa.
                                                                              and nn.
Glossopharyngeal n. (CN IX)

Internal jugular v.

Vagus n. (CN X)

Internal carotid a.   External carotid a.

FIGURE 8.74 Nerves and Vessels of the Cranial Base. (From *Netter's atlas of human anatomy,* ed 8, Plate 82; S-71.)

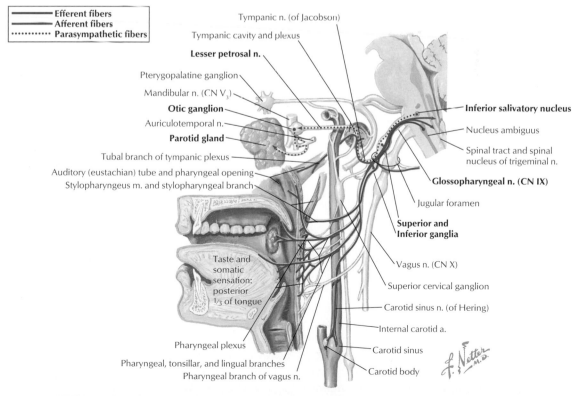

Efferent fibers
Afferent fibers
Parasympathetic fibers

                                              Tympanic n. (of Jacobson)
                                    Tympanic cavity and plexus

Lesser petrosal n.

Pterygopalatine ganglion   Inferior salivatory nucleus

Mandibular n. (CN V₃)
                                                                              Nucleus ambiguus
Otic ganglion
Auriculotemporal n.   Spinal tract and spinal
                                                                              nucleus of trigeminal n.
Parotid gland
                                                                              Glossopharyngeal n. (CN IX)
Tubal branch of tympanic plexus
Auditory (eustachian) tube and pharyngeal opening   Jugular foramen
Stylopharyngeus m. and stylopharyngeal branch
                                                                              Superior and
                                                                              Inferior ganglia
                             Taste and
                             somatic
                             sensation: Vagus n. (CN X)
                             posterior
                             ⅓ of tongue   Superior cervical ganglion

                                                                              Carotid sinus n. (of Hering)

                                                                              Internal carotid a.

Pharyngeal plexus   Carotid sinus

Pharyngeal, tonsillar, and lingual branches   Carotid body
Pharyngeal branch of vagus n.

FIGURE 8.75 Pathway Summary for CN IX. (From *Netter's atlas of human anatomy,* ed 8, Plate 152; S-67.)

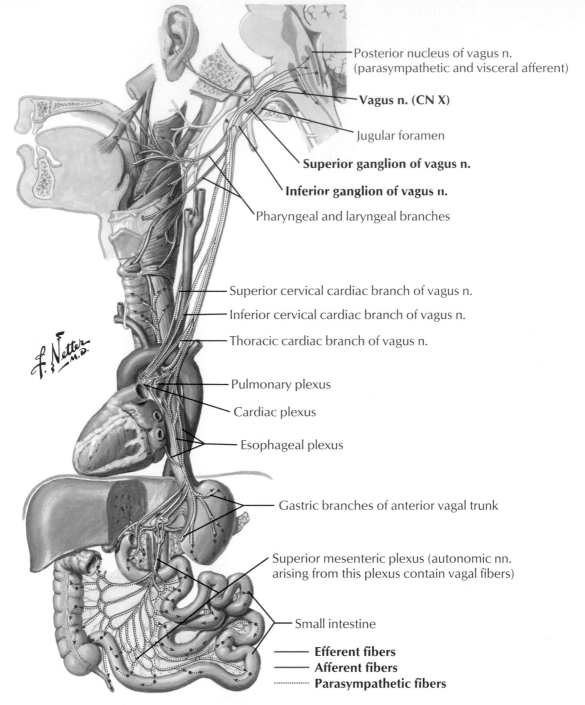

Posterior nucleus of vagus n.
(parasympathetic and visceral afferent)

Vagus n. (CN X)

Jugular foramen

Superior ganglion of vagus n.

Inferior ganglion of vagus n.

Pharyngeal and laryngeal branches

Superior cervical cardiac branch of vagus n.

Inferior cervical cardiac branch of vagus n.

Thoracic cardiac branch of vagus n.

Pulmonary plexus

Cardiac plexus

Esophageal plexus

Gastric branches of anterior vagal trunk

Superior mesenteric plexus (autonomic nn.
arising from this plexus contain vagal fibers)

Small intestine

—— **Efferent fibers**
—— **Afferent fibers**
············· **Parasympathetic fibers**

FIGURE 8.76 Pathway Summary for CN X. (From *Netter's atlas of human anatomy,* ed 8, Plate 153; S-68.)

evolutionary adaptation to terrestrial life. The original six pairs of arches develop into four pairs, with a cranial nerve, the muscles it innervates, a cartilage/bone element, and an aortic arch associated with each arch (Figs. 8.78 and 8.79). The muscles associated with each pharyngeal arch (also referred to as *branchiomeric or branchial muscles* muscles

because they are associated with the development of the gill arches) include the following groups (Fig. 8.79):

- **Arch 1:** muscles of mastication, mylohyoid muscle, anterior belly of the digastric muscle, tensor tympani muscle, and tensor veli palatini muscle; all innervated by **CN V₃**.

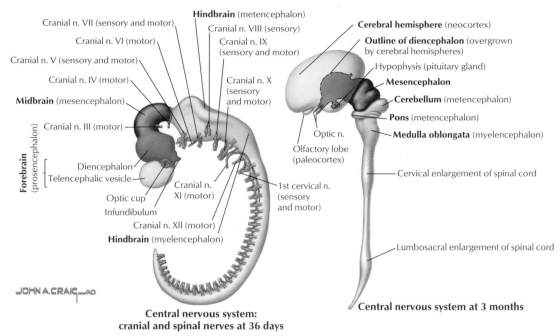

FIGURE 8.77 Brain Development at 5 Weeks and 3 Months.

Adult Derivatives of the Forebrain, Midbrain, and Hindbrain			
Forebrain	Telencephalon	Cerebral hemispheres Olfactory cortex Hippocampus Basal ganglia/corpus striatum Lateral and 3rd ventricles	Nerves: Olfactory (I)
	Diencephalon	Optic cup/nerves Thalamus Hypothalamus Mammillary bodies Part of 3rd ventricle	Optic (II)
Midbrain	Mesencephalon	Tectum Cerebral aqueduct Red nucleus Substantia nigra Crus cerebelli	Oculomotor (III) Trochlear (IV)
Hindbrain	Metencephalon	Pons Cerebellum	Trigeminal (V) Abducens (VI)
	Myelencephalon	Medulla oblongata	Facial (VII) Vestibulocochlear (VIII) Glossopharyngeal (IX) Vagus (X) Hypoglossal (XII)

- **Arch 2:** muscles of facial expression, posterior belly of digastric muscle, stylohyoid muscle, and stapedius muscle; all innervated by **CN VII.**
- **Arch 3:** stylopharyngeus muscle; only muscle innervated by **CN IX.**
- **Arch 4:** muscles of the palate (except the tensor muscle), pharyngeal constrictor muscles, and all the muscles of the larynx; all innervated by **CN X.**

Also derived from each of these pharyngeal arches are the bones, cartilages, and ligaments associated with each particular arch. These are summarized in Fig. 8.79.

Internally, each arch is also associated with an endoderm-derived **pharyngeal pouch,** an outpocketing of the *foregut* in the head and neck. Pharyngeal pouch development begins about the third to fourth week of embryonic development (Fig. 8.80) as an elaboration of bilateral *endoderm-derived* structures, which include the following:

- **Pouch 1:** auditory tube and middle ear.
- **Pouch 2:** tonsillar fossa and the epithelium of the palatine tonsils (the lymphoid tissue of the tonsil is derived from mesoderm).

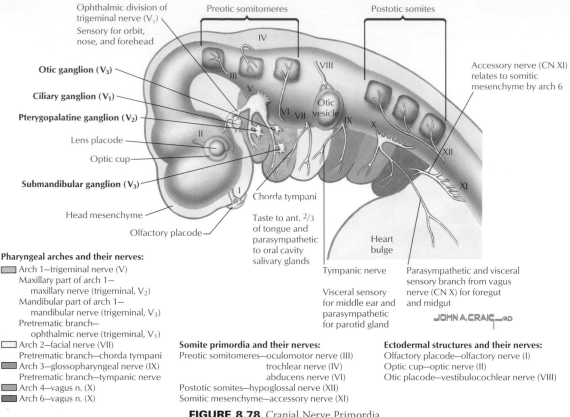

Pharyngeal arches and their nerves:

Arch 1—trigeminal nerve (V)
Maxillary part of arch 1—
maxillary nerve (trigeminal, V_2)
Mandibular part of arch 1—
mandibular nerve (trigeminal, V_3)
Pretrematic branch—
ophthalmic nerve (trigeminal, V_1)
Arch 2—facial nerve (VII)
Pretrematic branch—chorda tympani
Arch 3—glossopharyngeal nerve (IX)
Pretrematic branch—tympanic nerve
Arch 4—vagus n. (X)
Arch 6—vagus n. (X)

Somite primordia and their nerves:
Preotic somitomeres—oculomotor nerve (III)
trochlear nerve (IV)
abducens nerve (VI)
Postotic somites—hypoglossal nerve (XII)
Somitic mesenchyme—accessory nerve (XI)

Ectodermal structures and their nerves:
Olfactory placode—olfactory nerve (I)
Optic cup—optic nerve (II)
Otic placode—vestibulocochlear nerve (VIII)

FIGURE 8.78 Cranial Nerve Primordia.

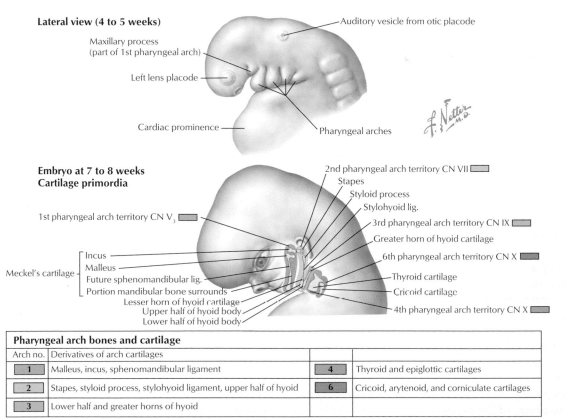

FIGURE 8.79 Pharyngeal Arches.

Pharyngeal arch bones and cartilage				
Arch no.	Derivatives of arch cartilages			
1	Malleus, incus, sphenomandibular ligament	4	Thyroid and epiglottic cartilages
2	Stapes, styloid process, stylohyoid ligament, upper half of hyoid	6	Cricoid, arytenoid, and corniculate cartilages
3	Lower half and greater horns of hyoid		

Sagittal section

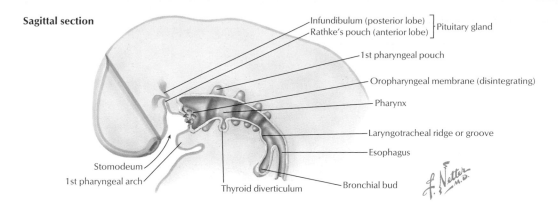

Pharynx (anterior view of left side)

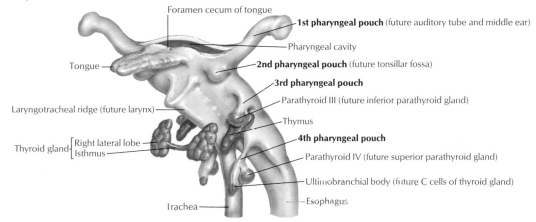

FIGURE 8.80 Pharyngeal Pouch Derivatives.

- **Pouch 3:** inferior parathyroid glands and thymus gland.
- **Pouch 4:** superior parathyroid glands and C cells (parafollicular cells; calcitonin-secreting cells) of the thyroid gland.

Clinical Focus 8.46 provides a composite summary of some of the more common clinical anomalies of the pharyngeal arch and pouch derivatives.

Facial and Palatal Development

The face develops primarily from the **neural crest** by the fusion of an unpaired frontonasal prominence and paired **nasal placodes**, with **bilateral maxillary and mandibular prominences** that meet in the midline (Fig. 8.81). Initially, the eyes develop laterally, but as the face begins to grow, the eyes move medially to their definitive anterior positions.

Internally, the common oral-nasal cavity becomes subdivided by a horizontal plate separating the oral cavity from the nasal cavity (Fig. 8.82). Fusion of the medial nasal processes gives rise to an intermaxillary segment called the **primary palate.** Swellings of the maxillary prominence of the face

form **palatine shelves** that project medially and fuse along the midline to form the **secondary palate.** These primary and secondary palatal tissues fuse, and all meet at the site of the *incisive foramen* (see Fig. 8.42). As this occurs, a midline **nasal septum** that divides the nose into right and left halves extends downward from the roof of the nasal cavity and fuses with the palate below.

Salivary Gland and Tooth Development

The salivary glands develop as solid epithelial buds of the oral cavity that grow into the underlying mesenchyme (primitive mesoderm). The paired **parotid glands** develop first about the sixth week; they arise from oral ectoderm, differentiate and canalize, and then begin serous (watery) secretion of saliva at 18 weeks of development. The **submandibular glands** appear late in the sixth week of development as endoderm-derived buds lateral to the tongue. They begin to secrete mixed serous and mucous saliva around the 16th week and continue to grow postnatally. The **sublingual glands** appear about the eighth week of

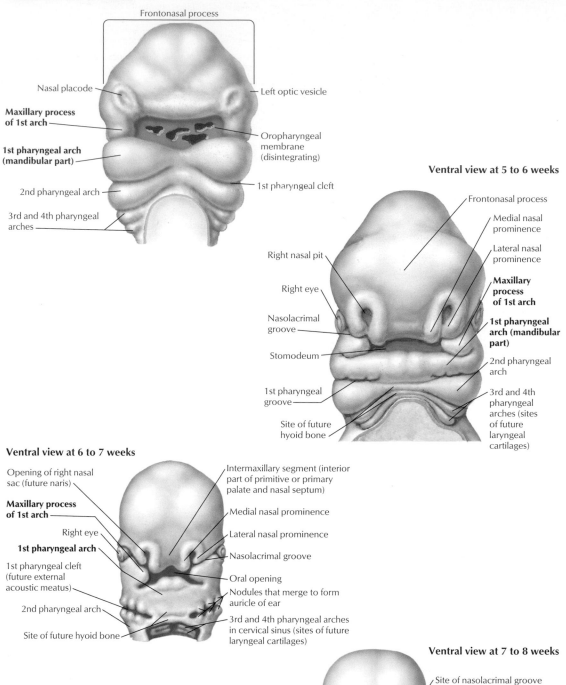

Ventral view at 4 to 5 weeks

Frontonasal process

Nasal placode

Maxillary process
of 1st arch

1st pharyngeal arch
(mandibular part)

2nd pharyngeal arch

3rd and 4th pharyngeal
arches

Left optic vesicle

Oropharyngeal
membrane
(disintegrating)

1st pharyngeal cleft

Ventral view at 5 to 6 weeks

Frontonasal process

Medial nasal
prominence

Lateral nasal
prominence

Maxillary
process
of 1st arch

1st pharyngeal
arch (mandibular
part)

2nd pharyngeal
arch

3rd and 4th
pharyngeal
arches (sites
of future
laryngeal
cartilages)

Right nasal pit

Right eye

Nasolacrimal
groove

Stomodeum

1st pharyngeal
groove

Site of future
hyoid bone

Ventral view at 6 to 7 weeks

Opening of right nasal
sac (future naris)

Maxillary process
of 1st arch

Right eye

1st pharyngeal arch

1st pharyngeal cleft
(future external
acoustic meatus)

2nd pharyngeal arch

Site of future hyoid bone

Intermaxillary segment (interior
part of primitive or primary
palate and nasal septum)

Medial nasal prominence

Lateral nasal prominence

Nasolacrimal groove

Oral opening

Nodules that merge to form
auricle of ear

3rd and 4th pharyngeal arches
in cervical sinus (sites of future
laryngeal cartilages)

Ventral view at 7 to 8 weeks

Site of nasolacrimal groove
(fusion of lateral nasal
and maxillary processes)

Site of fusion of medial nasal
and maxillary processes
(site of cleft lip)

Auricle of ear

Philtrum of upper lip (fusion
of medial nasal processes)

FIGURE 8.81 Development of the Face.

Roof of stomodeum (inferior view; 6 to 7 weeks)

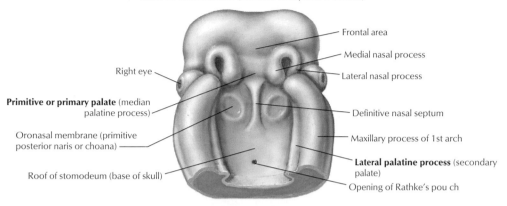

Frontal area

Medial nasal process

Lateral nasal process

Right eye

Primitive or primary palate (median palatine process)

Definitive nasal septum

Oronasal membrane (primitive posterior naris or choana)

Maxillary process of 1st arch

Lateral palatine process (secondary palate)

Roof of stomodeum (base of skull)

Opening of Rathke's pouch

Palate formation (inferior view; 7 to 8 weeks)

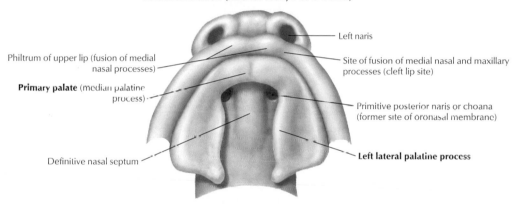

Left naris

Philtrum of upper lip (fusion of medial nasal processes)

Site of fusion of medial nasal and maxillary processes (cleft lip site)

Primary palate (median palatine process)

Primitive posterior naris or choana (former site of oronasal membrane)

Definitive nasal septum

Left lateral palatine process

Roof of oral cavity (inferior view; 8 to 10 weeks)

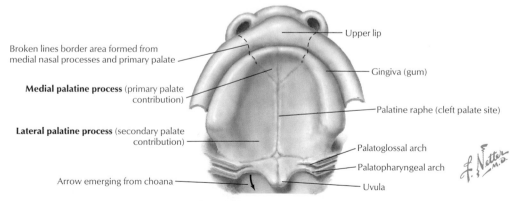

Upper lip

Broken lines border area formed from medial nasal processes and primary palate

Gingiva (gum)

Medial palatine process (primary palate contribution)

Palatine raphe (cleft palate site)

Lateral palatine process (secondary palate contribution)

Palatoglossal arch

Palatopharyngeal arch

Arrow emerging from choana

Uvula

FIGURE 8.82 Development of Hard Palate.

Craniosynostosis

As the brain grows, so does the neurocranium, by bone deposition along suture lines. If this process is interrupted (for unknown reasons or because of genetic factors), the cranium may compensate by depositing more bone along other sutures. If the sagittal suture closes prematurely, growth in width is altered, so growth occurs lengthwise and leads to a long, narrow cranium; coronal and lambdoid suture closure results in a short, wide cranium. The disorder occurs in about 1 in 2000 births and is more common in males than in females.

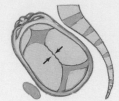

Limitation of growth of sagittal suture

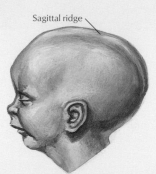

Sagittal ridge

Scaphocephaly due to sagittal craniosynostosis

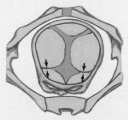

Limitation of growth of coronal sutures

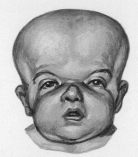

Brachycephaly due to coronal craniosynostosis

JOHN A. CRAIG—AD

Congenital Anomalies of the Oral Cavity

Because the face and oral cavity develop largely by midline fusion of various prominences, incomplete or failed fusion can lead to **cleft formation** (lips and palate) or anomalous features (ankyloglossia, torus formations). The etiology is multifactorial, but genetics appears to play some role.

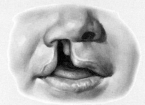

Unilateral cleft lip—partial

Unilateral cleft of primary palate—complete, involving lip and alveolar ridge

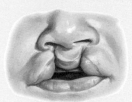

Bilateral cleft lip

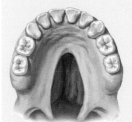

Partial cleft of palate

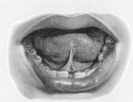

Ankyloglossia—restricted tongue movement from a short lingual frenulum

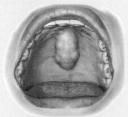

Torus palatinus—bone deposition on palate

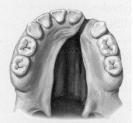

Complete cleft of secondary palate and unilateral cleft of primary palate

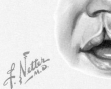

Clinical Focus 8.46

Pharyngeal Arch and Pouch Anomalies

Most anomalies of the pharyngeal apparatus involve fistulas, cysts, or ectopic glandular tissue. Some common anomalies and their sources from the associated pharyngeal pouch or wall are shown here in this *composite illustration.*

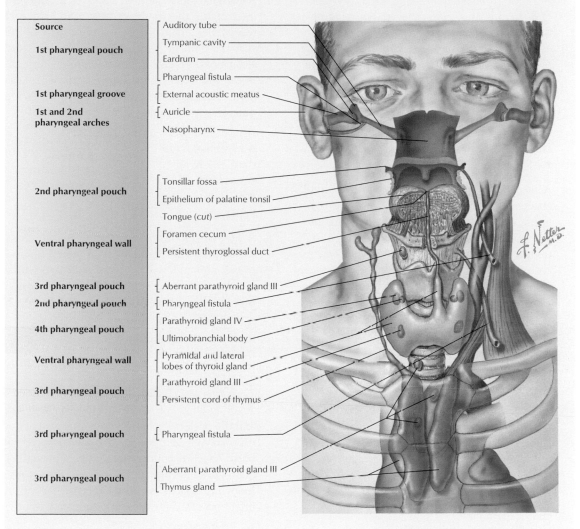

Source	
1st pharyngeal pouch	Auditory tube
	Tympanic cavity
	Eardrum
	Pharyngeal fistula
1st pharyngeal groove	External acoustic meatus
1st and 2nd pharyngeal arches	Auricle
	Nasopharynx
2nd pharyngeal pouch	Tonsillar fossa
	Epithelium of palatine tonsil
	Tongue (*cut*)
Ventral pharyngeal wall	Foramen cecum
	Persistent thyroglossal duct
3rd pharyngeal pouch	Aberrant parathyroid gland III
2nd pharyngeal pouch	Pharyngeal fistula
4th pharyngeal pouch	Parathyroid gland IV
	Ultimobranchial body
Ventral pharyngeal wall	Pyramidal and lateral lobes of thyroid gland
3rd pharyngeal pouch	Parathyroid gland III
	Persistent cord of thymus
3rd pharyngeal pouch	Pharyngeal fistula
3rd pharyngeal pouch	Aberrant parathyroid gland III
	Thymus gland

development from multiple endodermal buds that differentiate into 10 to 12 ducts. These glands also secrete a seromucous saliva, but it is thicker because of a greater proportion of mucus.

The **teeth** develop from oral ectoderm, mesoderm, and neural crest cells. The oral ectoderm gives rise to the **enamel,** the *hardest substance in the human body.* Mesenchyme, derived from the neural crest, and mesoderm give rise to the other components of the tooth (dentine, pulp cavity). Development begins with the formation of tooth buds in the anterior mandibular region and then progresses posteriorly in both the maxilla and the mandible, under the regulation of *HOX* genes.

Challenge Yourself Questions

1. A 2-month-old infant presents with no evidence of a thymus and some uncertainty regarding the number of parathyroid glands and location of parathyroid tissue. Which of the following pharyngeal pouches may be responsible for these findings?

   A. First pouch
   B. Second and third pouches
   C. Third pouch
   D. Third and fourth pouches
   E. Fourth pouch

2. A 46-year-old woman presents with painful erythematous vesicular eruptions over the right upper eyelid and forehead and spreading into her hairline over the squamous portion of the temporal bone. She is diagnosed with herpes zoster (shingles). Which of the following nerves is most likely responsible for transmitting this virus?

   A. Auriculotemporal nerve
   B. Greater petrosal nerve
   C. Nasociliary nerve
   D. Supraorbital nerve
   E. Zygomatic nerve

3. A 31-year-old man is diagnosed with a benign pituitary adenoma that has impinged on the right aspect of the cavernous sinus. Which of the following clinical signs is most likely to be evident in this patient?

   A. Bilateral painful ophthalmoplegia
   B. Left-sided diplopia
   C. Left-sided complete ptosis
   D. Right-sided pupillary dilation
   E. Right-sided dry eye

4. A teenage gang member receives a knife cut inferior to the angle of the mandible and receives emergency care for the repair of the vascular damage, cleansing of the wound, and closing of the incision. Unknown to the resident in the ER, the victim's hypoglossal nerve was completely severed. Which of the following muscles would mostly likely be affected?

   A. Anterior belly of the digastric
   B. Genioglossus
   C. Geniohyoid
   D. Mylohyoid
   E. Palatoglossus
   F. Stylohyoid

5. A 56-year-old woman presents in the clinic with diplopia of the left eye, complete left-sided ptosis, and an absent corneal reflex. At which location would one most likely find a lesion that would account for this presentation?

   A. Foramen ovale
   B. Foramen rotundum
   C. Inferior orbital fissure
   D. Optic canal
   E. Superior orbital fissure

6. A young child falls while sucking on a lollipop, and the stick lacerates the posterior wall of her oropharynx, stopped by a cervical vertebral body. As a precaution, the physician prescribes a broad-spectrum antibiotic. Which of the following spaces is most likely to harbor an infection after this type of puncture wound?

   A. Epidural space
   B. Mediastinum
   C. Pretracheal space
   D. Retropharyngeal space
   E. Subdural space

Multiple-choice and short-answer review questions available online; see inside front cover for details.

7. A baseball player is hit in his left eye and orbital region by a fastball that results in a blow-out fracture. The left orbital contents show evidence of an inferior herniation into which of the following spaces?

   A. Cavernous sinus
   B. Ethmoid sinus
   C. Frontal sinus
   D. Maxillary sinus
   E. Sphenoid sinus

8. An internist suspects a patient has an infection in the cavernous sinus. If the infection enters the infraorbital veins, it can next pass directly into which of the following venous channels and endanger the inferior alveolar and lingual nerves?

   A. Facial
   B. Infraorbital
   C. Pterygoid plexus
   D. Retromandibular
   E. Superficial temporal

9. A traumatic injury to the right side of the neck requires significant surgical attention. The patient has a hoarse voice, which will not resolve with time. Which of the following nerves was most likely damaged by this injury?

   A. Ansa cervicalis
   B. Hypoglossal
   C. Recurrent laryngeal
   D. Superior laryngeal
   E. Sympathetic trunk

10. An elderly woman stumbles while walking down her basement stairs but catches herself before falling. On examination by her physician, she presents with diplopia when looking inferiorly. Which of the following nerves is most likely affected?

    A. Abducens
    B. Oculomotor
    C. Ophthalmic (V_1)
    D. Optic
    E. Trochlear

11. A tumor compresses the sympathetic trunk in the lower neck. Which of the following muscles is most likely affected?

    A. Ciliary
    B. Geniohyoid
    C. Orbicularis oculi
    D. Pupillary constrictor
    E. Superior tarsal

12. The rupture of a berry aneurysm affecting the anterior communicating artery of the circle of Willis results in significant bleeding. Into which space will this bleeding occur?

    A. Cavernous sinus
    B. Epidural space
    C. Lateral ventricle
    D. Subarachnoid space
    E. Subdural space

13. A congenital malformation affecting the malleus and incus in the middle ear would be associated with the maldevelopment of which of the following structures?

    A. First pharyngeal arch
    B. Frontonasal process
    C. Pharyngotympanic tube
    D. Second pharyngeal arch
    E. Second pharyngeal pouch

14. A 56-year-old woman has had significant pain deep in her jaw, which has become localized to her temporomandibular joint (TMJ). Examination reveals that she has an inflamed TMJ. Which of the following muscles is most likely involved in this inflammatory process?

    A. Buccinator
    B. Lateral pterygoid
    C. Masseter
    D. Medial pterygoid
    E. Temporalis

For each condition described below (15-25), select the nerve from the list (A-Q) that is most likely responsible for the condition or affected by it.

(A) Abducens	(J) Nerve of pterygoid
(B) Accessory	canal
(C) Chorda tympani	(K) Oculomotor
(D) Deep petrosal	(L) Olfactory
(E) Facial	(M) Optic
(F) Glossopharyngeal	(N) Trigeminal
(G) Greater petrosal	(O) Trochlear
(H) Hypoglossal	(P) Vagus
(I) Lesser petrosal	(Q) Vestibulocochlear

_____ 15. A patient presents with diplopia and an inability to abduct the left eye.

_____ 16. Trauma to the right middle cranial fossa results in ipsilateral pupillary constriction and partial ptosis.

_____ 17. Sharp trauma to the left infratemporal fossa results in the ipsilateral loss of taste on the anterior two-thirds of the tongue.

_____ 18. A 21-year old woman presents with a drooping of her left eyelid and an asymmetrical smile.

_____ 19. During a routine examination, when the patient is asked to say "ah," the soft palate and uvula are elevated asymmetrically.

_____ 20. A fracture of the middle cranial fossa, just along the anterior base of the petrous portion of the temporal bone, results in a decreased secretion of the ipsilateral parotid gland.

_____ 21. You are talking and chewing gum at the same time and inadvertently bite your cheek. The site of injury is painful and begins to swell. You ask yourself, "What nerve mediates this pain?"

_____ 22. During a routine tonsillectomy, a complication results in the loss of taste and sensation on the posterior third of the tongue.

_____ 23. A severe bacterial infection of the left sphenoid sinus erodes into the bony floor of the sinus, resulting in an ipsilateral dry eye and dry nasal passage.

_____ 24. A small child screams in pain following a bee sting on his upper lip.

_____ 25. A blow to the head results in the rupture of the middle meningeal artery, causing an epidural hematoma, which is extremely painful.

26. A newborn infant presents with an underdeveloped mandible (hypoplasia), cleft palate, and ear abnormalities. Which of the following pharyngeal arches is most likely involved in these congenital defects?
    - **A.** First
    - **B.** Second
    - **C.** Third
    - **D.** Fourth
    - **E.** Sixth

27. A 54-year-old man presents with tic douloureux (trigeminal neuralgia), which results in episodic bouts of severe pain over the midface. Which of the following ganglia harbors the sensory nerve cell bodies that mediate this pain?
    - **A.** Geniculate
    - **B.** Inferior vagal
    - **C.** Otic
    - **D.** Pterygopalatine
    - **E.** Semilunar

28. An elderly gentleman slips on the ice and hits his head. Examination reveals a hematoma in the "danger space" of the scalp; it is observed spreading to his forehead and eyelid. This hematoma lies within which of the following layers of the scalp?
    - **A.** Aponeurotic layer (galea aponeurotica)
    - **B.** Loose connective tissue
    - **C.** Periosteum (pericranium)
    - **D.** Skin
    - **E.** Subcutaneous (connective) tissue

29. A 24-year-old woman presents with an abscess on the left side of her neck, which is surgically removed. Following surgery, the woman notices that she has difficulty turning her head to the opposite side and her shoulder is drooping. Which of the following nerves was most likely injured during the surgery?
    - **A.** Accessory
    - **B.** Ansa cervicalis
    - **C.** Facial
    - **D.** Hypoglossal
    - **E.** Posterior auricular

30. A 69-year-old man is admitted to the hospital with a hemorrhagic stroke. The hematoma lies within the immediate vicinity of the superior cerebellar artery. Which of the following cranial nerves is most likely to be affected by this hematoma?
    - **A.** Abducens
    - **B.** Facial
    - **C.** Glossopharyngeal
    - **D.** Trochlear
    - **E.** Vestibulocochlear

31. A 41-year-old man presents with severe infection in his mastoid air cells (mastoiditis); it

appears to be in the process of eroding into his posterior cranial fossa. Which of the following venous structures is most at risk of infection should this abscess erode through the thin bony wall?

A. Cavernous sinus
B. Inferior sagittal sinus
C. Pterygoid plexus of veins
D. Sigmoid sinus
E. Straight sinus

32. A hard blow to the head at the union of the frontal, parietal, sphenoid, and temporal bones is extremely dangerous; the resulting fracture can lead to an intracranial hemorrhage. Which of the following terms describes this unique area of the skull?

A. Asterion
B. Coronal suture
C. External occipital protuberance
D. Lambdoid suture
E. Pterion

33. Aberrant parathyroid glands are not uncommon; they can be found throughout the lower neck and even in the superior mediastinum, often in association with the thymus gland. Which of the following pharyngeal pouches most likely gives rise to these aberrant parathyroid glands?

A. First
B. Second
C. Third
D. Fourth
E. Sixth

34. During the act of swallowing, the tongue is raised and the bolus of food is passed up against the hard palate and then back into the oral pharynx. Which of the following muscles assists the styloglossus muscle in raising the tongue during swallowing?

A. Buccinator
B. Medial pterygoid
C. Mylohyoid
D. Stylohyoid
E. Thyrohyoid

For each description below (35-41), select the muscle from the list (A-P) that best fits the description.

(A) Buccinator
(B) Cricothyroid
(C) Lateral pterygoid
(D) Lateral rectus
(E) Levator palpebrae superioris
(F) Masseter
(G) Omohyoid
(H) Posterior cricoarytenoid
(I) Stapedius
(J) Stylopharyngeus
(K) Superior oblique
(L) Superior rectus
(M) Temporalis
(N) Tensor tympani
(O) Tensor veli palatini
(P) Thyrohyoid

_____ 35. It helps to tense the vocal folds.

_____ 36. In neutral gaze, it abducts the eyeball.

_____ 37. When contracted, it helps dampen loud noises; it is innervated by CN VII.

_____ 38. It is innervated by a nerve that also provides taste to the posterior third of the tongue.

_____ 39. This muscle is innervated by a nerve only after it has passed through the stylomastoid foramen.

_____ 40. Damage to the nerve innervating this muscle leads to a hoarse voice.

_____ 41. It possesses a smooth muscle at its distal insertion.

For each structure described below (42-45), select the name (A-I) on the radiograph of the skull that best fits the description.

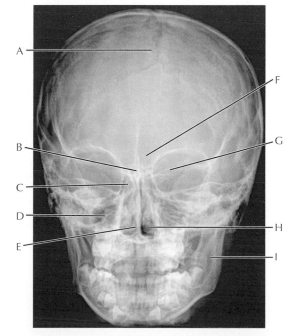

____ 42. This structure drains into the semi-lunar hiatus.

____ 43. This is the anterior attachment point for the falx cerebri.

____ 44. The optic nerve passes through a foramen in this bone.

____ 45. Branches of the nasociliary nerve innervate the mucosa in this structure.

Answers to Challenge Yourself Questions

1. **C.** The thyroid gland appears healthy, so we can assume that the C cells of the thyroid gland developed normally, along with the superior parathyroid glands of the fourth pouch. The third pharyngeal pouch, however, gives rise to the thymus gland and the inferior parathyroid glands, so this is the pouch most likely affected.

2. **D.** The supraorbital nerve is a branch of the ophthalmic division of the trigeminal nerve, and its distribution matches the description of the skin eruptions. The virus responsible for herpes resides in the sensory ganglia of nerves, in this case the semilunar ganglion of CN V.

3. **D.** The expansion to the right side will affect the right eye and orbit, and in this case it will affect the oculomotor nerve (CN III). The following nerves pass in close association with the cavernous sinus and can be affected by an expanding mass in this region: CN III, IV, V₁, V₂, and VI. The dilated pupil results from the unopposed sympathetic innervation of the dilator muscle; the constrictor of the pupil is affected by the compression on CN III, which carries the parasympathetics to the ciliary ganglion and this muscle.

4. **B.** Of the listed muscles, only the genioglossus muscle is innervated by CN XII. The other two muscles innervated by CN XII are the hyoglossus and styloglossus muscles.

5. **E.** These signs and symptoms are compatible with a lesion to CN III (denervation of four extraocular muscles and the levator palpebrae superioris muscle of the eyelid) and sensation over the cornea (ophthalmic division of the trigeminal nerve). Both of these nerves enter the orbit via the superior orbital fissure.

6. **D.** The retropharyngeal space lies between the buccopharyngeal (visceral) fascia and the prevertebral fascia (specifically the alar layer) and extends from the base of the cranium to the posterior mediastinum. Infections in this space can easily spread superiorly or inferiorly via the contractions of the pharyngeal muscles and esophagus, which can "knead" the bacteria along the space.

7. **D.** The floor of the orbit is the roof of the underlying maxillary sinus. Fractures in this area can result in the partial herniation of the orbital contents inferiorly, especially the orbital fat (the eye may droop but is tethered by the optic nerve and extraocular muscles).

8. **C.** From the inferior ophthalmic veins, the infection could spread in several directions, but to involve the inferior alveolar and lingual nerves, it would need to spread to the pterygoid plexus of veins draining the infratemporal region.

9. **C.** The recurrent laryngeal (inferior laryngeal) nerve passes through the neck in the tracheoesophageal groove as it ascends to innervate the muscles of the larynx. If injured, the only pair of abductors of the vocal folds would be compromised ipsilaterally (hemiparalysis of the posterior cricoarytenoids), leading to a hoarse voice.

10. **E.** The trochlear nerve (CN IV) innervates the superior oblique muscle, and the affected eye will be elevated and adducted. The patient will have difficulty looking inferiorly and medially as she steps down stairs or off curbs and will present with diplopia.

11. **E.** The superior tarsal muscle is the only muscle on the list innervated by the sympathetic fibers; when denervated, it will result in a partial ptosis ipsilaterally. This small smooth muscle connects to the superior tarsal plate. Complete ptosis is more often associated with denervation of the levator palpebrae superioris muscle by CN III. Compression of the sympathetic trunk would result in Horner's syndrome, and the patient would present not only with partial ptosis but also with miosis, anhidrosis, and flushed skin (vasodilation) ipsilaterally.

12. **D.** Bleeding from the cerebral arteries would occur in the subarachnoid space. Subdural hematomas usually occur from bleeding associated with the bridging veins passing to the superior sagittal dural venous sinus. Epidural bleeds are associated with bleeding from the middle meningeal artery or one of its many branches.

13. **A.** The first pharyngeal arch gives rise to Meckel's cartilage, and derivatives of this arch cartilage include the ossified mandible, malleus, incus, and sphenomandibular ligament. The sensory innervation comes from the mandibular division of the trigeminal nerve.

14. **B.** The lateral pterygoid muscle, in part, inserts into the articular disc of the TMJ and is the most likely muscle to be involved with this infection. Together, this pair of muscles help protrude the mandible and depress the chin in the initial act of opening the jaw.

15. **A.** Inability to abduct the eye without other movement impairment suggests that the lateral rectus muscle is affected, and it is innervated by the abducens nerve (CN VI).

16. **D.** Partial ptosis (denervation of the superior tarsal muscle) and pupillary constriction (absence of pupillary dilation) suggest an injury to the sympathetic system somewhere along its pathway to the head. Of the listed nerves, only the deep petrosal (postganglionic fibers from the superior cervical ganglion) nerve would show exclusively sympathetic involvement as it courses on the intracranial portion of the internal carotid artery.

17. **C.** If taste is the only sense affected, the answer is the chorda tympani, which is damaged before joining the lingual nerve (apparently sensation on the anterior tongue is intact). One might also expect that some parasympathetics to the submandibular ganglion would also be affected, but this may not be immediately obvious. The chorda tympani carries taste fibers and preganglionic parasympathetic fibers.

18. **E.** These signs indicate a problem or weakness related to the muscles of facial expression, innervated by the facial nerve (CN VII). Clinically known as Bell's palsy, this can occur anywhere along the pathway of the facial nerve; in this instance, it probably is a lesion of the nerve below its exit from the stylomastoid foramen (see Clinical Focus 8.18).

19. **P.** An ipsilateral asymmetrical elevation of the soft palate and uvula suggests that the levator veli palatini muscle is affected; the muscle is innervated by the vagus nerve.

20. **I.** The lesser petrosal nerve is found in this area and carries preganglionic parasympathetic secretory fibers to the otic ganglion, where the fibers synapse. Postganglionic fibers from the otic ganglion then join the auriculotemporal nerve to innervate the parotid gland. The lesser petrosal nerve arises from the tympanic plexus of CN IX (glossopharyngeal nerve).

21. **N.** The pain is mediated by the large "sensory" nerve of the head, the trigeminal nerve. Specifically, this buccal pain is mediated by the buccal branch of the mandibular division of CN V.

22. **F.** The glossopharyngeal nerve innervates one muscle (the stylopharyngeus muscle) and then passes into the posterior third of the tongue to provide general sensation and the special sense of taste to this portion of the tongue. As it does so, CN IX passes adjacent to the tonsillary fossa. For this reason, CN IX may be damaged during a tonsillectomy.

23. **J.** The nerve of the pterygoid canal (vidian nerve) runs in the floor of the sphenoid sinus and conveys postganglionic sympathetic fibers (from the deep petrosal nerve) and preganglionic parasympathetic fibers (from the greater petrosal nerve). In this case, the parasympathetics to the pterygopalatine ganglion are affected, and the lacrimal gland and nasal mucous glands have been denervated by the infection to this nerve.

24. **N.** Sensation on the upper lip is conveyed by the trigeminal nerve. Specifically, it will be by a superior labial sensory branch of the maxillary division of CN V.

25. **N.** The great sensory nerve of the head is the trigeminal nerve. CN V provides sensory innervation to most of the dura mater; the vagus nerve contributes some sensation to the posterior dura mater. The arachnoid mater and pia mater do not possess sensory innervation.

26. **A.** The first pharyngeal arch gives rise to the muscles innervated by the mandibular division of the trigeminal nerve and to Meckel's cartilage, which ultimately forms a portion of the mandible, the malleus and incus of the middle ear, and the sphenomandibular ligament.

27. **E.** Trigeminal neuralgia (tic douloureux) usually affects the maxillary and mandibular divisions of CN V, and the sensory ganglion of that nerve is the trigeminal (semilunar, gasserian) ganglion. CN V is the major "sensory" nerve of the head.

28. **B.** The hematoma will spread in the loose connective tissue layer of the scalp, which is also known as the "danger space" of the scalp. It lies between the aponeurotic and periosteal layers.

29. **A.** The accessory nerve (CN XI) has been damaged where it runs in close relationship to the sternocleidomastoid muscle; it innervates this muscle and the trapezius muscle. Ipsilateral weakness in shrugging the shoulders and turning the head to the opposite side would be evident with such damage.

30. **D.** The superior cerebellar artery is found at the terminal end of the basilar artery, just posterior to the oculomotor nerve. It passes around the cerebral peduncle close to the trochlear nerve (the only cranial nerve to arise from the dorsum of the brainstem), so this choice is the best of the options. The oculomotor nerve might also be affected, but it is not one of the options.

31. **D.** If the infection breaks through the thin wall of the mastoid air cells, it will pass into the posterior cranial fossa adjacent to the sigmoid sinus. This sinus loops downward, connecting the transverse dural sinus with the origin of the internal jugular vein at the jugular foramen.

32. **E.** The point at which these skull bones meet is called the pterion. It lies in close relationship to the middle meningeal artery running on the inner aspect of the sphenoid and temporal bones. The squamous portion of the temporal bone in this region is relatively thin.

33. **C.** The third pharyngeal pouch gives rise to the thymus and inferior parathyroid glands. As the thymus descends, one or more inferior parathyroid glands may follow its descent into the lower neck or superior mediastinum (see Clinical Focus 8.46).

34. **C.** The mylohyoid muscle assists the styloglossus muscle in raising the hyoid bone, the floor of the mouth, and the tongue during swallowing.

35. **B.** The cricothyroid muscle tilts the cricoid cartilage anteriorly and tenses the vocal folds.

36. **D.** The lateral rectus muscle is a pure abductor of the eyeball when the eye is in the neutral position. The superior rectus and inferior rectus muscles elevate and depress the eyeball when it is abducted.

37. **I.** The stapedius muscle dampens the vibrations of the stapes in the middle ear when it contracts during loud noises; it is innervated by CN VII. The tensor tympani muscle does the same for the eardrum by attaching to the malleus, but it is innervated by CN V_3.

38. **J.** The stylopharyngeus muscle is the only muscle innervated by the glossopharyngeal nerve, which also conveys taste fibers from the posterior third of the tongue to its inferior sensory ganglion.

39. **A.** The buccinator is a muscle of facial expression and is innervated by the motor branches of CN VII to these muscles after it exits the stylomastoid foramen (the stapedius is innervated by CN VII *before* it exits the foramen). The terminal motor branches of CN VII to the muscles of facial expression are the temporal, zygomatic, buccal, marginal mandibular, and cervical branches.

40. **H.** The posterior cricoarytenoid muscle is the only muscle that abducts the vocal folds. All of the intrinsic muscles of the larynx are innervated by the recurrent (inferior) branch of the vagus nerve. If damaged unilaterally, one's voice will sound hoarse.

41. **E.** The levator palpebrae superioris muscle elevates the upper eyelid. At its distal end lies the superior tarsal muscle, a smooth muscle innervated by postganglionics from the superior cervical ganglion. Partial ptosis occurs when the sympathetics are interrupted, and complete ptosis occurs if the levator palpebrae superioris muscle is denervated (it is innervated by CN V_1).

42. **F.** The frontal sinus drains into the semilunar hiatus of the middle meatus beneath the middle turbinate.

43. **B.** The crista galli is the anterior attachment point for the falx cerebri, a double fold of dura mater that separates the two cerebral hemispheres.

44. **G.** The lesser wing of the sphenoid bone contains the optic canal. The optic nerve (CN II) and the ophthalmic artery pass through this canal to enter the orbit.

45. **C.** The mucosa of the ethmoid sinus is innervated by the ethmoid branches of the nasociliary nerve, from CN V_1.

Index

Page numbers followed by "*f*" indicate
figures, "*t*" indicate tables, "*b*" indicate
boxes, and "*e*" indicate online content.